Thyroid and Parathyroid Diseases

Tamer Özülker • Mine Adaş
Semra Günay
Editors

Thyroid and Parathyroid Diseases

A Case-Based Guide

Springer

Editors
Tamer Özülker
University of Health Sciences (SBÜ)
Okmeydanı Training and Research
Hospital
Istanbul
Turkey

Mine Adaş
University of Health Sciences (SBÜ)
Okmeydanı Training and Research
Hospital
Istanbul
Turkey

Semra Günay
University of Health Sciences (SBÜ)
Okmeydanı Training and Research
Hospital
Istanbul
Turkey

ISBN 978-3-030-08708-1 ISBN 978-3-319-78476-2 (eBook)
https://doi.org/10.1007/978-3-319-78476-2

Softcover re-print of the Hardcover 1st edition 2019

This Springer imprint is published by the registered company Springer Nature Switzerland AG
The registered company address is: Gewerbestrasse 11, 6330 Cham, Switzerland

Preface

The overall incidence and prevalence of thyroid disease, particularly thyroid cancer, have both been increasing globally, mostly due to the scientific development and technological advances in diagnostic and therapeutic tools providing early detection and increased survival.

This increase is evident primarily in low-risk differentiated thyroid carcinomas, which confronts the clinician with the dilemma of performing overtreatment versus jeopardizing the patient while choosing a conservative approach. Guidelines which have been prepared to standardize and clarify the approaches to the thyroid diseases, depending on the researches that have been made over the last two decades yielded a paradigm shift in favor of behaving less invasive regarding surgery and radioiodine therapy. However, as we discussed the daily cases in our endocrine multidisciplinary meeting, we have recognized that the application of recommendations made in these current evidence-based clinical practice guidelines to the real cases with their unique features was not always as easy as it was thought. So, this observation gave us the inspiration to compile this case-based book with the hope that the cases might serve as a model in the solution of clinical situations that a clinical practitioner may face. Moreover, the effectuality of the case-based articles as a learning tool has been well known and we think that the cases in this book will provide a brief review of the literature.

This book also covers the cases with parathyroid diseases emphasizing the utility of innovative modalities like ^{18}F-Choline PET/CT in the localization and minimally invasive and endoscopic parathyroid surgery in the surgical excision of parathyroid adenomas.

All cases are from the daily practice of the renowned experts in nuclear medicine, clinical endocrinology, and endocrine surgery.

Thyroid and Parathyroid Diseases: A Case-Based Guide is divided into three parts. In Part I problems of benign thyroid diseases are discussed. Part II covers the various clinical issues confronted in the diagnosis and care of thyroid cancer. Part III is dedicated to the management of parathyroid diseases. We would like to thank all the contributors to the book. We thank our colleagues who have provided support to the evaluation of the cases, but who are not mentioned as authors in this book. We also wish to cordially thank Corinna Hauser and Rakesh Kumar Jotheeswaran from Springer for their assistance and input in the preparation of this book.

We hope nuclear medicine, clinical endocrinology, oncology, and general surgery specialists and residents who take care of patients with thyroid and parathyroid diseases will benefit from this book.

Istanbul, Turkey

Tamer Özülker
Mine Adaş
Semra Günay

Contents

Part III Parathyroid Diseases

Editors

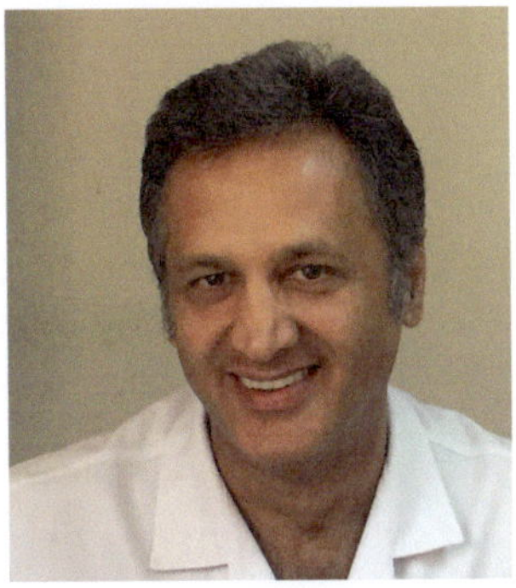

Tamer Özülker, MD is Associate Professor of Nuclear Medicine at the University of Health Sciences (SBÜ), Okmeydanı Training and Research Hospital, İstanbul, Turkey. He is a graduate of the Medical School of the University of Hacettepe, Ankara, and completed his nuclear medicine residency at Okmeydanı Training and Research Hospital. Dr. Özülker has published a number of peer-reviewed scientific articles in high-impact journals and is a co-editor of the 2015 Springer book *Atlas of PET-CT Imaging in Oncology: A Case-Based Guide to Image Interpretation* as well as a previous *Atlas of Bone Scintigraphy*. He serves as associate editor of the *Okmeydanı Medical Journal*. His clinical and research interests include PET-CT, PET-MRI, and thyroid diseases. tozulker@gmail.com.

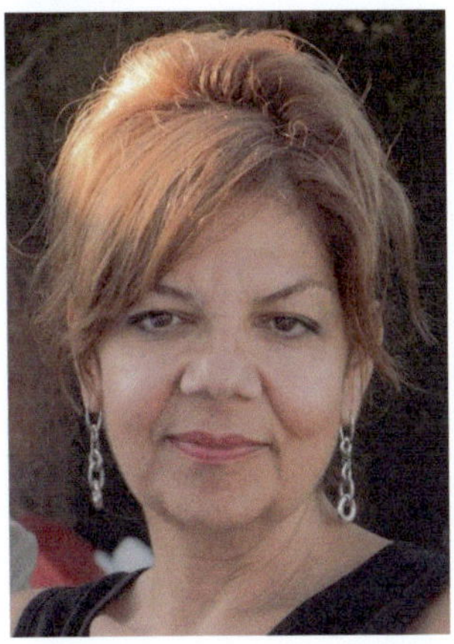

Semra Günay, MD is a specialist in breast and endocrine surgery who currently works at the University of Health Sciences (SBÜ), Okmeydanı Training and Research Hospital, İstanbul, Turkey. She is a graduate of the Istanbul University School of Medicine and completed her general surgery residency in the same faculty. She has published a number of peer-reviewed scientific articles and is one of the authors of the Turkish language book *Trauma* (ISBN 9789756395240). Dr. Günay has participated in the educational work of the Turkish Surgical Association and has worked as an instructor on postgraduate training courses in the field of endocrine surgery. She is coordinator and founder of İstanbul Endocrine Meetings (ISTET) and is a member of the editorial board of *Okmeydanı Medical Journal*. gunaysemra@gmail.com.

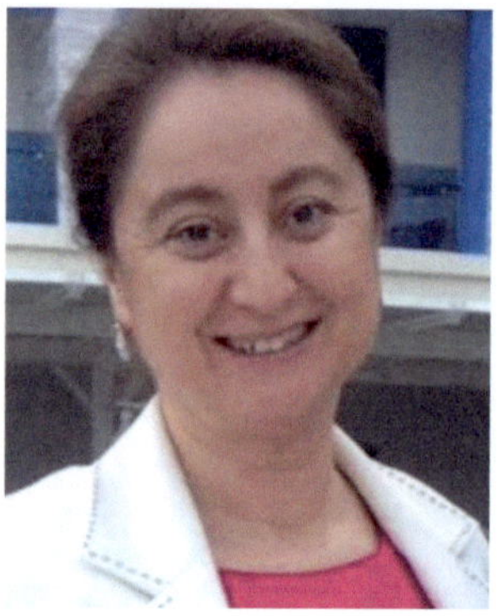

Mine Adaş, MD is Associate Professor of Endocrinology and Metabolism at the University of Health Sciences (SBÜ), Okmeydanı Training and Research Hospital, İstanbul, Turkey. She is a graduate of the Istanbul University School of Medicine. She completed her internal medicine residency at Okmeydanı Training and Research Hospital and then undertook her endocrinology training at Istanbul University School of Medicine, where she became a qualified endocrinologist in the year 2000. Dr. Adas has published a number of peer-reviewed scientific articles. Her clinical and research interests include thyroid, parathyroid, and suprarenal diseases. She is a member of the Turkish Society of Endocrinology and Metabolism, the Stem Cell and Stem Cell Therapy Association, and the European Society of Endocrinology and Endocrine Society. mineadas@yahoo.com.

Contributors

Mohammad Abuqbeitah Department of Nuclear Medicine, Cerrahpaşa Medical Faculty, Istanbul University, Istanbul, Turkey

Gökhan Adaş University of Health Sciences (SBÜ), Haseki Training and Research Hospital, Istanbul, Turkey

Mine Adaş University of Health Sciences (SBÜ), Okmeydanı Training and Research Hospital, Istanbul, Turkey

Tamer Akça Division of Breast and Endocrine Surgery, University of Mersin, Mersin, Turkey

Department of Medical History and Ethics, Mersin University, Mersin, Turkey

Burcu Esen Akkaş Department of Nuclear Medicine, University of Health Sciences (SBÜ) Dr. Abdurrahman Yurtaslan Ankara Oncology Training and Research Hospital, Ankara, Turkey

Nihat Aksakal Division of Endocrine Surgery, Istanbul University, Istanbul, Turkey

Betül Uğur Altun Department of Endocrinology, Başkent University Medical School, Ankara, Turkey

Başkent University Istanbul Hospital, Istanbul, Turkey

Nurcihan Aygün Şişli Hamidiye Etfal Training and Research Hospital, Department of General Surgery, Istanbul, Turkey

Banu Bilezikçi Department of Pathology, Güven Hospital, Ankara, Turkey

Betül Bozkurt Division of Endocrine and Breast Surgery, Hitit University Medical Faculty General Surgery Department, Çorum, Turkey

Güldeniz Karadeniz Çakmak Division of Breast and Endocrine Surgery, Bülent Ecevit Üniversity, Zonguldak, Turkey

Nuh Zafer Cantürk Division of Breast and Endocrine Surgery, Kocaeli University, Kocaeli, Turkey

Zeynep Cantürk Division of Endocrinology and Metabolism, Department of Internal Medicine, Kocaeli University, Kocaeli, Turkey

Mehmet Çelik Department of Endocrinology, Trakya University Medical Faculty, Edirne, Turkey

Tevfik Fikret Çermik University of Health Sciences, İstanbul Training and Research Hospital, Clinic of Nuclear Medicine, Istanbul, Turkey

Bülent Çitgez Division of Breast and Endocrine Surgery, General Surgery Department, Şişli Hamidiye Etfal Training and Research Hospital, Istanbul, Turkey

Hakan Demir Department of Nuclear Medicine, School of Medicine, Kocaeli University, Kocaeli, Turkey

B. Büşra Demirel Department of Nuclear Medicine, University of Health Sciences (SBÜ) Dr. Abdurrahman Yurtaslan Ankara Oncology Training and Research Hospital, Ankara, Turkey

Seher Demirer Ankara University, School of Medicine, Department of Surgery, Ankara, Turkey

Uğur Deveci Division of Breast and Endocrine Surgery, General Surgery Department, Maltepe University, Istanbul, Turkey

Ali Uğur Emre Division of Endocrine Surgery, Bülent Ecevit University, Zonguldak, Turkey

Yeşim Erbil Division of Endocrine Surgery, Istanbul University, Istanbul, Turkey

Serap Erel General Surgery, Ankara Education and Research Hospital, University of Health Sciences, Ankara, Turkey

Nurhan Ergül University of Health Sciences, İstanbul Training and Research Hospital, Clinic of Nuclear Medicine, Istanbul, Turkey

Ali İlker Filiz Department of General Surgery, İstanbul Okan University, Faculty of Medicine, Istanbul, Turkey

Nursel Gamsız Bilgin Division of Forensic Medicine, University of Mersin, Mersin, Turkey

Sertaç Ata Güler Division of Breast and Endocrine Surgery, Kocaeli University, Kocaeli, Turkey

Bahadır M. Güllüoğlu Marmara University, School of Medicine, Department of General Surgery, Istanbul, Turkey

Semra Günay University of Health Sciences (SBÜ), Okmeydanı Training and Research Hospital, Division of Breast and Endocrin Surgery, Okmeydanı, Istanbul, Turkey

Emin Gürleyik Department of Surgery, Düzce University, Düzce, Turkey

Günay Gürleyik Department of Surgery, Haydarpaşa Numune Training and Research Hospital, Istanbul, Turkey

Seyfettin Ilgan Department of Nuclear Medicine, Güven Hospital, Ankara, Turkey

Levent Kabasakal Department of Nuclear Medicine, Cerrahpaşa Faculty of Medicine, İstanbul University, Istanbul, Turkey

Abut Kebudi Division of Breast and Endocrine Surgery, General Surgery Department, Okan University, Istanbul, Turkey

Türkay Kırdak Division of Endocrine Surgery, Department of Surgery, Uludag University Faculty of Medicine, Bursa, Turkey

Taner Kıvılcım Department of General Surgery, Istanbul Okan University, Faculty of Medicine, Istanbul, Turkey

Mehmet Ali Koç Ankara University, School of Medicine, Department of Surgery, Ankara, Turkey

Akın Fırat Kocaay Ankara University, School of Medicine, Department of Surgery, Ankara, Turkey

Belma Koçer Department of Breast and Endocrine Surgery, Sakarya University, Faculty of Medicine, Sakarya, Turkey

Neslihan Kurtulmuş Department of Endocrinology, Acibadem University, Istanbul, Turkey

Özer Makay Division of Endocrine Surgery, Ege University, İzmir, Turkey

Meral Mert Department of Endocrinology and Metabolism, Bakirkoy Dr. Sadi Konuk Training and Research Hospital, Health Sciences University (SBÜ), Istanbul, Turkey

Bala Başak Öven Department of Medical Oncology, Haydarpaşa Numune Training and Research Hospital, Istanbul, Turkey

Serdar Özbaş Department of Surgery, Güven Hospital, Ankara, Turkey

Zehra Özcan Department of Nuclear Medicine, Ege University School of Medicine, Izmir, Turkey

Beyza Özçınar Division of Breast and Endocrine Surgery, Istanbul University, Istanbul, Turkey

Murat Özdemir Division of Endocrine Surgery, Ege University, İzmir, Turkey

Elgin Özkan Department of Nuclear Medicine, Medical Faculty of Ankara University, Ankara, Turkey

Sibel Özkan Gürdal Division of Breast and Endocrine Surgery, Tekirdağ Namık Kemal Üniversity, Tekirdağ, Turkey

Filiz Özülker Department of Nuclear Medicine, University of Health Sciences (SBÜ), Okmeydanı Training and Research Hospital, Istanbul, Turkey

Tamer Özülker Department of Nuclear Medicine, University of Health Sciences (SBÜ), Okmeydanı Training and Research Hospital, Istanbul, Turkey

Arzu Poyanlı Radiology and Interventional Radiology, Istanbul Medical Faculty, Istanbul, Turkey

Sait Sager Department of Nuclear Medicine, Cerrahpaşa School of Medicine, Istanbul University, İstanbul, Turkey

Onur Erdem Şahin Department of Nuclear Medicine, Cerrahpaşa Faculty of Medicine, İstanbul University, Istanbul, Turkey

Serpil Salman Istinye University Medical Faculty, Department of Internal Medicine, Istanbul, Turkey

Haluk B. Sayman Nuclear Medicine, Cerrahpaşa Medical Faculty, Istanbul University, Istanbul, Turkey

Yasemin Giles Şenyürek Division of Endocrine Surgery, Istanbul University, Istanbul Medical Faculty, Istanbul, Turkey

Atakan Sezer Department of Surgery, Trakya University Medical Faculty, Edirne, Turkey

Turgay Şimşek Division of Breast and Endocrine Surgery, Kocaeli University, Kocaeli, Turkey

Murat Sipahi Department of Nuclear Medicine, Bakirkoy Dr. Sadi Konuk Training and Research Hospital, Istanbul, Turkey

İsmail Cem Sormaz Division of Endocrine Surgery, Istanbul University, Istanbul Medical Faculty, Istanbul, Turkey

Çiğdem Soydal Department of Nuclear Medicine, Ankara University School of Medicine, Ankara, Turkey

Mehmet Tarık Tatoğlu Department of Nuclear Medicine, Göztepe Training and Research Hospital, Istanbul Medeniyet University, İstanbul, Turkey

Fatih Tunca Istanbul University Medical Faculty, Department of General Surgery, Istanbul, Turkey

Gülin Uçmak Department of Nuclear Medicine, University of Health Sciences (SBÜ) Dr. Abdurrahman Yurtaslan Ankara Oncology Training and Research Hospital, Ankara, Turkey

M. Ümit Uğurlu Marmara University, School of Medicine, Department of General Surgery, Istanbul, Turkey

Mehmet Uludağ Sisli Hamidiye Etfal Training and Research Hospital, Department of General Surgery, Istanbul, Turkey

Lebriz Uslu Beşli Department of Nuclear Medicine, Istanbul University Cerrahpaşa Medical Faculty, Istanbul, Turkey

Ayşe Kubat Üzüm Division of Endocrinology and Metabolism, Department of Internal Medicine, Istanbul Faculty of Medicine, Istanbul University, Istanbul, Turkey

Orhan Yalçın University of Health Sciences (SBÜ), Okmeydanı Training and Research Hospital, Department of Breast and Endocrine Surgery, Istanbul, Turkey

Gülşah Yenidünya Yalın Department of Endocrinology, Başkent University Istanbul Hospital, Istanbul, Turkey

Ülkem Yararbaş Department of Nuclear Medicine, Ege University School of Medicine, Izmir, Turkey

Dilek Yazıcı Department of Endocrinology, Koç University Medical School, Section of Endocrinology and Metabolism, Istanbul, Turkey

Nami Yeyin Department of Nuclear Medicine, Cerrahpaşa Medical Faculty, Istanbul University, Istanbul, Turkey

Part I

Benign Thyroid Diseases

1 Amiodarone-Induced Thyrotoxicosis in a Patient with Multinodular Goiter

Serpil Salman

Abstract

An old male who presented with atypical symptoms was diagnosed with thyrotoxicosis. He had multinodular goiter and was taking amiodarone (probably intermittently for a long time) for atrioventricular arrhythmias. The findings were interpreted in favor of amiodarone thyroiditis, but it was difficult to distinguish the type of amiodarone-induced thyrotoxicosis (AIT) because findings of both type 1 and 2 AIT were observed. Combined antithyroid drug (methimazole 20 mg/day) and corticosteroid (prednisolone 40 mg/day) were administered to treat both types of AIT. Normal thyroid hormone levels were found in the second week of treatment. Hepatotoxicity and decreasing platelet count developed as side effects of methimazole; therefore, the drug was stopped. Prednisolone was continued at the same dosage for 4 weeks and tapered to 6–10 mg every 4 weeks. Meanwhile, liver enzyme levels and platelet count returned to acceptable levels, but there was a risk of exacerbation. The patient was operated during the fourth month of follow-up when his cardiac problems were stable.

1.1 Case Presentation

A 74-year-old male was referred from a cardiology clinic because his thyroid-stimulating hormone (TSH) level was low during evaluation of a relapsed atrial fibrillation (AF) episode. He presented with weakness, fatigue, depressive mood, and palpitation. No typical hyperthyroidism symptoms, such as weight loss, sweating, and tremor, were observed. Oral amiodarone treatment was administered for 2 years and withdrawn 1.5 years ago. Since withdrawal, some infusions were administered at different medical centers for recurrent episodes of cardiac arrhythmia. Following a new AF episode with fast ventricular response, oral amiodarone of 200 mg/day was administered for 2 months. He had multinodular goiter (MNG) for a few years. He had no history of thyroid dysfunction, and he underwent his last checkup 1 year ago. Coronary artery bypass graft operation was performed 14 years ago. He was receiving aspirin 100 mg o.d., candesartan 16 mg o.d., and bisoprolol 5 mg b.i.d.

On physical examination, the patient was conscious and oriented but looked depressed and pale. His body mass index was 35.5 kg/m^2 (105 kg/172 cm), blood pressure was 130/80 mmHg, and arrhythmic heart rate was 110 beats/min. The thyroid gland was enlarged, bilateral nodules measuring 1–2 cm. There was no sign of thyroid eye disease or pretibial myxedema.

S. Salman
Istinye University Medical Faculty,
Department of Internal Medicine, Istanbul, Turkey

T. Özülker et al. (eds.), *Thyroid and Parathyroid Diseases*, https://doi.org/10.1007/978-3-319-78476-2_1

Laboratory test in the cardiology clinic revealed TSH levels of 0.054 (0.27–4.20) uIU/mL, free triiodothyronine (fT3) of 3.41 (2.0–4.4) pg/mL, and free thyroxine (fT4) of 1.92 (0.93–1.70) ng/dL. The cardiologist advised continuing amiodarone treatment.

1.2 Discussion

1.2.1 Evaluation and Diagnosis

The initial laboratory workup in the cardiology clinic showed mild hyperthyroidism, but after 5 days, the levels worsened as follows: TSH level of <0.001 (0.27–4.20) uIU/mL, total T3 level of 237 (83–200) ng/dL, fT3 level of 4.96 (2.0–4.40) pg/mL, and fT4 level of 4.11 (0.93–1.70) ng/dL. An effective treatment for thyrotoxicosis was needed because it is an important factor for the redevelopment of atrioventricular arrhythmias and exacerbation of ischemic heart disease or heart failure particularly in old age [1].

Detailed investigation of every patient is essential for an appropriate treatment plan for thyrotoxicosis. In addition to toxic MNG, other main causes of thyrotoxicosis accompanying euthyroid MNG should be considered in the present patient; these include autoimmune thyroid disease (Graves' disease), subacute thyroiditis, and intake of exogenous thyroxine and/or iodine (including amiodarone, iodine radiocontrast agent, and supplements). For initial workup, thyroid function tests, thyroid ultrasonography, and if possible thyroid uptake/scan are necessary [2]. Thyroglobulin testing works only in patients suspected of factitiously taking thyroxine whose scintigraphy test shows no uptake. Thyroglobulin testing is not needed for the diagnosis of other causes of thyrotoxicosis [2].

As previously mentioned, at first visit, the TSH level was low, and thyroid hormone levels (particularly FT4 levels) were high. Laboratory results revealed no abnormality except for a mildly decreased platelet count: TSH receptor antibody (TRAb) 0.37 (<1.75) IU/L, anti-thyroperoxidase (anti-TPO) level of 11 (<34) IU/mL, anti-thyroglobulin (anti-Tg) level of 10 (<115) IU/mL, aspartate aminotransferase (AST) level of 29 (0–40) U/L, alanine aminotransferase (ALT) level of 37 (0–41) U/L, alkaline phosphatase (ALP) level of 50 (40–130) U/L, total bilirubin level of 0.71 (0.20–1.10) mg/dL, creatinine level of 0.75 (0.70–1.20) mg/dL, erythrocyte sedimentation rate (ESR) of 18 (0–20) mm/h, C-reactive protein level of 3.25 (0–5) mg/L, white blood cell count of 4800/mm^3, hemoglobin level of 14.0 g/dL, and platelet count of 136,000/mm^3 (163,000–337,000). On thyroid ultrasonography, bilaterally enlarged thyroid gland with mixed nodules (maximum 27 mm in diameter) was observed, and color-flow Doppler sonography revealed no hypervascularity. Technetium-99m pertechnetate scan showed no uptake (0%).

According to these results, this was a case of thyrotoxicosis with an absent radioactive iodine uptake (RAIU) over the neck. The causes of normal or elevated RAIU, such as Graves' disease, toxic MNG, and resistance to thyroid hormone, were excluded [2]. Normal levels of thyroid antibodies, namely, TRAb, anti-TPO, and anti-Tg, were the other reasons for excluding Graves' disease. A near-absent RAIU can be associated with amiodarone-induced thyroiditis, painless (silent) thyroiditis, subacute (granulomatous, de Quervain's) thyroiditis, palpation thyroiditis, iatrogenic thyrotoxicosis, factitious ingestion of thyroid hormone, struma ovarii, acute thyroiditis, and extensive metastases from follicular thyroid cancer. In the present study, most of the possibilities were excluded according to history, physical examination, and laboratory results: Subacute thyroiditis is one of the main causes of low-uptake thyrotoxicosis, but it is generally painful, and high ESR is characteristic. Painless thyroiditis is mostly observed in women during postpartum period who have a personal or family history of autoimmune thyroid disease and typically have anti-TPO positivity. Struma ovarii is a disease that occurs in women (our patient was an old man). Our patient had no history of high-pressure neck palpation or taking thyroid hormone. Acute thyroiditis and extensive metastases from follicular thyroid cancer are very rare. In our case, RAIU was reported as to be low as 0%. It is rarely

<1% unless the iodine exposure is reoccurring, such as during amiodarone treatment [2]. Our patient was administered some drug infusions for the refractory arrhythmias in the last 1.5 years, and these were probably amiodarone infusions. Besides, the patient had long-term oral amiodarone use in the period before the 1.5 years and in the near past. Based on history, clinical, and laboratory findings, AIT was the most likely diagnosis.

Amiodarone is a commonly used antiarrhythmic drug worldwide. It is a benzofuran compound that contains approximately 37% iodine by weight; therefore, a patient taking a standard 200 mg oral daily dose of amiodarone ingests 75 mg of organic iodine each day [3]. Amiodarone infusion is also an option for medical therapeutic management of severe arrhythmias as it is a rich source of iodine. It is very lipophilic and accumulates in the adipose tissue, cardiac and skeletal muscles, and thyroid gland. An initial 50% reduction in plasma concentration 3–10 days after cessation of chronic therapy is followed by a longer terminal half-life of 13–142 days as tissue stores deplete [4].

To verify iodine load due to amiodarone, spot urine sample (creatinine corrected) was sent to the laboratory, but the assay results could not be obtained within 1 week. Thus, treatment had to be planned empirically (the result was found to be very high at 3799 mcg/g creatinine on the fifth day of treatment).

There are two types of AIT. Differentiating between the types is necessary because their therapies differ. In type 1, the problem is increased synthesis of thyroid hormone due to substrate (i.e., iodine) load. This type may occur in patients with underlying MNG or latent Graves' disease. High vascularity in color-flow Doppler sonography, T4/T3 ratio of <4, normal/slightly increased serum interleukin-6 (IL-6) level, and normal/increased thyroidal RAIU indicate a type 1 AIT. In addition, antibodies test positive if type 1 AIT is related to Graves' disease. In type 2, there is an excess release of T4 and T3 due to destructive thyroiditis caused by direct amiodarone toxicity on follicular cells. Clinical features of type 2 AIT are small, diffuse, firm, and occasionally tender gland on palpation, absent vascularity in color-flow Doppler sonography, T4/T3 ratio of >4, profoundly increased serum IL-6 level, and low/absent thyroidal RAIU [2, 5, 6].

In the present case, IL-6 level was found to be 7.1 (normal: <5.9) ng/mL, indicating type 1 AIT. The patient had features of both type 1 (nodular goiter, T4/T3 ratio of <4, and slightly increased IL-6 level) and type 2 (absent thyroid uptake, no vascularity) AIT. Therefore, the type of AIT could not be determined based on these results. Differentiating between the two types of AIT can frequently be difficult because most criteria are not highly specific and thyroid evaluation by Doppler requires an experienced sonographer. Indeed, both conditions may also coexist in a person. Combined antithyroid drug and corticosteroid therapy should be used to treat patients in whom the etiology of thyrotoxicosis cannot be unequivocally determined [2].

The clinical manifestations of hyperthyroidism were not prominent in our patient as expected to be seen in old age [1]. Amiodarone use can also mask symptoms in two ways: its beta-blocking activity minimizes adrenergic manifestations of excess thyroid hormone, and amiodarone metabolites may block binding of T3 to its nuclear receptor [7].

The time of amiodarone toxicity occurrence is unpredictable. Toxicity can occur in both short- and long-term uses as well as after drug withdrawal. According to Tomisti et al., the factors associated with a shorter time of onset are type 1 AIT, larger thyroid volume, and larger body surface area [8]. In our patient, AIT developed after a long time-irregular drug use. He was obese and had a large goiter. There was no information about his thyroid hormone levels from the previous year until the recent evaluation, which suggested the necessity for checkup at 3–6-month intervals [6], even after amiodarone withdrawal for at least 2 years [8].

1.2.2 Management

One question was whether amiodarone treatment could be continued. The recommendation of

2016 American Thyroid Association (ATA) Guideline [2] for the need to discontinue amiodarone states that "It is controversial because (1) this drug is frequently the only medication able to control cardiac arrhythmia, (2) the effects of this fat-soluble drug may persist for many months, (3) amiodarone may have T3-antagonistic properties at the cardiac level and inhibit T4 to T3 conversion in the heart such that withdrawal may actually aggravate cardiac manifestations of thyrotoxicosis. Deaths from ventricular fibrillation have occurred after stopping amiodarone in patients with AIT. In addition, type 2 AIT typically responds to treatment even if amiodarone therapy is continued, but continuation may lead to a more prolonged time to recovery and a higher rate of future recurrences of AIT." An alternative is dronedarone, which is a non-iodinated benzofuran derivative of amiodarone. It is relatively safe but does not sufficiently replicate the effects of amiodarone [5], and it is not available in our country. Thus, there was no effective alternative drug for our patient, and amiodarone was continued at a low dose of 200 mg because of his refractory arrhythmias.

For thyrotoxicosis, methimazole 20 mg and prednisone 40 mg were started, although the suggested starting dosage of methimazole is higher (40 mg/day) [2]. On the second week of treatment, the total T3, fT3, and fT4 levels normalized, but liver enzyme (such as AST, ALT, and GGT) levels were 3–4 times higher than the upper limit, and platelet count decreased from 136,000 to 55,000/mm^3. Bilirubin level remained in the normal range. Both hematology and hepatology consultations suggested discontinuation of aspirin and methimazole treatments. Therefore, both drugs were stopped. Two weeks later, liver enzyme and platelet levels normalized, and fT3 and/or fT4 levels were not increasing. The rapid response indicated type 2 AIT; prednisolone 40 mg/day was continued for another 4 weeks and was tapered to 6–10 mg every 4 weeks. Meanwhile, a new exacerbation of atrioventricular arrhythmia developed. Transthoracic Doppler echocardiography revealed diffuse hypokinesis of the left ventricle where the ejection fraction decreased from 52% to 38% and pulmonary arterial pressure increased from 45 to 56 mmHg compared with evaluation at attendance. No thrombus was noted on transesophageal echocardiography. A successful cardioversion was performed, and warfarin treatment was started.

During the fourth month of follow-up, his thyroid hormone levels were again at the upper limit, his urinary iodine was 932 mcg/g creatinine, and he was on sinus rhythm. A permanent solution was needed because, in case of a new thyroid exacerbation, there is no reliable treatment option, such as antithyroid medication or plasmapheresis (having platelets at the lower limit). Moreover, RAI therapy, which is usually not feasible in patients with AIT, because of low RAIU [9], was not applicable to our patient. Thyroidectomy was a valid option and was not delayed considering the risk of hemodynamic status deterioration [10].

1.2.3 Follow-Up and Outcome

At the end of the fourth month, the patient's cardiac problems, platelet count (137,000/mm^3), and thyroid function test results had stabilized, and total thyroidectomy was performed under steroid management. After the surgery, it is a routine procedure to wait for the pathological report and to endogenously check the stimulated thyroglobulin level during the third week for detecting any malignancy before starting thyroxine replacement. However, thyroxine replacement was given just after thyroidectomy because of cardiac risk. On pathological examination, one of the nodules showed tumor with a low risk (6 mm, follicular variant papillary, T1NxMx). Thyroxine replacement was continued and targeted at TSH level of 0.5–2.0 uIU/mL in accordance with the 2015 ATA Guideline [11]. During his last visit, his thyroglobulin level was <0.1 ng/mL, and his TSH level was 1.2 uIU/mL.

1.2.4 Future

There is a need to improve the decisive criteria for differentiating between type 1 and type 2 AIT.

What Can We Learn from This Case?

- The clinical manifestations of hyperthyroidism are not typical in old age, particularly in amiodarone users.
- During the evaluation of thyrotoxicosis in patients with underlying cardiac rhythm problem, even though there is no information about amiodarone use, the possibility of AIT should be investigated because some patients do not inform about any medication they took during heart attacks.
- Differentiating between the two types of AIT is important, even though it can frequently be difficult, and both conditions may coexist.
- If differentiation is not possible, treating both with antithyroid medication and steroids to control symptoms is necessary.

References

1. Samuels MH, Franklyn JA. Hyperthyroidism in aging. In: De Groot LJ, Chrousos G, Dungan K, Feingold KR, Grossman A, Hershman JM, Koch C, Korbonits M, McLachlan R, New M, Purnell J, Rebar R, Singer F, Vinik A, editors. Source endotext [internet]. South Dartmouth, MA: MDText.com, Inc.; 2000. Available at http://www.ncbi.nlm.nih.gov/books/NBK278986/.
2. Ross DS, Burch HB, Cooper DS, Greenlee MC, Laurberg P, Maia AL, et al. 2016 American Thyroid Association guidelines for diagnosis and management of hyperthyroidism and other causes of thyrotoxicosis. Thyroid. 2016;26:1343–421.
3. Zipes DP, Prystowsky EN, Heger JJ. Amiodarone: electrophysiologic actions, pharmacokinetics and clinical effects. J Am Coll Cardiol. 1984;3:1059–71.
4. Vassallo P, Trohman RG. Prescribing amiodarone: an evidence-based review of clinical indications. JAMA. 2007;298:1312–22.
5. Narayana SK, Woods DR, Boos CJ. Management of amiodarone-related thyroid problems. Ther Adv Endocrinol Metab. 2011;2:115–26. https://doi.org/10.1177/2042018811398516.
6. Jabrocka-Hybel A, Bednarczuk T, Bartalena L, Pach D, Ruchała M, Kamiński G, et al. Amiodarone and the thyroid. Endokrynol Pol. 2015;66:176–86. https://doi.org/10.5603/EP.2015.0025.
7. van Beeren HC, Bakker O, Wiersinga WM. Structure-function relationship of the inhibition of the 3,5,3′-triiodothyronine binding to the alpha1- and beta1-thyroid hormone receptor by amiodarone analogs. Endocrinology. 1996;137:2807–14.
8. Tomisti L, Rossi G, Bartalena L, Martino E, Bogazzi F. The onset time of amiodarone-induced thyrotoxicosis (AIT) depends on AIT type. Eur J Endocrinol. 2014;171:363–8. https://doi.org/10.1530/EJE-14-0267.
9. Czarnywojtek A, Czepczynski R, Ruchala M, Wasko R, Zgorzalewicz-Stachowiak M, Szczepanek E, et al. Radioiodine therapy in patients with amiodarone-induced thyrotoxicosis (AIT). Neuro Endocrinol Lett. 2009;30:209–14.
10. Pierret C, Tourtier JP, Pons Y, Merat S, Duverger V, Perrier E. Total thyroidectomy for amiodarone-associated thyrotoxicosis: should surgery always be delayed for pre-operative medical preparation? J Laryngol Otol. 2012;126:701–5. https://doi.org/10.1017/S0022215112000722.
11. Haugen BR, Alexander EK, Bible KC, Doherty GM, Mandel SJ, Nikiforov YE, et al. 2015 American Thyroid Association management guidelines for adult patients with thyroid nodules and differentiated thyroid cancer: the American Thyroid Association guidelines task force on thyroid nodules and differentiated thyroid cancer. Thyroid. 2016;26:1–133. https://doi.org/10.1089/thy.2015.0020.

Factitious Hyperthyroidism

2

Ayşe Kubat Üzüm and Gülşah Yenidünya Yalın

Abstract

Hyperthyroidism is generally characterized by symptoms of anxiety, fatigue, palpitations, tremor, heat intolerance, increased perspiration, and weight loss. The most common cause of endogenous hyperthyroidism is Graves' disease. However, the presence of exogenous hyperthyroidism should also be considered in the presence of hyperthyroidism symptoms in patients who are receiving levothyroxine replacement therapy. The term "exogenous hyperthyroidism" is used to describe hyperthyroidism caused by ingestion of excessive amounts of thyroid hormone. This is generally due to high dose of levothyroxine replacement which is aimed for TSH suppression during the treatment of thyroid carcinoma. However, it may also occur in patients with psychiatric disorders when they take excessive doses of thyroid hormone intentionally, especially when they aim to draw attention. This condition is termed "thyrotoxicosis factitia." We hereby present a case with thyrotoxicosis factitia and the challenges during the process of diagnosis.

A. K. Üzüm
Division of Endocrinology and Metabolism, Department of Internal Medicine, Istanbul Faculty of Medicine, Istanbul University, Istanbul, Turkey

G. Y. Yalın (✉)
Department of Endocrinology, Başkent University Istanbul Hospital, Istanbul, Turkey

2.1 Case Presentation

A 19-year-old female patient was admitted to our endocrinology outpatient clinic with symptoms of palpitation, tremor, heat intolerance, increased perspiration, and weight loss. She had been practicing as a nursing student, and her complaints had started 2 months ago after she had started a new educational program in the cardiology department. On her physical examination, her skin was warm and moist, heart rate was 122/min, and blood pressure was 145/80 mmHg. Cardiopulmonary and abdominal examination was unremarkable. The thyroid gland was non-palpable and painless. No sign of thyroid orbitopathy or pretibial edema was noted. Laboratory results were as follows: TSH, <0.001 mIU/L (0.27–4.2 mIU/L); free T4, 46 pmol/L (12–22 pmol/L); free T3, 9.3 pmol/L (3.1–6.8 pmol/L); anti-TPO, 10 IU/mL (0–34 IU/mL); anti-Tg, 32 IU/mL (0–115 IU/mL); thyroid stimulating immunoglobulin (TSI) < 1 U/L (negative); WBC, 5600/μL; Hgb, 12 g/dL; Hct, 36%; Plt, 160000/μL; ALT, 28 U/L; erythrocyte sedimentation rate, 10 mm/h; CRP < 5 mg/L; and β-HCG < 0.1 mLU/mL. Thyroid ultrasonography (USG) showed a homogenous parenchymal structure with normal gland size and vasculature. Scintigraphy of thyroid gland demonstrated low technetium-99m uptake (1%). The patient denied the presence of any prior medication or treatment that may have affected thyroid functions and had no known

T. Özülker et al. (eds.), *Thyroid and Parathyroid Diseases*, https://doi.org/10.1007/978-3-319-78476-2_2

previous iodine administration in her history. The initial diagnosis was presumed as silent thyroiditis, and beta-blocker treatment with propranolol 40 mg b.i.d. was initiated to ameliorate patient's symptoms. However, her condition gradually deteriorated, and free T4 levels continued to rise without any evident reason (fT4: 54 pmol/L). The patient denied consuming meat products which made ingestion of desiccated thyroid tissue and "hamburger hyperthyroidism" unlikely. Struma ovarii and factitious hyperthyroidism were also considered in the differential diagnosis. In order to rule out factitious hyperthyroidism, plasma thyroglobulin (Tg) level was assessed, and the result was extremely low (Tg < 0.1 ng/mL) despite the presence of hyperthyroidism. This finding confirmed factitious hyperthyroidism. On confrontation, the patient once again denied using any medication including levothyroxine. The patient was isolated to a private room with 24-h surveillance to ensure the cessation of levothyroxine ingestion. Cholestyramine treatment 4 × 4 g was initiated in order to prevent absorption of possible recent L-thyroxine ingestion, and the patient was consulted with the psychiatrists. After 7 days of cholestyramine treatment, fT4 levels decreased gradually (fT4:27 pmol/L).

2.2 Discussion

2.2.1 Evaluation and Diagnosis

The classic symptoms of hyperthyroidism are weight loss, heat intolerance, tremor, palpitations, anxiety, increased frequency of bowel movements, and shortness of breath. Factitious hyperthyroidism is a form of exogenous hyperthyroidism caused by the surreptitious use of thyroid hormone. As there is no de novo thyroid hormone secretion from the thyroid gland, it is considered that this condition should, in fact, be called "thyrotoxicosis factitia" [1]. The symptoms and signs in patients who take excessive doses of thyroid hormone are also similar to those in patients with hyperthyroidism due to other etiological factors such as Graves' disease. However, the laboratory findings may simply lead the physician to the accurate diagnosis when a cautious clinical evaluation is performed.

In a patient with symptoms of palpitations, tremor, heat intolerance, increased perspiration, and weight loss such as in our case, thyroid function tests should always be evaluated. Presence of diffuse goiter, ophthalmopathy, and pretibial myxedema may be indicative of Graves' disease which is the most common cause of endogenous hyperthyroidism [2]. Presence of thyroid bruit on auscultation, a greater increase in fT3 levels with respect to fT4 levels, and TRAB positivity are supportive findings for Graves' disease [3]. Radioactive iodine uptake (RAIU) is high on thyroid scintigraphy in Graves' disease indicating de novo synthesis of thyroid hormone [3]. Low RAIU may be associated with thyroiditis, iodine contamination (due to radiocontrast agents or medications like amiodarone), struma ovarii, or factitious hyperthyroidism. Therefore, uptake with thyroid scintigraphy can be helpful in the differential diagnosis by distinguishing presence of de novo synthesis of thyroid hormone (normal or high uptake) or release of preformed hormone into the circulation from destruction of thyroid tissue (low uptake) or an extrathyroidal source of thyroid hormone as in factitious hyperthyroidism (nearly absent uptake) [4].

In this patient, lack of diffuse goiter and thyroid orbitopathy with negative autoantibody levels helped exclude the diagnosis of Graves' disease. Serum β-HCG level was low, eliminating the possibility of gestational thyrotoxicosis. Therefore, a thyroid scintigraphy was performed after pregnancy was ruled out. Presence of pregnancy should always be ruled out in hyperthyroid young women who are at the reproductive age before thyroid scintigraphy is performed [4]. Low technetium-99m uptake results in thyroid scintigraphy could be associated with subclinical thyroiditis, iodine exposure, silent thyroiditis, "hamburger thyroiditis" [5], struma ovarii, or factitious hyperthyroidism [4]."Hamburger thyroiditis" is a novel form of exogenous hyperthyroidism caused by the ingestion of bovine thyroid tissue which is inadvertently consumed with the hamburger meat that consists of bovine thyroid gland in ground beef [5]. Normal acute phase reactants and lack of neck pain and tenderness on thyroid palpation eliminated the possibility of subacute thyroiditis. As the patient denied iodine exposure and consuming red meat recently, iodine exposure and hamburger thyroiditis were ruled out. Silent thyroiditis was presumed in the initial diagnosis, and beta-blocker treatment was administered to control symptoms. However, patient's symptoms and fT4 levels increased gradually and as silent thyroiditis is generally associated with mild hyperthyroidism which lasts shorter than 2 months. Struma ovarii and factitious hyperthyroidism were also suspected. The primary finding of exogenous hyperthyroidism is undetectable Tg levels in the presence of high thyroid hormone levels [4]. Tg is released along with thyroid hormone secretion during endogenous hyperthyroidism, whereas its release is suppressed in the setting of exogenous thyroid hormone administration [4]. As Tg levels would be high in struma ovarii due to ectopic thyroid hormone synthesis in ovarian tissue, this diagnosis was excluded. Furthermore, clinical and biochemical features of hyperthyroidism are generally uncommon in women with struma ovarii. Diagnosis of factitious hyperthyroidism was established in this patient based on small thyroid gland size, negative autoantibody levels, low uptake on thyroid scintigraphy, and undetectable Tg levels despite the presence of hyperthyroidism. However, it should also be kept in mind that anti-Tg levels should always be measured as well, whenever it is necessary to evaluate Tg levels, because high antibody titers may cause falsely decreased levels of Tg measurements in immunometric assays. In this patient, anti-Tg levels were also low eliminating any interference during the immunometric assays. For difficult cases where thyrotoxicosis factitia is suspected but Tg is either not suppressed probably because of goiter, or suppressed but not reliable due to the presence of high anti-Tg antibodies, fecal T4 measurement is reported to be useful. In one study, fecal T4 values were approximately 0.8 μg/g (1 nmol/g) in normal subjects, and the levels increased twofold in patients with Graves' hyperthyroidism and 12–24-fold in patients with exogenous hyperthyroidism [6].

2.3 Management

Treatment for factitious hyperthyroidism is simply the cessation of the exogenous use of thyroid hormone. Therefore, it is essential to keep this diagnosis in mind during the differential diagnosis of hyperthyroidism as antithyroid medications (thionamides) or other conservative treatment methods would fail as long as the patient kept on taking levothyroxine surreptitiously. Usually, withdrawal treatment alone is sufficient for patients with mild to moderate hyperthyroidism [7]. After the discontinuation of levothyroxine, serum T4 levels decrease by 50% in 7 days, and T3 is cleared even more rapidly as serum half-life time is about 1–2 days [7]. However, additional therapy may be beneficial in more symptomatic patients. Beta-adrenergic antagonist drugs relieve many of the symptoms of hyperthyroidism promptly by inhibiting the peripheral conversion of T4 to T3. Radiographic contrast agents like ipodate or iopanoic acid may also inhibit T4 conversion to T3. However, these drugs are not routinely preferred because of their adverse effects on bone marrow tissue [1]. It is generally recommended that these agents should not be used longer than 7 days in patients with factitious hyperthyroidism [1].

In patients who are surreptitiously taking T4, cholestyramine can be given to bind T4 and T3 in the intestine, thereby interrupting the physiological absorption and enterohepatic circulation of the two hormones [8]. The usual dose is 4 g four times a day. Patients with more severe hyperthyroidism and vigorous symptoms (such as atrial fibrillation or congestive heart failure) due to massive thyroid hormone overdose may benefit from plasmapheresis and exchange transfusion [9]. However, in general, conservative management is usually sufficient in the management of patients with mild to moderate hyperthyroidism [10].

One important aspect in the follow up of these patients after the cessation of levothyroxine is to be alert for the development of transient hypothyroidism. As the TSH levels are suppressed, these patients usually experience a brief period of transient hypothyroidism after the discontinuation of levothyroxine [1], and levothyroxine replacement may be necessary in physiological doses until the recovery of the pituitary-thyroid axis.

What Can We Learn from This Case?

- The classic symptoms of hyperthyroidism are weight loss, heat intolerance, tremor, palpitations, anxiety, increased frequency of bowel movements, and shortness of breath. In the presence of these symptoms, thyroid function tests should always be evaluated.
- Factitious hyperthyroidism is a form of exogenous hyperthyroidism caused by the surreptitious use of thyroid hormone. Factitious ingestion of thyroid hormone can be distinguished from other causes of thyrotoxicosis by a low serum thyroglobulin level and a near-zero RAIU.
- Antithyroid medications (thionamides) or other conservative treatment methods would fail as long as the patient continues to use levothyroxine. Therefore, it is substantial to keep factitious hyperthyroidism in mind for the differential diagnosis of hyperthyroidism.
- Physicians should be cautious during the follow up of these patients for the onset of transient hypothyroidism until the recovery of the thyroid-pituitary axis.

References

1. Cohen JH, Ingbar SH, Braverman LE. Thyrotoxicosis due to ingestion of excess thyroid hormone. Endocr Rev. 1989;10:113–24.
2. Brent GA. Clinical practice. Graves' disease. N Engl J Med. 2008;358:2594–605.
3. Trzepacz PT, Klein I, Roberts M. Graves disease: an analysis of thyroid hormone levels and hyperthyroid signs and symptoms. Am J Med. 1989;87:558–61.
4. Ross DS, Burch HB, Cooper DS, Greenlee M, Laurberg P, Maia AL. American Thyroid Association guidelines for diagnosis and management of hyperthyroidism and other causes of thyrotoxicosis. Thyroid. 2016;26:1343–421.
5. Hedberg CW, Fishbein DB, Janssen RS. An outbreak of thyrotoxicosis caused by the consumption of bovine thyroid gland in ground beef. N Engl J Med. 1987;316:993–8.
6. Bouillon R, Verresen L, Staels F. The measurement of fecal thyroxine in the diagnosis of thyrotoxicosis factitia. Thyroid. 1993;3:101–3.
7. Ross DS, Cooper DS, Mulder JE. Exogenous hyperthyroidism. https://www.uptodate.com. Accessed 14 Sept 2017.
8. Shakir KM, Michaels RD, Hays JH, Potter BB. The use of bile acid sequestrants to lower serum thyroid hormones in iatrogenic hyperthyroidism. Ann Intern Med. 1993;118:112–3.
9. Jha S, Waghdhare S, Reddi R, Bhattacharya P. Thyroid storm due to inappropriate administration of a compounded thyroid hormone preparation successfully treated with plasmapheresis. Thyroid. 2012;22:1283–6.
10. Kinney JS, Hurwitz ES, Fishbein DB, et al. Community outbreak of thyrotoxicosis: epidemiology, immunogenetic characteristics, and long-term outcome. Am J Med. 1988;84:10–8.

3 Management of Resistant Hyperthyroidism Following Obesity Surgery

Mehmet Çelik and Atakan Sezer

Abstract

The number of bariatric surgical procedures performed in recent years has increased significantly, because bariatric surgery is still the most effective and permanent treatment for severe obesity. A comprehensive surgical screening by a multidisciplinary team of bariatric surgical patients is important in order to prepare patients for successful outcomes. Although postoperative thyrotoxicosis is rarely seen in morbidly obese patients, hyperthyroidism has not been reported. Bariatric surgery, especially malabsorptive type, may result in mineral deficiency and malabsorption of medications used in treatment, about which clinicians must be alert.

In this report, we aimed to present the difficulties in oral medical replacement treatment after thyroid surgery for hyperthyroidism in a patient with previous bariatric surgery.

M. Çelik (✉)
Department of Endocrinology, Trakya University Medical Faculty, Edirne, Turkey

A. Sezer
Department of Surgery, Trakya University Medical Faculty, Edirne, Turkey

3.1 Case Presentation

A 44-year-old female patient was admitted to the outpatient clinic with palpitation, tremor in the hands, and elevated blood glucose level. The medical history of the patient revealed an ileal interposition surgery 3 years ago when the patient has a body mass index of 42.1 kg/m^2. After obesity surgery, the patient lost 40 kg during 2 years. Physical examination on admission demonstrated as blood pressure, 120/80 mm/Hg; pulse, 105/min; body height, 165 cm; body weight, 70 kg (BMI, 25.7); Hertel exophthalmometer value, 18 mm; and NO SPECS 2 exophthalmos. Laboratory examination findings were as follows: TSH, 0.001 (*n*, 0.55–4.78 μIU/ml); FT4, 2.84 (*N*, 0.8–1.8 ng/dl); FT3, 10.48 (*N*, 2–4.2 pg/ml); anti-thyroglobulin antibody, 30.5(0–60 IU/ml); anti-TPO antibody, 830.9 (0–60 IU/ml); TSH receptor antibody (+); glucose, 354 (70–105 mg/dl); creatinine, 0.61 (0.57–1.11 mg/dl); albumin, 3.9 (3.2–5.2 g/dl); calcium, 8.6 (8.4–10.2 mg/dl); phosphorus, 4.9 (2.3–4.7 mg/dl); intact parathyroid hormone, 277.4 (14–72 pg/ml); 25-OH-vitamin D, 3 (24–50 Ng/ml); and HbA1C, 11.5 (3.6–5.8%). Bolus-basal insulin treatment four times a day was prescribed for blood glucose regulation. The hyperthyroidism symptoms had been first diagnosed in the first postoperative year, and propyl-

T. Özülker et al. (eds.), *Thyroid and Parathyroid Diseases*, https://doi.org/10.1007/978-3-319-78476-2_3

thiouracil 3 × 3 and propranolol 2 × 1 per day had been prescribed for the treatment. Although normoglycemia was achieved, the patient had still hyperthyroidism symptoms despite 1.5 years of high-dose oral antithyroid treatment. The patient's neck ultrasonography (USG) examination revealed thyroid gland with increased lobulated borders and parenchymal heterogeneity. There was a 10 × 11 × 14 mm sized hypoechoic nodule in the left lobe with undefined borders and peripheral vascularization. Technetium-99m pertechnetate thyroid scintigraphy showed diffusely enlarged thyroid gland with increased uptake and normoactive nodule, which was, detected on the neck USG examination. Vitamin B12, vitamin D deficiency, and refractory hyperthyroidism were observed in the patient, although replacement therapy was done and malabsorption of medical treatment was considered. In addition, cholestyramine 3 × 4 g/day treatment was commenced due to elevated liver enzymes and persistent hyperthyroidism despite high-dose antithyroid medication. The Dunhill procedure was used to preserve endogenous thyroid hormone secretion in the patient. The patient was discharged on the second postoperative day. The patient was euthyroid at 6 weeks postoperatively. The patient was scheduled for thyroid surgery and underwent Dunhill procedure to maintain endogen thyroid hormone secretion. The patient was discharged on second day postoperative uneventfully, and on the first month postoperative visit, the patient was in euthyroid state.

3.2 Discussion

Obesity is defined as the accumulation of extraordinary or excessive fat tissue, which impairs fitness, ensuing in cardiovascular pathologies, diabetes mellitus, metabolic syndrome, musculoskeletal disorders, and psychiatric issues [1, 2]. The National Health and Nutrition Examination Survey (2007–2010) established the prevalence of obesity as 40.8% between 65 and 74 years in adult US citizens. Currently approximately 30% of people are overweight (body mass index (BMI) > 25) or obese (BMI > 30) around the world [3–9].

Even though right strategies to check frame fats exist, the measurement of body fat with the aid of those techniques is pricey and is frequently not conveniently available to most clinicians. Surrogate measures are critical in evaluating body fat, body mass index (BMI) (Table 3.1), and waist circumference (Table 3.2) [10–12].

A comprehensive and detailed history of the patient's obesity should be taken, and the following situations should be questioned. Obesity should be learned from the age of onset, duration, and application. The family history of obesity and related diseases (such as type 2 diabetes, HT, CVD, dyslipidemia, and OSAS) in the family and among first-degree relatives should be questioned. A detailed nutritional history (e.g., eating lunch) should be taken, including eating habits and eating behavior. Alcohol consumption, smoking, and drug habit should be questioned. Drugs and illnesses leading to secondary obesity should be asked. If there is no evidence of endocrine disease in history and physical examination, endocrine examination and investigation are not recommended.

It is important to prevent weight gain and detect concomitant other factors in subjects with BMI ≥25 kg/m^2 or waist circumference above

Table 3.1 Classifications for BMI [10]

Classifications	BMI (kg/m^2)
Underweight	<18.5
Normal weight	18.5–24.9
Overweight	25–29.9
Obesity (class 1)	30–34.9
Obesity (class 2)	35–39.9
Extreme obesity (class 3)	≥40

Table 3.2 Waist circumference values specific to the populations used for the diagnosis of obesity [11, 12]

	Waist circumference (cm)	
Society/ethnic group	Man	Woman
USA	102	88
Europe	94	80
Turkey	100	90
China	90	80
Japan	85	90

80 cm for females and 94 cm for males. In the evaluation of obese patients, obesity-related history should be taken, and physical examination should be performed to determine the degree and type of obesity; the reasons for secondary obesity and obesity-related complications should be evaluated. The treatment of obesity aims to reduce obesity-related morbidity and mortality risks, to get patient adopt an adequate and balanced nutrition habit and enhance the quality of life. In the course of obesity treatment, 10% weight loss achieved during the first 6-month period provides an important benefit in the prevention of obesity-related health problems. The first step of the management is to comprehend current situation of obese patient and to create a comprehensive program. Diet program should be individualized and be prepared by nutritionists and dietitians. Increasing physical activity is very important both in the treatment of obesity and maintaining ideal weight. The aim of increasing physical activity in obese patients is to permanently modify lifestyle and ensure a less sedentary and more active life. In general, a moderate level physical activity (for any age group, about 30–45 min/day in each day of the week, if possible) should be recommended. Recommendations for increasing physical activity must be individualized, and sustainability must be checked. The most important factors affecting the success of obesity treatment are constant monitorization, effective and long-term social and psychological support, and behavioral therapy. The primary condition of permanent and effective weight loss is to motivate patient by convincing him/her of success. Pharmacological therapy should be considered for patients with BMI >30 kg/m^2, who failed to lose weight with diet, exercise, and life changes; patients with BMI 27–29.9 kg/m^2 who have comorbidities (type 2 diabetes, coronary artery disease, cerebrovascular disease, hypertension, dyslipidemia); and patients with BMI 25–29.9 kg/m^2 and waist circumference of >101 cm for men and >87 cm in women. The main groups of drugs used in the treatment of obesity include centrally acting drugs affecting food intake, drugs that interfere peripheral food absorption, and drugs which increase energy expenditure. In case of ineffective treatment, surgical treatment may be considered in patients with BMI >40 kg/m^2, BMI >35 kg/m^2, and obesity-related comorbidities (e.g., type 2 diabetes, OSAS, severe HT) uncontrolled by medical treatment and lifestyle changes and in cases who have failed to lose weight with nonsurgical methods. Obesity surgery (bariatric surgery) methods include:

1. Restrictive method limiting food intake: Vertical banded gastroplasty (VBG) and laparoscopic adjustable gastric band (LAGB)
2. Surgery for malabsorption: Jejunoileal bypass (JİB) and duodenal switch (DS)
3. Restrictive and malabsorptive combined procedures: Roux-en-Y gastric bypass (RYGB), biliopancreatic diversion (BPD), and biliopancreatic diversion/duodenal switch (BPD/DS) [13–20]

The aim of surgical treatment is to reduce obesity-related morbidity and mortality and correct metabolic and organ functions. Despite important developments in technical issues, nursing and follow-up after bariatric operations, risk, and perioperative complications are still encountered. Therefore, selecting suitable patient and technique is very important. RYGB, SG, and AGB are recently the most preferred surgical techniques. Weight loss is more pronounced in surgical techniques aiming malabsorption. Patients with significant cardiovascular risk should be monitored during the first 24 h after operation. In postoperative period, antihypertensive and antidiabetic medications should be revised, and dose reduction should be considered. During this period, prophylaxis for deep vein thrombosis is given, and pulmonary rehabilitation is carried out to restore pulmonary functions. Nutrition intake is commenced under supervision of a dietician, and 1.5 L/day oral liquid intake (with gradually increasing the amount) should be ensured. The most common complications seen in this period are pulmonary embolism and intestinal leak. In addition, some other complications such as secondary hyperparathyroidism, stomal obstruction, short bowel syndrome, hypercalcemia, marginal ulcerations, distension of gastric remnant, cholelithiasis, hernia, renal failure, hepatic abnormalities, damping syndrome, gastric prolapse, vomiting, esophagitis, and reflux may be seen depending on the type of bariatric surgery. The patient is given a detailed diet program before discharge. Patients are discharged on postoperative fourth to sixth day under normal conditions. Soft foods are commenced after 2 weeks, and solid foods are gradually added.

A diet program including 60–120 mg protein should be given to prevent protein malnutrition. All patients should be motivated by moderate-intensity physical activity (30 min daily, at least 150 min/week) after discharge. Folic acid and vitamin A, E, and K deficiencies may develop in the course of time. 1200–1500 mg/day calcium and 400–800 U/day vitamin D are required to meet daily requirements. Alcohol should be avoided during the first 6–12 months after operation.

Before therapy, the clinician must keep in mind that the effect of various bariatric surgical procedures on drug absorption and metabolism are scarce. Then again, malabsorptive techniques that extensively exclude the proximal part of the small gut lower the surface area in which most drug absorption takes place and can result in a reduction in systemic bioavailability. Nonsteroidal anti-inflammatory capsules should be avoided entirely after bariatric surgical procedure, if possible because they were implicated in the improvement of anastomotic ulcerations/perforations. Definitive restoration of asymptomatic abdominal wall hernias may be deferred until weight loss stabilization, and dietary status is stepped forward to allow adequate recuperation (12–18 months after bariatric surgery).

Follow-up visits were scheduled at the end of the 1st, 3rd, 6th, and 12th month. Pre- and postoperative workup included physical examination, detailed laboratory (complete blood count, liver and renal function tests, electrolyte levels) and transabdominal ultrasonography, and psychological evaluation. Clinicians should be alert for mineral deficiency, anemia, and osteoporosis that may develop in the long term [13–20].

The clinical issue arises in patients who underwent bariatric surgery and has been previously diagnosed with hyperthyroidism. The main surgical treatment approach for hyperthyroidism is to remove all thyroid gland to prevent recurrences. The problem is how to maintain euthyroid state with exogenous thyroid supplement in patients who had bariatric surgery. The malabsorption in ileal interposition surgery may cause inadequate absorption of L-thyroxine and may result in continuous hypothyroidism. Low-level evidence-based clinical trials demonstrated that decreased postoperative levothyroxine requirements are needed after bariatric surgery, but among them, no patients were included in those trials with surgery for hyperthyroidism. On this point, clinicians should be alert on absorption of L-thyroxine from intestine and stomach for thyroid hormone replacement. But in bariatric surgery, ileal interposition surgery ends with malabsorption and uncontrolled thyroid hormone replacement. Although the gold standard is total thyroidectomy for hyperthyroidism, Dunhill procedure is an option for hyperthyroidism control in patients with bariatric surgery.

3.2.1 The Future

Clinical management simulating the results of surgical procedure might be hired efficiently; it may arise out of the modern genetic paintings. It can ultimately, within the next decades or so, replace the surgical remedy of significant obesity.

What Can We Learn from This Case?

- Obesity is an increasingly serious health problem.
- Intentional weight loss offers considerable advantages to sufferers and is related to a universal discount in mortality.
- Bariatric surgical treatment may be efficiently used to obtain sustainable weight loss in morbidly obese sufferers.
- The management of post-thyroidectomy complications such as hypocalcemia, hypothyroidism in patients with bariatric surgery may be exceedingly difficult.
- Bariatric surgery concurrently brings forth important functional outcomes on nutrient deficiencies and drug absorption that clinicians must be aware of.
- The Hartley-Dunhill procedure is an important site for patients who do not have good access to thyroid hormone and may maintain adequate thyroid function up to 60% of patients without thyroid hormone supplementation.

References

1. Garrow JS. Obesity and related diseases. London: Churchill Livingstone; 1988. p. 1–16.
2. Blackburn GL, Kanders BS. Medical evaluation and treatment of the obese patients with cardiovascular disease. Am J Cardiol. 1987;60:55–8.
3. Fakhouri TH, Ogden CL, Carroll MD, Kit BK, Flegal KM. Prevalence of obesity among older adults in the United States, 2007–2010 (no. 106). Hyattsville, MD: US Department of Health and Human Services, Centers for Disease Control and Prevention, National Center for Health Statistics; 2012.
4. Ng M, Fleming T, Robinson M, Thomson B, Graetz N, Margono C, et al. Global, regional, and national prevalence of overweight and obesity in children and adults during 1980–2013: a systematic analysis for the Global Burden of Disease Study 2013. Lancet. 2014;384:766–81.
5. Domienik-Karlowicz J, Dzikowska-Diduch O, Lisik W, Chmura A, Pruszczyk P. Short-term cardio metabolic risk reduction after bariatric surgery. Hell J Cardiol. 2015;56:61–5.
6. World Health Organization. Controlling the global obesity epidemic. 2003. Available: http://www.who.int/nutrition/topics/obesity/en/. Accessed 3 June 2014.
7. Prospective Studies Collaboration, Whitlock G, Lewington S, Sherliker P, Clarke R, et al. Body-mass index and cause-specific mortality in 900 000 adults: collaborative analyses of 57 prospective studies. Lancet. 2009;373:1083–96.
8. Berrington de Gonzalez A, Hartge P, Cerhan JR, Flint AJ, Hannan L, MacInnis RJ, et al. Body-mass index and mortality among 1.46 million white adults. N Engl J Med. 2010;363:2211–9.
9. Poirier P, Cornier MA, Mazzone T, Stiles S, Cummings S, Klein S, et al. Bariatric surgery and cardiovascular risk factors: a scientific statement from the American Heart Association. Circulation. 2011;123:1683–701.
10. WHO Expert Committee. Physical status: the use and interpretation of anthropometry. Report of a WHO Expert Committee. WHO technical report series: 854. Geneva: WHO; 1995. p. 1–452.
11. World Health Organization. Waist circumference and waist-hip ratio: report of a WHO expert consultation, Geneva, 8–11 December 2008. Geneva: WHO; 2011.
12. Sonmez A, Bayram F, Barcin C, Ozsan M, Kaya A, Gedik V. Waist circumference cutoff points to predict obesity, metabolic syndrome, and cardiovascular risk in Turkish adults. Int J Endocrinol. 2013;2013:767202. https://doi.org/10.1155/2013/767202.
13. Clinical guidelines on the identification, evaluation and treatment of overweight and obesity in adults. The evidence report. National Institute of health. Obes Res. 1998;6(Suppl. 2):51–209.
14. Willett WC, Dietz WH, Colditz GA. Guidelines for healthy weight. N Engl J Med. 1999;341:427–34.
15. Nguyen NT, Magno CP, Lane KT, Hinojosa MW, Lane JS. Association of hypertension, diabetes, dyslipidemia, and metabolic syndrome with obesity: findings from the national health and nutrition

examination survey, 1999 to 2004. J Am Coll Surg. 2008;207:928–34.
16. Tsigos C, Hainer V, Basdevant A, Finer N, Fried M, Mathus-Vliegen E, et al. Obesity management task force of the European association for the study of obesity. Management of obesity in adults: European clinical practice guidelines. Obes Facts. 2008;1:106–16.
17. Lau DC, Douketis JD, Morrison KM, Hramiak IM, Sharma AM, Ur E, Obesity Canada Clinical Practice Guidelines Expert Panel. 2006 Canadian clinical practice guidelines on the management and prevention of obesity in adults and children [summary]. CMAJ. 2007;176:1–13.
18. Lyznicki JM, Young DC, Riggs JA, Davis RM, Council on Scientific Affairs, American Medical Association. Obesity: assessment and management in primary care. Am Fam Physician. 2001;63:2185–96.
19. Villareal DT, Apovian CM, Kushner RF, Klein S, American Society for Nutrition, NAASO, The Obesity Society. Obesity in older adults: technical review and position statement of the American Society for Nutrition and NAASO, The Obesity Society. Am J Clin Nutr. 2005;82:923–34.
20. NICE clinical guideline 43 Obesity: guidance on the prevention, identification, assessment and management of overweight and obesity in adults and children. Issue date: December 2006. pp. 1–84. http://www.nice.org.uk/nicemedia/pdf/CG43NICEGuideline.pdf.

4 Toxic Multinodular Goiter in a Patient Who Has Been Followed Up with the Diagnosis of Hashimoto Thyroiditis and Has Normal TSH Values

Betül Uğur Altun and Gülşah Yenidünya Yalın

Abstract

Nodular thyroid disease arises from the increased proliferation rate of thyroid cells. Thyroid scintigraphy is considered as the gold standard imaging method for the diagnosis of thyroid nodules with autonomous function. Autonomously functioning thyroid nodules (AFTN) are defined as palpable nodules that are larger than 1 cm on ultrasonography demonstrating a focally increased uptake on thyroid scintigraphy. Practicing technetium scintigraphy for thyroid nodules is only recommended in the presence of suppressed or subnormal plasma TSH levels. However, this may result in underdiagnosis of these nodules in iodine-deficient countries. We hereby present a case with AFTN despite the presence of normal TSH values.

B. U. Altun
Başkent University Medical School, Ankara, Turkey

G. Y. Yalın (✉)
Department of Endocrinology, Başkent University Istanbul Hospital, Istanbul, Turkey

4.1 Case Presentation

A 52-year-old female patient was admitted to endocrinology outpatient clinic. She had been diagnosed with subclinical hypothyroidism for 3 years, and levothyroxine 50 mcg/day had been initiated at the time of diagnosis. However, the patient had stopped taking medication for the last 2 years. Medical and family history was otherwise normal except for the presence of autoimmune thyroid disease in two of her first-degree relatives. Her laboratory results were as follows: thyroid-stimulant hormone (TSH), 0.8 (0.4–4 μU/ml); free T4 (fT4), 1.38 (0.7–1.48 ng/dl); and antithyroid peroxidase (anti-TPO), 600 (0–34 IU/ml). Her TSH level had been 5.27 μU/mL 3 years ago when levothyroxine treatment had been initiated.

Thyroid ultrasonography (USG) demonstrated minimally increased thyroid size and heterogeneous background echogenicity. There were multiple 9 × 5 × 6 mm and 12 × 10 × 9 mm isoechoic nodules with regular margins on the right lobe, and the larger nodule (12 mm) included peripheral and central vascularization. There was an isoechoic 11 × 10 × 9 mm nodule with regular margins and prominent central and peripheral vascularization on the left lobe. Tc-99m pertechnetate scintigraphy revealed parenchymal hyperplasia and bilateral hyperactive nodules with increased Tc-99m uptake (Fig. 4.1).

T. Özülker et al. (eds.), *Thyroid and Parathyroid Diseases*, https://doi.org/10.1007/978-3-319-78476-2_4

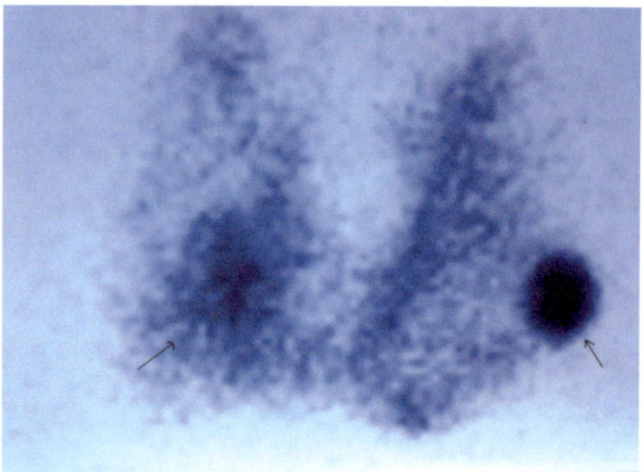

Fig. 4.1 Bilateral hyperactive nodules with increased uptake on thyroid Tc-99m pertechnetate scintigraphy (arrows)

The patient was diagnosed with autonomously functioning thyroid nodules (AFTN) with autoimmune thyroid disease in the background. She remained under surveillance once a year, and onset of subclinical hyperthyroidism was detected on her follow-up visit 1 year later.

4.2 Discussion

Plasma TSH and thyroid hormone levels should be measured in the initial evaluation of thyroid functions. Thyrotoxicosis is associated with increased thyroid hormones in the presence of suppressed plasma TSH levels. Etiology may not always be evident in clinical and laboratory findings. Thyroid scintigraphy is a valuable method in the differential diagnosis of benign and malign thyroid disorders. Thyroid scintigraphy is useful for (a) differential diagnosis of hyperthyroidism (low, diffuse, and nodular uptake patterns in patients with thyrotoxicosis are associated with subacute thyroiditis, Graves' disease, and toxic adenoma/multinodular goiter, respectively), (b) differential diagnosis of congenital hypothyroidism (thyroid agenesis, dyshormonogenesis, incomplete thyroid migration), and (c) before fine-needle aspiration biopsy (FNAB) for a thyroid nodule.

FNAB is only recommended for hypoactive nodules and is not recommended for hyperactive nodules. However, nodules which are smaller than 1 cm may not be visualized optimally during thyroid scintigraphy. Palpable nodules which are larger than 15 mm are more eligible for evaluation with thyroid scintigraphy. The activity uptake is also essential in the visualization of thyroid nodules, and hyperactive nodules are more easily detected than hypoactive nodules during thyroid scintigraphy. Nodule localization, neck position, and obesity may also affect the quality of the thyroid images [1].

Thyroid scintigraphy with Tc-99m pertechnetate or I-123 has been used with safety for a very long time. Nodular thyroid disease arises from the increased proliferation rate of thyroid cells. Increased rate of cell proliferation does not always result in hyperfunctioning thyroid nodules, and structural changes may also present with hypofunction. Scintigraphy is used in the detection of these functional changes in the parenchymal thyroid tissue. Thyroid scintigraphy is considered the gold standard imaging method for the diagnosis of thyroid nodules with autonomous function. USG, which is very useful in the structural evaluation of thyroid nodules, is not convenient for the assessment of nodule functions. Thyroid USG findings (size, echogenicity, vascularization) are not correlated with TSH levels in AFTN [2]. However, AFTN generally present as isoechoic nodules with peripheral and central vascularization (type III vascularization). Similarly, in the presented case, size of AFTN was not related to plasma TSH values, and plasma TSH level was not suppressed.

In some of the recent guidelines, the use of thyroid scintigraphy in clinical practice is only recommended for the diagnosis of hyperactive nodule/nodules and the evaluation of ectopic or residual thyroid gland [3]. Determination of hyperactive or hot nodules is not only necessary during the evaluation of thyroid function, but it is also essential in the differentiation of malign/

benign features in a thyroid nodule. Hot nodules have a low risk of malignancy, and thyroid biopsy or other invasive procedures are generally not recommended in the clinical practice. However, practicing thyroid scintigraphy for each thyroid nodule is not suggested by some of the clinical guidelines. These guidelines recommend practicing thyroid scintigraphy only in the presence of suppressed or subnormal plasma TSH levels [3]. However, these recommendations may not be applicable in all parts of the world. Maps on global iodine status affect guideline recommendations on this aspect. It is reported that low-normal TSH levels may also be an indication for the evaluation of hyperactive nodule/nodules especially in iodine-deficient regions [4–6]. The basis of this recommendation depends on the fact that the relationship between TSH and thyroid nodule autonomy may be different in iodine-deficient regions and that nodule autonomy may be present with non-suppressed, normal TSH levels in these areas. Furthermore, the presence of activating TSH receptor mutations in hot nodules may also be an additional risk factor for the development of thyrotoxicosis in iodine-deficient areas [7]. Because the USA is not one of the iodine- deficient countries, thyroid scintigraphy is only recommended in patients with low TSH levels [3]. However, iodine deficiency is also reported in some European countries such as Poland, Norway, Greece, Romania, and Turkey [8]. WHO reported that frequency of low urinary iodine excretion (<100 μg/L) is 56.9%, 9.8% and 42.6% in Europe, USA, and Africa, respectively [9]. Therefore, different recommendations for indication of thyroid scintigraphy have come into consideration in the current guidelines. Thyroid scintigraphy may be performed even in the presence of low-normal or normal TSH levels [5]. Administration of I^{131} during thyroid scintigraphy is not recommended in iodine-deficient areas.

AFTN is defined as a palpable nodule that is larger than 1 cm on USG demonstrating a focally increased uptake on thyroid scintigraphy [4]. Theoretically, TSH is expected to be low in these patients; however, in the presence of iodine deficiency, TSH levels may be normal in up to 49% of patients [6]. Therefore, a significant amount of AFTN may be underdiagnosed when only presence of low TSH levels is considered to suspect AFTN. Presence of iodine deficiency may prevent TSH suppression as it was the case in the patient presented above. Although FNAB is not recommended for AFTN, it is known that nearly 15% is investigated with FNAB [10]. FNAB results may be confusing due to benign follicular proliferative changes in hyperactive nodules which may be interpreted as malignancy, leading to false-positive results and unnecessary surgical interventions [4]. Therefore, evaluation with thyroid scintigraphy may be useful for preventing unnecessary procedures. Furthermore, the presence of normal TSH levels with AFTN implies a risk for the development of future hyperthyroidism. And every year, 4% of nontoxic thyroid nodules differentiate into toxic nodules. The relative increase of mortality is nearly 1.41 in subclinical hyperthyroidism, compared with euthyroid patients [11]. Therefore, it must be emphasized that patient surveillance is critical. In almost half of all the AFTN patients (24–80%), TSH is in normal ranges [4, 6, 12]. The gain of function mutations in TSHR or GNAS genes is considered as the main pathological factor in the development of AFTN.

Although rare, single nodule gaining autonomic function in a patient with Graves' disease is also reported. The toxic nodule is referred to as "Plummer syndrome," and presence of toxic nodule with background Graves' disease is called "Marine-Lenhart syndrome." Autonomous nodule and background autoimmune thyroiditis should be considered as two separate entities in this rare syndrome [13]. Although it is rare, this syndrome is mentioned in this section for its educational significance.

What Can We Learn from This Case?

- During the initial evaluation of thyroid functions, TSH should be used as the first-line laboratory test, and thyroid hormones should be measured when necessary.
- USG and TSH may not always be sufficient in the functional-structural evaluation of thyroid tissue leading to misdiagnosis of AFTN in iodine-deficient areas. Although indication for thyroid scintigraphy is limited to patients with low TSH levels in some guidelines, this recommendation may not apply to iodine-deficient regions, and it may lead to underdiagnosis of AFTN.
- Hot nodule or AFTN may cause false-positive pathology results leading to unnecessary surgical interventions.
- Iodine deficiency is a worldwide common public health problem, and some regions in Europe are still considered as iodine deficient.
- AFTN is more common than it is anticipated, and TSH levels may be normal in a considerable amount of these patients. It should also be kept in mind that AFTN may eventually differentiate into overt hyperthyroidism in these patients.

References

1. Sarkar S. Benign thyroid disease: what is the role of nuclear medicine? Semin Nucl Med. 2006;36:185–93.
2. Lanni F, Perotti G, Prete A, Pargliola RM, Ricciato MP, Carrozza C, et al. Thyroid scintigraphy: an old tool is still the gold standard for an effective diagnosis of autonomously functioning thyroid nodules. J Endocrinol Investig. 2013;36:233–6.
3. Haugen BR, Alexander EK, Bible KC, Doherty GM, Mandel SJ, Nikiforov YE, et al. American Thyroid Association management guidelines for adult patients with thyroid nodules and differentiated thyroid cancer. Thyroid. 2016;26:1–178.
4. Tregelia G, Trimboli P, Verburg FA, Luster M, Giovanella L. Prevalence of normal TSH value among patients with autonomously functioning thyroid nodule. Eur J Clin Investig. 2015;45:739–44.
5. Gharib H, Papini E, Garber JR, Duick DS, Harrell RM, Hegedüs L, et al. American Association of Clinical Endocrinologists, American College of Endocrinology, and Associazione Medici Endocrinologi medical guidelines for clinical practice for the diagnosis and management of thyroid nodules--2016 update. Endocr Pract. 2016;22:622–39.
6. Chami R, Moreno-Reyes R, Corvilain B. TSH measurement is not an appropriate screening test for autonomous functioning thyroid nodules: a retrospective study of 368 patients. Eur J Endocrinol. 2014;170:593–9.
7. Meller J, Becker W. The continuing importance of thyroid scintigraphy in the era of high-resolution ultrasound. Eur J Nucl Med Mol Imaging. 2002;29:425–38.
8. Vitti P, Delange F, Pinchera A, Zimmermann M, Dunn JT. Europe is iodine deficient. Lancet. 2003;361:1226–33.
9. Benoist B, Andersson M, Takkouche B, Egli I. Prevalence of iodine deficiency worldwide. Lancet. 2003;362:1859–60.
10. Mazzaferri EL. Management of solitary thyroid nodules. N Engl J Med. 1993;328:553–65.
11. Haentjens P, Van Meerhaeghe A, Poppe K, Velkeniers B. Subclinical thyroid dysfunction and mortality: an estimate of relative and absolute excess all-cause mortality based on time-to-event data from cohort studies. Eur J Endocrinol. 2008;159:329–41.
12. Giovanella L, D'Aurizio F, Campenni A, Ruggeri RM, Baldari S, Verburg FA, et al. Searching for the most effective thyrotropin (TSH) threshold to rule-out autonomously functioning thyroid nodules in iodine deficient regions. Endocrine. 2016;54:757–61.
13. Biersack HJ, Biermann K. The Marine-Lenhart syndrome revisited. Wien Klin Wochenschr. 2011;123:459–62.

5 Acute Suppurative Thyroiditis

Zeynep Cantürk

Abstract

The thyroid gland is remarkably resistant to infectious agents owing to several protective mechanisms; therefore, acute suppurative thyroiditis is rarely seen. The most common agents are *Staphylococcus* and *Streptococcus*. In this chapter, we report a man who presented with sudden onset left-sided neck swelling with pain and redness. His physical and laboratory examinations suggested acute suppurative thyroiditis due to a rare microorganism *Burkholderia cepacia* and treated successfully with appropriate antimicrobial therapy. Acute suppurative thyroiditis is a rare disease but should be kept in mind in any patient with acute painful neck swelling around thyroid gland. Although most common organisms are *Staphylococcus* and *Streptococcus*, physicians should be aware of the probability of other rare microorganisms.

Z. Cantürk
Division of Endocrinology and Metabolism, Department of Internal Medicine, Kocaeli University, Kocaeli, Turkey

5.1 Case Presentation

Case: 34-year-old male patient admitted to our clinic with sudden onset left-sided neck swelling with pain and redness (Fig. 5.1). There was no history of chronic disease, recent upper respiratory tract infection, or trauma. A painful nodule was palpated on the left lob of his thyroid gland. Otolaryngologic examination was normal. There were slight leukocytosis, 12,000 (4600–10,200); increased sedimentation rate, 52 mm/h (<20 mm/h); and C-reactive protein (CRP) level, 14.2 mg/dl (0–0.5). Thyroid hormones were within normal limits. Neck ultrasonography (USG) revealed 6 × 5 cm high-density cystic complex nodule, increased vascularity of left lobe, and reactive lymph nodes localized at the left jugular area. There was intense, heterogeneous cystic lesion compatible with infection or hemorrhage into the nodule on computerized tomography (CT) of the neck (Fig. 5.2). Based on the clinical and laboratory findings, the diagnosis was made as acute suppurative thyroiditis. Fine-needle aspiration from the cystic nodule and blood culture were performed for the microbiological identification. Amoxicillin-clavulanic acid treatment was started. Ciprofloxacin- and amikacin-sensitive *Burkholderia cepacia* was identified on the cystic nodule aspiration at the seventh day of the treatment. Antibiotic treatment switched to the ciprofloxacin. All the symptoms of the disease

T. Özülker et al. (eds.), *Thyroid and Parathyroid Diseases*, https://doi.org/10.1007/978-3-319-78476-2_5

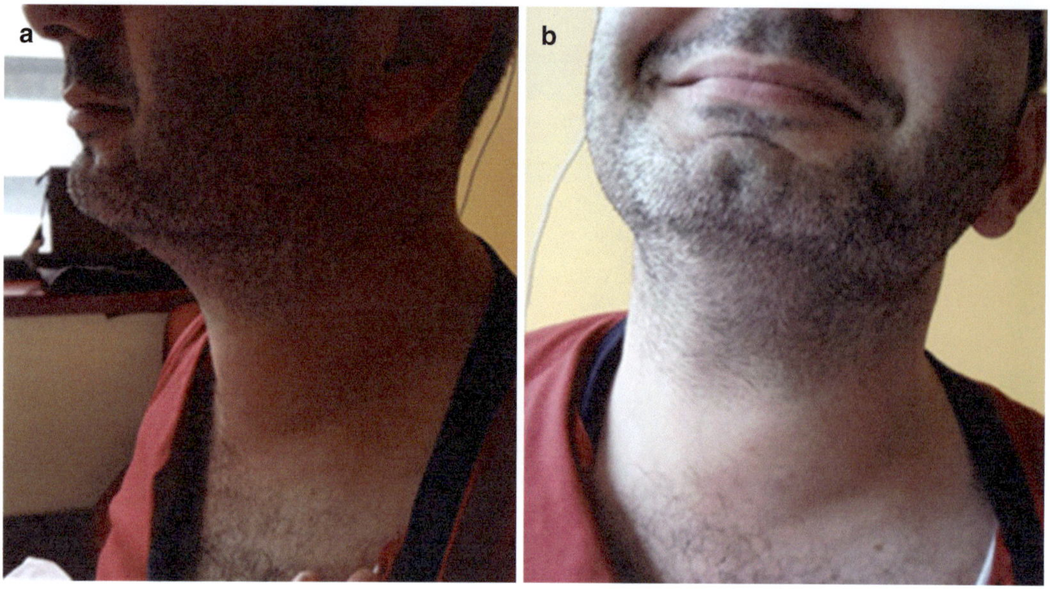

Fig. 5.1 Left-sided neck swelling with redness

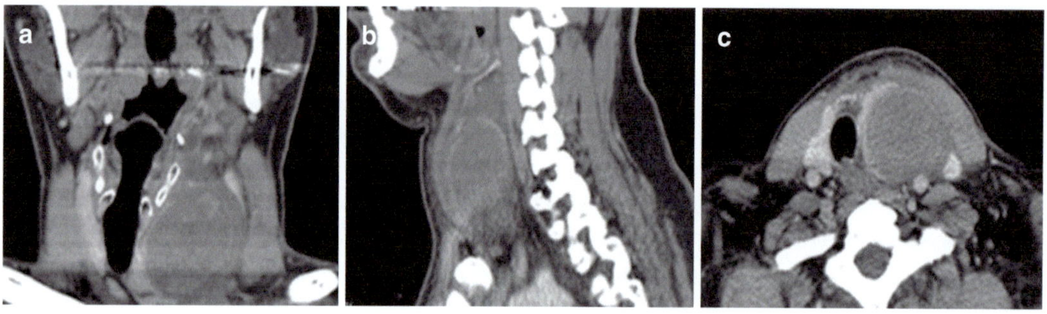

Fig. 5.2 Coronal (**a**), sagittal (**b**), and axial (**c**) slices of computerized tomography (CT) of the neck showing heterogeneous cystic lesion

were regressed, and sedimentation and CRP rates normalized at the twentieth day of the ciprofloxacin treatment.

5.2 Discussion

5.2.1 Evaluation and Diagnosis

In this chapter, we have presented a case of acute suppurative thyroiditis caused by a rare infectious agent.

Acute suppurative thyroiditis (AST) is a rare clinical entity, caused by an infection of the thyroid gland. Thyroid abscess and AST represent only 0.1–0.7% of surgically treated thyroid disorders. If AST is left untreated, it can be life-threatening, with 12% or higher mortality [1]. The thyroid is a well-known gland that resists infections. The rarity of thyroid infection has been attributed to the presence of high amounts of iodine within the gland, ample supply of blood and lymphatics, the fact that hydrogen peroxide is generated within the gland as a requirement for the synthesis of thyroid hormone, and its normal encapsulated position away from external structures. All of these features make the thyroid gland relatively resistant to infection by direct extension from contiguous sites [2].

Thyroidal infections are most commonly bacterial in origin, fungi, parasitic organisms, and mycobacteria being isolated much less frequently and more chronic; and these infections occur more frequently in immunocompromised patients [3].

Virtually any type of bacterium can infect the thyroid gland. Gram-positive bacteria including *Streptococcus* and *Staphylococcus* species are the most common causative organisms. In that case, *Burkholderia cepacia* (*B. cepacia*) was isolated in culture. *B. cepacia*, formerly known as *Pseudomonas cepacia* as it belonged to the *Pseudomonas* genus, is a Gram-negative aerobic bacillus. *B. cepacia* is known to cause opportunistic infections in immunocompromised hosts. It is highly virulent and often causes a necrotizing invasive infection. It is also highly resistant to antimicrobial agents [4]. Only one case from Korea has been reported as a cause of AST. A 54-year-old male with benign thyroid nodule had been infected by *B. cepacia* after acupuncture on his neck for the treatment and had been successfully treated [5].

Acute suppurative thyroiditis is a rare condition, and two-thirds of the cases are related to structural abnormalities [6]. In adults, the routes of infection are predominantly hematogenous or lymphatic; however, it can also spread via direct traumatic inoculation from an adjacent infection [7]. Patients with preexisting thyroid diseases have a greater predisposition for AST. Simple goiter, nodular goiter, Hashimoto's thyroiditis, or thyroid carcinoma have been observed in up to two-thirds of women and one-half of men with infective thyroiditis [8]. Other predisposing factors, especially in childhood, are pyriform sinus fistula; third and fourth arch abnormalities; immunocompromised states; rarely, endocarditis; tooth abscess; and fine-needle aspiration biopsy. In most cases, recurrent ASTs are usually due to congenital abnormalities located in the left lobe [1, 9]. In the present case, there was no predisposing factor. However, in some situations, such as persistence of pyriform sinus fistula, thyroid gland becomes susceptible to infection and abscess formation which is more commonly seen in children and young adults between 20 and 40 years of age. 92% of the affected patients are children, and there is no gender preference [10].

5.2.2 Clinical Manifestations

Acute bacterial thyroiditis is the most common cause of infectious thyroiditis, and more than 90% of patients will present with thyroidal pain, tenderness, fever, and local compression resulting in dysphagia and dysphonia. The pain may radiate to the mandible or ear on the same side. Signs or symptoms of systemic toxicity may be present. The thyroid with unilateral and bilateral lobar enlargement is tender to palpation and is associated with erythema and warmth of the skin. Abscess formation is detected by fluctuance; it is important to know that a firm nodule may progress to fluctuance in the course of 1–3 days, and so repeated physical examinations must be done carefully. Cervical lymphadenopathy may be present but is not a prominent feature unless there is predisposing pharyngitis [8].

Thyrotoxicosis does not typically accompany an episode of AST, but in some cases, it can be seen transiently and explained by the release of pre-synthesized and stored thyroid hormone into the circulation as a result of inflammation and disruption of the thyroid follicles. If this happens, thyroid hormone levels return to normal in most patients within 1–3 months [7].

In the present case, thyroid hormone levels were within normal limits.

Differential diagnosis of such a patient should focus on the differentiation between thyroidal and nonthyroidal causes. Essentially all the nonthyroidal causes are infectious in origin and present as discrete painful masses: infected thyroglossal duct cyst, infected branchial cleft cyst, infected cystic hygroma, cervical adenitis, and cellulitis of the anterior neck. Thyroidal causes of the painful anterior neck mass are subacute granulomatous thyroiditis, acute hemorrhage into a cyst, acute hemorrhage into a benign or malignant nodule, rapidly enlarging thyroid carcinoma, painful Hashimoto's thyroiditis, and radiation thyroiditis. Subacute granulomatous thyroiditis is the most common cause of the painful thyroid and often results in both local and systemic symptoms similar to those with infectious thyroiditis [8].

The diagnosis of AST can be supported by laboratory investigations. The serum thyroxine (T4), triiodothyronine (T3), and thyroid-stimulating hormone (TSH) are generally normal, although thyrotoxicosis and hypothyroidism have been reported in less than one-third of patients. In contrast, overt thyroid dysfunction frequently occurs in patients with subacute granulomatous thyroiditis. Leukocytosis, elevated erythrocyte sedimentation rate, and elevated C-reactive protein are usually present in AST. An elevated erythrocyte sedimentation rate is also seen in subacute granulomatous thyroiditis [8, 11].

It is suggested to evaluate patients with suspected AST with an ultrasound of the neck. In AST, the ultrasound often reveals unilobular swelling and/or abscess formation. These findings assist in the differentiation of AST from other causes of anterior neck pain and fever. Sonography of AST generally reveals a unifocal perithyroidal hypoechoic space and effacement of the plane between the thyroid and perithyroid tissues. Atrophy and an unclear hypoechoic or low-density area in and around the affected lobe are observed in the late inflammatory stage [12]. Alternatively, the sonoelastography may reveal very stiff lesions corresponding to the areas of the thyroid which are especially painful during acute phases of the AST episode which soften significantly as the patient responds to treatment [13]. The CT scan can be useful imaging modality due to findings. They also vary with the stage of AST. In the early inflammatory phase, nonspecific low-density areas in the swollen thyroid along with potential tracheal displacement may be seen. During the acute inflammatory stage, a CT can also demonstrate edema of the ipsilateral hypopharynx and abscess formation. In the late inflammatory stage, deformity of the thyroid, atrophy of the affected lobe, and scarring of the perithyroidal tissues may be observed [12]. However, during the early stage, features on ultrasound and CT scans may lead to an erroneous diagnosis of subacute thyroiditis, resulting in the prescription of prednisolone, which will have an adverse impact. Therefore, a careful ultrasonographical examination should be performed to detect characteristic findings during the early stage. If suspected, imaging with barium swallow study or fine-needle aspiration combined with a cytological examination and bacterial culturing might confirm the correct diagnosis of AST [12].

FNA is the best laboratory test for the evaluation of infectious thyroiditis and also is diagnostic for the most cases, especially if the tenderness is limited to a solitary nodule or a localized area and subacute granulomatous thyroiditis has been ruled out [8]. FNA performed during the acute phases of AST is important as the FNA has a superior ability to differentiate the patient with AST from those with subacute thyroiditis by cytological criteria and also provides appropriate bacteriologic specification for allowing accurate antibiotic selection for the patient with AST [1]. The aspiration material should be cultured also for aerobic and anaerobic bacteria, fungi, and mycobacteria. Gram and acid-fast stains should be performed, but a negative Gram stain does not exclude bacterial infection [11]. On the other hand, transcutaneous aspiration of the infectious material can be performed to relieve pressure on a displaced trachea in patients with a compromised airway [1, 8]. For all children and younger patients with recurrent or left-sided thyroiditis, a careful evaluation is recommended for pyriform sinus fistula. It's also suggested for patients with unexplained AST. Pyriform sinus fistula may be identified by a barium swallow, a possible fistulous tract located on the left side between the pyriform sinus and the thyroid gland. The barium swallow has very good sensitivity in detecting the presence of the fistula tracts as 89–97% of those examined in early and acute stages of AST were confirmed with this technique [12]. Transnasal flexible fiber optic laryngoscopy also has been used to visualize the internal sinus tract and is an effective technique [1, 14].

The present case matched most of the criteria of acute suppurative thyroiditis.

5.3 Management

Treatment of AST usually requires admission to the hospital, if necessary, drainage of any abscess is mandatory, and parenteral antimicrobial therapy must be used aimed at the causative agent. Gram stain and culture of the aspirate will reveal the causative organism in more than 90% of cases [8]. Due to a wide range of different bacteria that can be involved in this infection, broad coverage of antimicrobial agents is indicated, at least until culture results are available. Empiric antimicrobial therapy should provide adequate coverage for *S. aureus* and *S. pyogenes* [15].

For initial empiric treatment, an antibiotic regimen that provides coverage for aerobic and anaerobic organisms including *S. aureus*, *S. pyogenes*, Gram-negative anaerobic bacilli, and *Peptostreptococcus* is recommended. Appropriate antibiotic regimens include clindamycin alone, or the combination of penicillin and a beta-lactamase inhibitor, or the combination of metronidazole and a macrolide [11].

The antibiotic regimen is then adjusted based on the results of the culture and sensitivity test. Early administration of treatment with antibiotics can prevent most cases of AST from progressing to suppuration. However, once fluctuation occurs, antibiotic therapy alone is generally not sufficient. Surgical drainage is indicated when antibiotic therapy fails to control the infection promptly, as evidenced by leukocytosis, continued fever, and progressive signs of local inflammation. Drainage of the abscess is helpful in promoting resolution. It should be carried out if clinical examination or radiographical findings by ultrasound/CT scan are consistent with an abscess or if there is evidence of gas formation. If extensive necrosis or persistence of infection in spite of antibiotics is demonstrated, lobectomy may be required. Debridement of necrotic tissue should be done, and wound is allowed to heal by secondary intention [15]. CT-guided percutaneous drainage may be an effective and safe alternative to surgical treatment. The removal of the fistula is also necessary in recurrent infections [16]. If no clinical improvement occurs after 36–48 h of therapy, a reassessment of therapy is needed.

Nowadays, less invasive management is recommended during active inflammation and infection [1]. For very mild disease or after substantial clinical improvement, treatment with oral antibiotics may be possible [11].

5.4 Follow-Up and Outcome

Acute suppurative thyroiditis is a rare infectious disease. When the clinician encounters acute suppurative thyroiditis, abscess aspiration culture and blood culture for the microbiological identification and antibiogram should be performed because rare microorganisms would be the causative agent of existing acute suppurative thyroiditis. In this case, we present acute suppurative thyroiditis caused by *B. cepacia*, which is a rare infectious agent in adults. Isolation of microorganism was made by FNA material after amoxicillin-clavulanic acid treatment was started. Ciprofloxacin- and amikacin-sensitive *B. cepacia* is identified on the cystic nodule aspiration at the seventh day of the treatment. Antibiotic treatment switched to the ciprofloxacin. All the symptoms of the disease regressed, and sedimentation and CRP rates normalized at the twentieth day of the ciprofloxacin treatment. The disease didn't recur.

What Can We Learn from This Case?

- Although acute suppurative thyroiditis is rare, it should be suspected in any febrile patient with an acute painful anterior neck swelling.
- Patients generally present with the acute onset of pain and tender swelling in the anterior aspect of the neck that develops over days to a few weeks, often associated with fever and leukocytosis.
- Gram-positive bacteria including staphylococcal and streptococcal species are the most common causative organisms.
- Since this disease can be associated with anatomic abnormalities such as pyriform sinus fistula, it must be ruled out especially in younger, recurrent, and left-sided cases.
- Patients with suspected suppurative thyroiditis should be evaluated with ultrasonography. This will assess for abscess formation and possible extension of the infection into adjacent structures.
- Ultrasound-guided fine-needle aspiration can be helpful. The specimen should be stained and cultured for aerobic and anaerobic bacteria, fungi, and mycobacteria.
- All patients with presumed suppurative thyroiditis should be treated promptly with antibiotics.
- In cases where an abscess forms, surgical drainage may be necessary.
- With early diagnosis treatment is easy, and with proper treatment, abscess formation can be prevented.

References

1. Paes JE, Burman KD, Cohen J, et al. Acute bacterial suppurative thyroiditis: a clinical review and expert opinion. Thyroid. 2010;20:247–50.
2. Shah SS, Baum SG. Diagnosis and Management of Infectious Thyroiditis. Curr Infect Dis Rep. 2000;2:147–53.
3. Burman KD. Overview of thyroiditis. UpToDate. Topic 7824; vers.14.0.
4. Lee JH, Lee SH, Hong SJ, Choi YC, Hwang EG. A case of lung abscess caused by Burkholderia cepacia in healthy child. Korean J Pediatr. 2007;50:89–92.
5. Kim TY, Yang HM, Hwang JK, Cho YM, Park YJ, Park DJ, et al. A case of acute suppurative thyroiditis as a complication of acupuncture in patient with a benign thyroid nodule. J Korean Soc Endocrinol. 2002;17:576–82.
6. Unluturk U, Ceyhan K, Corapcioglu D. Acute suppurative thyroiditis following fine-needle aspiration biopsy in an immunocompetent patient. J Clin Ultrasound. 2014;42:215–8.
7. Dunham B, Nicol TL, Ishii M, Basaria S. Suppurative thyroiditis. Lancet. 2006;368:1742.
8. Farwell AP. Infectious thyroiditis. In: Braverman LE, Utiger RD, editors. Werner and Ingbar's the thyroid: a fundamental and clinical text. 8th ed. Philadelphia: Lippincott Williams and Wilkins; 2000. p. 1044–50.
9. Lazarus J, Henessey J. Acute and subacute and Riedel's thyroiditis. In: De Groot LJ, editor. The thyroid and its diseases. 6th ed. New York: Elsevier; 1996.
10. Pearce E, Farewell P, Braverman LE. Thyroiditis. NEJM. 2003;348:2646–55.
11. Brook I. Suppurative thyroiditis in children and adolescents. UpToDate. Topic 5822; vers. 12.0.
12. Masuoka H, Miyauchi A, Tomoda C, Inoue H, Takamura Y, Ito Y, et al. Imaging studies in sixty patients with acute suppurative thyroiditis. Thyroid. 2011;21:1075–80.
13. Ruchala M, Szczepanek-Parulska E, Zybek A, Moczko J, Czarnywojtek A, Kaminski G, et al. The role of sonoelastography in acute, subacute and chronic thyroiditis – a novel application of the method. Eur J Endocrinol. 2012;166:425–32.
14. Smith SL, Pereira KD. Suppurative thyroiditis in children: a management algorithm. Pediatr Emerg Care. 2008;24:764–7.
15. Brook I. Microbiology and management of acute suppurative thyroiditis in children. Intl J Pediatr Otorhinolaryngol. 2003;67:447–51.
16. Ghaemi N, Sayedi J, Bagheri S. Acute suppurative thyroiditis with thyroid abscess: a case report and review of the literature. Iran J Otorhinolaryngol. 2014;26:51–5.

Graves' Ophthalmopathy

6

Lebriz Uslu Beşli

Abstract

A 45-year-old female patient was diagnosed with Graves' ophthalmopathy. She was euthyroid under methimazole treatment, and thyroid scan revealed bilateral diffuse hyperplasia of the thyroid gland. Orbital MRI revealed a symmetrical increase in the volume of all extraocular muscles as well as the expansion of retro-orbital fat tissue, which are in concordance with the presence of bilateral exophthalmos. TRAb level was moderately elevated, and CAS score was 1. The patient received 15 mCi (555 MBq) radioiodine with oral glucocorticoids, to avoid exacerbation of orbital inflammation. Hyperthyroidism resolved within 6 months without progression of the ophthalmopathy. Graves' ophthalmopathy is an important clinical problem, as treatment of hyperfunctioning thyroid gland without triggering or exacerbating eye disease can be challenging. The presence and severity of orbital inflammation cannot be foreseen easily, and reversal of orbital damage cannot always be maintained. Several imaging modalities, biochemical parameters, and clinical assessment methods have been proposed to differentiate Graves' patients with active orbital inflammation from the patients with the inactive stage of the disease. To date, orbital MRI, serum TRAB level assessment, and CAS score are the most common methods to assess ophthalmopathy activity.

L. U. Beşli
Department of Nuclear Medicine,
Istanbul University Cerrahpaşa Medical Faculty,
Istanbul, Turkey

6.1 Case Presentation

A 45-year-old female patient was referred to our hospital for radioiodine therapy for treatment of hyperthyroidism. She was diagnosed with Graves' disease 2 years ago and was under methimazole treatment. She had cosmetic-related complaints about ophthalmopathy, which had started 6 months after the onset of hyperthyroidism. She had quit smoking 1 year ago. Her current serum thyroid-stimulating hormone (TSH) level was 0.55 μIU/ml (normal range: 0.4–4.2 μIU/ml), free triiodothyronine (fT3) level was 2.9 pg/ml (normal range: 1.8–4.2 pg/ml), and free thyroxine (fT4) level was 1.2 ng/dl (normal range: 0.7–1.9 ng/dl) under methimazole (6 tablets/day) treatment. Antithyroglobulin and antithyroid peroxidase (anti-TPO) antibody levels were low (15.8 IU/ml (normal range <34 IU/ml) and 3.3 IU/ml (normal range <115 IU/ml), accordingly), whereas anti-TSH receptor antibody (TRAb) level was moderately elevated (6.4 IU/ml, normal range <1.1 IU/ml). TRAb level 1 year ago was found as 18 IU/ml.

T. Özülker et al. (eds.), *Thyroid and Parathyroid Diseases*, https://doi.org/10.1007/978-3-319-78476-2_6

Thyroid ultrasonography (USG) revealed symmetrically enlarged thyroid gland with heterogenous reduced echogenicity. Bilaterally increased vascularity was observed in Doppler study. After 1 week discontinuation of methimazole treatment, thyroid scintigraphy with Tc-99m pertechnetate showed bilaterally diffuse hyperplasia of the thyroid gland, and radioactive iodine uptake (RAIU) test with 0.37 MBq I-131 revealed 17% and 34% uptake at the 2nd and 24th hours, respectively.

Orbital magnetic resonance imaging (MRI) revealed a symmetrical increase in the volume of all extraocular muscles, particularly inferior and medial rectus muscles, as well as the expansion of retro-orbital fat tissue (Fig. 6.1). The distance between the interzygomatic line and anterior edge of the globe was 21 mm, which indicates the presence of proptosis. All MRI findings were in concordance with thyroid ophthalmopathy. Eye examination revealed the presence of bilateral proptosis, lid retraction, and swelling of the eyelids. The clinical activity score (CAS) was 1.

The patient was given oral 15 mCi (555 MBq) radioiodine treatment, with oral prednisone (0.5 mg/kg for 1 month). Methimazole and propranolol were also prescribed.

6.2 Discussion

Graves' disease is an autoimmune disease, where autoantibodies against thyroid antigens cause hyperthyroidism [1]. It has a classical triad of hyperthyroidism, exophthalmos, and pretibial myxedema [2]. It is the most common cause of hyperthyroidism in areas with adequate iodine intake, and it is six to eight times more common in women [3]. The onset of the disease is generally 30–50 years of age. Although Graves' disease is not common in the population, Graves' ophthalmopathy can be seen in nearly half of all Graves' disease patients, having a severe course in 3–5% [4].

Several immunological factors are present in the pathogenesis of the disease: activation of specific T and B lymphocytes targeting TSH receptors is the leading cause of the disease, whereas lymphocytes targeting other autoantigens, such as thyroglobulin, thyroid peroxidase, and sodium-iodine symporter, also contribute in the pathogenesis of the disease [1]. Antibodies targeting TSH receptors stimulate thyroid gland and lead to hyperthyroidism and related symptoms, such as tachycardia, palpitation, nervousness, heat intolerance, hyperactivity, tremor, increase in appetite, systolic hypertension, and weight loss

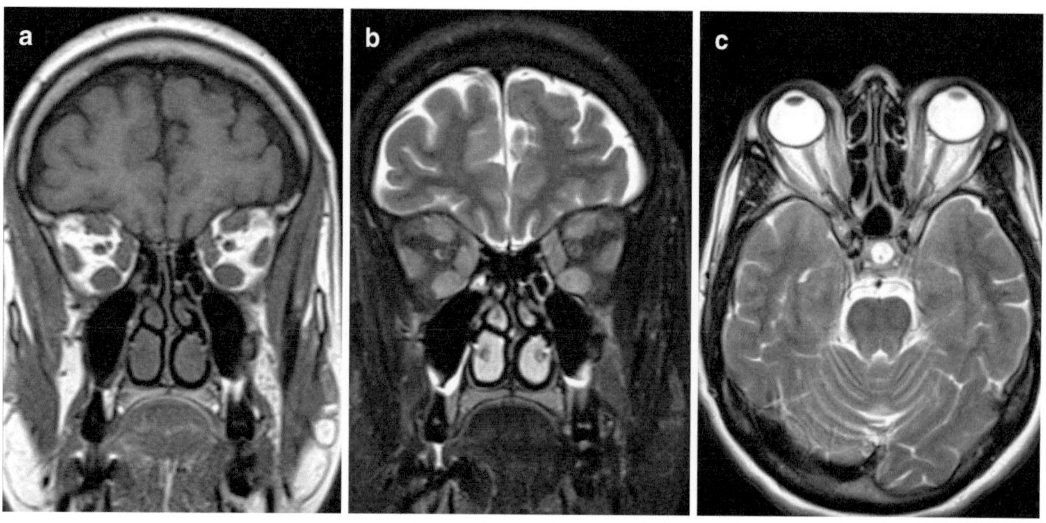

Fig. 6.1 Orbital MRI of the patient revealed bilateral symmetrically increased volume of orbital rectus muscles; on T1-weighted (**a**) and T2-weighted (**b**) coronal images. Proptosis and expansion of retro-orbital fat tissue can be observed on axial T2-weighted MRI images (**c**)

[3]. Inflammatory cells triggered by various cytokines and autoantibodies migrate to orbit and accumulate in retro-ocular tissue, causing an increase in orbital fat and fibrous tissue and extraocular muscle volume, resulting in Graves' ophthalmopathy [5]. Other factors, such as proliferation of fibroblasts stimulated by platelet-derived growth factors (PDGF A and B), mast cells, monocytes and macrophages, hyaluronic acid and interleukin-6 production of the stimulated fibroblasts, overexpression of insulin-like growth factor-1 (IGF-1) receptors in the fibroblasts, various cytokines, and increased oxidative stress, are the other contributors in the pathogenesis of Graves' ophthalmopathy [6]. Orbital muscles are generally spared in the initial phase of the disease, but they are infiltrated by mast cells and T and B lymphocytes in the course of the disease, resulting in increased muscle thickness [6].

Several genetic and environmental factors contribute to the development of Graves' ophthalmopathy. First- and second-degree relatives of Graves' disease patients have increased incidence of Graves' disease [7], and disease penetrance is 30% in identical twins [3]. The most significant environmental factor in Graves' ophthalmopathy development is smoking: ophthalmopathy is more common and more severe in smokers compared to nonsmoker Graves' patients [3]. Although Graves' disease is more common in females, ophthalmopathy is generally more severe in males. Smoking was a significant risk factor for our patient for development and worsening of the eye disease. Unfortunately, our patient refused to quit smoking until progression of the eye disease occurred.

Our patient was euthyroid under methimazole treatment. Thyroid hormone status is another important factor in the development of Graves' ophthalmopathy. Ophthalmopathy can be more severe in patients with thyroid dysfunction [8]; therefore, early treatment of hyperthyroidism is recommended in Graves' patients [9].

Although exophthalmos started concomitant with the onset of hyperthyroidism in our patient, which is the most common presentation, Graves' ophthalmopathy does not always start together with the onset hyperthyroidism; but it can start later in the course of the disease or even before the onset of hyperthyroidism. In 10–15% of Graves' patients, ophthalmopathy is seen with hypothyroidism [10]. Similar to other autoimmune diseases, ophthalmopathy has a dynamic course, including an initial progressive deterioration (active progressive phase), a plateau phase and a regression phase, and finally an inactive static phase, which was first described by Rundle in 1945 (Fig. 6.2) [11]. This process generally lasts nearly 1 year but may be prolonged to 3 years. In the active phase, classical signs of inflammation, including redness, pain, swelling, and impaired function, are seen, which lead to spontaneous retrobulbar pain, pain on eye movement, redness of the eyelids and conjunctiva, swelling of eyelids, inflammation of caruncle and plica, and conjunctival edema. The features are assessed in the scoring of the ophthalmopathy activity, which is called clinical activity score (CAS) (Table 6.1) [9]. The severity of ophthalmopathy is related to anatomical changes in the orbita. Swelling and redness of the eyelids, redness and edema of the conjunctiva, inflammation of the caruncle and plica, exophthalmos, eye muscle, and corneal or optic nerve involvements are evaluated for assessment of disease severity (Table 6.2) [9].

Medial and inferior orbital rectus muscles are the most commonly involved extraocular muscles. Although symmetrical involvement is generally seen, an asymmetrical involvement of the extraocular muscles can also be observed. MRI is currently the modality of choice for assessment of active orbital inflammation and evaluation of treatment response [12]. MRI signal intensity of inflamed extraocular muscles is related to CAS score, and inflammatory edema within the extraocular muscles can be detected measuring T2 relaxation time [12]. CT scan can also be used to assess extraocular muscle thickness. Ultrasonography [12] and scintigraphy using Ga-67 citrate [13], In-111 octreotide [14], Tc-99m HYNIC TOC [15], Ga-68 DOTA NOC [16], and F-18 FDG PET [17] are also other suggested alternatives for the detection of active ophthalmopathy, but these imaging modalities are not routinely used in the clinical practice for Graves' patients.

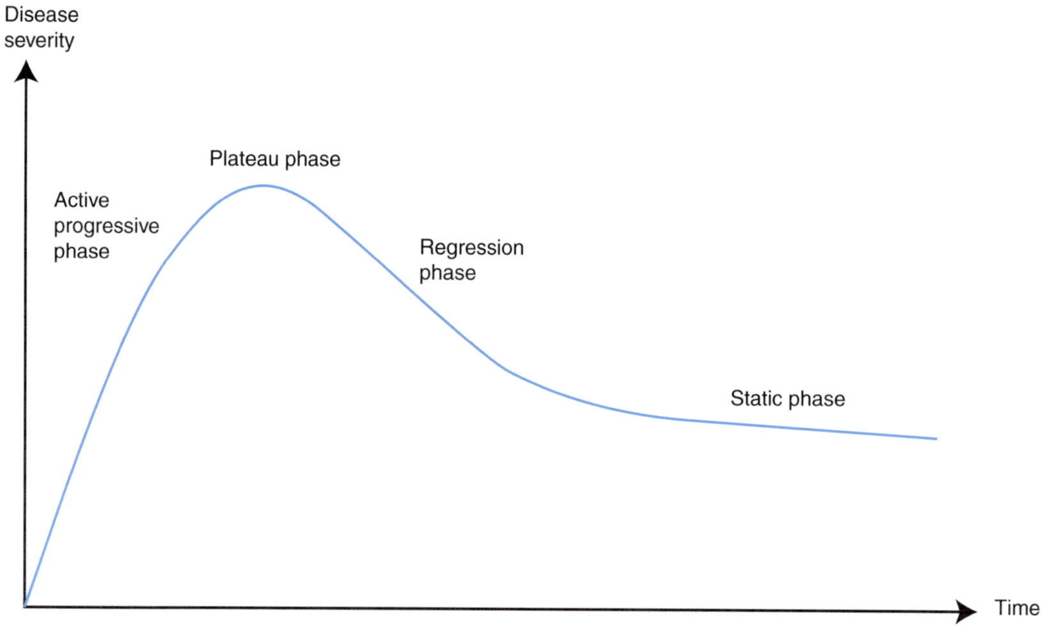

Fig. 6.2 Rundle curve describing the course of Graves' ophthalmopathy. The disease has an initial dynamic phase, where the severity of the disease increases progressively lasting for months after a sudden onset; a plateau phase where the progression ends lasting for months; and a regression phase, where slow improvement can be seen continuing for months to years. Finally, an inactive static phase is reached. Although rare, during the static phase, autoimmune activation may be triggered causing reactivation of the ophthalmopathy

Table 6.1 Clinical activity score for assessment of ophthalmopathy activity [10]. Each item in the list has 1 point, and ≥3/7 points indicate active Graves' ophthalmopathy

Spontaneous retrobulbar pain
Pain on attempted up- or downgaze
Redness of the eyelids
Redness of the conjunctiva
Swelling of the eyelids
Inflammation of the caruncle and/or plica
Conjunctival edema

Table 6.2 Severity measures of Graves' ophthalmopathy [10]

Lid aperture (in mm)
Swelling of the eyelids (absent/equivocal, moderate, severe)
Redness of the eyelids (absent/present)
Redness of the conjunctivae (absent/present)
Conjunctival edema (absent/present)
Inflammation of the caruncle or plica (absent/present)
Exophthalmos (measured in mm with Hertel exophthalmometer)
Subjective diplopia score (0 = no diplopia, 1 = intermittent, 2 = inconstant, 3 = constant)
Eye muscle involvement
Corneal involvement (absent/punctate keratopathy/ulcer)
Optic nerve involvement (visual acuity, color vision, optic disk, relative afferent pupillary defect, visual fields)

Treatment of hyperthyroidism is vital for Graves' ophthalmopathy patients, as thyroid dysfunction can aggravate the orbital inflammation. Antithyroid drugs, radioiodine therapy, and thyroidectomy are used for the treatment of hyperthyroidism. Among those treatment options, radioactive iodine has been postulated to activate and worsen the ophthalmopathy, which can be prevented by concomitant usage of oral or intravenous steroids [9, 18]. Local treatment modalities, such as lubricant eye drops, prisms to correct diplopia, or botulinum toxin for upper lid retraction, are recommended if the ophthalmopathy is mild, and intravenous steroids and/or radiotherapy is spared for moderate-to-severe active ophthalmopathy [9]. Somatostatin analogs, nonsteroidal anti-inflammatory drugs (NSAIDs), intravenous immunoglobulins, selenium, DNA synthesis inhibitors, and tumor necrosis factor-α (TNF-α) are the other options suggested for treatment of Graves' ophthalmopathy [19]. Cessation of smoking should be advised, as smoking is an important risk factor for the development of ophthalmopathy. For patients with moderate-to-severe inactive ophthalmopathy, rehabilitative surgery can be performed.

Assessment of ophthalmopathy activity is essential for treatment planning, as radioiodine treatment itself could exacerbate eye involvement. Exophthalmos had started 2 years ago in our patient, which suggests that ophthalmopathy has probably reached the inactive static phase. Only mildly elevation of TRAB levels also supports the inactive phase of the disease. However, MRI findings show that in addition to retro-orbital fat tissue expansion, extraocular muscle volume is increased, and T2 relaxation time is prolonged, suggesting that disease may still be in the active stage. Although MRI findings and CAS score generally correlate with each other, controversies can also occur, as seen in our case. Therefore, we have suggested to give radioiodine therapy with oral glucocorticoids to avoid any radioiodine-related exacerbation of the disease.

6.3 Follow-Up and Outcome

One month after radioiodine therapy, serum TSH was 0.4 μIU/ml, and both fT3 and fT4 were within normal limits under methimazole (4 tablets/day) treatment. On third-month follow-up, TSH was 0.9 μIU/m and fT3 and fT4 were within normal limits under one tablet/day methimazole treatment. On sixth-month follow-up, TSH level increased to 5 μIU/ml, and l-thyroxine supplementation (37 mcg/day) was initiated. No significant change was observed in the eye examination, and CAS score remained one during 6-month follow-up.

What Can We Learn from This Case?

- Euthyroid status and cessation of smoking should be maintained to avoid progression of Graves' ophthalmopathy.
- Assessment of ophthalmopathy activity is needed for treatment planning of patients.
- MRI and CAS score are generally used to assess ophthalmopathy activity.
- Corticosteroids or radiotherapy are spared for active ophthalmopathy.
- Radioiodine can exacerbate ophthalmopathy in the active phase unless given with corticosteroids.

References

1. Davies TF. The pathogenesis of Graves' disease. In: Braverman LE, Utiger RD, editors. Werner & Ingbar's the thyroid: a fundamental and clinical text. 9th ed. Philadelphia: Lippincott Williams & Wilkins; 2005. p. 458.
2. Franklyn JA, Boelaert K. Thyrotoxicosis. Lancet. 2012;379:1155–66.
3. Prabhakar BS, Bahn RS, Smith TJ. Current perspective on the pathogenesis of Graves' disease and ophthalmopathy. Endocr Rev. 2003;24:802–35.
4. Wiersinga WM, Bartalena L. Epidemiology and prevention of Graves' ophthalmopathy. Thyroid. 2002;12:855–60.
5. Orgiazzi J, Ludgate M. Pathogenesis. In: Wiersinga WM, Kahaly GJ, editors. Graves' Orbitopathy: a multidisciplinary approach - questions and answers. 2nd ed. Basel: Karger Verlag; 2010. p. 40–56.
6. Naik VM, Naik MN, Goldberg RA, Smith TJ, Douglas RS. Immunopathogenesis of thyroid eye disease: emerging paradigms. Surv Ophthalmol. 2010;55:215–26.
7. Ploski R, Szymanski K, Bednarczuk T. The genetic basis of graves' disease. Curr Genomics. 2011;12:542–63.
8. Tallstedt L, Lundell G, Blomgren H, Bring J. Does early administration of thyroxine reduce the development of Graves' ophthalmopathy after radioiodine treatment? Eur J Endocrinol. 1994;130:494–7.
9. Bartalena L, Baldeschi L, Dickinson A, Eckstein A, Kendall-Taylor P, Marcocci C, et al. Consensus statement of the European Group on Graves' orbitopathy (EUGOGO) on management of GO. Eur J Endocrinol. 2008;158:273–85.

10. Lazarus JH. Epidemiology of Graves' orbitopathy (GO) and relationship with thyroid disease. Best Pract Res Clin Endocrinol Metab. 2012;26:273–9.
11. Rundle FF, Wilson CW. Development and course of exophthalmos and ophthalmoplegia in Graves' disease with special reference to the effect of thyroidectomy. Clin Sci. 1945;5:177–94.
12. Kirsch E, Hammer B, von Arx G. Graves' orbitopathy: current imaging procedures. Swiss Med Wkly. 2009;139:618–23.
13. Konuk O, Atasever T, Unal M, Ayvaz G, Yetkin I, Cakir N, et al. Orbital gallium-67 scintigraphy in Graves' ophthalmopathy: a disease activity parameter that predicts the therapeutic response to immunosuppressive treatment. Thyroid. 2005;15:358–63.
14. Postema PT, Krenning EP, Wijngaarde R, Kooy PP, Oei HY, van den Bosch WA, et al. [111In-DTPA-D-Phe1] octreotide scintigraphy in thyroidal and orbital Graves' disease: a parameter for disease activity? J Clin Endocrinol Metab. 1994;79:1845–51.
15. Kainz H, Bale R, Donnemiller E, Gabriel M, Kovacs P, Decristoforo C, et al. Image fusion analysis of 99m Tc-HYNIC-octreotide scintigraphy and CT/MRI in patients with thyroid-associated orbitopathy: the importance of the lacrimal gland. Eur J Nucl Med Mol. 2003;30:1155–9.
16. Pichler R, Sonnberger M, Dorninger C, Assar H, Stojakovic T. Ga-68-DOTA-NOC PET/CT reveals active Graves' orbitopathy in a single extraorbital muscle. Clin Nucl Med. 2011;36:910–1.
17. Garcia-Rojas L, Adame-Ocampo G, Alexanderson E, Tovilla-Canales JL. 18-Fluorodeoxyglucose uptake by positron emission tomography in extraocular muscles of patients with and without Graves' ophthalmology. J Ophthalmol. 2013;2013:529187.
18. Traisk F, Tallstedt L, Abraham-Nordling M, Andersson T, Berg G, Calissendorff J, et al. Thyroid-associated ophthalmopathy after treatment for Graves' hyperthyroidism with antithyroid drugs or iodine-131. J Clin Endocrinol Metab. 2009;94:3700–7.
19. Marcocci C, Marino M. Treatment of mild, moderate-to-severe and very severe Graves' orbitopathy. Best Pract Res Clin Endocrinol Metab. 2012;26:325–37.

Surgery in Graves' Disease

7

Belma Koçer

Abstract

Graves' disease (GD) is an autoimmune disorder associated with hyperthyroidism, diffuse goiter, ophthalmopathy, dermopathy, and thyroid acropachy. Hyperthyroidism in GD is caused by stimulatory autoantibodies to TSH-receptor antibody. Typical signs and symptoms of thyrotoxicosis, ophthalmopathy, elevated thyroid hormone levels, and decreased serum TSH levels with or without the presence of serum thyroid antibodies confirm the diagnosis of GD. Thyroid ultrasound also provides useful prognostic information in terms of thyroid volume and vascularity. Radionuclide imaging is helpful in situations where thyroiditis cannot be distinguished from Graves' hyperthyroidism.

Treatment options for GD are medication, radioactive iodine treatment (RAT), or thyroidectomy. Antithyroid drugs (ATD) are often chosen as a primary treatment, and they are also used as pretreatment in selected patients prior to definitive treatment. For the management of resistant thyrotoxicosis, surgery or RAT is the treatment option. RAT is indicated in women planning a pregnancy in later than 4–6 months and patients with contraindication to ATD use or failure to medical therapy with ATDs. Surgery is usually considered for patients who have a large goiter, compressive symptoms, and a risk for malignancy and for women desiring pregnancy within 4–6 months or having significant ophthalmopathy. Total and near-total thyroidectomy is the recommended operation for patients undergoing surgery for GD. Nodular lesions are also detected in GD and would be managed in a similar manner as that in patients without this disorder. Papillary thyroid cancer might also coexist with GD. We present a case that highlights management options in patients with resistant thyrotoxicosis. Radioactive iodine and surgery are definitive modes of treatment, while beta-blockers, glucocorticoids, Lugol's solution, and cholestyramine can be used for rapid preoperative preparation in patients with resistant GD and to achieve euthyroidism.

7.1 Case Presentation

A 27-year-old woman attended the endocrine clinic with complaints of tachycardia, tremor, heat intolerance, weight loss, and fatigue for 6 months after the first labor. On presentation, her blood pressure was 140/80 mm Hg, and pulse was 120 beats per minute. Her electrocar-

B. Koçer
Department of Breast and Endocrine Surgery, Sakarya University, Faculty of Medicine, Sakarya, Turkey

T. Özülker et al. (eds.), *Thyroid and Parathyroid Diseases*, https://doi.org/10.1007/978-3-319-78476-2_7

diogram was consistent with sinus tachycardia. Her physical examination was remarkable for mild bilateral exophthalmos, tremor, and a diffusely enlarged and firm goiter. The serum TSH level was <0.05 mU/I (normal range 0.35–4.94 mU/I), and the serum-free triiodothyronine (FT3) and serum-free thyroxine (FT4) levels were elevated (FT3, 22.9 pmol/I, range 2.62–5.69 pmol/I; FT4, 40.7 pmol/L; normal range 9.00–19.04 pmol/I). Serum anti-TSH-receptor antibodies (TRAb) were markedly increased to 20 IU/L (range 0–1.5 IU/L), whereas antithyroglobulin antibodies (Tg-Ab) and anti-peroxidase antibodies (TPO-Ab) were absent. Serum beta-hCG was negative. Ultrasonography of the thyroid gland revealed mild diffuse enlargement, with the parenchyma showing heterogeneous echogenicity (Fig. 7.1). Hypervascularity was detected on Doppler USG (Fig. 7.2). A hyperechogenic nodule measuring 4 × 3 mm was detected in the left lobe. Fine needle aspiration biopsy (FNAB) was not performed because of the size of the nodule and the unsuspicious appearance. Technetium-99

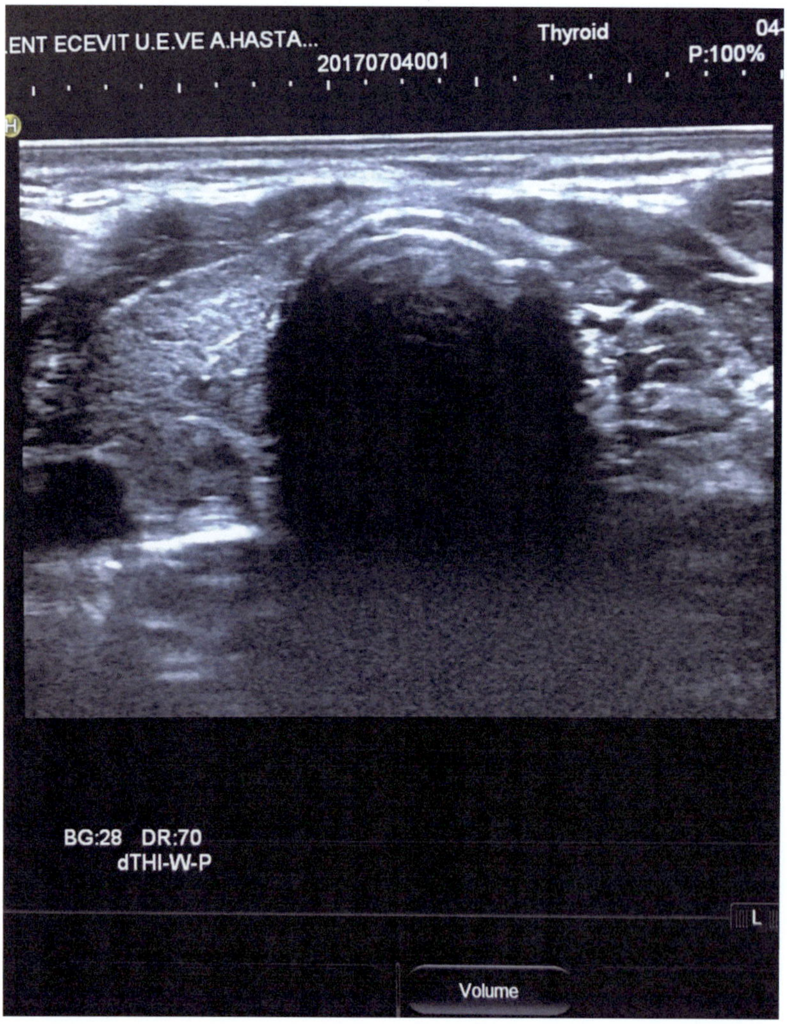

Fig. 7.1 Ultrasonographic appearance of the thyroid gland of the patient. The parenchyma shows heterogeneous echogenicity

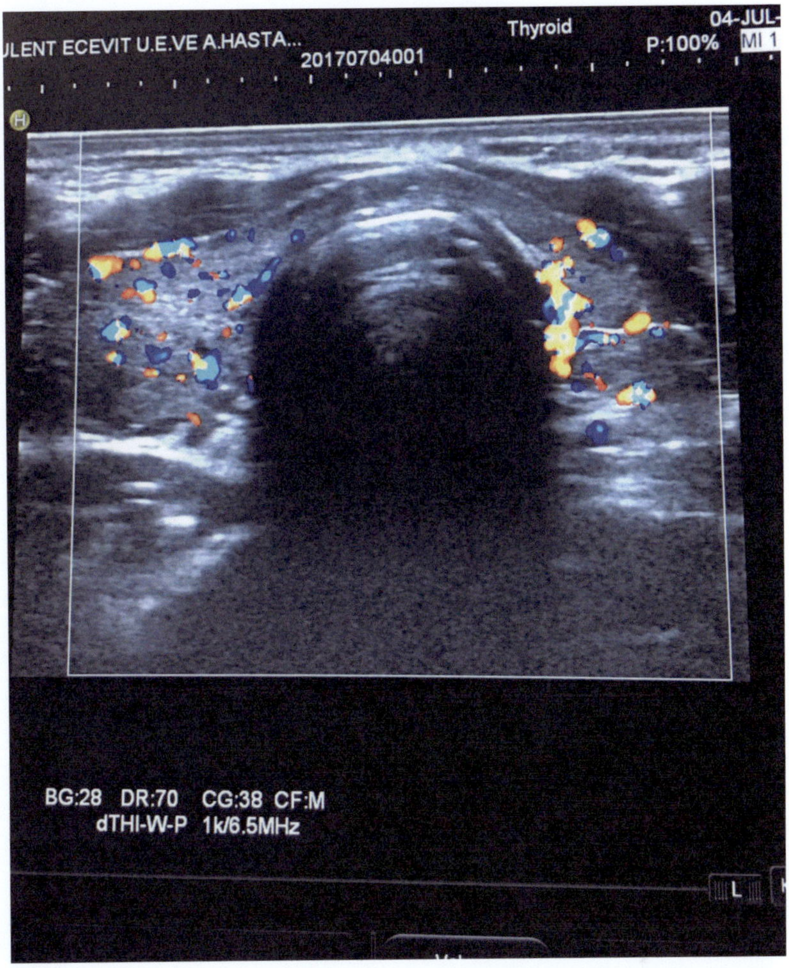

Fig. 7.2 Hypervascularity in the thyroid gland on Doppler USG

Pertechnetate scan of the thyroid gland showed diffuse enlargement with inhomogeneously increased activity, with uptake of 7.07% (Fig. 7.3). Based on the clinical presentation and laboratory findings, we diagnosed the condition as thyrotoxicosis due to Graves' disease (GD) with a nodular variant. Treatment with methimazole [MMI (30 mg/day) with divided doses] was started along with propranolol (40 mg/dL with divided doses); however, methimazole was increased up to 60 mg/day as there was no improvement in symptoms despite 3 months of treatment. The patients didn't get response to maximum doses of methimazole. High doses of prednisolone (1 mg/kg/day) along with cholestyramine (4 g every 6 h) for 2 weeks were then given to the patient. In addition, daily treatment with 0.5 mL (7 drops–375 mg) of Lugol's solution was also given for the last 7 days. After treatment with steroids, cholestyramine, and Lugol's solution, the patient showed progressive improvement of symptoms and signs of thyrotoxicosis with normalization of FT3 and FT4 levels. A total thyroidectomy was performed without any complication. Histopathological findings were conclusive for 5-mm papillary microcarcinoma (PTC) and follicular variation on the left lobe, with no lymphovascular invasion and extrathyroidal invasion (Fig. 7.4).

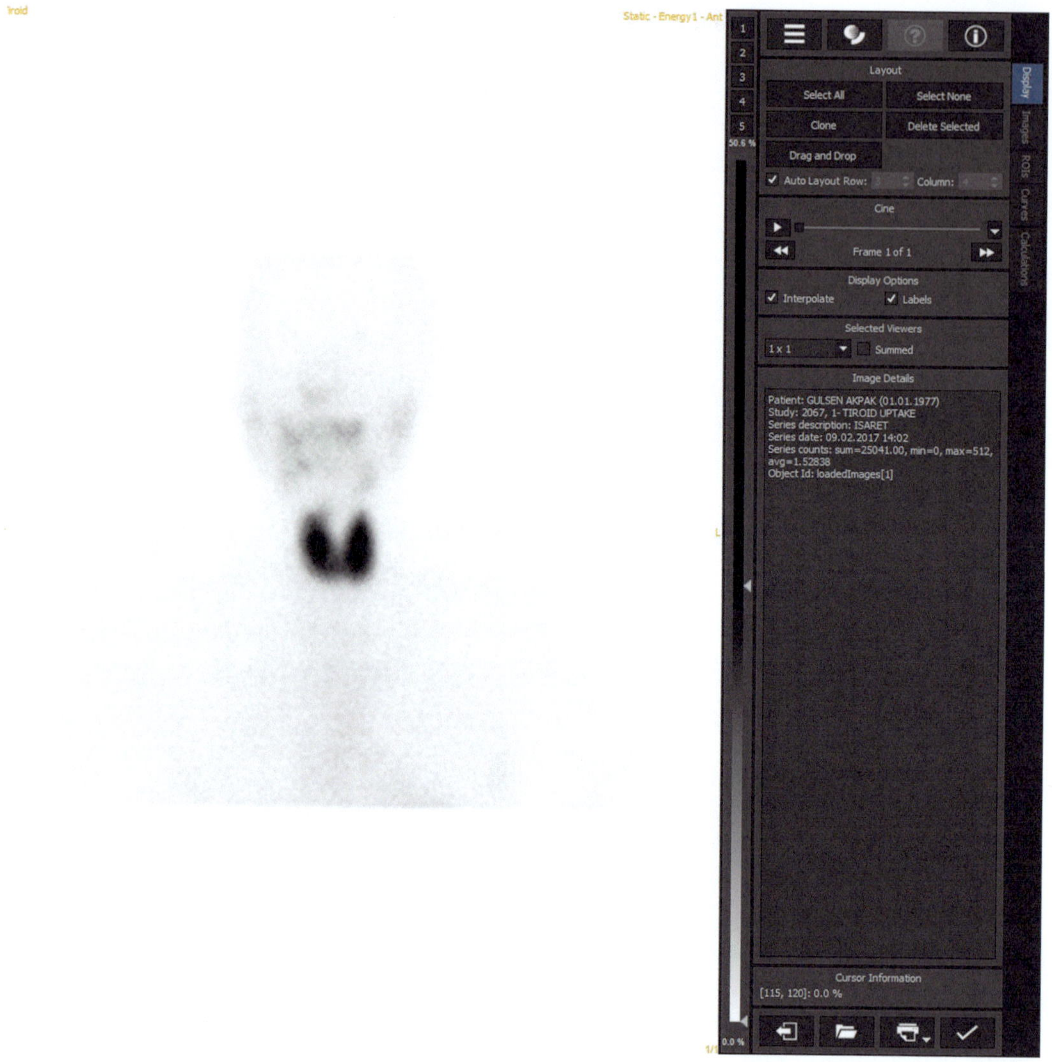

Fig. 7.3 Technetium-99 Pertechnetate scan of the patient. The thyroid gland shows diffuse enlargement with inhomogeneously increased activity, with an uptake of 7.07%

7.2 Discussion

7.2.1 Evaluation and Diagnosis

We report a case of thyrotoxicosis in a patient with GD that was resistant to antithyroid drugs but successfully responded to additional treatment with high-dose steroids, cholestyramine, and Lugol's solution prior to thyroidectomy so that surgery could be administered later.

GD is an autoimmune disorder characterized by hyperthyroidism, diffuse goiter, ophthalmopathy, and, in rare cases, dermopathy and thyroid acropachy. TRAb is responsible for causing hyperthyroidism. Thyroid dermopathy that comprises 1% of all GD cases consists of pretibial cutaneous nodules or diffuse thickening. Graves' ophthalmopathy (GO) is clinically relevant in approximately 25–50% of patients with GD, of whom about 3–5% have severe ophthalmopathy. Smoking, the level of thyroid dysfunction, the presence of persistently elevated TRAb levels, and the type of the treatment (RAT) influence the development and course of the GO [1].

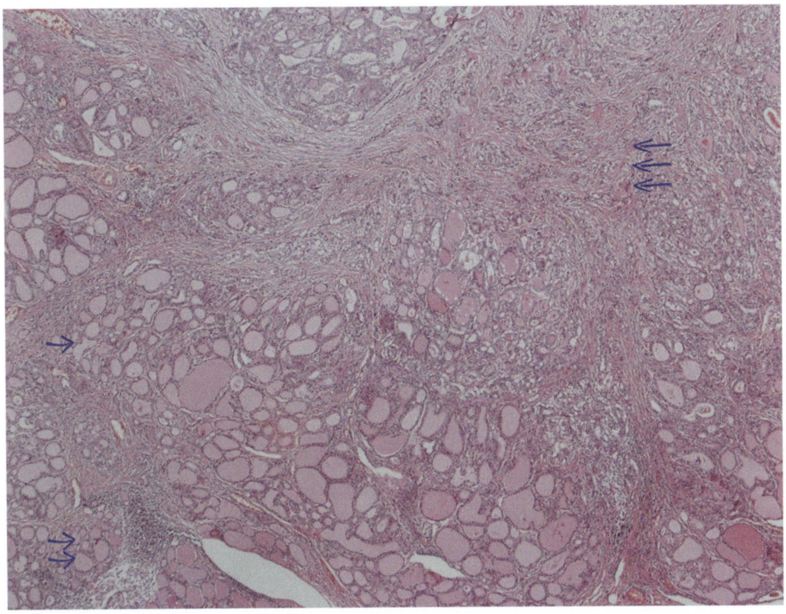

Fig. 7.4 Histopathological image of the patient's thyroid gland. Histological findings of GD are usually hyperplastic and dilated follicles of variable size with scalloping of the colloid in the follicle. Papillary microcarcinoma is shown by three arrows. ↑, normal thyroid tissue; ↑↑, lymphocytic inflammatory cell infiltration; ↑↑↑, papillary carcinoma

Diagnosis of GD depends on the presence of cardinal signs and symptoms of thyrotoxicosis, ophthalmopathy, elevated free or total thyroid hormone levels, and reduced serum TSH levels with or without the documented presence of serum thyroid antibodies. Thyroid ultrasound also provides useful prognostic information in terms of thyroid volume and vascularity. Radionuclide imaging is not essential for the diagnosis, but it is helpful in situations where thyroiditis cannot be distinguished from Graves' hyperthyroidism [2].

7.3 Management

GD is managed with medication, RAT, or thyroidectomy (Table 7.1). Several factors are considered in providing recommendations and choosing the treatment modality. Pharmacologic therapy is often chosen as first-line therapy for GD treatment. GD can be treated with medications that block thyroid hormone synthesis using drugs such as methimazole and carbimazole and also those that block peripheral T4 to T3 conversion using propylthiouracil. However, these drugs have well-known side effects; the most serious potential side effect are agranulocytosis, and hepatotoxicity, along with other side effects such as loss of taste, gastrointestinal upset, arthralgia, and most commonly rash, which can be severe. Antithyroid drugs can be used as primary treatment, and they are also used as initial treatment in selected patients prior to RAT and in surgery. Using antithyroid drugs, cure can be achieved for 12–18 months, which is sustained in around 40–50% of patients [3, 4].

A second possibility is radioactive iodine treatment that is indicated in women planning a pregnancy in later than 4–6 months and patients with contraindication to ATD uses or failure to achieve euthyroidism with ATDs or recurrent hyperthyroidism. Factors favoring pursuit of RAT over surgery include patients with a previously operated neck or externally irradiated necks or lack of access to a high-volume thyroid surgeon and those with comorbidities that increase the operative risks. RAT results in hypothyroidism in 80–85% of patients [5, 6]. Contraindications to RAT include pregnancy, lactation, and coexisting presence of thyroid cancer and patients with moderate to severely active GO [6]. The use of RAT therapy allows 15–30% risk of inducing or aggravating Graves' orbitopathy [6, 7]. A recent guideline recommended corticosteroid prophylaxis with RAT in patients with mild to moderate

Table 7.1 Treatment modality for Graves' disease: advantages, disadvantages, and success of treatment

Modality	Advantages	Disadvantages	Success of treatment
Antithyroid drugs	No ablative therapy	– Minor side effects <5% – Major side effects 0.2–0.3%	40–50% remission
Radioactive iodine treatment (I-131)	– Definitive treatment – Few side effects	– Recurrent thyrotoxicosis – Hypothyroidism time is less predictable – Lifelong thyroid hormone replacement – Radiation thyroiditis – Avoids pregnancy for 4–6 months – Contraindicated in pregnancy or breastfeeding – Prolonged increase in TRAb levels – Inducing or aggravating Graves' orbitopathy (15–30%)	80–85% permanent hypothyroidism
Surgery	– Rapid control of thyrotoxicosis – Definitive histology results – Immediate relief of the pressure symptoms in those with a large gland – Performed during pregnancy (second trimester) – Reduced need for regular follow-up – Rapid decline of TRAb levels	– Requires lifelong replacement therapy – Risk of hypoparathyroidism and recurrent laryngeal nerve injury	– Definitive treatment (100%)

GO and in patients who have risk factor worsening disease (such as tobacco smoking) and in patients with moderate Graves' orbitopathy [6].

Another option is surgery, which is often considered in cases of recurrence or intolerance of GD after medical therapy. Surgery is recommended in patients with symptomatic compression or large goiters (>80 g), risk for malignancy (e.g., suspicious or indeterminate cytology), and large thyroid nodules, especially if >4 cm or if nonfunctioning or hypofunctioning nodules on I^{123} or $Tc^{99}m$ pertechnetate scanning, associated with hyperparathyroidism; women desiring a pregnancy within 4–6 months, especially if TRAb levels are particularly high; and patients with moderate to severely active GO. Pregnancy is a relative contraindication, and surgery should only be used in the patients who cannot be adequately treated with antithyroid medications (i.e., those who develop an allergic reaction to the drugs) or resistance to ATDs or in circumstance when rapid control of hyperthyroidism is required. Optimally, thyroidectomy is performed in the second trimester [6, 8]. Our patient had mild bilateral exophthalmos and desired pregnancy in the near future; therefore, we chose surgery as a definitive treatment modality.

In European countries, ATDs tend to be the first-line treatment. Failure or intolerance of medical therapy is the most common reason for patients requiring definitive treatment for GD [9]. In the USA, endocrinologists favor RAT in 58.6% of the patients with GD, antithyroid drugs in 40.5%, and less than 1% for surgery [10].

Different approaches have been used for the management of resistant thyrotoxicosis, while surgery or radioiodine therapy is the treatment option. However, achieving a euthyroid state before definitive treatment is often necessary. TSH levels usually remain suppressed due to prolonged hyperthyroidism in patients who have otherwise normalized their T4 and T3 levels with therapy. Beta-blockers and high-dose glucocorticoids inhibit the peripheral conversion of T4 to T3, while inorganic iodide (Lugol's solution) and iopanoic acid decrease the synthesis and release of thyroid hormone [11], and cholestyramine enhances the enterohepatic excretion of thyroxine [12]. High-dose glucocorticoids can be added to antithyroid drugs in the management of thyroid crisis and for rapid preoperative preparation of resistant thyrotoxicosis. These agents could be recommended preoperatively in patients with GD with failed medical treatment, especially if side effects of antithyroid drugs have occurred [13]. Our patient had achieved euthyroidism after addition of steroids, cholestyramine, and Lugol's solution to high-dose thionamides and β-blocker treatment.

Antithyroid drug therapy resulted in a higher rate of adverse reactions (17.3%) than that with RAI (1.2%) and surgery (5.7%). This led to the discontinuation of ATDs and a change in therapy in 58% of these patients [4]. Patients may be switched from one drug to another when necessary due to minor side effects, but 30–50% of patients have a similar reaction to each drug. ATD therapy has also been associated with a higher relapse rate (48%) than that with RAI therapy (8%), whereas surgery has a 100% success rate [14].

Surgery provides definitive control of hyperthyroidism; it protects against the side effects of RAT and the potential side effects of ATD. The rates of surgical complications have been reported to be higher in patients with GD after thyroid surgery. Complications of surgery include transient and permanent hypoparathyroidism and recurrent laryngeal nerve damage in approximately 1–4% of patients. In a meta-analysis potential complications of thyroidectomy for GD were reported as hypocalcemia (32.5% temporary, 2.6% permanent), recurrent laryngeal nerve injury (3.43% temporary, 1.46% permanent), and immediate postoperative bleeding (<1%) among eight studies. In addition, new or worsened GO (15–33%), especially in smokers and those with radiation thyroiditis (1%), were common RAT complications identified by their analysis [14]. Vincent et al. reported that the complication rate of surgery was higher compared to the RAT group (36.9% vs. 2.7%); however, all the complications were transient [5]. High-volume thyroid surgeons who regularly perform thyroid surgery encounter lower surgical complication rates [15].

The recommended surgery for GD is total thyroidectomy as subtotal thyroidectomy carries a significant risk of recurrent thyrotoxicosis, which has been reported to occur in up to 30% of patients, and moreover, reoperative completion thyroid surgery is associated with a higher complication rate [16]. Total and near-total thyroidectomy is a safe and effective method of treating GD [6].

Diffuse thyroid enlargement is most frequent, but several patients with GD who live in iodine-deficient regions have coexisting nodular goiter. The prevalence of palpable thyroid nodules in patients with GD is around 15% [17] and fivefold higher than that in the general population [18]. Nodular lesions in GD could be managed in a similar manner as that in patients without this disorder, i.e., FNAB of the sonographically suspicious nodules and preferably hypoechoic solid nodules. The patients with GD more frequently showed atypical PTC findings on ultrasonography. The frequency of perinodular hypervascularity was significantly higher, and the frequency of hypoechogenicity was significantly lower in PTC patients with GD than that in PTC patients without GD [19].

FNAB is now accepted as a standard procedure for identifying neoplastic nodules arising in GD and is highly specific in PTC diagnosis; however, cytological and architectural atypia was commonly observed in nonneoplastic nodules arising in GD, especially in patients who underwent antithyroid treatment and prior RAT. The rate of indeterminate diagnoses has been reported to be significantly high (39.1%) [20]. Total thyroidectomy is recommended for FNAB diagnosis of PTC and suspicious PTC [21].

Papillary thyroid cancer also coexists with GD. The American Thyroid Association states that the frequency of thyroid cancer in patients with GD is 2% or less [6]; however, Staniforth JUL reported a meta-analysis showing that carcinoma occurred in 23% of GD cases with nodules, the proportion of carcinoma was only 5% in patients with no nodules, and 38% of the malignancy associated with the nodules was papillary microcarcinoma [18]. PTC was the most frequently reported cancer type. In several cases, the carcinomas are found incidentally during postoperative histological examination of the thyroid, and the majority of them are low-risk papillary thyroid microcarcinomas without lymph node metastasis or lymphovascular and extrathyroidal invasion. In one study, patients with GD and microcarcinomas showed a longer disease-free survival and an excellent prognosis compared with those in euthyroid patients with cancer of equal size [22]. However, Pellegriti et al. reported that nonoccult DTCs occurring in patients with GD caused increased disease-specific mortality compared to that with DTCs in matched euthyroid control patients [17]. Further studies are needed to fully clarify the prognosis of thyroid carcinoma occurring in patients with GD.

What Can We Learn from This Case?

- Failed medical therapy or intolerance of antithyroid drugs is the most common reason for patients requiring definitive treatment for GD.
- Thyrotoxic patients should be as close as possible to clinical and biochemical euthyroidism before going to surgery.
- Beta-blockers, high-dose glucocorticoids, Lugol's solution, and cholestyramine can be used for the rapid preoperative preparation of resistant thyrotoxicosis.
- Total thyroidectomy should be the optimal surgical treatment for GD.
- GD might be coexisting with papillary thyroid cancer.
- DTC associated with GD should be treated and followed up according to the ATA guideline for DTC.

7.4 Follow-Up and Outcome

Serum thyroglobulin measurements with thyroglobulin antibodies and neck USG were performed as part of the early postoperative evaluation in our patient. The patient has been evaluated as showing an excellent response (no clinical, biochemical, or structural evidence of disease) and not requiring RAI ablation. According to the ATA guidelines for DTC, RAI ablation is not routinely recommended after lobectomy or total thyroidectomy for patients with unifocal papillary microcarcinoma in the absence of other adverse features. The patient was started on a replacement dose of thyroid hormone, and her TSH levels were maintained between 0.5 and 2 mU/L [21].

References

1. Bartalena L, Fatourechi V. Extrathyroidal manifestation of Graves' disease: a 2014 update. J Endocrinol Investig. 2014;37:691–700. https://doi.org/10.1007/s40618-014-0097-2.
2. Okosieme OE, Chan D, Price SA, Lazarus JH, Premawardhana LD. The utility of radioiodine uptake and thyroid scintigraphy in the diagnosis and management of hyperthyroidism. Clin Endocrinol. 2010;72:122–7. https://doi.org/10.1111/j.1365-2265.2009.03623.x.
3. Abraham P, Avenell A, McGeoc SC, Clark LF, Bevan JS. Antithyroid drug regimen for treating Graves' hyperthyroidism. Cochrane Database Syst Rev. 2010:CD003420. https://doi.org/10.1002/14651858.CD003420.pub3.
4. Sundaresh V, Brito JP, Wang Z. Comparative effectiveness of therapies for Graves' hyperthyroidism: a systematic review and network meta-analysis. J Clin Endocrinol Metab. 2013;98:3671–7. https://doi.org/10.1210/jc.2013-1954.

5. Wu VT, Lorenzen AW, Beck AC, Reid VJ, Sugg SL, Howe JR, et al. Comparative analysis of radioactive iodine versus thyroidectomy for definitive treatment of Graves' disease. Surgery. 2017;161:147–55. https://doi.org/10.1016/j.surg.2016.06.
6. Ross DS, Burch HB, Cooper DS, Greenlee C, Laurberg P, Mala AL, et al. 2016 American Thyroid Association guidelines for diagnosis and management of hyperthyroidism and other causes of thyrotoxicosis. Thyroid. 2016;26:1343–14210. https://doi.org/10.1089/thy.2016.0229.
7. Traisk F, Tallstedt L, Abraham-Nordling M, Andersson T, Berg G, Calissendorff J, Thyroid Study Group of TT 96, et al. Thyroid-associated ophthalmopathy after treatment for Graves' hyperthyroidism with antithyroid drugs or iodine-131. J Clin Endocrinol Metab. 2009;94:3700–7. https://doi.org/10.1210/jc.2009-0747.
8. Burch HB, Cooper DS. Management of Graves' disease: a review. JAMA. 2015;314:2544–54. https://doi.org/10.1001/jama.2015.16535.
9. Bartalena L, Burch HB, Burman KD, Kahaly GJA. A 2013 European survey of clinical practice patterns in the management of Graves's disease. Clin Endocrinol. 2016;84:115–20. https://doi.org/10.1111/cen.12688.
10. Burch HB, Burman KD, Cooper DSA. A 2011 survey of clinical practice patterns in the management of Graves' disease. J Clin Endocrinol Metab. 2012;97:4549–58. https://doi.org/10.1210/JC.2012-2802.
11. Pearce EN. Diagnosis and management of thyrotoxicosis. BMJ. 2006;332:1369–73. https://doi.org/10.1136/bmj.332.7554.1369.
12. Tsai WC, Pei D, Wang TF, Wu DA, Li JC, Wei CL, et al. The effect of combination therapy with propylthiouracil and cholestyramine in the treatment of Graves' hyperthyroidism. Clin Endocrinol. 2005;62:521–4. https://doi.org/10.1111/j.1365-2265.2005.02249.x.
13. Langley RW, Burch HB. Perioperative management of the thyrotoxic patient. Endocrinol Metab Clin N Am. 2003;32:519–34. https://doi.org/10.1016/S0889-8529(03)00010-0.
14. Sundaresh V, Brito JP, Thapa P, Bahn RS, Stan MN. Comparative effectiveness of treatment choices for Graves' hyperthyroidism: a historical cohort study. Thyroid. 2017;27:497–505. https://doi.org/10.1089/thy.2016.0343.
15. Hassan I, Koller M, Kluge C, Hoffman S, Zielke A, Rothmund M. Supervised surgical trainees performed thyroid surgery for Graves' disease safely. Langenbeck's Arch Surg. 2006;391:597–602. https://doi.org/10.1007/s00423-006-0077-x.
16. Guo Z, Yu P, Liu Z, Si Y, Jin M. Total thyroidectomy vs bilateral subtotal thyroidectomy in patients with GD: a meta-analysis of randomized clinical trials. Clin Endocrinol. 2013;79:739–46. https://doi.org/10.1111/cen.12209.
17. Pellegriti G, Mannarino C, Russo M, Terranova R, Marturano I, Vigneri R, et al. Increased mortality in patients with differentiated thyroid cancer associated with Graves' disease. J Clin Endocrinol Metab. 2013;98:1014–21. https://doi.org/10.1210/jc.2012-2843.
18. Staniforth JUL, Erdirimanne S, Eslick GD. Thyroid carcinoma in Graves' disease: a meta-analysis. Int J Surg. 2016;27:118–25. https://doi.org/10.1016/j.ijsu.2015.11.027.
19. Chung JO, Cho DH, Chung DJ, Chung MY. Ultrasonographic features of papillary thyroid carcinoma in patients with Graves' disease. Korean J Intern Med. 2010;25:71–6. https://doi.org/10.3904/kjim.2010.25.1.71.
20. Hang JF, Lilo MT, Bishop JA, Ali SZ. Diagnostic accuracy of fine needle aspiration in thyroid nodules arising in patients with Graves' disease. Acta Cytol. 2017;61:117–24. https://doi.org/10.1159/000464094.
21. Haugen BR, Alexander EK, Bible KC, Caturegli P, Doherty GM, Mandel SJ, et al. 2015 American Thyroid Association management guidelines for adult patients with thyroid nodules and differentiated thyroid cancer: the American Thyroid Association guidelines task force on thyroid nodules ND differentiated thyroid cancer. Thyroid. 2016;26:1–133. https://doi.org/10.1089/thy.2015.0020.
22. Kikuchi S, Noguchi S, Yamashita H, Uchino S, Kawamoto H. Prognosis of small thyroid cancer in patients with Graves' disease. Br J Surg. 2006;93:434–9. https://doi.org/10.1002/bjs.5279.

Surgery in Hyperthyroidism: Toxic Adenoma and/or Multinodular Goiter

8

Türkay Kırdak

Abstract

Toxic multinodular goiter is observed in areas of endemic iodine deficiency and commonly in elderly individuals. Diagnosis and assessment are made easily by physical examination, serum thyroid function tests, ultrasonography, and scintigraphy. The disease presents with subclinical hyperthyroidism in a significant part of the patients. Radioactive iodine therapy and surgery are two basic treatment methods of the disease with specific advantages and disadvantages. Selection of the treatment method is made upon factors about the disease, patient, and physician. This paper presents a case with toxic nodular goiter and discusses treatment options.

8.1 Case Presentation

A 64-year-old female patient has presented with complaints of swelling and pressure in the cervical region for 10 years, fatigue, and palpitations. She has been using propylthiouracil 100 mg/day for 3–4 years due to hyperthyroidism. The patient had been recommended to have surgery due to hyperthyroidism previously with a pre-diagnosis of toxic multinodular goiter (TMNG), but she had abstained from the operation. She presented to our clinics due to exacerbation of her complaints.

Physical examination revealed an easily detectable and palpable, significantly grown, painless, asymmetric thyroid gland with mild retrosternal extension and moderate stiffness, including various-sized nodules on the surface. No enlarged lymph node was detected on palpation. No significant ophthalmopathy was observed. The remaining systemic examinations were normal.

Laboratory analyses included thyroid-stimulating hormone (TSH), free T3 and free T4, which were measured to be 0.125 μIU/mL (normal range: 0.350–4.940), 2.23 pg/mL (normal range: 1.71–3.71), and 1.20 ng/dL (normal range: 0.70–1.48), respectively. The level of thyroglobulin was slightly over the normal range. The level of 25-OH vitamin D was 12 μg/L. Complete blood count and biochemical analyses, level of TSH receptor antibodies, and electrocardiography examination were normal. The patient, who had been receiving antihypertensive medication for hypertension, had no family history of goiter or thyroid cancer.

Cervical ultrasonography (USG) revealed an enlarged thyroid gland with bilateral retrosternal extension, more significant on the right. Many

T. Kırdak
Division of Endocrine Surgery, Department of Surgery, Uludag University Faculty of Medicine, Bursa, Turkey
e-mail: tkirdak@uludag.edu.tr

T. Özülker et al. (eds.), *Thyroid and Parathyroid Diseases*, https://doi.org/10.1007/978-3-319-78476-2_8

nodules were detected bilaterally, the largest being a regular bordered isoechoic nodule located in the inferior aspect of the right lobe with a 4 cm longitudinal length, which included an area of cystic degeneration. A 2-cm-sized, partially irregular bordered, hypoechoic nodule was notable in the inferior aspect of the left lobe as well. No lymph node of pathological size was observed in the cervical region.

The thyroid scintigraphy performed with Tc-99m pertechnetate revealed that the thyroid gland was greater than its normal size and included a hyperactive nodule of 4 cm in the right lobe and a smaller hyperactive nodule in the superior aspect of the left lobe. Suppressed areas were also notable.

Atypia of undetermined significance was reported for the fine needle aspiration (FNA) biopsy obtained from the suspicious nodule located in the inferior aspect of the left thyroid lobe. The patient underwent total thyroidectomy. The blood parathormone and total calcium levels measured at the postoperative 12 h were 12 pg/mL (normal range: 15–68.3) and 7.8 mg/dL (normal range: 8.4–10.2), respectively, and oral calcium and vitamin D treatment was begun for the patient and discharged in the first day postoperative. No complication was observed. The pathology report revealed benign nodular colloidal goiter. Thyroid hormone replacement was begun. Calcium and vitamin D replacements were stopped during the follow-up period. The blood parathormone and calcium levels were found to be within normal ranges in the sixth month postoperatively.

8.2 Discussion

8.2.1 Evaluation and Diagnosis

Nodular goiter is frequent among areas of endemic iodine deficiency [1]. In these cases, hyperplasia and nodule formation are observed in the thyroid gland in time as a result of chronic stimulation. As the stimulation continues, the number and sizes of the nodules, as well as the sizes of the thyroid gland, increased over time, and nontoxic multinodular goiter (MNG) subsequently develops. In these cases, the volume of the thyroid gland is increased directly proportional to the age and duration of goiter. It has been reported that the increase in the volume of the gland is approximately 4.5% annually [2]. If MNG is not treated, some of the nodules may gain autonomy with the effect of somatic mutations in time, and TMNG may appear due to the excessive amount of thyroid hormone they secrete. In these cases, hyperthyroidism appears subclinically at the beginning and turns into clinical type [3, 4]. Eventually, the thyroid gland may reach extremely large sizes in cases with TMNG in years. Almost half of the cases are asymptomatic, and symptoms related to airway compression or swallowing may appear in 15% of the cases [5]. The transition from nontoxic MNG to TMNG necessitates a certain period. Díez [6] reported that 91% of their cases had been diagnosed within the last 10 years of life. Therefore, the incidence of TMNG-dependent hyperthyroidism is higher in the elderly [1, 6]. The median age of the patients was found to be 68, and 85% was found to be older than 55 years [2]. Our case was older than 60 years of age as well and had a nodular thyroid gland considerably enlarged in time along with hyperthyroidism, which were consistent with the data above.

In cases with hyperthyroidism treated with radioactive iodine (RAI), the all-cause mortality, morbidity, and mortality related to cardiovascular and cerebrovascular causes or fractures have been observed to increase [7, 8]. Cardiac complications are observed in 32% of the cases [5]. It was previously believed that mortality was independent from the etiology of hyperthyroidism [2]. However, it has recently been reported that the mortality rates among patients with TMNG were higher compared to those of patients with Graves' disease [8]. Therefore, hyperthyroidism-related complications should be investigated in patients with TMNG. In our case, no important complication was observed except for hypertension.

Subclinical hyperthyroidism (suppressed TSH and normal T4) has been determined in 82% of the cases with TMNG [9]. The clinical outcomes of subclinical hyperthyroidism are minimal, and the issue of whether it should be treated or not is under debate. However, treatment is recommended in case of a TSH level of <0.1 mIU/L and when the age of the patient is >65, or when the patients have comorbidities such as cardiovascular disease or osteoporosis [10, 11]. Since subclinical hyperthyroidism may be a messenger of clinical hyperthyroidism (suppressed TSH and high T4), patients who are not treated should be closely followed up.

In cases of hyperthyroidism with nodular gland, toxic nodular goiter should be the first prediagnosis to be made. However, physical examination and USG may not be sufficient for the differential diagnosis. Thyroid scintigraphy is important in the differential diagnosis of hyperthyroidism [12]. In our case, TMNG was considered due to our observation of bilateral hot nodules on the scintigraphy and normal TSH receptor antibody levels.

The incidence of thyroid cancer is similar among cases with TMNG, toxic adenoma (TA), and MNG, which varies between 4% and 11% [13, 14]. However, Smith et al. [15] determined a rate of incidental cancer of 18% in toxic nodular goiter. Furthermore, they reported that the incidental cancer rate among cases with TMNG (21%) was significantly higher compared to that of cases with TA (4.5%). However, most of the cancer types determined in these cases are micropapillary [14, 15]. No matter what the rate of the cancer is, evaluation of the nodules in TMNG is similar to that of MNG. However, as known, thyroid scintigraphy is facilitative in detecting hyperfunctioning nodules with low malignancy risk (hot) and hypofunctioning nodules with high malignancy risk (cold) in cases with TMNG. Therefore, the concurrent presence of scintigraphic findings with USG findings has been recommended for the decision of nodules to undergo FNA biopsy in cases with hyperthyroidism [16]. In our case, the decision of biopsy was made since the 2 cm nodule located in the inferior pole of left thyroid lobe was sonographically suspicious, and it was not hyperfunctioning according to the scintigraphic findings. The biopsy report revealed atypia of undetermined significance. The biopsy was not repeated since a decision for total thyroidectomy was made already due to TMNG. In these cases, cytological evaluation is not always necessary if there is no doubt of cancer in thyroid nodules smaller than 1 cm [16].

Preparation of patients with hyperthyroidism for surgery is important. In order to minimize the risk of thyrotoxic goiter in patients with TMNG, the T3 and T4 levels should be kept within normal ranges in the preoperational period. Surgery is not inconvenient in the presence of subclinical hyperthyroidism. In the presence of an accompanying disease, sufficient evaluation and preparation should be made prior to anesthesia. In these cases, the use of beta-blockers prior to surgery may reduce the symptoms. Our patient had subclinical and controlled hyperthyroidism and was receiving antithyroid medication. The decision of surgery could be made nonproblematically.

8.2.2 Management

Long-term medication with antithyroid drugs is not recommended in toxic nodular disease due to its side effects. The latest ATA guidelines recommend surgery or RAI therapy for precise treatment of TMNG or TA [12]. However, these methods have advantages and disadvantages as well. The recurrence risk of hyperthyroidism is almost none following surgical treatment, and the disease is controlled within days. However, all patients need thyroid hormone replacement in the postoperative period. Furthermore, complications such as permanent hypocalcemia or recurrent nerve injury specific to thyroidectomy may be observed although as low as 2% [5, 9]. There is no risk of surgery-related complication following RAI. Patients remain euthyroid in the long-term, and hyperthyroidism develops in 72% of the patients within 26 years [17]. On the other hand, a longer time is needed for control of the hyperthyroidism (mean: 5.4 months) following RAI, and control may not be provided in 15–22% of the patients despite the therapy [5, 18]. Furthermore, although not frequent, some of the patients may refuse to receive treatment due to the long-term carcinogenic effects of radioactivity. Therefore, various criteria should be considered for the decision of therapy selection. For example, surgery should be the first-line therapy for the presence of malignant or suspicious nodules in TMNG. Thyroidectomy also provides rapid elimination of compressive symptoms just after the surgery in cases with large and retrosternal goiter. However, RAI therapy provides a regression in the thyroid volume in 38% of the cases [5]. Furthermore, the regression in thyroidal volume is limited and is approximately 40% [19]. Therefore, compressive symptoms may not completely disappear. In cases with previous thyroidectomy or cervical surgery, in elderly individuals and those with serious accompanying disease, RAI may be the first-line therapy. On the other hand, if surgery is planned for patients with TMNG, it has been recommended that surgery should be performed by thyroid surgeons who have a large patient volume in order to reduce the risk of complications [20]. In the absence of an experienced surgeon, the patient may be referred for RAI therapy. The patient choice is another important factor in therapy selection. Therefore, the treatment selection should be made upon the common decision of the patient and the doctor. In our case, surgery was selected due to the presence of a large goiter that led to compressive symptoms, the absence of an accompanying disease that could increase the risk of the surgery, and absence of a previous cervical operation or a suspicious thyroid nodule.

The recommended surgical approach was total/almost total thyroidectomy in cases with TMNG and hemithyroidectomy in cases with TA [21]. In this case, the risk of recurrence is almost zero. Subtotal thyroidectomy is not currently preferred due to its high risk of morbidity in case of a recurrence or a need for a reoperation. The blood TSH levels of the patients undergoing hemithyroidectomy should be followed up in the postoperative period due to the risk of hypothyroidism.

A careful and precise surgery is important in avoiding complications during thyroidectomy. The strap muscles may be surgically cut when needed in order to provide a good exploration. The vascular structures should be carefully bound. The thyroid capsule should be set free via dissection, bilateral recurrent laryngeal nerves should be visualized, and the parathyroid glands should be protected with their vascular pedicles. Unprotected parathyroid glands should be implanted into sternocleidomastoid muscle. The superior laryngeal nerve should be visualized. If it cannot be visualized, medial capsular dissection and close and separate binding of the vessels to the thyroid gland are recommended in the upper pole due to the close relationship of the vessels and nerves in the upper pole [22, 23].

8.3 The Future

There are also local treatment methods for TMNG and TA such as ethanol injection or radiofrequency ablation. Although successful outcomes of percutaneous treatment methods have been reported, these methods have not been introduced as routine methods used in the treatment of toxic nodular disease yet. Thus, percutaneous methods are generally recommended in patients not proper for surgery or RAI. Further studies are needed in order to introduce percutaneous methods into routine algorithms of toxic nodular disease.

What Can We Learn from This Case?

- The thyroid gland may reach extremely large size in cases with TMNG in years.
- The toxic nodular disease should be treated due to its local, as well as its systemic, effects.
- RAI and surgery are two different methods of therapy with their advantages and disadvantages. Selection of the treatment method should be made upon factors related to the disease, the patient, and the physician.

References

1. Bülow Pedersen I, Knudsen N, Jørgensen T, Perrild H, Ovesen L, Laurberg P. Large differences in incidences of overt hyper- and hypothyroidism associated with a small difference in iodine intake: a prospective comparative register-based population survey. J Clin Endocrinol Metab. 2002;87:4462–9.
2. Nyirenda MJ, Clark DN, Finlayson AR, Read J, Elders A, Bain M. Thyroid disease and increased cardiovascular risk. Thyroid. 2005;15:718–24.
3. Berghout A, Wiersinga WM, Smits NJ, Touber JL. Interrelationships between age, thyroid volume, thyroid nodularity, and thyroid function in patients with sporadic nontoxic goiter. Am J Med. 1990;89:602–8.
4. Miller JM, Block MA. Functional autonomy in multinodular goiter. JAMA. 1970;214:535–9.
5. Kang AS, Grant CS, Thompson GB, van Heerden JA. Current treatment of nodular goiter with hyperthyroidism (Plummer's disease): surgery versus radioiodine. Surgery. 2002;132:916–23.
6. Díez JJ. Hyperthyroidism in patients older than 55 years: an analysis of the etiology and management. Gerontology. 2003;49:316–23.
7. Franklyn JA, Maisonneuve P, Sheppard MC, Betteridge J, Boyle P. Mortality after the treatment of hyperthyroidism with radioactive iodine. N Engl J Med. 1998;338:712–8.
8. Giesecke P, Rosenqvist M, Frykman V, Friberg L, Wallin G, Höijer J. Increased cardiovascular mortality and morbidity in patients treated for toxic nodular goiter compared to Graves' disease and nontoxic goiter. Thyroid. 2017;27:878–85.
9. Porterfield JR Jr, Thompson GB, Farley DR, Grant CS, Richards ML. Evidence-based management of toxic multinodular goiter (Plummer's disease). World J Surg. 2008;32:1278–84.
10. Surks MI, Ortiz E, Daniels GH, Sawin CT, Col NF, Cobin RH, et al. Subclinical thyroid disease: scientific review and guidelines for diagnosis and management. JAMA. 2004;291:228–38.
11. Donangelo I, Suh SY. Subclinical hyperthyroidism: when to consider treatment. Am Fam Physician. 2017;95:710–6.
12. Ross DS, Burch HB, Cooper DS, Greenlee MC, Laurberg P, Maia AL, et al. 2016 American Thyroid Association guidelines for diagnosis and management of hyperthyroidism and other causes of thyrotoxicosis. Thyroid. 2016;26:1343–421.
13. Negro R, Valcavi R, Toulis KA. Incidental thyroid cancer in toxic and nontoxic goiter: is TSH associated with malignancy rate? Results of a meta-analysis. Endocr Pract. 2013;19:212–8.
14. Gelmini R, Franzoni C, Pavesi E, Cabry F, Saviano M. Incidental thyroid carcinoma (ITC): a retrospective study in a series of 737 patients treated for benign disease. Ann Ital Chir. 2010;81:421–7.
15. Smith JJ, Chen X, Schneider DF, Nookala R, Broome JT, Sippel RS, et al. Toxic nodular goiter and cancer: a compelling case for thyroidectomy. Ann Surg Oncol. 2013;20:1336–40.
16. Haugen BR, Alexander EK, Bible KC, Doherty GM, Mandel SJ, Nikiforov YE, et al. 2015 American Thyroid Association management guidelines for adult patients with thyroid nodules and differentiated thyroid cancer: the American Thyroid Association guidelines task force on thyroid nodules and differentiated thyroid cancer. Thyroid. 2016;26:1–133.
17. Holm LE, Lundell G, Israelsson A, Dahlqvist I. Incidence of hypothyroidism occurring long after iodine-131 therapy for hyperthyroidism. J Nucl Med. 1982;23:103–7.
18. Schneider DF, Sonderman PE, Jones MF, Ojomo KA, Chen H, Jaume JC, et al. Failure of radioactive iodine in the treatment of hyperthyroidism. Ann Surg Oncol. 2014;21:4174–80.
19. Nygaard B, Hegedüs L, Ulriksen P, Nielsen KG, Hansen JM. Radioiodine therapy for multinodular toxic goiter. Arch Intern Med. 1999;159:1364–8.
20. Adam MA, Thomas S, Youngwirth L, Hyslop T, Reed SD, Scheri RP, et al. Is there a minimum number of thyroidectomies a surgeon should perform to optimize patient outcomes? Ann Surg. 2017;265:402–7.
21. Bron LP, O'Brien CJ. Total thyroidectomy for clinically benign disease of the thyroid gland. Br J Surg. 2004;91:569–74.
22. Bliss RD, Gauger PG, Delbridge LW. Surgeon's approach to the thyroid gland: surgical anatomy and the importance of technique. World J Surg. 2000;24: 891–7.
23. Kark AE, Kissin MW, Auerbach R, Meikle M. Voice changes after thyroidectomy: role of external laryngeal nerve. Br Med J (Clin Res Ed). 1984;289: 1412–5.

9 A Case of Sarcoidosis, Differentiated Thyroid Carcinoma, and Graves' Disease in the Thyroid Gland

Filiz Özülker and Tamer Özülker

Abstract

Sarcoidosis is an idiopathic chronic, systemic, and noncaseating granulomatous disease involving multiple systems. There have been reports indicating that there might be an association between autoimmune thyroid diseases and sarcoidosis. Pulmonary sarcoidosis has also been known to coexist with malignancies including differentiated thyroid cancer. It is not clear whether patients with sarcoidosis tend to develop malignancies or malignancies induce sarcoidosis. Overlapping of clinical and radiological findings between malignancies and sarcoidosis causes a difficulty in the management. We present a case of a 49-year-old female patient who had sarcoidosis, autoimmune thyroid disease, and differentiated thyroid cancer.

9.1 Case Presentation

A 49-year-old female patient who had been suffering from unexplained fever, weight loss, weakness, fatigue, and a dry, hacking cough for the last 6 months was referred to the chest diseases department. On examination there was no significant finding other than a palpable thyroid gland.

Laboratory examination results were as follows: TSH 0.01 (0.27–4.20) μIU/mL, free triiodothyronine (fT3) 10.3 (2.0–4.4) pg/mL, free thyroxine (fT4) 2.48 (0.93–1.70) ng/dL, anti-thyroglobulin antibody (anti-Tg) 124.5 (<115) IU/mL, antithyroid peroxidase (anti-TPO) 279 (<34) IU/mL, calcium 10.67 (8.6–10) mg/dL, parathormone (PTH) 32 (8–51) pg/mL, urinary calcium 150 (20–275) mg/24 h, angiotensin-converting enzyme (ACE) 72 IU/L (range, 8–52 IU/L), WBC 12 (4.1–11.2) × 10^3/μL, hemoglobin 14.7 (11.7–15.5) g/dL, and thrombocyte 374 (160–390) × 10^3/μL. Computerized tomography (CT) of the chest revealed bulky lymphadenopathy throughout the chest, including bilaterally hilar, subcarinal, aortopulmonary window and paratracheal lymph nodes. ^{18}F-FDG positron emission tomography (PET)/CT which was carried out for metabolic characterization of mediastinal lymph nodes and exploring any possible malignancy revealed intense accumulation of ^{18}F-FDG in the conglomerated mediastinal lymph nodes (SUVmax 27.6). Heterogenous FDG uptake with moderate intensity was also noted in the thyroid gland (Fig. 9.1). Sputum smear and sputum culture for bacteria and fungus were negative. Sputum and bronchoalveolar lavage (BAL) fluid did not

F. Özülker · T. Özülker (✉)
Department of Nuclear Medicine, University of Health Sciences (SBÜ), Okmeydanı Training and Research Hospital, Istanbul, Turkey

T. Özülker et al. (eds.), *Thyroid and Parathyroid Diseases*, https://doi.org/10.1007/978-3-319-78476-2_9

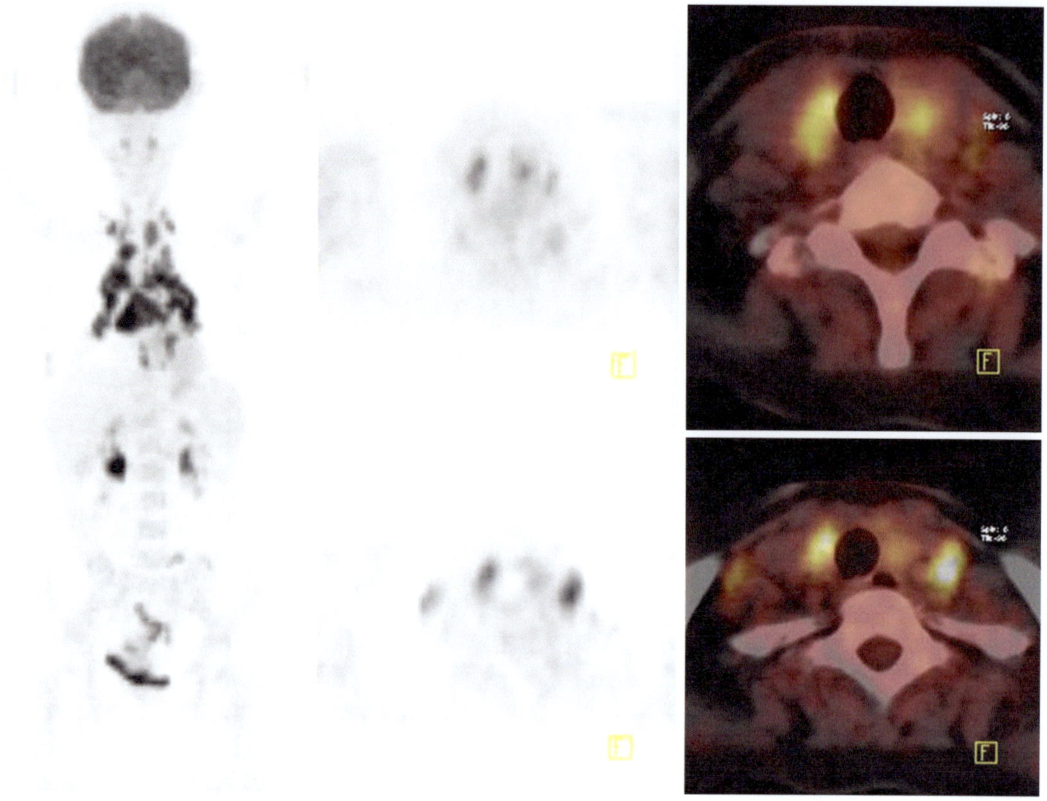

Fig. 9.1 ^{18}F-FDG PET/CT study showing hypermetabolic mediastinal lymph nodes in MIP images (left column), increased heterogenous FDG uptake in the thyroid gland on axial PET and fusion images (right column)

reveal any foreign body. Tubercle bacilli test or viral and immune serum tests were normal. Transbronchial lung biopsy, transbronchial needle aspiration of subcarinal and paratracheal lymph nodes, and bronchoalveolar lavage were performed, and histological analysis of the mediastinal lymph node biopsy showed a chronic, noncaseating, granulomatous inflammation. The ultrasonography (USG) of the thyroid gland revealed two hypoechoic nodules 6 mm in diameter and an enlarged gland with a heterogeneous, hypoechoic echotexture suggestive of autoimmune thyroid disease. Thyroid scintigraphy with 99mTc-pertechnetate showed a substantially increased diffuse uptake in both lobes and hypoactive area at the inferior pole of the right lobe adjacent to the isthmus, corresponding to a thyroid nodule (Fig. 9.2).

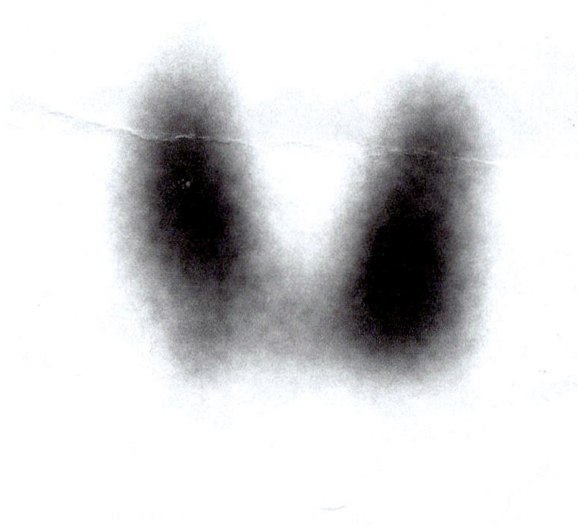

Fig. 9.2 Thyroid scintigraphy with 99mTc-pertechnetate showed a substantially increased diffuse uptake in both lobes and hypoactive area at the inferior pole of the right lobe adjacent to the isthmus, corresponding to a thyroid nodule

In the light of these findings, the patient was diagnosed with sarcoidosis and autoimmune thyroid disease (Graves' disease); oral prednisolone and methimazole were prescribed. The symptoms of the patient gradually receded with the administration of corticosteroid, and the patient became euthyroid. Two years later, a repeat USG revealed an enlargement in the two right-sided hypoechoic thyroid nodules with sizes of 12.2 × 7 and 10 × 7.5 mm, showing microcalcifications, irregular margins, and increased internal vascularization.

There were also newly developed subcentimeter hypoechoic nodules in the left thyroid lobe. Fine needle aspiration biopsy (FNAB) came out as papillary thyroid carcinoma (Bethesda VI). The patient underwent total thyroidectomy, and histopathology revealed multifocal papillary thyroid carcinoma with $BRAF^{V600E}$ mutated and showed five foci in both lobes, largest one being 2 cm in diameter. There was no vascular invasion, extrathyroidal extension, or metastatic lymph node involvement. The pathologic stage of the patient was pT1bN0M0 (Stage I) per the AJCC/TNM VIII system [1], and it was in intermediate risk group according to ATA guideline (2015) [2]. The patient was given 100 mCi (3700 MBq) 131-I, and the uptake at the remnant thyroid tissue in the neck without any other pathological uptake at the other sites of the body was detected in the posttreatment 131-I whole-body scintigraphy (Fig. 9.3).

9.2 Discussion

Sarcoidosis (S) is an idiopathic chronic, systemic, and noncaseating granulomatous disease involving multiple systems [3]. Almost all organs can be affected from S, but pulmonary sarcoidosis is the most commonly seen type. The liver, skin, and eyes are among other commonly involved organ systems [4].

Although the etiopathogenetic of the disease has not yet been fully understood, the suggested pathophysiologic mechanism is an autoimmune reaction triggered by a wide variety of stimuli, including bacteria, dust, viruses, foreign bodies, malignancy, metabolites, and chemicals. Normally, the inflammation formed during this process vanishes as the foreign stimulus is removed, but in patients with S who are supposed to be genetically susceptible, granulomatous inflammation persists probably because of the failure of the immune regulatory mechanisms to restrict the duration of the inflammatory process [5, 6]. There are characteristic clinical radiological features and histopathological findings of noncaseating granulomas which are suggestive of S, but since none of them are exclusively seen in S, the diagnosis is mostly made by ruling out the other alternative diagnoses [7]. The typical bilateral hilar lymphadenopathy can be detected on chest X-ray which has been the most widely used radiological imaging modality for diagnostic purposes of S. The characteristic appearance on computerized tomography (CT) is diffuse pulmonary perilymphatic micronodules which are distributed in peri-lobular and fissural areas predominantly in upper and posterior parts of the lung [8]. CT and magnetic resonance imaging (MRI) are equally effective in the evaluation of extrathoracic involvement, although MRI outperforms CT in the assessment of neurosarcoidosis and cardiac sarcoidosis [9]. Nuclear medicine procedures also have a role in the assessment of the extent and activity of the disease, thus guiding the biopsy. The accumulation of ^{67}Ga in intrathoracic lymph nodes forms a shape resembling the Greek letter lambda (lambda sign) and a symmetrical accumulation in bilateral parotid and lacrimal glands named as panda sign because of its resemblance to a panda face [10]. In recent years, ^{18}F-FDG PET/CT has proved to be useful in assessing disease extent and activity, treatment planning, and evaluating therapy response [9].

In our case, the metabolic activity of the subcarinal and paratracheal lymph nodes on ^{18}F-FDG PET/CT guided the transbronchial needle aspiration. ^{18}F-FDG PET also has a crucial role in the assessment of disease activity and monitoring therapy response in patients with cardiac sarcoidosis [11]. Somatostatin receptor imaging

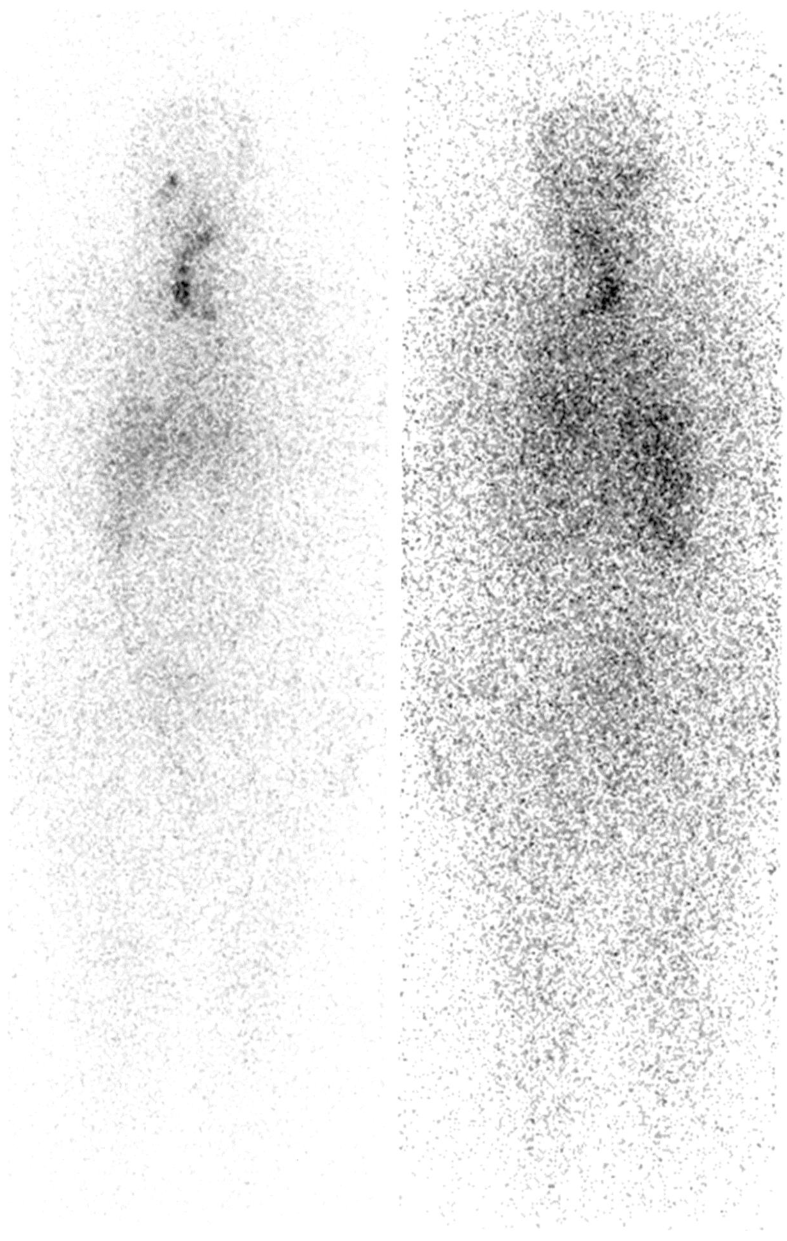

Fig. 9.3 Posttreatment 131-I whole-body scintigraphy showing uptake at the remnant thyroid tissue in the neck without any other pathological uptake at the other sites of the body

with ^{68}Ga-DOTATOC-PET/CT showed promising results in the assessment of the extent of the disease and directing peptide receptor radionuclide therapy (PRRT) with ^{177}Lu-DOTATOC in patients with otherwise treatment-refractory disease [12].

In the index case, ^{18}F-FDG PET/CT study conducted for the initial evaluation of the disease had shown heterogeneously increased metabolic activity in the thyroid gland, a finding raising the suspicion of the diagnosis of autoimmune thyroid disorder, which was also supported by laboratory findings and clinic of the patient. There have been numerous studies showing a significantly increased risk for hypothyroidism, antithyroid peroxidase antibodies (TPOAb), and thyroid autoimmunity, in female patients with S [6]. There have been preliminary reports pointing out that there might be an association between autoimmune thyroid diseases and sarcoidosis [13, 14].

Papadopoulos et al. examined a series of Swedish patients with sarcoidosis and found that 20% of the patients had endocrine autoimmunity, and evidence of thyroid autoimmunity was detected in 13 out of 89 patients, 8 of whom had clinical autoimmune thyroid disease (ATD) (2 with Graves' disease and 6 with autoimmune thyroiditis) [15]. Antonelli et al. detected a highly significant association of S and thyroid autoimmunity and concluded that thyroid function, TPOAb antibodies, and USG should be tested as part of the clinical profile in female S patients [16]. Fallahi et al. investigated the prevalence of other autoimmune disorders among 3069 patients with ATD and found that in these patients, the prevalence of autoimmune disorders including sarcoidosis increased significantly compared to control subjects [17]. Since ATDs are very commonly seen in comparison with S, it is stated that it is not necessary to investigate for S in patients with ATD, but it may be wise to check for ATD in patients with S [6].

There have been also few cases of direct involvement of thyroid gland with S in the literature [18, 19].

The patient in the index case underwent FNAB of the thyroid nodule, for the nodule had well-known USG features of malignancy; hypoechogenicity, microcalcifications, irregular margins, and increased internal vascularization. Enlargement of the thyroid nodules during the 2-year follow-up also raised suspicion for malignancy. Thyroid scintigraphy was used as a guide to determine which nodule to biopsy, for the malignancy risk in hyperactive nodules, is extremely low rendering the FNAB unnecessary. FNAB of the hypoactive nodule at the inferior pole of the right lobe adjacent to isthmus carrying the malignancy features on USG turned out to be malignant.

There have been two retrospective case series, indicating that 4–14% of all patients with malignancy can show some histopathological evidence of sarcoidosis [20, 21]. Whether the patients with pulmonary sarcoidosis are predisposed to develop malignancies or malignancies induce sarcoidosis continues to be a matter of debate [22]. The coexistence of thyroid cancer and S has been previously described in individual case reports [23]. Myint and Chow reported a case of sarcoidosis mimicking metastatic thyroid cancer following radioactive iodine therapy. The authors draw attention to the inability of clinical presentation and radiological evaluation, including PET and CT scans to discriminate between cancer recurrence and S. Sarcoid, or sarcoid-like reactions, should be kept in mind while evaluating the FDG-avid lesions any time after antineoplastic therapy including RAT [24]. Bruins et al. reported the development of papillary thyroid carcinoma in a patient with sarcoidosis following treatment with minocycline [25].

9.3 Follow-Up and Outcome

The chest radiography and CT performed at 7-month follow-up confirmed a remission of S. Currently, our patient is being monitored with regular follow-up under L-thyroxin suppression and is not receiving steroids.

What Can We Learn from This Case?

- Sarcoidosis can be associated with autoimmune diseases including Graves' disease.
- Differentiated thyroid carcinoma and sarcoidosis can coexist causing a difficulty in the diagnosis and therapeutic management since the clinical presentation and radiological findings may overlap between malignancy and S.

Acknowledgment We would like to thank Professor Dr. Kerim Sönmezoğlu for kindly providing Fig. 9.1 from the archive of Cerrahpasa School of Medicine, Department of Nuclear Medicine, İstanbul, Turkey.

References

1. Amin MB, Edge SB, Greene FL, Compton CC, Gershenwald JE, Brookland RK, et al., editors. AJCC cancer staging manual. 8th ed. New York: Springer; 2017.

2. Haugen BR, Alexander EK, Bible KC, Doherty GM, Mandel SJ, Nikiforov YE, et al. 2015 American Thyroid Association management guidelines for adult patients with thyroid nodules and differentiated thyroid cancer: the American Thyroid Association guidelines task force on thyroid nodules and differentiated thyroid cancer. Thyroid. 2016;26:1–133. https://doi.org/10.1089/thy.2015.0020.
3. Harder H, Büchler MW, Fröhlich B, Ströbel P, Bergmann F, Neff W, et al. Extrapulmonary sarcoidosis of liver and pancreas: a case report and review of literature. World J Gastroenterol. 2007;13:2504–9. https://doi.org/10.3748/wjg.v13.i17.2504.
4. Baughman RP, Lower EE. Sarcoidosis. In: Longo DL, editor. Harrison's principles of internal medicine. 18th ed. New York: McGraw-Hill; 2012. p. 2805–13.
5. Baughman RP, Culver DA, Judson MA. A concise review of pulmonary sarcoidosis. Am J Respir Crit Care Med. 2011;183:573–81. https://doi.org/10.1164/rccm.201006-0865CI.
6. Fazzi P, Fallahi P, Ferrari SM. Sarcoidosis and thyroid autoimmunity. Front Endocrinol (Lausanne). 2017;8:177. https://doi.org/10.3389/fendo.2017.00177. eCollection 2017. Review.
7. Baughman RP, Drent M, Kavuru M, Judson MA, Costabel U, Du BR, et al. Infliximab therapy in patients with chronic sarcoidosis and pulmonary involvement. Am J Respir Crit Care Med. 2006;174:795–802.
8. Valeyre D, Bernaudin JF, Uzunhan Y, Kambouchner M, Brillet PY, Soussan M, et al. Clinical presentation of sarcoidosis and diagnostic work-up. Semin Respir Crit Care Med. 2014;35:336–51. https://doi.org/10.1055/s-0034-1381229. Epub 2014 Jul 9. Review.
9. Larici AR, Glaudemans AW, Del Ciello A, Slart RH, Calandriello L, Gheysens O. Radiological and nuclear medicine imaging of sarcoidosis. Q J Nucl Med Mol Imaging. 2018;62:14–33. https://doi.org/10.23736/S1824-4785.17.03046-1. Epub 2017 Nov 30.
10. Yoshimizu T, Suga K, Orihashi N, Soejima K, Kaneko T, Kawamura M, et al. The appearance of "lambda" and "panda" sign on Ga-67 scintigraphy in sarcoidosis. Kaku Igaku. 1991;28:1151–7.
11. Skali H, Schulman AR, Dorbala S. 18F-FDG PET/CT for the assessment of myocardial sarcoidosis. Curr Cardiol Rep. 2013;15:352. https://doi.org/10.1007/s11886-013-0352-8. Review.
12. Lapa C, Kircher M, Hänscheid H, Schirbel A, Grigoleit GU, Klinker E, et al. Peptide receptor radionuclide therapy as a new tool in treatment-refractory sarcoidosis - initial experience in two patients. Theranostics. 2018;8:644–9. https://doi.org/10.7150/thno.22161. eCollection 2018.
13. Cooke R. Sarcoidosis of thyroid. Proc R Soc Med. 1959;52:174–5.
14. Karlish AJ, MacGregor GA. Sarcoidosis, thyroiditis, and Addison's disease. Lancet. 1970;2:330–3. https://doi.org/10.1016/S0140-6736(70)92871-0.
15. Papadopoulos KI, Hörnblad Y, Liljebladh H, Hallengren B. High frequency of endocrine autoimmunity in patients with sarcoidosis. Eur J Endocrinol. 1996;134:331–6. https://doi.org/10.1530/eje.0.1340331.
16. Antonelli A, Fazzi P, Fallahi P, Ferrari SM, Ferrannini E. Prevalence of hypothyroidism and Graves disease in sarcoidosis. Chest. 2006;130:526–32. https://doi.org/10.1378/chest.130.2.526.
17. Fallahi P, Ferrari SM, Ruffilli I, Elia G, Biricotti M, Vita R, et al. The association of other autoimmune diseases in patients with autoimmune thyroiditis: review of the literature and report of a large series of patients. Autoimmun Rev. 2016;15:1125–8. https://doi.org/10.1016/j.autrev.2016.09.009.
18. Kmieć P, Lewandowska M, Dubaniewicz A, Mizan-Gross K, Antolak A, Wołyniak B. Two cases of thyroid sarcoidosis presentation as painful, recurrent goiter in patients with Graves' disease. Arq Bras Endocrinol Metabol. 2012;56:209–14.
19. Zimmermann-Belsing T, Christensen L, Hansen HS, Kirkegaard J, Blichert-Toft M, Feldt-Rasmussen U. A case of sarcoidosis and sarcoid granuloma, papillary carcinoma, and Graves' disease in the thyroid gland. Thyroid. 1997;7:901–3.
20. Brincker H. Sarcoid reactions in malignant tumors. Cancer Treat Rev. 1986;13:147–56.
21. Llombart A Jr, Escudero JM. The incidence and significance of epithelioid and sarcoid-like cellular reaction in the stromata of malignant tumours: a morphological and experimental study. Eur J Cancer. 1970;6:545–51.
22. Krawczyk BP, Gryglicka B, Kieszko R, Korobowicz E, Sojczuk S. Malignant neoplasms and pulmonary sarcoidosis—a case report. New Med. 2004;7:94–6.
23. Ergin AB, Nasr CE. Thyroid cancer & sarcoidosis. Sarcoidosis Vasc Diffuse Lung Dis. 2014;31:239–43.
24. Myint ZW, Chow RD. Sarcoidosis mimicking metastatic thyroid cancer following radioactive iodine therapy. J Community Hosp Intern Med Perspect. 2015;5:26360. https://doi.org/10.3402/jchimp.v5.26360. eCollection 2015.
25. Bruins NA, Oswald JE, Morreau H, Kievit J, Pavel S, Smelt AH. Papillary thyroid carcinoma in a patient with sarcoidosis treated with minocycline. Neth J Med. 2007;65:185–7.

A Patient Presenting with an Incidentally Found Hypermetabolic Thyroid Nodule on FDG-PET/CT

10

Bala Başak Öven and Mehmet Tarık Tatoğlu

Abstract

The prevalence of thyroid lesions on FDG-PET was reported as 4%, and the malignancy rate in these nodules was found to be 14–50%. We reported a case of thyroid incidentaloma, detected during follow-up of known primary malignancy. Thyroid nodule was detected in FDG PET/CT of a 68-year-old woman with known breast cancer during follow-up. Because of suspicious USG findings and high SUVmax value, fine needle aspiration biopsy (FNAB) was performed and the result came out as suspicious in terms of papillary carcinoma oncocytic variant (Bethesda Category V). If the thyroid nodule is detected with FDG uptake, the cytological examination is necessary to differentiate benign nodule from malignant ones and figure out whether it is a thyroid metastasis from primary cancer or not.

B. B. Öven
Department of Medical Oncology, Haydarpaşa Numune Training and Research Hospital, Istanbul, Turkey

M. T. Tatoğlu (✉)
Department of Nuclear Medicine, Goztepe Training and Research Hospital, Istanbul Medeniyet University, İstanbul, Turkey

10.1 Case

A 68-year-old female patient with stage II (T2N1M0) breast cancer was operated 3 years ago after receiving anthracycline, cyclophosphamide, and docetaxel as neoadjuvant chemotherapy. Radiotherapy, hormonotherapy, and trastuzumab were given as adjuvant therapy. Vertebra fracture because of metastasis was detected during the follow-up period, and trastuzumab, an aromatase inhibitor, and zoledronic acid treatment were planned. Meanwhile, a positron emission tomography with 2-deoxy-2-[fluorine-18]fluoro-D-glucose integrated with computed tomography (^{18}F-FDG PET/CT) performed during routine follow-up revealed intensely hypermetabolic nodular lesion at left thyroid lobe adjacent to the isthmus (SUVmax: 9.8) (Fig. 10.1a–c). Correlation with thyroid and neck ultrasonography (USG) and histopathologic examination were suggested because of this finding.

In the history of the patient, thyroid nodule, familial thyroid cancer, radiotherapy to the neck region, MEN2, PTEN hamartoma tumor syndrome (Cowden disease), FAP, Carney complex, and Werner syndrome were absent. The pathologic cervical lymph node was not detected in neck examination and USG. Serum thyroid-stimulating hormone (TSH) levels were within normal limits. USG-guided fine needle aspiration biopsy (FNAB) was performed to the nodular

T. Özülker et al. (eds.), *Thyroid and Parathyroid Diseases*, https://doi.org/10.1007/978-3-319-78476-2_10

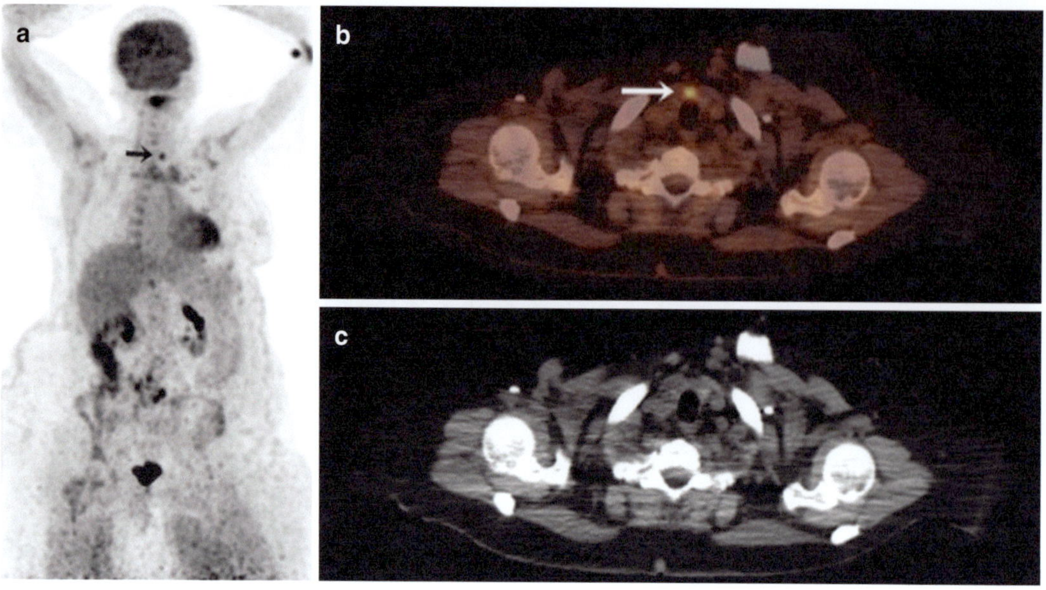

Fig. 10.1 MIP (**a**), axial fusion (**b**) and axial CT (**c**) images of ^{18}F-FDG PET/CT showing focal FDG uptake in the thyroid gland

lesion measuring 8.9 mm in size located in the left lobe-isthmus junction of the thyroid. The pathology of the nodular lesion was reported as suspicious in terms of papillary carcinoma oncocytic variant (Bethesda Category V).

10.2 Discussion

Thyroid nodules are commonly encountered in clinical practice. Nonpalpable thyroid nodules incidentally detected by anatomic imaging methods during the investigation of other diseases are called incidentaloma. Normal thyroid tissue is not observed in ^{18}F-FDG PET images. During the ^{18}F-FDG PET/CT examination, which is usually performed to diagnose malignant and some nonmalignant diseases, incidental focal or diffuse uptake can be detected in the thyroid gland. In this case, we detected a hypermetabolic thyroid nodule on PET/CT, which was performed to evaluate the therapeutic response in the patient. In a meta-analysis including 22 studies with ^{18}F-FDG PET/CT examinations, the incidence of focal thyroid uptake was reported to be 1.6%, while diffuse thyroid uptake was 2.1%, and 35% of these incidentally found focal lesions turned out to be malignant [1]. Focal FDG uptake in the thyroid gland is usually detectable in benign or malignant nodular lesions, whereas diffuse thyroid uptake may be associated with Graves', Hashimoto's disease, or other infectious/inflammatory, benign thyroid diseases [2].

According to the guidelines published by the American Thyroid Association (ATA) in 2015, USG-confirmed >1 cm thyroid nodules with focal uptake on ^{18}F-FDG PET/CT are suggested to be evaluated with USG-guided FNAB due to potential malignancy. In a patient with ultrasonographically and clinically confirmed chronic lymphocytic thyroiditis, there is no need to proceed with FNAB when diffuse FDG uptake in the thyroid gland is detected on ^{18}F-FDG PET/CT. It is recommended that thyroid nodules with <1 cm with high-risk features on USG or show focal FDG uptake on ^{18}F-FDG PET/CT should be followed up [3].

In the guidelines published by the American Association of Clinical Endocrinologists (AACE) in 2016, FNAB is recommended because of the high risk of malignancy in thyroid nodules that are presented with focal FDG uptake on ^{18}F-FDG PET/CT. If Tc99m MIBI uptake is detected in thyroid nodules as in the case of ^{18}F-FDG PET/

CT, USG-guided FNAB is also recommended for high risk of malignancy [4].

Are et al. reported that malignancy had been detected in 24 out of 57 patients (42%), with FNAB performed on 263 out of 8800 patients and with 16,300 ^{18}F-FDG PET studies, with abnormal FDG uptake in the thyroid gland [5]. In this article, USG-guided FNAB is recommended because of the high risk of malignancy in patients with focal or unilateral F18-FDG uptake in the thyroid gland [5].

It is known that benign thyroid tumors may show FDG uptake and FDG affinity may be low or negative in well-differentiated thyroid tumors; therefore, ^{18}F-FDG PET imaging is not recommended for staging of well-differentiated thyroid papillary carcinoma [1, 3, 5].

When a thyroid nodule is detected, it is necessary to question the information that may be related to thyroid cancer: previous head and neck irradiation; exposure to nuclear fallout, e.g., from Chernobyl; family history of medullary thyroid carcinoma or multiple endocrine neoplasia type 2; family history of papillary thyroid carcinoma; familial polyposis coli; Cowden's or Gardner's syndrome; recent onset of hoarseness, dysphonia, dysphagia, or dyspnea; and past medical history of thyroid cancer [6]. Our case had no history of risk factor for thyroid cancer. Although thyroid nodule in our case is <1 cm, FNAB was performed to rule metastasis from breast cancer.

The structure of the gland and the presence of the nodules should be examined by palpation. Subcentimetric-sized nodules may not be detected by palpation.

When diffuse or focal increased ^{18}F-FDG uptake is detected in the thyroid gland, it is essential to evaluate with USG. The presence of associated cervical lymph nodes, USG characteristics of thyroid nodules suggesting of malignancy (hypoechogenicity, solid composition, irregular margin, fine microcalcification, absence of halo, shape tall more than wide, central rather than peripheral blood flow on Doppler USG) should be taken into account [7].

When thyroid nodules are detected, TSH level should be measured. Thyroid nodules are more likely to be malignant in patients with elevated TSH levels, while patients with subclinical or apparent hyperthyroidism with lower TSH levels are less likely to have malignancy [8, 9]. In patients with low TSH levels, thyroid scintigraphy may be performed with Tc99m pertechnetate for evaluation of the nodule regarding its functional status.

It should be kept in mind that other than thyroid gland primary malignancy, metastases from tumors such as thyroid lymphoma, malign melanoma, renal cell carcinoma, lung, breast, esophagus, stomach, colon, and uterus cancers and rarely nasopharyngeal carcinoma, choriocarcinoma, malignant phyllodes, and osteosarcoma can be detected [5, 10, 11].

In the guideline published by ATA in 2015, sonographic patterns were defined as five groups based on the estimated risk of malignancy. Fine needle aspiration guidance for thyroid nodules and FNAB recommendation was determined according to their malignancy risks.

Our patient had solid hypoechoic thyroid nodule on USG, and with this feature, it was included in intermediate-suspicious group with a 10–20% of malignancy potential according to ATA 2015. FNAB is not recommended in nodules <1 cm unless there is a high-risk factor, and FNAB was performed in our patient due to the risk of metastasis from primary breast cancer.

It has been reported that the evaluation of thyroid nodule by USG elastography can contribute to conventional USG and can be utilized with high sensitivity in the assessment of primary thyroid malignancies. However, elastography is still operator dependent, lacking a standardized method for data reporting. Cystic nodules and nodules with calcified shells are not suitable for elastographic evaluation [4].

Computerized tomography (CT) and magnetic resonance imaging (MRI) examinations are not recommended in the routine evaluation of thyroid nodules. However, it is suggested that substernal extending nodules can be evaluated with the CT or MRI for the presence of airway compression. The use of contrast during CT examinations is not recommended because the contrasts are usually iodized and may reduce radioactive iodine uptake and may trigger hyperthyroidism [4, 12]. When evaluating these types of cases, MRI examination may be more appropriate. Ramos et al. reported that the SUV values at thyroid nodules above 5.69 (average uptake) and 8.5 (maximum uptake) may be related to the likelihood of malignancy. Choi et al. reported that SUV values above 4.1 (maximum uptake) may be significant for malignancy potential [13, 14].

Kim et al. and Are et al. reported that they did not detect either average or maximum SUV for benign and malignant lesions in their studies [5, 10]. Kim et al. reported that this was a possible reason for not setting a threshold value, as there may be cases of partial volume effect in small lesions, follicular lesions, or histologically undetected malignant lesions that are benign or Hürthle cell adenomas with high FDG uptake [10]. Our patient's thyroid nodule detected by PET/CT had SUVmax value of 9.8 which pointed out malignancy rather than benign etiologies.

It has been reported that the FNAB procedure is more reliable and reduces the nondiagnostic evaluation rate when it is guided by USG [4].

For the standardization of biopsies taken with FNAB, it is suggested to evaluate according to Bethesda System for Reporting Thyroid Cytopathology [3, 15]. Our patient's thyroid nodule's FNAB revealed Category 5 in respect to Bethesda system which was defined as suspicious for malignancy; malignancy risk is specified as 60–75%, and near-total thyroidectomy or surgical lobectomy is recommended.

Thyroidectomy operation is recommended when malignant cytology is detected, but it is reported that active surveillance can be applied instead of emergent surgery in cases with very low-risk nonaggressive cytology papillary microcarcinomas, patients with surgical risk due to comorbid conditions, patients with serious illnesses with short life expectancy (cardiopulmonary disease, malignancy, age), and those who had undergone thyroid surgery before [3].

10.3 Follow-Up and Outcome

In the present case, we did not repeat the biopsy and the patient was offered total thyroidectomy. However, no surgical procedures were performed due to comorbidities such as metastatic breast cancer, obesity, immobility, and heart failure, and it was decided to be followed up with current status.

What Can We Learn from This Case?

- For the thyroid nodules with focal uptake during ^{18}F-FDG PET/CT examination, further examination with FNAB under USG guidance is recommended due to malignancy risk.
- Before FNAB, malignancy risk factors in the history of the patient should be questioned.
- If focal FDG uptake is detected on PET/CT of patients with known malignancy, the metastasis of primary malignancy should be ruled out.
- Serum TSH level should be measured in each patient to be evaluated for thyroid nodule.
- Thyroid gland and neck should be evaluated with USG.
- If diffuse ^{18}F-FDG uptake is detected in the thyroid gland, evaluations with thyroid function tests, USG, and thyroid antibodies will be appropriate since findings are thought to be primarily related to Hashimoto, Graves', and other inflammatory thyroid diseases.

References

1. Soelberg KK, Bonnema SJ, Brix TH, Hegedüs L. Risk of malignancy in thyroid incidentalomas detected by 18F-fluorodeoxyglucose positron emission tomography: a systematic review. Thyroid. 2012;22:918–25. https://doi.org/10.1089/thy.2012.0005.
2. Salvatori M, Melis L, Castaldi P, Maussier ML, Rufini V, Perotti G, et al. Clinical significance of focal and diffuse thyroid diseases identified by (18) F-fluorodeoxyglucose positron emission tomography. Biomed Pharmacother. 2007;61:488–93. https://doi.org/10.1016/j.biopha.2007.05.001.
3. Haugen BR, Alexander EK, Bible KC, Doherty GM, Mandel SJ, Nikiforov YE, et al. 2015 American Thyroid Association management guidelines for adult patients with thyroid nodules and differentiated thy-

roid cancer: the American Thyroid Association guidelines task force on thyroid nodules and differentiated thyroid cancer. Thyroid. 2016;26:1–133. https://doi.org/10.1089/thy.2015.0020.

4. Gharib H, Papini E, Garber JR, Duick DS, Harrell RM, Hegedüs L, et al. American Association of Clinical Endocrinologists, American College of Endocrinology, and Associazione Medici Endocrinologi medical guidelines for clinical practice for the diagnosis and management of thyroid nodules. 2016 update. Endocr Pract. 2016;22:622–39. https://doi.org/10.4158/EP161208.GL.
5. Are C, Hsu JF, Schoder H, Shah JP, Larson SM, Shaha AR. FDG-PET detected thyroid incidentalomas: need for further investigation? Ann Surg Oncol. 2007;14:239–47. https://doi.org/10.1245/s10434-006-9181-y.
6. Aspinall SR, Ong SG, Wilson MS, Lennard TW. How shall we manage the incidentally found thyroid nodule? Surgeon. 2013;11:96–104. https://doi.org/10.1016/j.surge.2012.11.004.
7. Frates MC, Benson CB, Charboneau JW, Cibas ES, Clark OH, Coleman BG, et al. Management of thyroid nodules detected at US: Society of Radiologists in Ultrasound consensus conference statement. Radiology. 2005;237:794–800. https://doi.org/10.1148/radiol.2373050220.
8. Haymart MR, Repplinger DJ, Leverson GE, Elson DF, Sippel RS, Jaume JC, et al. Higher serum thyroid stimulating hormone level in thyroid nodule patients is associated with greater risks of differentiated thyroid cancer and advanced tumor stage. J Clin Endocrinol Metab. 2008;93:809–14. https://doi.org/10.1210/jc.2007-2215.
9. Boelaert K, Horacek J, Holder RL, Watkinson JC, Sheppard MC, Franklyn JA. Serum thyrotropin concentration as novel predictor of malignancy in thyroid nodules investigated by fine-needle aspiration. J Clin Endocrinol Metab. 2006;91:4295–301. https://doi.org/10.1210/jc.2006-0527.
10. Kim TY, Kim WB, Ryu JS, Gong G, Hong SJ, Shong YK. 18F-gluorodeoxyglucose uptake in thyroid from positron emission tomogram (PET) for evaluation in cancer patients: high prevalence of malignancy in thyroid PET incidentaloma. Laryngoscope. 2005;115:1074–8. https://doi.org/10.1097/01.MLG.0000163098.01398.79.
11. Lam KY, Lo CY. Metastatic tumors of the thyroid gland: a study of 79 cases in Chinese patients. Arch Pathol Lab Med. 1998;122:37–41.
12. Lee SY, Rhee CM, Leung AM, Braverman LE, Brent GA, Pearce EN. A review: radiographic iodinated contrast media-induced thyroid dysfunction. J Clin Endocrinol Metab. 2015;100:376–83. https://doi.org/10.1210/jc.2014-3292.
13. Choi JY, Lee KS, Kim HJ, Shim YM, Kwon OJ, Park K, et al. Focal thyroid lesions incidentally identified by integrated 18F-FDG PET/CT: clinical significance and improved characterization. J Nucl Med. 2006;47:609–15.
14. Ramos CD, Chisin R, Yeung HW, Larson SM, Macapinlac HA. Incidental focal thyroid uptake on FDG positron emission tomographic scans may represent second primary tumor. Clin Nucl Med. 2001;26:193e7.
15. Bongiovanni M, Spitale A, Faquin WC, Mazzucchelli L, Baloch ZW. The Bethesda system for reporting thyroid cytopathology: a meta-analysis. Acta Cytol. 2012;56:333–9. https://doi.org/10.1159/000339959.

11 Management of a Thyroid Nodule Which Is Hypoactive on Thyroid Scintigraphy and Has Eggshell Calcification on USG

Gülşah Yenidünya Yalın and Betül Uğur Altun

Abstract

Thyroid nodules arise from the increased proliferation rate of thyroid cells. The primary target when assessing thyroid nodules is to exclude the presence of thyroid cancer, which is present in approximately 4.0–6.5% of thyroid nodules. Thyroid ultrasound (USG) should be performed in all patients with a suspected thyroid nodule or nodular goiter on physical examination. The population who are more prone to have thyroid carcinoma are adults <30 or over 60 years old, patients with a history of head and neck irradiation, and patients with a family history of thyroid cancer. We hereby present a 43-year-old female patient who had a hypoactive thyroid nodule with eggshell calcification on thyroid ultrasonography.

G. Y. Yalın (✉) · B. U. Altun
Department of Endocrinology, Başkent University Istanbul Hospital, Istanbul, Turkey

11.1 Case

43-year-old female patient was admitted to the endocrinology outpatient clinic due to the presence of multinodular goiter. She denied having previous neck radiotherapy or familial thyroid carcinoma in her medical history. Her thyroid function tests were as follows: thyroid-stimulating hormone (TSH), 2.4 (0.4–4 mU/ml); free T4 (fT4), 1.1 (0.7–1.48 ng/dl); and antithyroid peroxidase (anti-TPO), 10 (0–34 IU/ml).

Neck USG revealed normal thyroid size with minimal heterogeneity on background echogenicity. On the right thyroid lobe, there were 4 × 3× 5 mm and 7 × 6 × 8 mm isoechoic nodules with well-defined regular borders and no sign of vascularization. On the left thyroid lobe, there was a 12 × 10 × 8 mm hypoechogenic nodule with regular borders and subtle peripheral vascularization. Presence of eggshell calcification was noted on the 1/3 outer rim of this nodule (Fig. 11.1).

Thyroid scintigraphy with Tc-99m which had been performed 1 year before demonstrated that the nodule on the left thyroid lobe was associated with a hypoactive region (Fig. 11.2). At that time fine needle aspiration biopsy (FNAB) was also performed twice at 6-month intervals. The first FNAB resulted with nondiagnostic material and the second one revealed benign histopathological results.

T. Özülker et al. (eds.), *Thyroid and Parathyroid Diseases*, https://doi.org/10.1007/978-3-319-78476-2_11

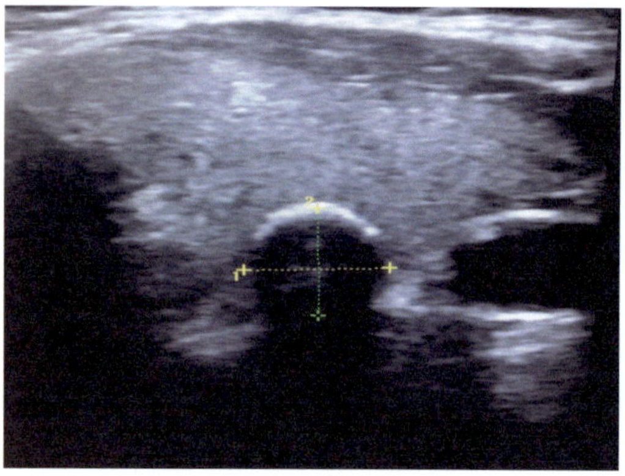

Fig. 11.1 Presence of eggshell calcification on the 1/3 outer rim of the thyroid nodule

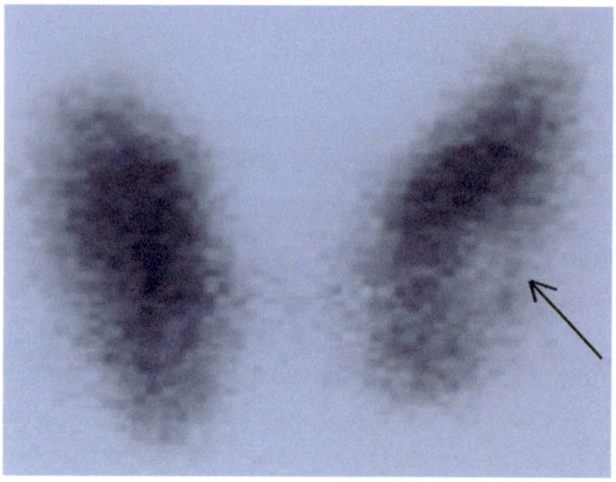

Fig. 11.2 Tc-99m thyroid scintigraphy demonstrating hypoactive nodule on left thyroid lobe

11.2 Discussion

Although thyroid nodule prevalence is high in general population, thyroid malignancy is relatively rare. There is no specific imaging modality that can provide the most accurate information about the characteristic features of every single nodule. High-resolution USG is the most sensitive, most feasible, and cost-effective diagnostic evaluation [1–3]. Nodules smaller than 1 cm are generally not detected with neck palpation. On the other hand, nodules which are even 1–2 mm in size can be detected with high-resolution USG. In autopsy series, multiple nodules and solitary nodules are reported as 37.3% and 12.2%, respectively, and malignancy rate is approximately 5% with 2–4/100,000 per year [4]. Thyroid cancer is reported as 1% of all of the malignancies and 0.5% of all cancer-related deaths [4].

Evaluation with neck USG is mandatory in the presence of thyroid nodule suspicion and during the follow-up period. USG provides information on the characteristic features of thyroid nodules which may be useful in predicting the presence of thyroid malignancy [5]. Thyroid nodules are classified as (a) high suspicion pattern for malignancy, (b) intermediate suspicion of malignancy, (c) low suspicion for malignancy, (d) very low suspicion for malignancy, and (e) benign pattern, according to findings on USG [1, 3]. FNAB should be performed in groups with high and intermediate suspicion for malignancy. Malignancy rate is reported as 70–90% and 10–20% in high suspicion and intermediate suspicion groups, respectively. Malignancy rates are 5–10%, 3%, and <1% in low suspicion, very low suspicion, and benign nodules, respectively [1, 4].

FNAB is the most valuable diagnostic method for the evaluation of thyroid nodules [1, 3]. There are some critical features that should always be evaluated with USG such as the presence of individually specified calcification patterns, irregular margins, the presence of hypoechogenicity in a solid nodule, and intranodular hypervascularization in a chaotic pattern. These findings are generally associated with malignancy [6]. Presence of cervical lymph node metastasis and extrathyroidal extension is also a strong malignancy indicator which is relatively rare. Spongiform nodules, purely or predominantly cystic nodules, the presence of hypoechogenic halo with a regular margin, and iso- and hyperechogenicity are generally considered as benign features. However, it should always be kept in my mind that neither of these USG features can eliminate the presence of malignancy with 100% accuracy. FNAB is considered as the most reliable method during the preoperative evaluation of a thyroid nodule. Calcifications in thyroid gland are merely classified as micro- and macrocalcifications [3, 7] or (a) microcalcification, (b) rim calcification, and (c) macrocalcification. Although calcifications are generally more common in malignant nodules, they can be observed in both benign and malignant nodules. As an example, intranodular calcification was reported as 47% and 31% in malignant and benign nodules, respectively [8]. In comparison with a noncalcified nodule, malignancy risk is increased by threefolds and twofolds in the presence of micro- and macrocalcification, respectively. The probability of malignancy should always be considered in the presence of calcification, regardless of the calcification pattern [2]. Microcalcification is observed as thin hyperechogenic spots that are approximately 1 mm either with an absent or a very thin acoustic shadow on USG image. Microcalcification is the calcified forms of necrosed papillary cells [7] which have a specificity of 76–94% for the diagnosis of papillary thyroid cancer [2, 7, 9, 10]. However, it may also be an indicator for medullary thyroid carcinoma [7]. Microcalcification may rarely be present in Graves' disease, lymphocytic thyroiditis, and hyperplastic nodular goiter, as well. Colloid and amyloid deposition may sometimes be confused with microcalcifications, and therefore the sensitivity is lower [7]. Macrocalcification is wider with a circumference >2 mm, and an acoustic shadow is always present. Macrocalcification may either be due to the calcification of degenerated follicles or liquefaction necrosis of malignant cells [7]. Macrocalcification is less specific for the presence of malignancy and is more common in benign multinodular goiter. However, the presence of macrocalcification in a single solitary nodule indicates a higher risk of malignancy. Presence of acoustic shadow is associated with dysmorphic and amorph accumulation of calcium on necrotic material or fibrous tissue.

Benign and malignant lesions range in a spectrum of round and ovoid-shaped nodules. Most of the nodules have regular margins. Eggshell calcification is classified under rim calcification. When it is complete with continuous borders, it is generally considered as benign and is usually present in patients with multinodular goiter. However, incomplete and thick eggshell calcifications are usually associated with papillary thyroid carcinoma and rarely follicular carcinoma necessitating evaluation with FNAB [7, 10, 11]. Presence of hypoechogenic halo with regular margins in an iso- or hyperechogenic nodule is associated with benign features. This appearance is probably due to the reflection of fibrous connective tissue as a pseudocapsule formation. Compressed adjacent thyroid tissue and vascular structures may also create this hypoechoic capsule image. Specificity of eggshell calcification as an indicator for benign nodules is reported as 96% [8]. Irregular halo structure may be present in up to 15–30% of malign thyroid lesions [2, 3]. In our case with multinodular goiter, the presence of thin eggshell calcification with continuous borders was detected in the largest nodule.

Thyroid vascularization is classified as peripheral or central vascularization. Peripheral vascularization is generally associated with benign lesions. Central and chaotic vascularization, on the other hand, is usually related to the presence of malignancy. Although avascular nodules are commonly considered as benign lesions, there may also be no sign of vascularization in more than 20% of malign nodules [2].

Nodules are classified as pure cystic, pure solid, predominantly cystic (>50% cystic), predominantly solid (>50% solid), and spongiform according to the ratio of their solid-cystic components. Malignant nodules are generally associated with the presence of predominantly solid components. The frequency of pure cystic nodules is <2%, and risk of malignancy is very low in these nodules. The cystic component may be present in 13–26% of thyroid cancers, and 6% of papillary thyroid cancers are reported as predominantly cystic nodules. The spongiform structure is also an indicator for benign features. Thyroid nodules with a spongiform component of more than 50% are generally benign nodules (with 99.7% accuracy) [2]. Thyroid nodules are demonstrated as hypo-, hyper-, or isoechoic nodules according to their echogenic features. Malignancy risk increases showing an inverse correlation with echogenicity pattern. Malignancy risk in a hyperechogenic solid nodule is 4%, and this ratio may increase up to 25% in isoechoic nodules [2].

Nodule size is not an indicator of malignancy. There is usually only one nodule with malignant features in a patient with multiple thyroid nodules. However, this nodule is not always the largest nodule on the USG. Therefore, the FNAB should be performed to the nodule with the most suspicious findings for malignancy rather than the nodule with the largest size [1–3].

Thyroid scintigraphy is an effective method for the diagnosis of autonomously functioning thyroid nodules [12]. However current guidelines do not recommend routine thyroid scintigraphy for the evaluation of thyroid nodules. The recommendation is to avoid FNAB for hyperactive nodules which are detected in the thyroid scintigraphy of patients with low or low-normal TSH levels [1, 3]. In this case, thyroid scintigraphy was not performed with the accurate indication as the scintigraphy uptake would not provide further information on the interpretation of laboratory results and also would not change the management of this patient.

FNAB should be considered in suspicious nodules even when they are as small as 5 mm; however, in low-risk and very low-risk nodules, the current recommendation is to perform FNAB when they are larger than 1.5 cm and 2 cm, respectively [1]. In our case, the thyroid nodule which was 12 mm on the largest diameter demonstrates benign features with eggshell calcification, vascularization pattern, and shape and regular margins, and the only reason for FNAB was the hypoechogenicity of the nodule.

USG findings should always be defined in detail including information about nodule echogenicity (anechoic, hyperechoic, isoechoic, hypoechoic), presence and type of halo (faint-definite, thin-thick), calcification patterns (macrocalcification, central/peripheral; microcalcification), capsular contact (absent, present), shape (oval, irregular, longitudinal length higher than horizontal size), content (solid, homogeneous/heterogeneous; mixed, predominantly solid/predominantly cystic; cystic, pure/with sediments, spongiform), margins (regular, irregular), other hyperechogenic punctuations (colloid punctuation), and vascularization patterns (absent, dominantly peripheral, dominantly central, diffuse) [13].

11.3 Follow-Up and Outcome

There is no indication for re-biopsy in this nodule with continuous, thin eggshell calcification which does not demonstrate any indicator of malignancy other than hypoechogenicity, and USG surveillance with 1–2 year intervals would be appropriate during the follow-up of this patient.

What Can We Learn from This Case?

- USG is a valuable method which provides information on the benign or malignant features during the evaluation of thyroid nodules. However, none of the findings excludes the presence of malignancy with 100% accuracy.
- Structural properties of the nodule such as shape and margins, echogenicity and vascularization pattern, and the presence of calcification and halo are important features. Although eggshell calcification is generally considered as a benign criterion, it should always be evaluated with other ultrasonographical features, and it should be kept in mind that it may also be associated with malignancy in rare circumstances.
- Thyroid scintigraphy is not recommended for the routine evaluation of thyroid nodules. Presence of hyperactive nodule on scintigraphy is considered as a benign criterion in patients with low or low-normal TSH levels.

References

1. Haugen BR, Alexander EK, Bible KC, Doherty GM, Mandel SJ, Nikiforov YE, et al. American Thyroid Association management guidelines for adult patients with thyroid nodules and differentiated thyroid cancer. Thyroid. 2016;26:1–178.
2. Anil G, Hedge A, Chang FHV. Thyroid nodules: risk stratification for malignancy with ultrasound and guided biopsy. Cancer Imaging. 2011;11:209–13.
3. Gharib H, Papini E, Garber JR, Duick DS, Harrell RM, Hegedüs L, AACE/ACE/AME Task Force on Thyroid Nodules, et al. American Association

of Clinical Endocrinologists, American College of Endocrinology, and Associazione Medici Endocrinologi medical guidelines for clinical practice for the diagnosis and management of thyroid nodules-2016 update. Endocr Pract. 2016;22:622–39.

4. Wong CKM, Wheeler MH. Thyroid nodules: rational management. World J Surg. 2000;24:934–41.
5. Burman DB, Wartofsky L. Thyroid nodules. N Engl J Med. 2015;373:2347–56.
6. Li Q, Chen S, Xiong H, Xu X, Li Z, Guo G. Papillary thyroid carcinoma on sonography. Clin Imaging. 2010;34:121–6.
7. Lacout A, Chevenet C, Thariat J, Marcy PY. Thyroid calcifications: a pictorial essay. J Clin Ultrasound. 2016;44:245–51.
8. Taki S, Terahata S, Yamashita R, Kinuya K, Nobata K, et al. Thyroid calcifications: sonographic patterns and incidence of cancer. Clin Imaging. 2004;28:368–71.
9. Kim BY, Choi YS, Kwon HY, Lee JS, Heo JJ, Han YJ, et al. Relationship between patterns of calcification in thyroid nodules and histopathologic findings. Endocr J. 2013;60:155–60.
10. Yaturu S, Rainer L. Thyroid nodule with eggshell calcification and oncocytic thyroid cancer. Med Sci Monit. 2010;16:25–8.
11. Yoon JH, Lee HS, Kim E, Moon HJ, Kwak JY. Malignancy risk stratification of thyroid nodules: comparison between the thyroid imaging reporting and data system and the 2014 American Thyroid Association management guidelines. Radiology. 2016;278:917–24.
12. Ianni F, Perotti G, Prete A, Paragliola RM, Ricciato MP, Carrozza C, et al. Thyroid scintigraphy: an old tool is still the gold standard for an effective diagnosis of autonomously functioning thyroid nodules. J Endocrinol Investig. 2013;36:233–6.
13. Russ G. Risk stratification of thyroid nodules on ultrasonography with the French TI-RADS: description and reflections. Ultrasonography. 2016;35:25–38.

Percutaneous Ethanol Injection (PEI) in a Patient with Cystic Thyroid Nodule

12

Sait Sager

Abstract

Percutaneous ethanol injection in a benign cystic thyroid nodule is an alternative procedure to surgical therapy. In this case, percutaneous ethanol injection method was performed in a 76-year-old female patient with a gross cystic thyroid nodule. There was no complication and recurrence after the therapy. This method is a safe and effective therapeutic tool for the treatment of benign cystic thyroid nodules.

12.1 Case Presentation

A 76-year-old female patient presented to our thyroid polyclinic for neck swelling. A thyroid function test demonstrated normal results. Thyroid ultrasound (USG) and thyroid scintigraphy were performed. A gross cystic thyroid nodule was seen in the thyroid USG (Fig. 12.1).

The volume of thyroid nodule was automatically calculated using the ellipsoid formula ([le ngth × width × height] × π/6). The width was measured as the maximum transverse diameter, and the height was measured as the maximum anterior-posterior diameter perpendicular to the width. The length of the thyroid nodule was measured as the maximum longitudinal diameter on longitudinal US images. The maximum diameters of the cystic nodule were measured as 44.9 × 36.7 × 35.7 mm, and the nodule volume was measured as 30.85 ml. Thyroid scintigraphy with Tc-99m pertechnetate was performed to evaluate the real volume of the nodule and to exclude the solid part of the nodule (Fig. 12.2).

This patient was wheelchaired and could not go to operation because of cardiac problems. She had respiratory problems because of the gross thyroid nodule. Percutaneous ethanol injection (PEI) therapy was recommended, and she

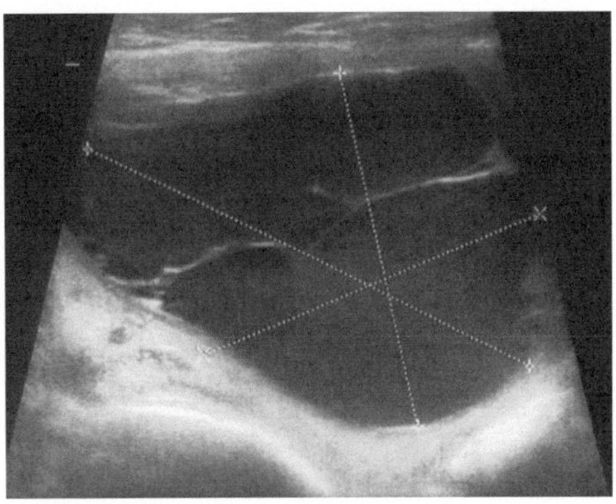

Fig. 12.1 Thyroid USG of the patient before percutaneous ethanol injection. Maximum diameters of the cystic nodule measured 44.9 × 36.7 × 35.7 mm

S. Sager
Department of Nuclear Medicine, Cerrahpaşa School of Medicine, Istanbul University, İstanbul, Turkey

T. Özülker et al. (eds.), *Thyroid and Parathyroid Diseases*, https://doi.org/10.1007/978-3-319-78476-2_12

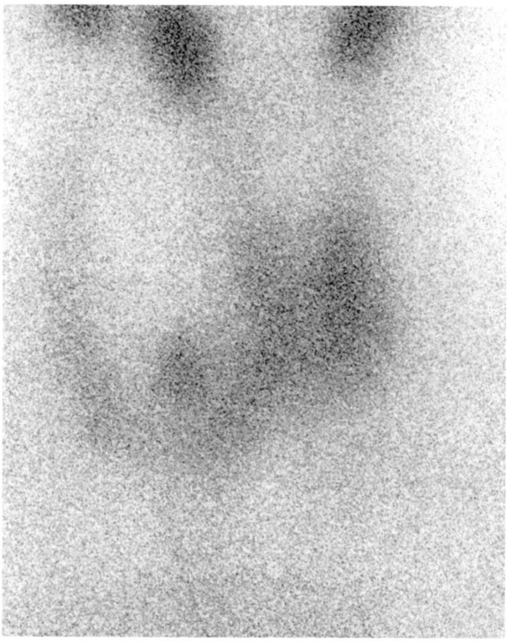

Fig. 12.2 Thyroid scintigraphy with Tc-99m pertechnetate. There is gross hypoactive thyroid nodule can be seen in the right thyroid lobe

accepted the therapy. After the evacuation of the cystic content of nodule, 95% ethanol was instilled under sonographic guidance with a 21-gauge needle. In our procedure, ethanol was not reevacuated. The amount of alcohol injected was about 50% of the amount of fluid aspirated. Gentle pressure was applied over the puncture site for 10–15 min, and the patient was watched for signs of any complication. Before ethanol injection intranodular local anesthesia was given to reduce pain. After the ethanol injection, the needle was washed with 1–2 ml of saline into the nodule. The saline rinse prevents ethanol leakage through the superficial tissues, which may cause intense pain to the patient. This procedure is so effective to reduce complications such as discomfort and pain. No major side effect was observed apart from a transient pain by the patient.

Thyroid USG was performed at every follow-up visit to assess the cyst volume. It was performed every week after ethanol injection for the first month. Four months after the therapy, the diameters of the nodule were measured as 24.7 × 25.6 × 24.2 mm, and nodule volume was measured as 8.01 ml (Fig. 12.3). Therapeutic success was defined as a noticeable reduction of volume and disappearance of clinical symptoms. Also, a complete esthetic satisfaction was reported by the patient.

12.2 Discussion

The objective of this case is to evaluate the efficacy and safety of PEI in the treatment of benign cystic thyroid nodules. Ethanol injection causes irreversible tissue damage through cellular dehydration, protein denaturation, and coagulative necrosis. PEI is used only for benign thyroid nodules and cystic or mixed cystic-solids with large fluid components. PEI method can be used in solitary thin-walled thyroid cysts larger than 10 mm, cystic big nodules with compression of neck organs in elderly and seriously ill patients to reduce the lesion volume. USG-guided PEI can be used for outpatients and is quite a low-cost, safe method of treatment.

PEI for the treatment of thyroid and parathyroid lesions was introduced into clinical practice in 1990 [1]. Ethanol injection causes irreversible tissue damage through cellular dehydration, protein denaturation, and coagulative necrosis. This technique was initially proposed as an alternative to surgery or radioiodine administration in thyroid nodules, but the use of PEI for this purpose has sensibly decreased. Ethanol has been successfully used in the treatment of cystic thyroid nodules for a long time.

Cystic thyroid lesions with a predominant fluid component are a frequent finding, representing up to 32% of all thyroid nodules [2]. Pure thyroid cysts are less frequent, corresponding to about 1% of thyroid nodules [3]. The majority of these nodules are asymptomatic. Sometimes they may cause compressive or cosmetic discomfort because of their size and location. Fine-needle aspiration (FNA) of the fluid content may reduce the lesion size; however, in 80% of the cases, thyroid cysts recur after aspiration [4]. Treatment of benign cystic thyroid nodules is usually undertaken for cosmetic reasons or local compressive

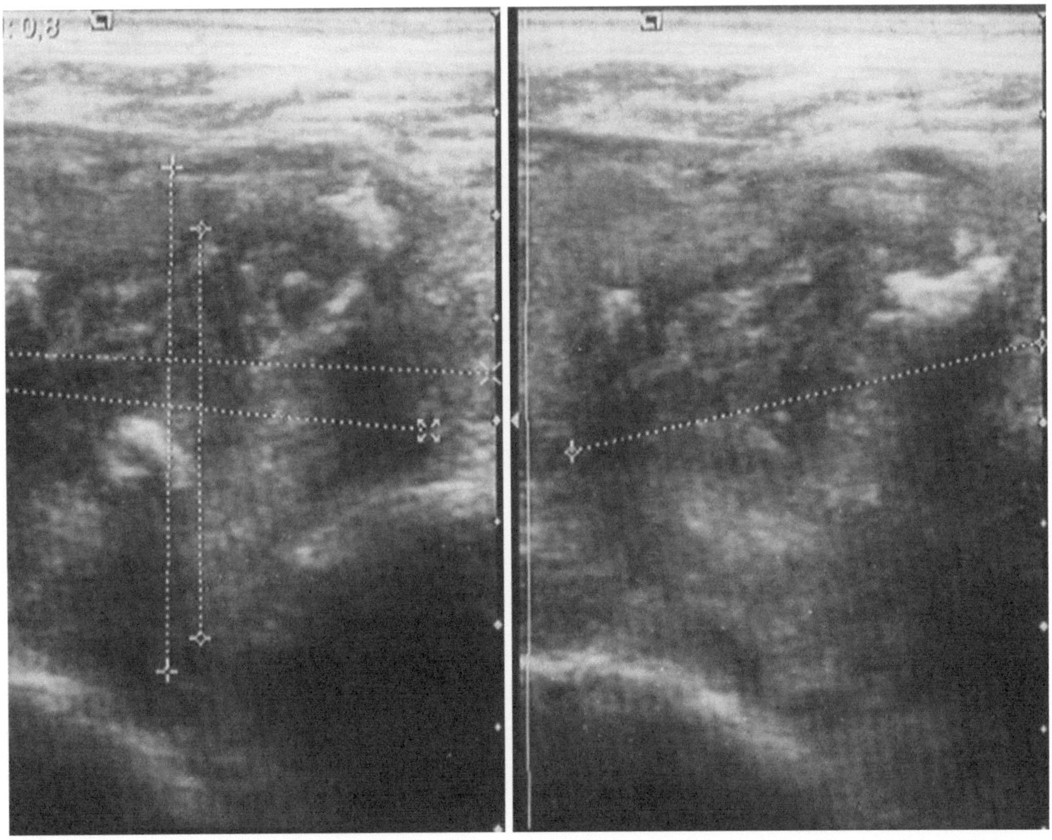

Fig. 12.3 Thyroid USG after the percutaneous ethanol injection. Four months after the therapy, diameters of the nodule measured 24.7 × 25.6 × 24.2 mm. The volume of the cystic nodule decreased from 30.85 to 8.01 ml

symptoms [5]. Surgery is curative but has disadvantages, such as general anesthesia-related complications, scar formation, and hypothyroidism. PEI therapy is effective in reducing size of cystic thyroid nodules. Ethanol volume to be introduced into the nodule is determined individually, depending on nodule size and nodule cyst content. In our case, the amount of alcohol injected was about 50% of the amount of fluid aspirated. In our procedure, ethanol was not reevacuated. Some authors claim that complete evacuation of infused ethanol avoids the risk of ethanol leakage and any related complications. Available data comparing the two different technics, there are no differences in term of successful results [6].

Cystic nodules with volumes >20 ccs may need more number of alcohol injections and longer follow-ups. Tarantino et al. and Zingrillo et al. showed that nodules with mean volume >38 ml showed significant reduction in size after 2 years [7, 8]. According to some researchers, successful PEI in thyroid nodules is characterized by a reduction in nodule size of 2–3 times with replacement by connective tissue within 6 months [9].

Ethanol sclerotherapy is also associated with some complications. Mild transient pain and a burning sensation at the site of injection are the most commonly seen side effects. The most frequently reported complaint is pain [10]. In most cases, pain is due to leakage of ethanol into subcutaneous tissue during needle extraction. This can be prevented by rinsing the needle tip with a small amount of saline before extracting the needle. Uncommon complications include hematoma, dyspnea, and vocal cord paralysis [10]. The most severe complication of PEI is unilateral cord paralysis due to the toxic action of absolute ethanol on the recurrent laryngeal nerve. Our patient did not show any complications or side effects.

Use of PEI is limited in multichambered cysts, multiple small cysts, or isoechoic nodules larger than 30 mm [11]. Particular attention should be paid when PEI is performed in the nodules located in the dorsal compartments of the thyroid lobes.

What Can We Learn from This Case?

- Ethanol sclerotherapy is an effective and safe nonsurgical treatment option for benign cystic thyroid nodules.
- Cystic nodules with volumes >20 ccs may need more number of alcohol injections and longer follow-up before results become evident.

References

1. Livraghi T, Paracchi A, Ferrari C, Bergonzi M, Garavaglia G, Raineri P, et al. Treatment of autonomous thyroid nodule with percutaneous ethanol injection: preliminary results. Radiology. 1990;175:827–9.
2. De Los Santos ET, Keyhani-Rofagha S, Cunningham JJ, Mazzaferri EL. Cystic thyroid nodules the dilemma of malignant lesions. Arch Intern Med. 1990;150:422–7.
3. Sheppard MC, Franklyn JA. Management of the single thyroid nodule. Clin Endocrinol. 1994;41:719–24.
4. Jensen F, Rasmussen SN. The treatment of thyroid cysts by ultrasonographically-guided fine needle aspiration. Acta Chir Scand. 1976;142:209–11.
5. Bennedbaek FN, Hegedüs L. Management of the solitary thyroid nodule: results of a North American survey. J Clin Endocrinol Metab. 2000;85:2493–8.
6. Kim DW, Rho MH, Kim HJ, Kwon JS, Sung YS, Lee SW. Percutaneous ethanol injection for benign cystic thyroid nodules: is aspiration of ethanol-mixed fluid advantageous? AJNR Am J Neuroradiol. 2005;26:2122–7.
7. Tarantino L, Antonio G, Nicola M, de Stefano G, Perrotta A, Aloisio V. Percutaneous ethanol injection of large autonomous hyperfunctioning thyroid nodules. Radiology. 2000;214:143–8.
8. Zingrillo M, Torlontano M, Chiarella R, Ghiggi MR, Nirchio V, Bisceglia M, et al. Percutaneous ethanol injection may be a definitive treatment for symptomatic thyroid cystic nodules not treatable by surgery: five-year follow-up study. Thyroid. 1999;9:763–7.
9. Kim DW, Rho MH, Park HJ, Kwag HJ. Ultrasonography-guided ethanol ablation of predominantly solid thyroid nodules: a preliminary study for factors that predict the outcome. Br J Radiol. 2012;85:930–6.
10. Lee SJ, Ahn M. Effectiveness of percutaneous ethanol injection therapy in benign nodular and cystic thyroid diseases: long-term follow-up experience. Endocr J. 2005;52:455–62.
11. Guglielmi R, Pacella CM, Bianchini A, Bizzarri G, Rinaldi R, Graziano FM, et al. Percutaneous ethanol injection treatment in benign thyroid lesions: role and efficacy. Thyroid. 2004;14:125–31.

Fibrin Injection in a Hemorrhagic Cystic Thyroid Nodule

13

Haluk B. Sayman

Abstract

In this case report, a new technique to be used in the treatment of hemorrhagic cystic thyroid nodules among the other historical therapeutical modalities was described. A two-component fibrin sealant, which contains two of the proteins—fibrinogen and thrombin—that make blood clot, was introduced into cyst cavity after punction by a syringe under ultrasonography guidance.

The follow-up ultrasonographies consequently showed the significant volumetric regression of the cyst in time. Hence, this method is recommended for the treatment of hemorrhagic cystic thyroid nodules as an alternative modality.

13.1 Case Presentation

A 26-year-old female patient presented with a left-sided neck swelling. A soft and firm thyroid nodule without pain was detected by palpation. Her neck ultrasonography (USG) revealed a cystic nodule having a single compartment. The rest of her thyroid had uniform echo pattern without any subsequent pathology.

An intervention is planned if the cyst fluid would be proven to be hemorrhagic after a fine needle aspiration. As this procedure was a new method, an approval of the hospital ethics committee and the written consent of the patient were obtained.

The patient laid neck extended, and the cyst was aspirated by a 21-gauge needle attached to a 20 cc syringe. By visual inspection, the fluid was pale red colored. The specimen was sent to pathological examination in the original syringe. After having confirmed that the cyst was hemorrhagic, the patient was called again, and a second neck USG was performed (Fig. 13.1). In this examination, it was seen that the cyst was filled again with dimensions of 18.1 × 23.9 × 26.7 mm, expressing the similar features as it was before. Then a second aspiration was performed, but without removing the needle, previously prepared fibrin solution according to the manufacturer's recommendations was administered inside the empty cyst cavity. After the operation site was dressed, the patient was sent home without any complications.

The follow-up USGs which were planned 3 days and 1 month after the application showed a progressive decrease in the volume of the nodule, and by time only a remnant of hyperechoic biological debris was seen on that site. The nodule

H. B. Sayman
Nuclear Medicine, Cerrahpaşa Medical Faculty, Istanbul University, Istanbul, Turkey

T. Özülker et al. (eds.), *Thyroid and Parathyroid Diseases*, https://doi.org/10.1007/978-3-319-78476-2_13

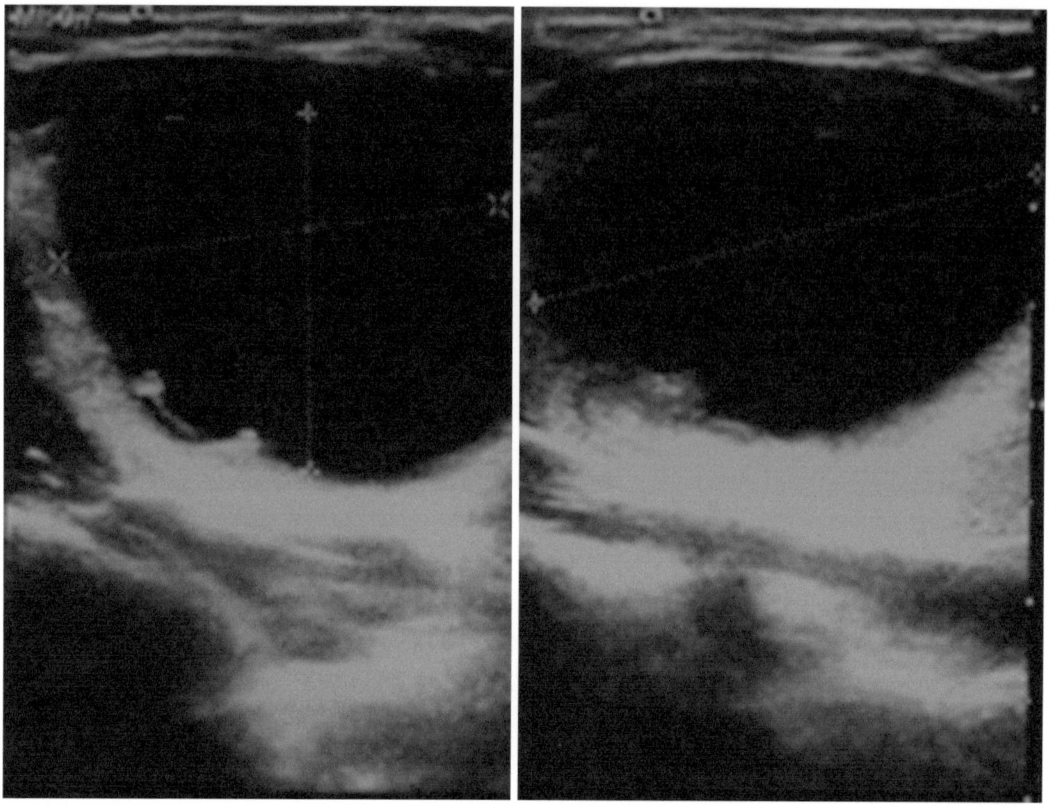

Fig. 13.1 Ultrasonographic images of transaxial and longitudinal sections of a cystic nodule on the left thyroid lobe at the initial presentation of a patient

dimensions calculated as 14.3 × 19.9 × 22.7 mm at the third day (Fig. 13.2) and 4.8 × 7.1 × 13.8 mm at first month (Fig. 13.3) showed a significant reduction in size.

13.2 Discussion

Thyroid nodules are a common pathological condition, and a large proportion of them have mixed cystic and solid components. A nodule is called a cyst only if it is predominantly cystic on USG. Thus, either mixed or pure cystic, up to 50% of thyroid nodules are cystic. Most of them recur after aspirated by fine needle. The appropriate evaluation and management of patients with cystic thyroid nodules is an area of controversy.

Although many of these nodules are detected as an incidental finding during a routine physical examination or imaging procedure, in some of them, sudden enlargement with hemorrhage or hemorrhagic infarction can result in a painful neck mass which brings the patient to a physician. Even relatively small hemorrhagic cysts of only 1–2 ml may be associated with considerable neck discomfort and dysphagia. More extensive hemorrhage may cause hoarseness and vocal cord paralysis and may compromise the airway, especially if the nodule is located within or below the thoracic inlet [1].

The majority of cystic thyroid nodules are benign degenerating thyroid adenomas. Purely cystic lesions rarely contain cancer cells, but the likelihood of cancer in complex (cystic and solid) nodules approaches that of solid nodules (5–10%). The likelihood of malignancy decreases as the proportion of the nodule that is cystic increases. Among the thyroid cancers that are associated with cysts, papillary thyroid cancer is

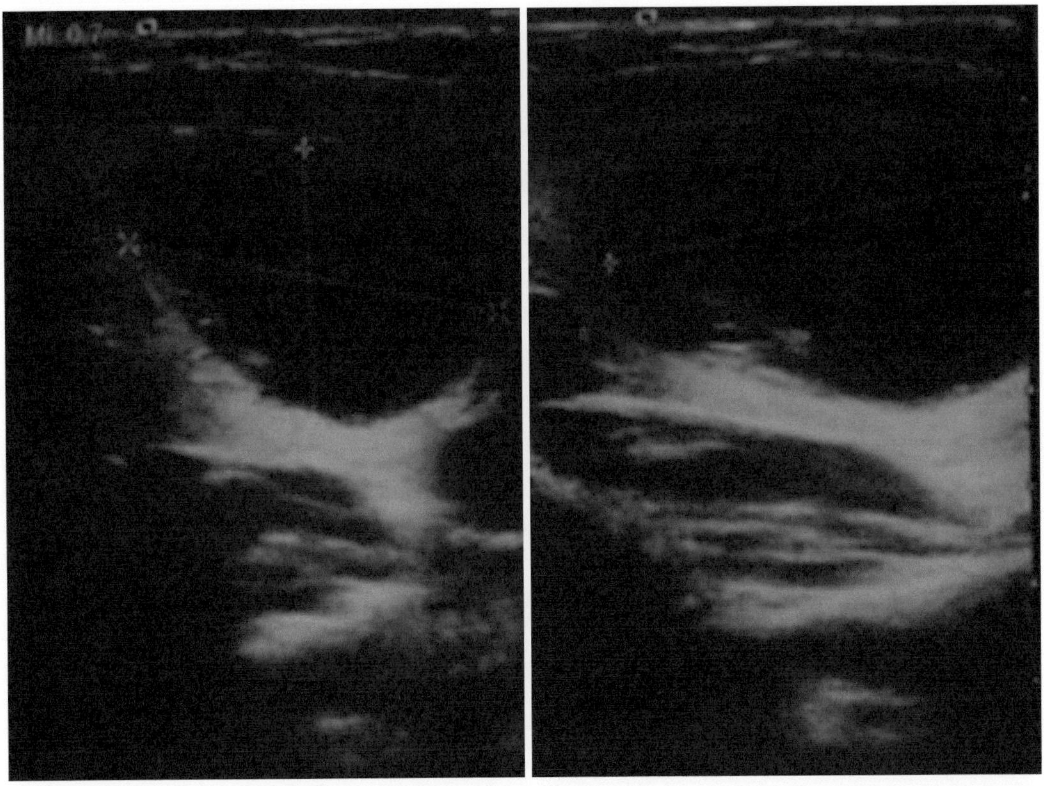

Fig. 13.2 Ultrasonographic images of transaxial and longitudinal sections of a cystic nodule on the left thyroid lobe at the third day after fibrin application

most common and is the one with the most favorable outcome [2, 3].

Thyroid USG should be performed in all patients with a suspected thyroid nodule on physical examination or with nodules incidentally noted on other imaging studies. The decision to biopsy a thyroid nodule should be based upon a combination of ultrasonographic features and increase in nodule size with time [4]. Purely cystic nodules (no mural component) do not require a diagnostic fine needle aspiration biopsy (FNAB).

The fluid from nodules that contain cancer is usually hemorrhagic or pink colored [5]. Chocolate-colored fluid suggests hemorrhage that occurred at least 1 week before aspiration. Straw-colored fluid is less likely to be associated with cancer [6].

FNAB alone may be curative in a minority of patients. Cancer is uncommon in cystic nodules that are no longer palpable after aspiration or substantially resolved on USG [7].

Despite benign cytology, many patients opt for surgical excision of cystic nodules if the nodule recurs after one or more successful aspirations or if there is continued enlargement or pain associated with fluid reaccumulation.

Thyroxine therapy was not beneficial in a small randomized trial of patients with cystic nodules where in one study, recurrences occurred in seven patients (70%) in both the placebo- and thyroid hormone-treated groups [8].

Other available treatment methods apart from open surgery for cystic nodules include ethanol [9] or tetracycline [10, 11] injections after aspiration of the cyst fluid. These approaches have not gained widespread acceptance because of potential complications, including occasional reports of prolonged pain after the procedure.

A two-component fibrin sealant, which contains two of the proteins that make blood clot, is in the market for many years to use during surgical interventions (Tisseel Lyo, Baxter AG, 1221

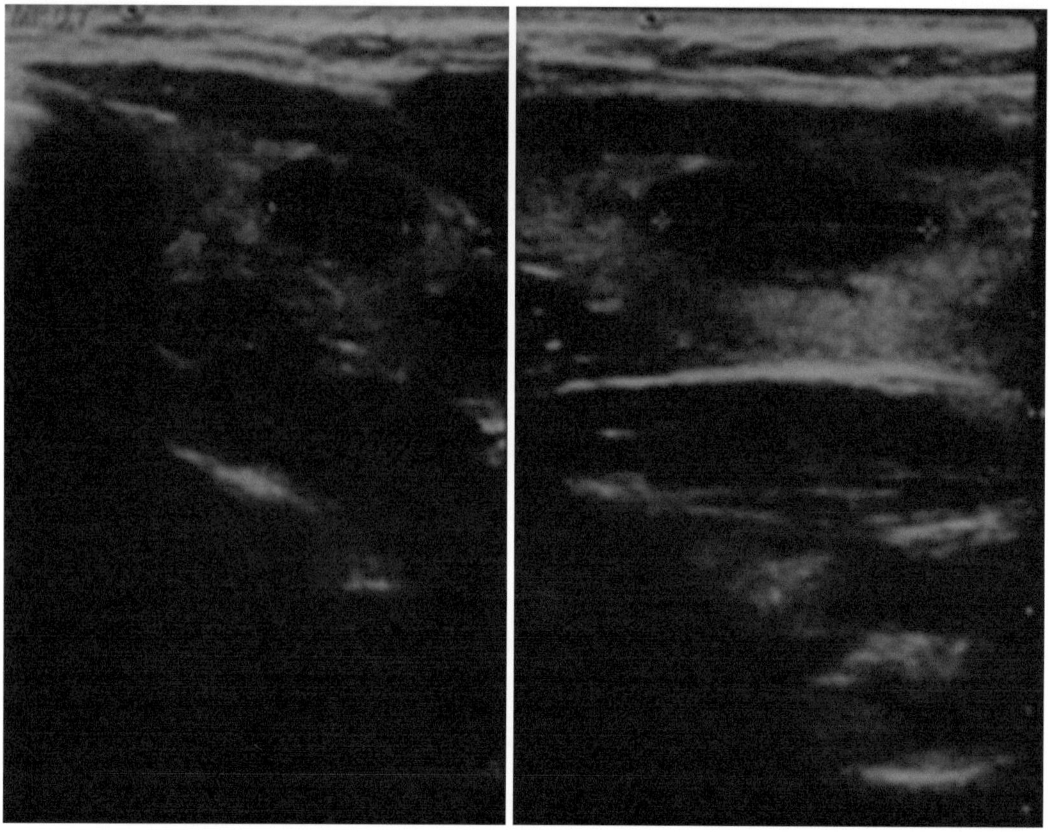

Fig. 13.3 Ultrasonographic images of transaxial and longitudinal sections of a cystic nodule on the left thyroid lobe at the first month after fibrin application

Vienna, Austria). These well-known proteins, fibrinogen and thrombin, when mixed are used mostly in hepatic surgery successfully where a clot formation is needed to control or stop bleeding. Depending on this fact, we proposed the idea of using the same product to detain bleeding into the cyst cavity in hemorrhagic thyroid nodules and designed this treatment modality.

Tisseel Lyo is a two-component fibrin sealant, and it contains two of the proteins that make blood clot. These proteins are called fibrinogen and thrombin. When these proteins mixed during application, they form a clot as a result of the last phase of physiological hemocoagulation. As it is in the cyst cavity, it forms a fibrin sealant which adheres the walls of the cyst to stop the further bleeding of capillaries. By the time passes, the fibrinolytic activity of the body overcomes the antifibrinolytic activity of aprotinin, which is present in Tisseel Lyo as an antifibrinolytic, and the resorption takes place by fibrinolysis and phagocytosis. This also causes the shrinkage of the nodule as illustrated by serial ultrasonographic examinations performed in this case.

What Can We Learn from This Case?

- Hemocoagulation by fibrin application may be considered as an alternative treatment modality for a subtype of cystic thyroid nodules.
- Fibrin injection into a thyroid cyst cavity is a safe and minimally invasive technique for those nodules proven to be as nonmalignant after cytological examination.

References

1. Massoll N, Nizam MS, Mazzaferri EL. Cystic thyroid nodules: diagnostic and therapeutic dilemmas. Endocrinologist. 2002;12:185–98.
2. Frates MC, Benson CB, Doubilet PM, Kunreuther E, Contreras M, Cibas ES, et al. Prevalence and distribution of carcinoma in patients with solitary and multiple thyroid nodules on sonography. J Clin Endocrinol Metab. 2006;91:3411–7. https://doi.org/10.1210/jc.2006-0690.
3. Lee MJ, Kim EK, Kwak JY, Kim MJ. Partially cystic thyroid nodules on ultrasound: probability of malignancy and sonographic differentiation. Thyroid. 2009;19:341–6. https://doi.org/10.1089/thy.2008.0250.
4. Cooper DS, Doherty GM, Haugen BR, Kloos RT, Lee SL, Mandel SJ, et al. American Thyroid Association (ATA) guidelines taskforce on thyroid nodules and differentiated thyroid Cancer, revised American Thyroid Association management guidelines for patients with thyroid nodules and differentiated thyroid cancer. Thyroid. 2009;19:1167–214. https://doi.org/10.1089/thy.2009.0110.
5. Rosen IB, Provias JP, Walfish PG. Pathologic nature of cystic thyroid nodules selected for surgery by needle aspiration biopsy. Surgery. 1986;100:606–13.
6. de los Santos ET, Keyhani-Rofagha S, Cunningham JJ, Mazzaferri EL. Cystic thyroid nodules. The dilemma of malignant lesions. Arch Intern Med. 1990;150:1422–7.
7. Melliere D, Massin JP, Calmettes C, Chigot JP, Savoie JC, Arnier H. The risk of malignancy in cold thyroid nodules. 607 operated cases. Presse Med. 1970;78:311–4.
8. McCowen KD, Reed JW, Fariss BL. The role of thyroid therapy in patients with thyroid cysts. Am J Med. 1980;68:853–5.
9. Del Prete S, Caraglia M, Russo D, Vitale G, Giuberti G, Marra M, et al. Percutaneous ethanol injection efficacy in the treatment of large symptomatic thyroid cystic nodules: ten-year follow-up of a large series. Thyroid. 2002;12:815–21. https://doi.org/10.1089/105072502760339398.
10. Treece GL, Georgitis WJ, Hofeldt FD. Resolution of recurrent thyroid cysts with tetracycline instillation. Arch Intern Med. 1983;143:2285–7.
11. Hegedüs L, Hansen JM, Karstrup S, Torp-Pedersen S, Juul N. Tetracycline for sclerosis of thyroid cysts a randomized study. Arch Intern Med. 1988;148:1116–8.

14 Should Calcitonin Be Measured in Every Thyroid Nodule?

Mine Adaş and Gökhan Adaş

Abstract

There are controversial suggestions in the literature about the routine measurement of calcitonin (Ct) in thyroid nodules. Barriers in front of measuring routine serum calcitonin are cost-effectiveness and the possibility of having elevated serum Ct in the absence of medullary thyroid carcinoma (MTC). Here we report a sporadic MTC patient with negative fine needle aspiration biopsy (FNAB) result whose diagnosis was made by preoperative calcitonin measurement. As we perform routine Ct measurement before surgery, the surgeon becomes aware of the MTC earlier, and this gives the opportunity of making an appropriate surgical procedure which is crucial for patients' outcome.

14.1 Case Presentation

A 45-year-old woman admitted to endocrinology outpatient clinic with a 4-week history of palpable cervical mass. Physical examination revealed grade 1b palpable thyroid gland with 1 cm nodules on both lobes. Other physical examination findings and family history were unremarkable. Thyroid function tests were within the normal limit. Anti-TPO was 117.6 IU/ml (<9 IU/ml). Neck ultrasound (USG) revealed bilateral hypoechoic thyroid nodules with irregular margins and microcalcifications. Fine needle aspiration biopsy (FNAB) from left-sided nodule was benign, while right-sided nodule showed Hurthle cell metaplasia with benign findings. We measured calcitonin (Ct) according to our routine practice. The serum calcitonin level was 4049 pg/ml (0–11.5 pg/ml). Repeated Ct level at another center was >1636 pg/ml (<10 pg/ml) again. Twenty-four-hour urine estimation of catecholamines, normetanephrine and plasma normetanephrine, serum calcium, and parathyroid hormone (PTH) was determined to identify or exclude pheochromocytoma and hyperparathyroidism. All were within the normal limits. RET protooncogene testing was negative. The patient underwent total thyroidectomy and central compartment node clearance (level VI). Postoperative histopathology confirmed thyroid medullary carcinoma of 1.2 cm in the right lobe, papillary microcarcinoma of 0.5 cm at three different foci at the left lobe, and metastatic medullary thyroid carcinoma in the resected lymph nodes. After thyroid operation serum Ct level was 10.3 pg/ml (0–11.5 pg/ml).

M. Adaş (✉)
University of Health Sciences (SBÜ), Okmeydanı Training and Research Hospital, Istanbul, Turkey

G. Adaş
University of Health Sciences (SBÜ), Haseki Training and Research Hospital, Istanbul, Turkey

T. Özülker et al. (eds.), *Thyroid and Parathyroid Diseases*, https://doi.org/10.1007/978-3-319-78476-2_14

14.2 Discussion

14.2.1 Evaluation and Diagnosis

The rate of MTC diagnosed only after thyroid operation is approximately 10–15% [1]. This delay in diagnosis can adversely affect the patient's outcome. Initial surgery is an important modality in the treatment and course of MTC. Diagnosis of MTC before surgery also has significance for the diagnosis of MEN syndromes especially accompanying life-threatening pheochromocytoma in index cases. There are controversial suggestions in the literature about the routine measurement of Ct in thyroid nodules. "The American Thyroid Association (ATA) Guideline for Thyroid Nodule and Differentiated Thyroid Cancer" does not recommend either for or against routine measurement of serum Ct (Recommendation 4) [2], while "The American Association of Clinical Endocrinologists (AACE), Associazione Medici Endocrinologi (AME), and European Thyroid Association (ETA) Thyroid Nodule Guidelines" recommend measurement of basal serum Ct level as a useful test in the initial evaluation of thyroid nodules [3]. The reasons for ATA recommendation are unresolved issues of assay performance, lack of pentagastrin availability in the United States, and potential biases in the cost-effectivity analysis [2]. The ATA recommendation and evidence quality about Ct are insufficient. There are false-negative and false-positive results of basal Ct measurement that cause misdiagnosis. Technical problems, (hook effect, heterophilic antibodies), some drugs (omeprazole), chronic renal failure, pernicious anemia, and lymphocytic thyroiditis are some reasons of false-positive results, while nonsecretory medullary thyroid carcinoma is the false-negative result [4]. If basal calcitonin level is increased, the test should be repeated, and if confirmed in the absence of modifiers, a pentagastrin or calcium stimulation test will increase the diagnostic accuracy [3]. However, pentagastrin is not available in every country, and there are problems with calcium stimulation test like cutoff levels, cost, assay performance, sensitivity, and specificity [2]. The main rationale for the recommendation of AACE, AME, and ETA concerning Ct measurement in the thyroid nodule is its higher sensitivity compared to FNAB [5–11]. As it is in our case, FNAB was not able to diagnose the MTC of the patient. If routine calcitonin had not been measured, the patient could be misdiagnosed.

Another problem in the routine measurement of basal calcitonin for every thyroid nodule is the cost-effectiveness of this screening. There are studies from the United States and European countries demonstrating that it is valuable to measure calcitonin level [12–14]. However, the costs of finding one patient with abnormal results and MTC are quite reasonable for routine basal Ct measurement, compared with the potential costs of missing the diagnosis of this treatable malignant condition [15].

14.2.2 Management

One of the important benefits of knowing preoperative Ct is the tailoring of surgical treatment. Central neck lymph node dissection is an important and necessary treatment modality in the management of MTC. As we perform routine Ct measurement before surgery, the surgeon becomes aware of the MTC earlier, and the procedure is at least total thyroidectomy and central neck lymph node dissection as it was in our case. Also, preoperative Ct measurement is effective in the detection of clinically occult MTC [5–8]. In addition, screening thyroid nodules with serum Ct measurement allows the diagnosis and treatment of MTC at an earlier stage, resulting in a better outcome compared with MTC not detected by serum Ct measurement [13].

14.3 Follow-Up and Outcome

The patient has been under follow-up for 6 years. Her postoperative serum calcitonin level was 10.3 pg/ml (0–11.5 pg/ml).After 5 years of follow-up, last serum calcitonin level was 13.56 pg/ml (0–6.4 pg/ml). Neck USG revealed nothing pathologic. The patient is on L-thyroxin replacement therapy.

14.3.1 The Future

Barriers in front of measuring routine serum Ct are cost-effectiveness and the possibility of having elevated serum Ct in the absence of an MTC. Other different diagnostic modalities can help us in this regard. Recent small studies have shown improved sensitivity with Ct measurement in FNA washout fluid with as high as 100% accuracy [16]. Procalcitonin, the precursor of Ct, has been reported as a potential MTC marker and could be a good candidate for a first-line screening test to exclude MTC in patients with suspicious thyroid nodules [17].

What Can We Learn from This Case?

- Ct measurement is an effective method for the diagnosis of MTC and is superior to FNAB concerning diagnosis of MTC.
- Recognition of MTC by preoperative calcitonin measurement increases the chance of curative therapy by diagnosing MTC in the early stages and then performing the appropriate surgical procedure.

References

1. Ahmed SR, Ball DW. Incidentally discovered medullary thyroid cancer: diagnostic strategies and treatment. J Clin Endocrinol Metab. 2011;96:1237–45.
2. Haugen BR, Alexander EK, Bible KC, Doherty GM, Mandel SJ, Nikiforov YE, et al. 2015 American Thyroid Association management guidelines for adult patients with thyroid nodules and differentiated thyroid cancer: the American Thyroid Association guidelines task force on thyroid nodules and differentiated thyroid cancer. Thyroid. 2016;26:1–133.
3. Gharib H, Papini E, Paschke R, Duick DS, Valcavi R, Hegedus L, et al. American Association of Clinical Endocrinologists, Associazione Medici Endocrinologi, and European Thyroid Association medical guidelines for clinical practice for the diagnosis and management of thyroid nodules: executive summary of recommendations. J Endocrinol Investig. 2010;33(5 Suppl):51–6.
4. Elisei R, Romei C. Calcitonin estimation in patients with nodular goiter and its significance for early detection of MTC: European comments to the guidelines of the American Thyroid Association. Thyroid Res. 2013;6(Suppl 1):S2.
5. Pacini F, Fontanelli M, Fugazzola L, Elisei R, Romei C, Di Coscio G, et al. Routine measurement of serum calcitonin in nodular thyroid diseases allows the preoperative diagnosis of unsuspected sporadic medullary thyroid carcinoma. J Clin Endocrinol Metab. 1994;78:826–9.
6. Rieu M, Lame MC, Richard A, Lissak B, Sambort B, Vuong-Ngoc P, et al. Prevalence of sporadic medullary thyroid carcinoma: the importance of routine measurement of serum calcitonin in the diagnostic evaluation of thyroid nodules. Clin Endocrinol. 1995;42:453–60.
7. Niccoli P, Wion-Barbot N, Caron P, Henry JF, de Micco C, Saint Andre JP, et al. Interest of routine measurement of serum calcitonin: study in a large series of thyroidectomized patients. The French Medullary Study Group. J Clin Endocrinol Metab. 1997;82:338–41.
8. Vierhapper H, Raber W, Bieglmayer C, Kaserer K, Weinhäusl A, Niederle B. Routine measurement of plasma calcitonin in nodular thyroid diseases. J Clin Endocrinol Metab. 1997;82:1589–93.
9. Kaserer K, Scheuba C, Neuhold N, Weinhäusel A, Vierhapper H, Haas OA. C-cell hyperplasia and medullary thyroid carcinoma in patients routinely screened for serum calcitonin. Am J Surg Pathol. 1998;22:722–8.
10. Ozgen AG, Hamulu F, Bayraktar F, Yilmaz C, Tüzün M, Yetkin E, et al. Evaluation of routine basal serum calcitonin measurement forearly diagnosis of medullary thyroid carcinoma in seven hundred seventy-three patients with nodular goiter. Thyroid. 1999;9:579–82.
11. Hahm JR, Lee MS, Min YK, Lee MK, Kim KW, Nam SJ, et al. Routine measurement of serum calcitonin is useful for early detection of medullary thyroid carcinoma in patients with nodular thyroid diseases. Thyroid. 2001;11:73–80.
12. Verga U, Ferrero S, Vicentini L, Brambilla T, Cirello V, Muzza M, et al. Histopathological and molecular studies in patients with goiter and hypercalcitoninemia: reactive or neoplastic C-cell hyperplasia? Endocr Relat Cancer. 2007;14:393–403.
13. Elisei R, Bottici V, Luchetti F, Di Coscio G, Romei C, Grasso L, et al. Impact of routine measurement of serum calcitonin on the diagnosis and outcome of medullary thyroid cancer: experience in 10,864 patients with nodular thyroid disorders. J Clin Endocrinol Metab. 2004;89:163–8.
14. Cheung K, Roman SA, Wang TS, Walker HD, Sosa JA. Calcitonin measurement in the evaluation of thyroid nodules in the United States: a cost-effectiveness and decision analysis. J Clin Endocrinol Metab. 2008;93:2173–80.
15. Turk Y, Makay O, Ozdemir M, Ertunc G, Demir B, Icoz G, et al. Routine calcitonin measurement in nodular thyroid disease management: is it worthwhile? Ann Surg Treat Res. 2017;92:173–8.
16. Hu MI, Ying AK, Jimenez C. Update on medullary thyroid cancer. Endocrinol Metab Clin N Am. 2014;43:423–42.
17. Lim SK, Guéchot J, Vaubourdolle M. Negative predictive value of procalcitonin in medullary thyroid carcinoma. Ann Biol Clin. 2016;74:213–8.

15 The Role of Thyroid Scintigraphy in the Evaluation of Thyroid Nodules in Patients with Normal TSH

Levent Kabasakal and Onur Erdem Şahin

Abstract

The widespread use of imaging modalities such as ultrasonography (USG), magnetic resonance imaging (MRI), and computer tomography (CT) has significantly increased thyroid nodule detection. Thyroid nodules are generally benign, but identification of malignant nodules is an important clinical problem. Nodules with hyperfunction on thyroid scintigraphy, also known as autonomously functioning thyroid nodules (AFTNs), are often considered as benign.

The American Thyroid Association (ATA) Guideline, revised in 2015, recommends thyroid scintigraphy only in conditions with subnormal TSH values. On the contrary, the American Association of Clinical Endocrinologists, American College of Endocrinology, and Associazione Medici Endocrinologi Medical (AACE/ACE/AME) guidelines recommend to perform thyroid scan in iodine-deficient regions, to exclude an autonomous thyroid nodule or MNG even when the TSH level is low-normal.

Especially in areas with iodine deficiency, it has been shown that AFTNs can be seen with the TSH values in the normal range. As in the cases from Turkey, an iodine deficiency area, AFTNs are detected, although TSH values are monitored in the normal range. Avoiding from thyroid scintigraphy in cases with normal TSH values in the direction of ATA guideline can cause some AFTNs to be missed. The unnecessary biopsies resulting from indeterminate reports like AUS and FLUS can lead to unnecessary operations. For these reasons, thyroid scintigraphy has an important role in the detection of AFTN, especially in iodine deficiency areas.

15.1 Case 1

The patient is a 64-year-old woman who was referred to our department by an orthopedist because of the thyroid nodule noted on a magnetic resonance imaging (MRI) for cervical herniation. There was a thyroid nodule in the right thyroid lobe measuring approximately 2 cm. She had no symptoms of hyperthyroidism or hypothyroidism. On visual inspection of the neck, the patient appears to have a slightly enlarged thyroid gland. She hasn't any radiation exposure history, relatives with thyroid cancer, or any abnormal medical history about thyroid. Thyroid studies revealed a TSH of 0.527 uIU/ml, free T3 of 3.31 pg/ml (ref range, 2–4.4 pg/ml), and free T4 of 1.03 ng/dl (ref range, 0.93–1.7 pg/ml). The thyroid ultrasonography (USG) reported a

L. Kabasakal (✉) · O. E. Şahin
Department of Nuclear Medicine, Cerrahpaşa Faculty of Medicine, İstanbul University, Istanbul, Turkey
e-mail: lkabasakal@tsnm.org

T. Özülker et al. (eds.), *Thyroid and Parathyroid Diseases*, https://doi.org/10.1007/978-3-319-78476-2_15

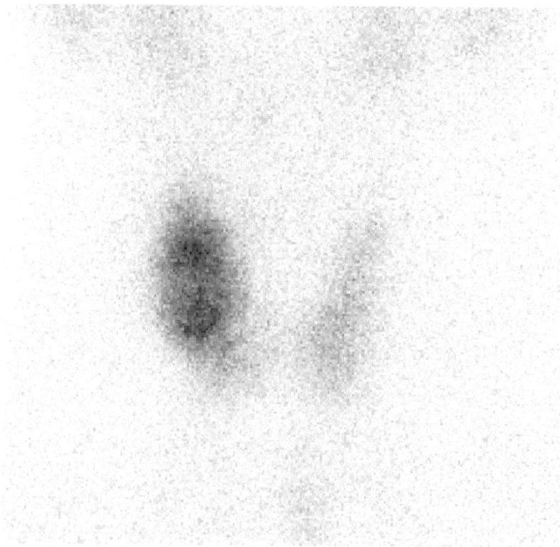

Fig. 15.1 Thyroid scan with Tc-99m pertechnetate showed hot nodule on the right base

29 × 18 × 14 mm well-defined, solid iso-hypoechoic thyroid nodule with microcalcification in the right mid-lobe. Additionally, color Doppler USG demonstrated intranodular and peripheral vascularity. Although the thyroid functioning tests are in normal range, we decided to request a thyroid scan. The thyroid scan showed that the nodule in the right lobe was hyperfunctioning (Fig. 15.1). We decided to follow the patient with USG and thyroid function tests. During the 2-year follow-up, thyroid nodule size hasn't changed, and thyroid function tests were in normal range.

15.2 Case 2

A 65-year-old man was referred to our department regarding enlarged thyroid gland and sweating. He had diabetes mellitus, hypertension, and hyperlipemia. He hadn't family history about thyroid disease. Also, he hadn't any suspicious finding or history of thyroid malignancy. In physical examination of the enlarged thyroid gland, the thyroid nodule was detected on the left lobe inferior pole. After that TSH assay and USG were requested. TSH level revealed 0.7 uIU/ml. The thyroid USG reported a 11 × 14 mm well-defined, mixed echoic, nodule with both solid-cystic areas and calcifications in the left lobe. Furthermore, a 5 × 6 mm well-defined hypoechoic nodule was reported in the right lobe. Thyroid scan was requested to evaluate the thyroid nodule. The nodule in the left lobe was visualized as a "hot spot" on the thyroid scan. The other nodule was visualized as a cold nodule. We decided to follow the patient with USG and thyroid function tests. In control USG done after 1 year, that nodule size was reported 17.4 × 14.9 mm. FNA biopsy was requested because of size enlargement, and biopsy result was reported as a benign lesion. During the 4-year follow-up, TSH levels remained in normal range.

15.3 Discussion

The term thyroid nodule refers to discrete lesions within the thyroid gland, radiologically distinct from surrounding thyroid parenchyma [1]. They may be discovered by palpation during a general physical examination or with chance during a cervical imaging procedure performed for medical evaluations, like USG computed tomography (CT), magnetic resonance imaging (MRI), or PET-CT scan. Thyroid nodules are extremely common. An estimated 4% of the population have a palpable thyroid nodule, and more than 50% have a nodule detectable by USG [2]. With increased sensitivity and widespread use of imaging modalities in clinical practice, incidental thyroid nodules are being found more frequently [3]. Generally, they are detected in euthyroid persons and don't cause any symptoms. Thyroid nodules are clinically important because of the risk of thyroid cancer. The reported prevalence of malignancy in thyroid nodules ranges 7–15% depending on age, gender, radiation exposure history, family history, and other factors [4, 5]. Therefore, a complete history and physical examination focusing on the thyroid gland and adjacent cervical lymph nodes are important to evaluate a thyroid nodule. Physical findings like vocal cord paralysis, cervical lymphadenopathy, fixation of the nodule to surrounding tissue, hoarseness, and the historical factors include a history of head and neck radiation therapy, exposure to ionizing radiation, and some genetic anomalies including Cowden's disease, FAP, Carney complex, and MEN 2 are increasing the possibility of malignancy [6, 7]. The American Thyroid Association (ATA) Guideline, revised in 2015, recommends measuring serum TSH during the initial evaluation of a patient with a thyroid nodule. If there are normal or elevated TSH levels, ATA guideline recommends ultrasound imaging for the decision of FNA [1]. Recommendation of diagnostic FNA depends on the size and suspicious ultrasound findings like irregular margins, microcalcifications, taller-than-wide shape, disrupted rim calcifications with small extrusive hypoechoic soft tissue component, and evidence of extrathyroidal extension. Also, if there is a subnormal TSH level, thyroid scan is recommended by the ATA guideline [1]. Thyroid scan provides information on the function of the thyroid nodule. Nodules detected by thyroid scan are classified according to their radionuclide uptake compared to normal thyroid parenchyma. Hypofunctioning (cold nodules) are more common, but the minority of thyroid nodules are hyperfunctioning (hot nodules), also known as autonomously functioning thyroid nodules (AFTNs). The ATA guideline does not suggest FNA biopsy for patients whose thyroid scan shows hot nodules, and it does not suggest thyroid scans either as long as the TSH value is within the normal range [1]. On the contrary, the American Association of Clinical Endocrinologists, American College of Endocrinology, and Associazione Medici Endocrinologi Medical (AACE/ACE/AME) guidelines recommend performing thyroid scan in iodine-deficient regions, to exclude autonomy of a thyroid nodule or MNG even when the TSH level is low-normal [8].

AFTNs are demonstrated by thyroid scan even if TSH values are in the normal range [9, 10]. The prevalence of AFTNs was higher in the iodine-deficient area [11]. Additionally, as we presented in our cases, serum TSH level may remain in the normal range in patients from iodine-deficient regions even if autonomy is present. The reason of that iodine deficiency effects thyroid gland, decreased proliferation rate of thyroid epithelial cells, and the low synthesis rate of thyroid hormones results in unsuppressed TSH levels [8]. Due to these reasons, using only TSH measurement is not an effective test to detect the presence of an AFTN [9, 10]. In our patients who live in Turkey, an iodine deficiency area, serum TSH measurement was not enough for the AFTN diagnosis; it could only be diagnosed with a thyroid scan. A thyroid scan is also useful to evaluate patients with multinodular goiter in iodine deficiency area. Detection of hot and cold nodules helps to prioritization for FNA biopsy in patients with MNGs [8]. Because of the ATA guideline recommendation, thyroid scan is rarely performed for a thyroid nodule in euthyroid patients. With only serum TSH monitoring, it's possible to miss some of the AFTNs. Those nodules may undergo unnecessary FNA biopsy. Indeterminate biopsy results like follicular lesion of undetermined significance (FLUS) cause to perform unnecessary thyroid surgery.

Although AFTNs are accepted as benign lesions, some case reports show thyroid malignancy in AFTNs [12]. Also, we know that the suspicious patterns defined by ATA guideline like microcalcifications, hypoechoic aspect, and perinodal and intranodular vascularization are higher in AFTNs than in cold nodules [13]. We need more studies to assess the risk of malignity in AFTNs and prevalence of malignancy.

What Can We Learn from This Case?

- Thyroid nodules are extremely common, and most of them are asymptomatic.
- The basis of thyroid nodule management is the categorization of malignancy risk.
- Complete medical history, physical examination, TSH assay, and USG are widely accepted as the first steps in evaluating the thyroid nodule.
- It's assumed that the risk of malignancy in an AFTN is generally very low.
- Using only TSH measurement is not an effective test to detect the presence of an AFTN.
- Especially in iodine deficiency regions, we may see unsuppressed serum TSH levels with AFTNs.

- Contrary to the ATA guideline recommendation, thyroid scan is an important detection instrument of AFTNs even if the TSH levels are in normal range.
- Additionally, we need more studies to evaluate malignancy possibility in AFTNs.

References

1. Haugen BR, Alexander EK, Bible KC, Doherty GM, Mandel SJ, Nikiforov YE, et al. 2015 American Thyroid Association management guidelines for adult patients with thyroid nodules and differentiated thyroid cancer: the American Thyroid Association guidelines task force on thyroid nodules and differentiated thyroid cancer. Thyroid. 2016;26:1–133. https://doi.org/10.1089/thy.2015.0020.
2. Levine RA. Current guidelines for the management of thyroid nodules. Endocr Pract. 2012;18:596–9. https://doi.org/10.4158/ep12071.co.
3. Dean DS, Gharib H. Epidemiology of thyroid nodules. Best Pract Res Clin Endocrinol Metab. 2008;22:901–11. https://doi.org/10.1016/j.beem.2008.09.019.
4. Hegedüs L. The thyroid nodule. N Engl J Med. 2004; 351:1764–71. https://doi.org/10.1056/NEJMcp031436.
5. Mandel SJ. A 64-year-old woman with a thyroid nodule. JAMA. 2004;292:2632–42. https://doi.org/10.1001/jama.292.21.2632.
6. Raza SN, Shah MD, Palme CE, Hall FT, Eski S, Freeman JL. Risk factors for well-differentiated thyroid carcinoma in patients with thyroid nodular disease. Otolaryngol Head Neck Surg. 2008;139:21–6. https://doi.org/10.1016/j.otohns.2007.10.021.
7. Pacini F, Vorontsova T, Demidchik EP, Molinaro E, Agate L, Romei C, et al. Post-Chernobyl thyroid carcinoma in Belarus children and adolescents: comparison with naturally occurring thyroid carcinoma in Italy and France. J Clin Endocrinol Metab. 1997;82:3563–9. https://doi.org/10.1210/jcem.82.11.4367.
8. Gharib H, Papini E, Garber JR, Duick DS, Harrell RM, Hegedüs L, et al. American Association of Clinical Endocrinologists, American College of Endocrinology, and Associazione Medici Endocrinologi medical guidelines for clinical practice for the diagnosis and management of thyroid nodules – 2016 update. Endocr Pract. 2016;22(Suppl 1):1–60. https://doi.org/10.4158/EP161208.GL.
9. Treglia G, Trimboli P, Verburg FA, Luster M, Giovanella L. Prevalence of normal TSH value among patients with autonomously functioning thyroid nodule. Eur J Clin Investig. 2015;45:739–44. https://doi.org/10.1111/eci.12456.
10. Chami R, Moreno-Reyes R, Corvilain B. TSH measurement is not an appropriate screening test for autonomous functioning thyroid nodules: a retrospective study of 368 patients. Eur J Endocrinol. 2014;170:593–9.
11. Belfiore A, Sava L, Runello F, Tomaselli L, Vigneri R. Solitary autonomously functioning thyroid nodules and iodine deficiency. J Clin Endocrinol Metabol. 1983;56:283–7. https://doi.org/10.1210/jcem-56-2-283.
12. Mirfakhraee S, Mathews D, Peng L, Woodruff S, Zigman JM. A solitary hyperfunctioning thyroid nodule harboring thyroid carcinoma: review of the literature. Thyroid Res. 2013;6:7. https://doi.org/10.1186/1756-6614-6-7.
13. Moreno-Reyes R, Kyrilli A, Lytrivi M, Bourmorck C, Chami R, Corvilain B. Is there still a role for thyroid scintigraphy in the workup of a thyroid nodule in the era of fine needle aspiration cytology and molecular testing? F1000Research. 2016;5:F1000 Faculty Rev-763. https://doi.org/10.12688/f1000research.7880.1.

16 Incidentally Detected Thyroid Follicular Adenoma on Myocardial Perfusion Scintigraphy with Tc-99m MIBI

Meral Mert and Murat Sipahi

Abstract

Technetium-99m sestamibi (Tc-99m MIBI) is a routinely used radiopharmaceutical for myocardial perfusion scintigraphy (MPS). Here, we present a case of a 76-year-old woman with mild transient chest pain but normal laboratory examination results who underwent Tc-99m sestamibi (MIBI) myocardial perfusion imaging, and an abnormal focal radionuclide uptake in the left lobe of the thyroid gland was detected. After that, the patient underwent left hemithyroidectomy, and the result of the pathology came out as follicular adenoma. In this case, we wanted to discuss the significance of MIBI uptake in thyroid nodules and discuss the importance of evaluating raw data images for the detection of noncardiac pathologies in myocardial perfusion scintigraphy.

M. Mert
Department of Endocrinology and Metabolism, Bakirkoy Dr. Sadi Konuk Training and Research Hospital, Health Sciences University (SBÜ), Istanbul, Turkey

M. Sipahi (✉)
Department of Nuclear Medicine, Bakirkoy Dr. Sadi Konuk Training and Research Hospital, Istanbul, Turkey

16.1 Case Presentation

A 76-year-old female patient without known thyroid disease and a history of thyroid disease-related drug use presented with a complaint of chest pain to cardiology outpatient clinic, and myocardial perfusion scintigraphy (MPS) has been requested. Abnormal focal technetium-99m-methoxyisobutylisonitrile (MIBI) uptake was seen in the area of the left thyroid gland when looking at the raw images of myocardial perfusion scintigraphy (Fig. 16.1). At the same session, no other pathological focus was detected on whole-body MIBI imaging (Fig. 16.2). Advanced examinations were suggested to the patient such as neck ultrasonography (USG), thyroid scintigraphy, and laboratory investigations. Thyroid scintigraphy couldn't be performed because the patient didn't want to undergo a second examination in the nuclear medicine clinic. In the left thyroid lobe, 29 × 36 × 41 mm-sized hypoechoic nodule was observed with thyroid USG (Fig. 16.3).

The patient was euthyroid according to her laboratory findings. A biopsy accompanied by USG was performed. The result of the biopsy was "suspicious for follicular neoplasm" (Bethesda 4), and the patient underwent left hemithyroidectomy. The result of the pathology was follicular adenoma.

T. Özülker et al. (eds.), *Thyroid and Parathyroid Diseases*, https://doi.org/10.1007/978-3-319-78476-2_16

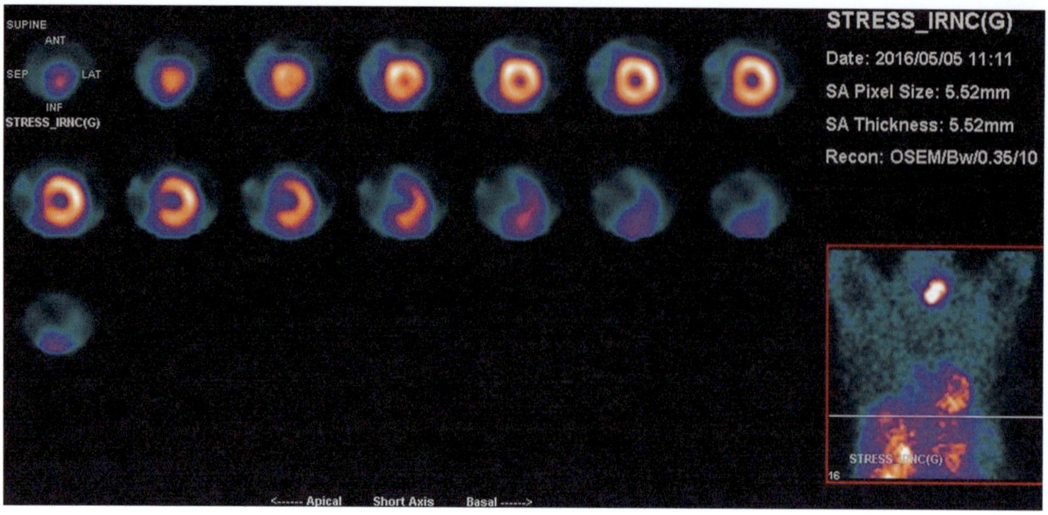

Fig. 16.1 Tc99m MIBI myocardial perfusion image. An abnormal focus of MIBI at the left thyroid lobe

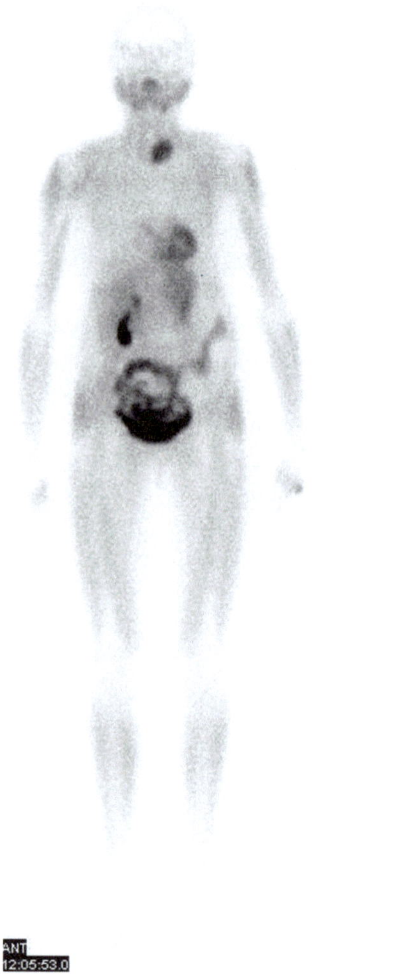

Fig. 16.2 Whole-body MIBI scan. No abnormal finding other than an abnormal focus of uptake at the left thyroid lobe

16.2 Discussion

MPS is a noninvasive imaging test that is used in the evaluation of coronary diseases. MIBI is a cationic molecule which is primarily used in MPS. Over the years, technetium-99m MIBI scintigraphy has also been used in the localization of parathyroid adenoma [1, 2].

technetium-99m MIBI accumulates in the cells which is associated with high proliferative activity and increased number of mitochondria. These features are typical in tumor cells [3]. For this reason, technetium-99m MIBI is has been used nonspecifically in the diagnosis of breast, thyroid, and lung cancers [3]. In a study of analysis of 330 MPS images, focal thyroid uptake was detected in 41 cases (12.4%) [4]. Thyroid nodules were observed in 25 of the 41 patients in the study group. Fine-needle aspiration biopsy (FNAB) of the thyroid was performed in 21 patients. One case of papillary thyroid carcinoma was determined and confirmed by histopathology after thyroidectomy [4].

In a study of analysis of technetium-99m pertechnetate and technetium-99m MIBI uptake in thyroid nodules, 28 of 77 nodules were observed cold both with technetium-99m pertechnetate and technetium-99m MIBI imaging; in 27 nodules which were observed cold with technetium-99m pertechnetate, technetium-99m MIBI and normal thyroid tissue were of similar

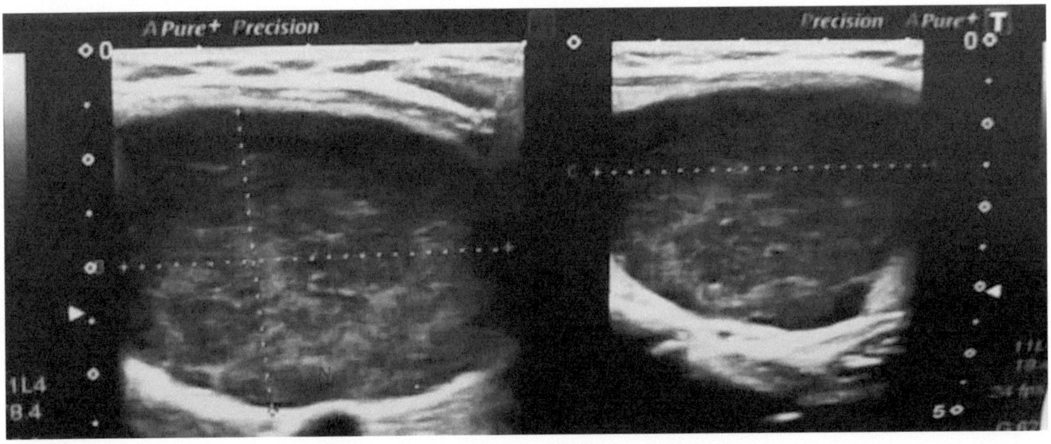

Fig. 16.3 A 29 × 36 × 41 mm-sized hypoechoic nodule in the left lobe in thyroid USG

intensity; five nodules which were cold with technetium-99m pertechnetate were observed hot with technetium-99m MIBI [5]. The histopathology of 34 surgically removed nodules proved that increased, normal, or decreased MIBI accumulation is not specific for thyroid malignancy [5].

Noncardiac findings can be detected in MPS. In this regard, in a comprehensive study of 12,256 patients, noncardiac findings have been identified in 207 patients, and thyroid uptake was present in seven patients. Three of seven patients could be followed-up, and thyroid pathology was not detected in any of them [6].

Technetium-99m MIBI can be used in the evaluation of thyroid nodules due to its positive predictive value; however, it cannot help to identify nodules which have Bethesda category III [atypia of undetermined significance (AUS) or follicular lesion of undetermined significance (FLUS)] and Bethesda category IV (suspicious for follicular lesions or follicular neoplasms) cytologies [3].

To date, indeterminate cytology (e.g., AUS/FLUS or SFN/FN) nodules prevalence ranges between 20% and 30%. Many published data showed that a malignant tumor could not have been identified in final histological diagnosis in 85% of patients with an indeterminate cytology [7, 8].

However, several researchers [9–11] have already done studies on ^{99}mTc-MIBI's possible role in the discrimination of malignancies in the thyroid nodules. In particular, MIBI has been reported to have quite high sensitivity and negative predictive value in the exclusion of malignancy. In their prospective research, Giovanella et al. [9] showed that negative MIBI scan had 100% sensitivity and negative predictive value in the exclusion of malignancy. Two years later, similar results were also published by Bruckner et al. [10]. In a meta-analysis, the diagnostic performance of technetium-99m MIBI scan was evaluated in terms of predicting the risk of malignancy in patients with solitary thyroid nodule or multinodular goiter. Sensitivity and specificity of Tc-MIBI scan in detecting malignant thyroid nodules were 85.1% and 45.7% [12].

This was based on the assumption that technetium-99m MIBI uptake within nodule reflects actively working of mitochondrial abundance and hence oxidative load: technetium-99m MIBI-positive nodules are more likely to be malignant when compared with negative nodules [12].

16.2.1 Follow-Up and Outcome

There were no problems in the follow-up after the lobectomy of the patient. Extra cardiac findings detected during MPS should always be taken into account, and advanced examination should be performed.

16.3 Future

A number of studies have been conducted for further diagnosis of thyroid incidentalomas. Recently published 2015 American Thyroid

Association's (ATA's) Management Guidelines for Adult Patients with Thyroid Nodules and Differentiated Thyroid Cancer has discussed the possible role of F-18 FDG-PET/CT in the differentiation of malignant from benign lesions [13]. For now, F-18 FDG-PET/CT isn't routinely recommended in thyroid nodules with indeterminate cytology; however, it is indicated to be useful.

What Can We Learn from This Case?

- In this case, we wanted to emphasize the importance of evaluating raw data images for the detection of noncardiac pathologies in MPS.
- Extracardiac findings detected during MPS are important, and further investigation is necessary.

References

1. McBiles M, Albert T, Cote M. Sestamibi parathyroid imaging. Semin Nucl Med. 1995;25:221–34.
2. Coakley A, Kettle AG, Wells CP, O'Doherety MJ, Collins RE. Technetium-99m-sestamibi: a new agent for parathyroid imaging. Nucl Med Commun. 1989;10:791–4.
3. Bucerius J, Ahmadzadehfar H, Biersack H. 99mTc-Sestamibi clinical applications. Berlin: Springer; 2012.
4. Giejda K, Piszczek S, Stembrowicz-Nowakowska Z, Saracyn M, Dziuk M, Kamiński G. Incidentally recognised thyroid focal uptake of 99mTc-sestamibi during stress myocardial perfusion scintigraphy. Endokrynol Pol. 2015;66:521–5. https://doi.org/10.5603/EP.2015.0064.
5. Földes I, Lévay A, Stotz G. Comparative scanning of thyroid nodules with technetium-99m pertechnetate and technetium-99m methoxyisobutylisonitrile. Eur J Nucl Med. 1993;20:330–3.
6. Williams KA, Hill KA, Sheridan CM. Noncardiac findings on dual-isotope myocardial perfusion SPECT. J Nucl Cardiol. 2003;10:395–402.
7. Cibas ES, Ali SZ. The Bethesda system for reporting thyroid cytopathology. Am J Clin Pathol. 2009;132:658–65. https://doi.org/10.1309/AJCPPHLWMI3JV4LA.
8. Trimboli P, Treglia G, Guidobaldi L, Saggiorato E, Nigri G, Crescenzi A, et al. Clinical characteristics as predictors of malignancy in patients with indeterminate thyroid cytology: a meta-analysis. Endocrine. 2014;46:52–9. https://doi.org/10.1007/s12020-013-0057-1.
9. Giovanella L, Suriano S, Maffioli M, Ceriani L, Spriano G. (99m)Tc-sestamibi scanning in thyroid nodules with nondiagnostic cytology. Head Neck. 2010;32:607–11. https://doi.org/10.1002/hed.21229.
10. Leidig-Bruckner G, Cichorowski G, Sattler P, Bruckner T, Sattler B. Evaluation of thyroid nodules—combined use of 99mTc-methylisobutylnitrile scintigraphy and aspiration cytology to assess risk of malignancy and stratify patients for surgical or nonsurgical therapy—a retrospective cohort study. Clin Endocrinol. 2012;76:749–58. https://doi.org/10.1111/j.1365-2265.2011.04292.x.
11. Saggiorato E, Angusti T, Rosas R, Martinese M, Finessi M, Arecco F, et al. 99mTc-MIBI imaging in the presurgical characterization of thyroid follicular neoplasms: relationship to multidrug resistance protein expression. J Nucl Med. 2009;50:1785–93. https://doi.org/10.2967/jnumed.109.064980.
12. Treglia G, Caldarella C, Saggiorato E, Ceriani L, Orlandi F, Salvatori M, et al. Diagnostic performance of (99m)Tc-MIBI scan in predicting the malignancy of thyroid nodules: a meta-analysis. Endocrine. 2013;44:70–8. https://doi.org/10.1007/s12020-013-9932-z.
13. Haugen BR, Alexander EK, Bible KC, Doherty GM, Mandel SJ, Nikiforov YE, et al. 2015 American Thyroid Association management guidelines for adult patients with thyroid nodules and differentiated thyroid cancer. Thyroid. 2016;26:1–133. https://doi.org/10.1089/thy.2015.0020.

17 Follicular Neoplasia

M. Ümit Uğurlu and Bahadır M. Güllüoğlu

Abstract

The term "follicular neoplasia" encompasses a spectrum of diseases ranging from benign to malignant nature. It includes benign follicular adenoma, follicular carcinoma, and follicular variant of papillary cancer. Since the preoperative diagnosis addresses both benign and malignant lesions, gray zones exist and diagnostic surgery is generally required for a definitive diagnosis. Herein, we focus on the clinical presentation, management strategies, and histopathologic architecture of a case with a preoperative diagnosis of "follicular neoplasia" taking into account the current guidelines, promising molecular markers and future directives.

17.1 Case Presentation

A 42-year-old woman was referred to endocrine surgery unit after an incidental finding of a thyroid nodule on MRI done for cervical lumbago. She suffered from neck pain radiating to the right shoulder for 5 years. The patient had no compressive symptoms, voice change, or any other complaints. In her physical examination, her vitals were within normal physiological limits for her age. She was a daily smoker with 20 packs/year. Her past medical history is nonsignificant, and she did not have any previous irradiation to the head and neck area. She had a family history of hypertension and diabetes mellitus in her parents, and she denied any family history of malignancy. On her neck examination, there was a non-tender palpable nodule in the right thyroid lobe. There were no palpable nodule(s) on the left thyroid lobe and no palpable cervical lymph nodes bilaterally. We asked for ECG (electrocardiogram), chest x-ray, serum TSH and free T4 analysis, a complete blood count, and a neck Doppler USG (ultrasound) examination. ECG and chest x-ray were normal. The patient was euthyroid, and the rest of the laboratory values was unremarkable. The USG revealed a circumscribed, heterogeneous, hyperechoic nodule on the right thyroid lobe which was 1.8 × 1.8 × 2 cm in size and had a cystic component. The nodule had a thin peripheral halo. On Doppler mode, the nodule had peripheral vascularity. The left thyroid lobe was normal. On USG guidance, we performed FNAB (fine needle aspiration biopsy). The microscopic evaluation of the Papanicolaou-stained FNAB smears showed hypercellular background, composed of abortive microfollicles with central dark colloid. The smear background was homogenous and revealed no other specific components other than these cellular groups. FNAB was reported as follicular neoplasm, Bethesda category IV (Fig. 17.1).

M. U. Uğurlu (✉) · B. M. Güllüoğlu
Marmara University, School of Medicine, Department of General Surgery, Istanbul, Turkey
e-mail: bmgulluoglu@superonline.com

T. Özülker et al. (eds.), *Thyroid and Parathyroid Diseases*, https://doi.org/10.1007/978-3-319-78476-2_17

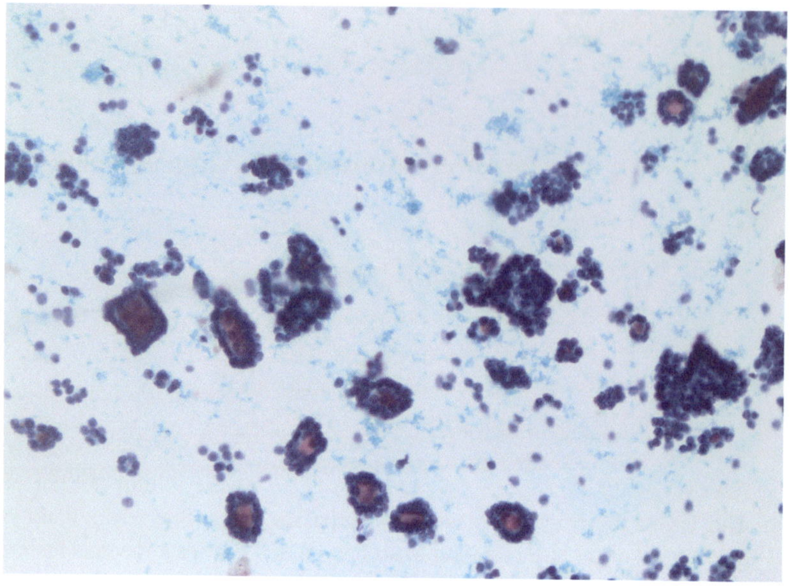

Fig. 17.1 The smear is cellular and consists of microfollicular groups. Most of them have compact colloid in the center of these groups. The cells are homogenous with dark and centrally located nuclei with well-defined nuclear borders (*Image courtesy of Pelin Bagci, MD*)

We informed the patient about the term "follicular neoplasia" and offered hemithyroidectomy and isthmusectomy for further evaluation. The surgery passed eventless; the right recurrent laryngeal nerve was seen and monitored during the surgery. The right superior and inferior parathyroid glands were seen and protected. The patient was discharged on postoperative day 1.

The macroscopic pathological examination of the lobectomy specimen revealed 1.8 × 2 cm nodule located on the right inferior thyroid pole. The nodule had a thick and regular capsule. The cut section of the nodule showed poor colloid compared to the adjacent thyroid parenchyma (Fig. 17.2). There were no other nodules or lesions in the rest of the specimen. The nodule was sampled totally. On the microscopic evaluation, there was no capsular and vascular invasion in the vessels of the capsule. The capsule was thick and homogenous. Nodule parenchyma was also homogenous and composed of microfollicles. The high-power examination showed compact colloid in the center of the florid-like microfollicles. There were no mitosis and necrosis. The cells lining these follicles were all homogenous, small, and cubic, and their nuclei were homogenous and vesicular. The adjacent thyroid tissue revealed no other specific feature (Fig. 17.3). The diagnosis was reported as follicular adenoma.

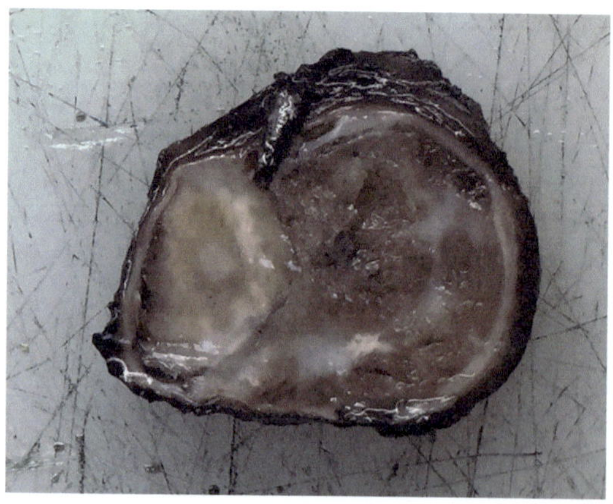

Fig. 17.2 The hemithyroidectomy specimen reveals 1.8 × 2 cm nodule with thick and regular capsule and poor colloid (*Image courtesy of Pelin Bagci, MD*)

17.2 Discussion

17.2.1 Evaluation and Diagnosis

The term "follicular neoplasm" encompasses a spectrum of diseases ranging from benign to

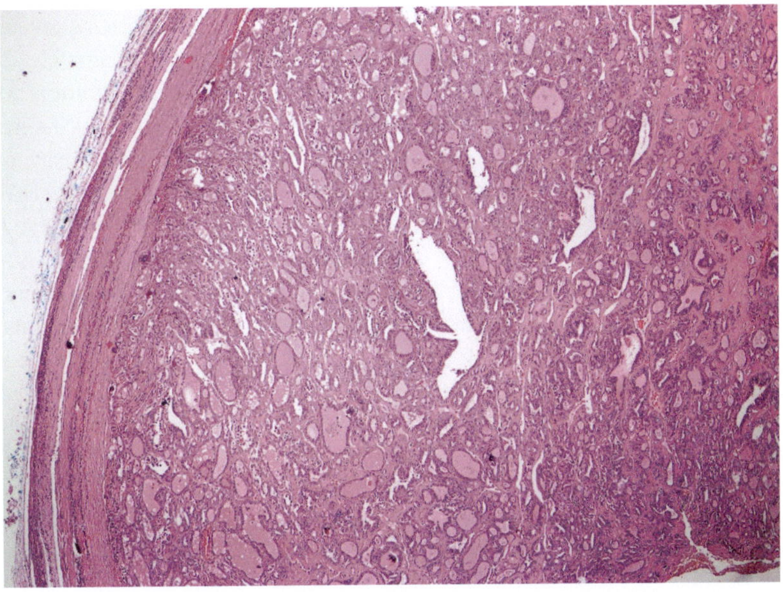

Fig. 17.3 H&E stained slide shows the fibrous and thick capsule. The tumor underlying the capsule is homogenous and microfollicular, each group with a central colloid. The capsule has been sampled thoroughly, and no capsular or vascular invasion is present (*Image courtesy of Pelin Bagci, MD*)

malignant nature. It includes benign follicular adenoma, follicular carcinoma, and follicular variant of papillary cancer. Patients with follicular adenoma or carcinoma are usually asymptomatic and present with a palpable nodule or non-palpable incidental nodule discovered in radiologic imaging. Symptomatic cases have larger nodules and can have complaints of compression, dyspnea, choking sensation, or hoarseness. There can be accompanying thyroiditis or nodular hyperplasia. Mostly patients are euthyroid, but 1% can have hyperthyroidism with a benign toxic adenoma, which is usually ≥3 cm in size [1]. Follicular carcinoma accounts for 10% of thyroid malignancies and is classified as minimally invasive follicular carcinoma and widely invasive follicular carcinoma by World Health Organization. It's more prevalent in iodine-deficient regions. Widely invasive type occurs most often in older women with a mean age of 60, and minimally invasive type is more common in young women. Rarely, at initial presentation, follicular carcinoma can make distant metastasis to the lung or bone via hematogenous route [2].

After a thorough physical examination, the evaluation of thyroid nodules continues with a neck ultrasound. Ultrasound examination shall include the bilateral thyroid glands and the bilateral cervical neck regions to seek for the presence of lymphadenopathies. Certain USG features can be predictors of malignancy. However, in context of follicular neoplasm, USG features of benign follicular adenoma and follicular carcinoma are very similar. Follicular carcinoma is usually solid, lacking cystic change, larger (>2 cm) compared to benign adenomas, unifocal, and isoechoic to hypoechoic with irregular margins, has a discontinued or lacking halo, and may have microcalcifications. Color Doppler USG can detect intranodular flow on follicular neoplasms. Positive predictive value and negative predictive value of increased internal vascularity to indicate follicular carcinoma were found to be 51% and 97%, respectively [3, 4]. Thyroid imaging reporting and data system (TIRADS) can help to stratify the risk of malignancy. TIRADS scores features such as component, echogenicity, margins, the presence of microcalcifications, and shape to predict malignancy. The score 4–5 is associated with increased probability of malignancy and make the patient a candidate for FNAB [5].

For the evaluation of thyroid nodules, FNAB is the next step diagnostic procedure. For decision making, whether to perform surgery or to follow up the patient, physicians use the findings of FNAB along with the clinical features and USG. Surgeons encounter the diagnosis as "follicular neoplasm or suspicious for follicular neoplasm" in 15–20% of the FNAB reports, which is termed to be the "gray zone" in cytopathology of thyroid nodules [6, 7]. The reason for the difficulty in the distinction of these lesions is that both the follicular adenoma and follicular carcinoma differentiates from follicular cells, and they both have a microfollicular architecture with monotonous population of follicles with minimal/absent background colloid lined by cuboidal epithelium. Nuclear atypia can be seen, which is not a diagnostic criterion of malignancy because follicular adenoma can have nuclear atypia. So, even though FNAB is very sensitive for the distinction of benign from malignant nodules, it has limited value in follicular lesions, because the hallmark of malignancy is the capsular and/or vascular invasion, and it cannot be assessed with FNAB [8]. Cytological diagnosis of follicular variant of papillary carcinoma on FNAB can also be problematic; the cytological criteria of papillary carcinoma may be lacking or not completely unequivocal [9]. Overall, the Bethesda system recognizes these lesions in FNAB as category IV, and 15–30% of follicular neoplasm is estimated to be malignant [10].

Some investigators suggested frozen sections for intraoperative decision making in the management of follicular lesions [11]. Despite the other literature suggesting the limited value of intraoperative frozen section of follicular lesions, surgeons still practice the frozen sectioning to progress from hemithyroidectomy to total thyroidectomy. The reason to advocate not performing a frozen section in follicular neoplasm is its infeasibility to get adequate sampling of the capsule to evaluate for capsular and/or vascular invasion [12]. Hence, frozen sectioning of follicular lesions is non-definitive in most of the cases to dictate total thyroidectomy rather than hemithyroidectomy, and it is not practical in the intraoperative setting.

Genetic tests are being investigated for differential diagnosis of follicular lesions in adjunct to cytology. At the time of aspiration, a small portion of the material is saved for molecular analysis. A seven-gene panel of mutations including RAS (H-RAS, K-RAS, N-RAS), BRAF, RET/PTC, and PAX8/PPARg was studied and identified in >70% of thyroid cancers. These genetic markers are adjunct to FNAB and associated with a sensitivity of 57–75%, specificity of 97–100%, positive predictive value of 87–100%, and negative predictive value of 79–86% in nodules with follicular neoplasm or suspicious for follicular neoplasm cytology [13, 14]. Also, the gene expression classifier was developed to identify benign nodules among patients who have cytology of follicular neoplasm or atypia of undetermined significance. Afirma (Veracyte, CA, USA) is a commercially available gene expression classifier test, which uses a mRNA expression panel of 142 genes to identify the benign signature. The Afirma test follows an algorithm for the analysis of gene expression profiles and reports the result as either "benign" or "suspicious." It's reported that the negative predictive value of Afirma for follicular neoplasm/suspicious for follicular neoplasm was 94%, with a 92% sensitivity and 52% specificity. Due to its low specificity, Afirma's true negativity rate was found to be 50%, and false positivity rate was found to be 50%; hence it's not specific enough to alter the management strategy [1, 2, 15, 16]. Hence, Afirma is particularly helpful as a "rule-out" test in thyroid nodules with Bethesda III and IV cytology. Even though it needs further studies, the ATA guidelines 2015 recommends (weakly) molecular testing as an adjunct method before proceeding to surgery.

17.2.2 Management

Due to the uncertainty of follicular lesions in FNAB, in conditions that the molecular testing is not performed or inconclusive, the guideline strongly recommends surgical excision for the management of thyroid nodules with follicular neoplasm and/or suspicious follicular neoplasm histology [17]. The type of surgery should, at minimum, be a thyroid lobectomy with isthmusectomy. In patients with a strong family history of thyroid cancer, multiple nodular goiter, personal history of head/neck radiation treatment, and worrisome USG features or in case of patients' preference, initial surgery can be as total thyroidectomy. If the final pathology is reported as follicular adenoma, the patient needs no further treatment. The encapsulated follicular variant of papillary thyroid cancer is recently reclassified as noninvasive follicular carcinoma with papillary features (NIFTP), and this can be followed carefully without completion thyroidectomy due to its excellent prognosis. Minimally invasive follicular cancer, which is characterized as a well-defined tumor with microscopic capsular and/or 1–4 foci of vascular invasion, also has an excellent prognosis. So, minimally invasive cancers can be simply followed especially in patients who are young with tumor size <4 cm [18]. However, in the National Comprehensive Cancer Network guideline for thyroid cancer (*vers 2.2017*), completion thyroidectomy is also recommended for patients who have minimally invasive follicular cancer on final histology after lobectomy with isthmectomy due to published deaths attributed to these lesions. When the final histopathologic evaluation reveals follicular carcinoma after lobectomy performed for follicular neoplasia and/or suspicious for follicular neoplasia, the decision for completion thyroidectomy depends on the features of the tumor. Patients having <1 cm tumor in size without extrathyroidal extension, metastasis to nodes (N1 disease) or metastasis to distant sites can be followed without completion thyroidectomy unless there is a history of prior head/neck irradiation or familial thyroid cancer. For tumors which are 1–4 cm in size, lobectomy may suffice, or completion thyroidectomy may be performed. For tumors >4 cm, the completion thyroidectomy will be the right management strategy [17]. If completion thyroidectomy is planned after hemithyroidectomy, it may be performed within 2 weeks of initial lobectomy procedure or 6–8 weeks later. Follicular cancer metastasizes to lymph nodes in <10% of the cases. Prophylactic central neck dissection should not be a routine practice during completion thyroidectomy [2].

17.3 Follow-Up and Outcome

This patient on the above case was diagnosed with "follicular adenoma." The patient was informed and reassured about the condition. No further surgical or medical evaluation was recommended. Since it's a benign lesion and the lobectomy is curative, the decision on the multidisciplinary meeting was to follow up this patient with annual physical examination and ultrasound.

17.3.1 The Future

The progress in the application of molecular markers to evaluate thyroid nodules parallels the expansion of knowledge on genetic mechanisms and the introduction of high-throughput genotyping techniques. Next-generation sequencing is very promising, which is used to find out genetic alterations on small FNAB samples. ThyroSeqv2 is an example of next-generation sequencing, which relies on detection of 14 mutations, 42 types of fusions, and expression of 16 genes. Recently it's shown that the "negative" ThyroSeq results in Bethesda III and IV nodules decrease the cancer risk to 3–4% [19]. Recent trials on new diagnostic tests like ThyGenX/ThyraMIR and Rosetta GX Reveal focus on miRNA markers. The results are promising to predict cancer and select the patients who are likely benefit from surveillance or surgical intervention [20]. The ongoing trials seem to focus on the molecular tests on patients with indeterminate FNAB results like follicular neoplasm.

What Can We Learn from This Case?

- Follicular neoplasm of thyroid includes benign follicular adenoma, minimally invasive follicular carcinoma, widely invasive follicular carcinoma, and follicular variant of papillary carcinoma.
- FNAB is a highly valuable tool in the evaluation of thyroid nodules; however, for follicular lesions, 15–30% of aspirates diagnosed as "follicular neoplasm/suspicious for follicular neoplasm" are actually carcinomas; the remaining 70–85% of nodules are benign.
- Only capsular and/or vascular invasion which is shown on microscopic examination of the surgical specimen can set the diagnosis as carcinoma.
- Molecular testing on FNAB aspirates may be useful in differential diagnosis of follicular neoplasm. In ATA 2015 guidelines, these tests are recommended as an adjunct method before proceeding to surgery whenever available.
- Surgical excision of Bethesda category IV nodules as lobectomy is also recommended for assessment of capsule and to obtain a definitive diagnosis.
- The intraoperative frozen section is impractical and is non-definitive in most of the cases to dictate total thyroidectomy.
- Molecular markers are a promising area and need further research to be proven as effective to differentiate benign from malignant follicular lesions.

References

1. McHenry CR, Phitayakorn R. Follicular adenoma, and carcinoma of the thyroid gland. Oncologist. 2011;16:585–93. https://doi.org/10.1634/theoncologist.2010-0405.
2. Mathur A, Olson MT, Zeiger MA. Follicular lesions of the thyroid. Surg Clin North Am. 2014;94:499–513. https://doi.org/10.1016/j.suc.2014.02.005.
3. Iared W, Shigueoka DC, Cristófoli JC, Andriolo R, Atallah AN, Ajzen SA, et al. Use of color Doppler ultrasonography for the prediction of malignancy in follicular thyroid neoplasms: systematic review and meta-analysis. J Ultrasound Med. 2010;29:19–25.
4. Kalra N, Ahuja CK, Dutta P, Rajwanshi A, Mittal BR, Bhansali A, et al. Comparison of Sonographically guided percutaneous sodium tetradecyl sulfate injection with ethanol injection in the treatment of benign nonfunctioning thyroid nodules. J Vasc Interv Radiol. 2014;25:1218–24. https://doi.org/10.1016/j.jvir.2014.04.026.
5. Kwak JY, Han KH, Yoon JH, Moon HJ, Son EJ, Park SH, et al. Thyroid imaging reporting and data system for US features of nodules: a step in establishing better stratification of cancer risk. Radiology. 2011;260:892–9. https://doi.org/10.1148/radiol.11110206.
6. Baloch ZW, Fleisher S, LiVolsi VA, Gupta PK. Diagnosis of "follicular neoplasm": a gray zone in thyroid fine-needle aspiration cytology. Diagn Cytopathol. 2002;26:41–4.
7. Baloch ZW, Cibas ES, Clark DP, Layfield LJ, Ljung BM, Pitman MB, et al. The National Cancer Institute Thyroid fine needle aspiration state of the science conference: a summation. Cytojournal. 2008;5:6. https://doi.org/10.1186/1742-6413-5-6.
8. Castro MR, Gharib H. Thyroid fine-needle aspiration biopsy: progress, practice, and pitfalls. Endocr Pract. 2003;9:128–36.
9. Lloyd RV, Erickson LA, Casey MB, Lam KY, Lohse CM, Asa SL, et al. Observer variation in the diagnosis of follicular variant of papillary thyroid carcinoma. Am J Surg Pathol. 2004;28:1336–40.
10. Baloch ZW, LiVolsi VA, Asa SL, Rosai J, Merino MJ, Randolph G, et al. Diagnostic terminology and morphologic criteria for cytologic diagnosis of thyroid lesions: a synopsis of the National Cancer Institute Thyroid Fine-Needle Aspiration State of the Science Conference. Diagn Cytopathol. 2008;36:425–37. https://doi.org/10.1002/dc.20830.
11. Paphavasit A, Thompson GB, Hay ID, Grant CS, van Heerden JA, Ilstrup DM, et al. Follicular and Hurthle cell thyroid neoplasms. Is frozen-section evaluation worthwhile? Arch Surg. 1997;132:674–8. discussion 678–80.
12. LiVolsi VA, Baloch ZW. Use and abuse of frozen section in the diagnosis of follicular thyroid lesions. Endocr Pathol. 2005;16:285–93.
13. Nikiforov YE, Ohori NP, Hodak SP, Carty SE, LeBeau SO, Ferris RL, et al. Impact of mutational testing on the diagnosis and management of patients with cytologically indeterminate thyroid nodules: a prospective analysis of 1056 FNA samples. J Clin Endocrinol Metab. 2011;96:3390–7. https://doi.org/10.1210/jc.2011-1469.
14. Nikiforov YE, Steward DL, Robinson-Smith TM, Haugen BR, Klopper JP, Zhu Z, et al. Molecular testing for mutations in improving the fine-needle aspiration diagnosis of thyroid nodules. J Clin Endocrinol Metab. 2009;94:2092–8. https://doi.org/10.1210/jc.2009-0247.
15. Alexander EK, Kennedy GC, Baloch ZW, Cibas ES, Chudova D, Diggans J, et al. Preoperative diagnosis

of benign thyroid nodules with indeterminate cytology. N Engl J Med. 2012;23(367):705–15. https://doi.org/10.1056/NEJMoa1203208.

16. Aragon Han P, Olson MT, Fazeli R, Prescott JD, Pai SI, Schneider EB, et al. The impact of molecular testing on the surgical management of patients with thyroid nodules. Ann Surg Oncol. 2014;21:1862–9. https://doi.org/10.1245/s10434-014-3508-x.
17. Haugen BR, Alexander EK, Bible KC, Doherty GM, Mandel SJ, Nikiforov YE, et al. 2015 American Thyroid Association management guidelines for adult patients with thyroid nodules and differentiated thyroid cancer: the American Thyroid Association guidelines task force on thyroid nodules and differentiated thyroid cancer. Thyroid. 2016;26:1–133. https://doi.org/10.1089/thy.2015.0020.
18. Goffredo P, Cheung K, Roman SA, Sosa JA. Can minimally invasive follicular thyroid cancer be approached as a benign lesion?: a population-level analysis of survival among 1,200 patients. Ann Surg Oncol. 2013;20:767–72. https://doi.org/10.1245/s10434-012-2697-4.
19. Nikiforov YE, Carty SE, Chiosea SI, Coyne C, Duvvuri U, Ferris RL, et al. Impact of the multi-gene ThyroSeq next-generation sequencing assay on Cancer diagnosis in thyroid nodules with atypia of undetermined significance/follicular lesion of undetermined significance cytology. Thyroid. 2015;25:1217–23. https://doi.org/10.1089/thy.2015.0305.
20. Nikiforov YE. Role of molecular markers in thyroid nodule management: then and now. Endocr Pract. 2017;23:979–88. https://doi.org/10.4158/EP171805.RA.

18 A Gray Zone in Thyroid Fine-Needle Aspiration Cytology: AUS-FLUS

Mehmet Ali Koç, Seher Demirer, and Akın Fırat Kocaay

Abstract

Thyroid nodules are a common finding in the adult population. Fine-needle aspiration biopsy (FNAB), when required, has an important role in the assessment of a thyroid nodule by assisting the triage of patients to surgery or surveillance. However, FNABs which are classified in the Bethesda category 3 (atypia of undetermined significance (AUS) or follicular lesion of undetermined significance (FLUS)) are difficult to manage because of the wide spectrum of cytopathologic findings in this category. While the Bethesda System for Reporting Thyroid Cytopathology recommends repeat FNAB for category 3, recent studies recommend molecular testing, if available. And also, surveillance or surgery is recommended especially if repeat FNAB cytology and/or molecular testing is not performed or inconclusive. In conclusion, unlike other categories in Bethesda classification, management of the AUS/FLUS category is still controversial.

M. Ali Koç · S. Demirer · A. F. Kocaay (✉)
Ankara University, School of Medicine,
Department of Surgery, Ankara, Turkey

18.1 Case Report

A 59-year-old female was admitted to the hospital with the complaint of swelling in the neck. She was a housewife and had two children. Physical examination revealed that there was a palpable nodule in the left thyroid lobe. The patient had no family history or radiation exposure. T4 and TSH levels were 10.84 pmol/L (range, 7–15.96 pmol/L) and 1.58 mIU/L (range, 0.38–5.33 mIU/L), respectively. Sonographically, only a 2 cm nodule was detected in the left lobe, and the right lobe was normal. No lymphadenopathy was detected in the neck. The nodule was hypoechogenic and solid. Fine-needle aspiration biopsy (FNAB) was performed. Cytology result was "follicular lesion of undetermined significance" (FLUS). Therefore repeat FNAB was performed. Repeat FNAB result was again FLUS. Because the patient's nodule was solid and hypoechogenic, surgery was performed. During surgery the left thyroid lobe and isthmus were removed. The specimen was sent to the pathologist for a frozen section. But pathologist could not differentiate the nodule if it was malignant or follicular neoplasm. After surgery, final pathology result was invasive encapsulated follicular variant of papillary thyroid carcinoma. Microscopically, the nodule was 2 cm in length and had a fibrous capsule. There were granular and oncocytic follicular epithelial cells with eosinophilic cytoplasm and irregular nucleus. There was no vascular invasion, but capsular invasion was detected. All surgical margins were negative.

T. Özülker et al. (eds.), *Thyroid and Parathyroid Diseases*, https://doi.org/10.1007/978-3-319-78476-2_18

Therefore, completion thyroidectomy was performed. The result of the second pathology after completion surgery was thyroid tissue composed of colloid-filled follicles. The patient was T1b N0 M0 according to AJCC/UICC TNM system.

18.2 Discussion

Thyroid nodules are a common finding in the adult population. As ultrasonography (USG), computerized tomography (CT), and magnetic resonance imaging (MRI) have been used widespread, many nonpalpable thyroid nodules have been found incidentally [1]. Although most nodules are asymptomatic, they should be assessed in detail by testing thyroid-stimulating hormone, USG, and FNAB when necessary [2].

FNAB has an important role in the assessment of a thyroid nodule. By estimating the risk of malignancy, FNAB assists the triage of patients to surgery or surveillance [3]. The Bethesda System for Reporting Thyroid Cytopathology (TBSRTC) classifies FNAB results into six categories that have been used generally in planning further management [4]. Each of these diagnostic categories has a suggested risk of malignancy and specific recommendations for subsequent management.

Fine-needle aspirations which can't be classified into the benign, suspicious, or malign categories in the Bethesda system are defined as "atypia of undetermined significance" (AUS) or FLUS (Bethesda category 3) [4].

AUS/FLUS is the most controversial category and heterogeneous group [5]. The wide spectrum of cytopathologic findings in this category ranges from sample preparation artifacts to focal features suggestive of papillary thyroid carcinoma [6]. Therefore, AUS/FLUS category should be used as a last resort, and its use should be limited up to approximately 7% of all thyroid FNABs [4].

The risk of malignancy of AUS/FLUS category according to Bethesda system is probably closer to 5–5% [4]. However, some recent studies have reported malignancy rates ranging from 6% to 81% [7–14]. According to another recent study, when evaluated separately, the rate of malignancy was 25.8% in nodules with AUS and 17.6% in nodules with FLUS [12]. According to these findings, the malignancy rates for AUS/FLUS, which is estimated in TBSRTC, might not be accurate, and since only a small fraction of patients with AUS/FLUS have been operated, the true incidence is unknown [15]. In our case, FNAB result was FLUS, and after diagnostic surgery, the final pathology result was malignant.

AUS/FLUS has various architectural or nuclear abnormalities that do not fit into any other category [16]. Several studies suggest that this category should be subclassified based on the presence of these abnormalities [17–20]. The popular opinion for the subclassification is the proposal to distinguish AUS/FLUS lesions according to their nuclear or architectural atypia. In a recent study, malignancy was diagnosed in 15.5% of nodules with architectural atypia and in 41.5% of nuclear atypia [17]. Another study showed that the malignancy rate for nodules with nuclear atypia was significantly higher than the rate for nodules with architectural atypia [18]. Chandra et al. showed that malignancy rate was higher in cases (24.1%) with atypical nuclear features in comparison to architectural atypia [19]. And Kim et al. found that the rate of neoplasm, which includes all malignancy and adenoma, showed a significant difference between cellular (51.8%) and architectural (25.2%) atypia [20].

TBSRTC recommends repeat FNAB for the further management of the category 3 FNAB results [4]. According to clinical and sonographic correlations, the American Thyroid Association guidelines recommend that nodules with AUS/FLUS cytology should be investigated by repeat FNAB and molecular testing. Although many authors have suggested performing repeat FNAB not sooner than 3 months, it is not necessary to wait especially when clinical or USG features are suspicious. And also, surveillance or surgery is recommended especially if repeat FNAB cytology and/or molecular testing is not performed or inconclusive [21]. Moreover, in a recent study, active surveillance is recommended after careful assessment of the patient and the nodule's characteristics [6]. In our case, we performed repeat FNAB. However, repeat FNAB result was again FLUS. In our institution, molecular analysis is not available. Thus, diagnostic surgery was performed because the nodule was solid and hypoechogenic sonographically.

Molecular analysis is one of the recommended methods for undetermined FNABs. Positive predictive value for thyroid cancer is high when *BRAF*, *NRAS*, *HRAS*, and *KRAS* point mutations and *PAX8*/*PPARG* and *RET*/*PTC* rearrangements are detected [22, 23]. Good predictive values have also been shown in several studies [24–26]. However, genetic tests are not available at many centers and expensive [27].

Sonographic malignancy criteria of the nodules are solid component, hypoechogenicity, irregular margins, microcalcifications, and a shape taller than wide measured on a transverse view [21, 28]. Recent studies which investigate sonographic malignancy features of the nodules that have FNAB results of AUS/FLUS also showed that irregular margins, taller-than-wide shape, and microcalcifications are associated with malignancy. But, nodule size is not a criterion for malignancy in patients with AUS/FLUS [1]. Our patient's nodule was hypoechogenic and solid. Although FNAB result was indeterminate, these sonographic findings were suspicious for malignancy.

The aim of the surgery for indeterminate nodules is to establish a histological diagnosis and provide treatment. Therefore, surgery is planned for the nodules with AUS/FLUS cytology if there is a suspicion for malignancy according to repeat FNAB or molecular analysis results or having sonographic malignancy criteria which are mentioned before [21]. Thyroid lobectomy should be the first choice of treatment for an indeterminate single nodule [21]. However clinical or sonographic characteristics, patient preference, and molecular testing may alter the choice of the surgical treatment.

Total thyroidectomy can be the initial treatment for the patients with a nodule of AUS/FLUS cytology when there are sonographic malignancy criteria or a history of familial thyroid cancer or radiation exposure [21]. Moreover, total or near total thyroidectomy can be preferred when the patient has bilateral multinodular disease or to avoid future contralateral thyroidectomy due to patients' request. Patients should undergo completion thyroidectomy if the tumor is >1 cm, or if the patient is older (>45), or if the patient has contralateral nodules or a family history of differentiated thyroid carcinoma or a history of radiation exposure to the head and neck [21]. In our case, FNAB result was inconclusive, and molecular analysis was not available; therefore diagnostic surgery was inevitable due to sonographic findings. As mentioned before, final pathology result was invasive encapsulated follicular variant of papillary thyroid carcinoma, and the 2 cm nodule had capsular invasion. Thus we performed completion thyroidectomy.

In conclusion, unlike other categories in Bethesda classification, management of the AUS/FLUS category is controversial due to a wide spectrum of cytopathologic finding ranges from sample preparation artifacts to focal features suggestive of papillary thyroid carcinoma. Therefore, several studies suggest subclassification of this category according to the nuclear or architectural atypia in cytology to triage the patients to surgery or surveillance. On the other hand, molecular analysis is a promising but an expensive method, and it is not available in many institutes. Under these circumstances, it is necessary to evaluate the cytologic findings considering the institutes own malignancy rates and the sonographic findings for the management of Bethesda category 3 nodules.

What Can We Learn from This Case?

- Repeat FNAB is recommended for the further management of the category 3 FNAB results.
- Molecular analysis is a recommended and promising method for undetermined FNABs. However, it is expensive and not available in many institutes.
- TBSRTC is a widely accepted classification method. But given the recent studies, a subclassification in the Bethesda category 3 might be useful for the management of the patients.
- Because of the wide range of differences among the malignancy risk of category 3 lesions in the literature, clinicians should consider the clinical and USG features and the malignancy rates of their institutions.

References

1. Kiernan CM, Solórzano CC. Bethesda category III, IV, and V thyroid nodules: can nodule size help predict malignancy? J Am Coll Surg. 2017;225:77–82.
2. Russ G, Leboulleux S, Leenhardt L, Hegedus L. Thyroid incidentalomas: epidemiology, risk stratification with ultrasound and workup. Eur Thyroid J. 2014;3:154–63.
3. Polyzos SA, Kita M, Avramidis A. Thyroid stepwise diagnosis and management. Hormones. 2007;6:101–19.
4. Cibas ES, Ali SZ, NCI Thyroid FNA State of the Science Conference. The Bethesda system for reporting thyroid cytopathology. Am J Clin Pathol. 2009;132:658–65.
5. Estrada Muñoz L, Díaz Del Arco C, Ortega Medina L, Fernández Aceñero MJ. Thyroid atypia/follicular lesion of undetermined significance: attitudes towards the diagnosis of Bethesda system III nodules. Acta Cytol. 2017;61:21–6.
6. Cohen O, Tzelnick S, Lahav Y, Schindel D, Halperin D, Yehuda M. Selection of atypia/follicular lesion of unknown significance patients for surgery versus active surveillance, without using genetic testing: a single institute experience, prospective analysis, and recommendations. Thyroid. 2017;27:928–35.
7. Kholova I, Ludvikova M. Thyroid atypia of undetermined significance or follicular lesion of undetermined significance: an indispensable Bethesda 2010 diagnostic category or waste garbage? Acta Cytol. 2014;58:319–29.
8. Kim SK, Hwang TS, Yoo YB, Han HS, Kim DL, Song KH, et al. Surgical results of thyroid nodules according to a management guideline based on the BRAF(V600E) mutation status. J Clin Endocrinol Metab. 2011;96:658–64.
9. Carr R, Ustun B, Chhieng D, Schofield K, Theoharis C, Hammers L, et al. Radiologic and clinical predictors of malignancy in the follicular lesion of undetermined significance of the thyroid. Endocr Pathol. 2013;24:62–8.
10. Crowe A, Linder A, Hameed O, Salih C, Roberson J, Gidley J, et al. The impact of implementation of the Bethesda system for reporting thyroid cytopathology on the quality of reporting, "risk" of malignancy, surgical rate, and rate of frozen sections requested for thyroid lesions. Cancer Cytopathol. 2011;119:315–21.
11. Bongiovanni M, Spitale A, Faquin WC, Mazzucchelli L, Baloch ZW. The Bethesda system for reporting thyroid cytopathology: a meta-analysis. Acta Cytol. 2012;56:333–9.
12. Topaloglu O, Baser H, Cuhaci FN, Sungu N, Yalcin A, Ersoy R, et al. Malignancy is associated with microcalcification and higher AP/T ratio in ultrasonography, but not with Hashimoto's thyroiditis in histopathology in patients with thyroid nodules evaluated as Bethesda Category III (AUS/FLUS) in cytology. Endocrine. 2016;54:156–68.
13. Gocun PU, Karakus E, Bulutay P, Akturk M, Akin M, Poyraz A. What is the malignancy risk for atypia of undetermined significance?. Three years' experience at a university hospital in Turkey. Cancer Cytopathol. 2014;122:604–10.
14. Park HJ, Moon JH, Yom CK, Kim KH, Choi JY, Choi SI, et al. Thyroid "atypia of undetermined significance" with nuclear atypia has high rates of malignancy and BRAF mutation. Cancer Cytopathol. 2014;122:512–20.
15. Turkyilmaz S, Ulusahin M, Celebi B, Cekic AB, Mungan S, Kucuktulu U, et al. Thyroid nodules classified as atypia or follicular lesions of undetermined significance deserve further research: analysis of 305 surgically confirmed nodules. Cytopathology. 2017;28:391–9.
16. Vanderlaan PA, Krane JF, Cibas ES. The frequency of 'atypia of undetermined significance' interpretations for thyroid fine-needle aspirations is negatively correlated with histologically proven malignant outcomes. Acta Cytol. 2011;55:512–7.
17. Rosario PW, Calsolari MR. Importance of cytological subclassification of thyroid nodules with Bethesda category III cytology (AUS/FLUS) into architectural atypia only and nuclear atypia: a prospective study. Diagn Cytopathol. 2017;45(7):604.
18. Gan TR, Nga ME, Lum JH, Wong WM, Tan WB, Parameswaran R, et al. Thyroid cytology-nuclear versus architectural atypia within the "atypia of undetermined significance/follicular lesion of undetermined significance" Bethesda category have significantly different rates of malignancy. Cancer. 2017;125:245–56.
19. Chandra S, Chandra H, Bisht SS. Malignancy rate in thyroid nodules categorized as atypia of undetermined significance or follicular lesion of undetermined significance: an institutional experience. J Cytol. 2017;34:144–8.
20. Kim SD, Han SH, Jeong WJ, Kim H, Ahn SH. Differences in clinical features between subcategories of "atypia/follicular lesion of undetermined significance". Endocr Pathol. 2017;28:247–52.
21. Haugen BR, Alexander EK, Bible KC, Doherty GM, Mandel SJ, Nikiforov YE, et al. 2015 American Thyroid Association management guidelines for adult patients with thyroid nodules and differentiated thyroid cancer: the American Thyroid Association guidelines task force on thyroid nodules and differentiated thyroid cancer. Thyroid. 2016;26:1–133.
22. Nikiforov YE, Ohori NP, Hodak SP, Carty SE, LeBeau SO, Ferris RL, et al. Impact of mutational testing on the diagnosis and management of patients with cytologically indeterminate thyroid nodules: a prospective analysis of 1056 FNA samples. J Clin Endocrinol Metab. 2011;96:3390–7.
23. Cantara S, Capezzone M, Marchisotta S, Capuano S, Busonero G, Toti P, et al. Impact of proto-oncogene mutation detection in cytological specimens from

thyroid nodules improves the diagnostic accuracy of cytology. J Clin Endocrinol Metab. 2010;95:1365–9.
24. Labourier E, Shifrin A, Busseniers AE, Lupo MA, Manganelli ML, Andruss B, et al. Molecular testing for miRNA, mRNA, and DNA on fine-needle aspiration improves the preoperative diagnosis of thyroid nodules with indeterminate cytology. J Clin Endocrinol Metab. 2015;100:2743–50.
25. Nikiforov YE, Carty SE, Chiosea SI, Coyne C, Duvvuri U, Ferris RL, et al. Impact of the multi-gene ThyroSeq next-generation sequencing assay on cancer diagnosis in thyroid nodules with atypia of undetermined significance/follicular lesion of undetermined significance cytology. Thyroid. 2015;25:1217–23.
26. Lithwick-Yanai G, Dromi N, Shtabsky A, Morgenstern S, Strenov Y, Feinmesser M, et al. Multicentre validation of a microRNA-based assay for diagnosing indeterminate thyroid nodules utilising fine needle aspirate smears. J Clin Pathol. 2017;70:500–7.
27. Wu JX, Lam R, Levin M, Rao J, Sullivan PS, Yeh MW. Effect of malignancy rates on cost-effectiveness of routine gene expression classifier testing for indeterminate thyroid nodules. Surgery. 2016;159:118–26.
28. Kwak JY, Han KH, Yoon JH, Moon HJ, Son EJ, Park SH, et al. Thyroid imaging reporting and data system for US features of nodules: a step in establishing better stratification of cancer risk. Radiology. 2011;260:892–9.

19 Is Surgery the Treatment of Choice for Every Thyroid Nodule?

Semra Günay and Orhan Yalçın

Abstract

The correct diagnosis of the thyroid nodule begins with clinical examination, interrogation, biochemical detection of the hormone level and ultrasonography (USG), and, if necessary, fine needle aspiration cytology (FNAC). The FNAC decision is based on the clinical and radiological (USG) characteristics of the nodule. At this stage, it is essential to classify the nodule according to current knowledge and guidelines regarding the risk of cancer. Thyroid nodule diagnosis is prevalent, but no surgical treatment is needed to treat all of them.

A 29-year-old male patient with a diagnosis of papillary microcarcinoma who underwent surgical resection for a solid thyroid nodule was presented. While describing the clinical process of this case, the limits of surgery (total thyroidectomy–hemithyroidectomy) were discussed.

The correct implementation of procedures for the operation decision, the evaluation of the results, and the place of concept of work multidisciplinary in the whole process were reviewed according to current guidelines.

S. Günay (✉) · O. Yalçın
University of Health Sciences (SBÜ), Okmeydanı Training and Research Hospital, Division of Breast and Endocrin Surgery, Okmeydanı, Istanbul, Turkey

19.1 Case Presentation

A 29-year-old male patient presented with a lump in his neck in January 2015, which he had realized approximately 3 months ago. In his physical examination, the left lobe of the thyroid gland was swollen with a soft mass approximately 3 cm in diameter and homogenous surfaced structure. There are no unusual findings in his neck area examination and general physical examination. His TSH level was measured as 2.2 mg/dl. Ultrasonographic examination of the thyroid gland revealed that the dimensions of the right lobe were 17 × 10 × 6 mm, left lobe 28 × 14 × 10 mm, and isthmus anteroposterior length 3 mm, and the parenchymal echo seemed normal. A macronodule of dimensions 39 × 29 × 27 mm, which appeared heterogeneously isoechoic in the left lobe with central location and vascular codings and cystic structures, was shown on USG (Fig. 19.1). In ultrasonographic neck examination of submental area, there were only a few lymph nodes which were <1 cm, and they seemed benign. The cytological findings of the fine needle aspiration biopsy (FNAB) were as follows: aspiration material was hypocellular but sufficient in amount, thyrocytes were uniform, and colloidal fluid was minimal. The diagnosis was benign cystic nodule of the thyroid (Bethesda 2). Although the nodule was benign, surgery decision was made due to the patient's risk factors and concerns, and hemithyroidectomy was performed.

T. Özülker et al. (eds.), *Thyroid and Parathyroid Diseases*, https://doi.org/10.1007/978-3-319-78476-2_19

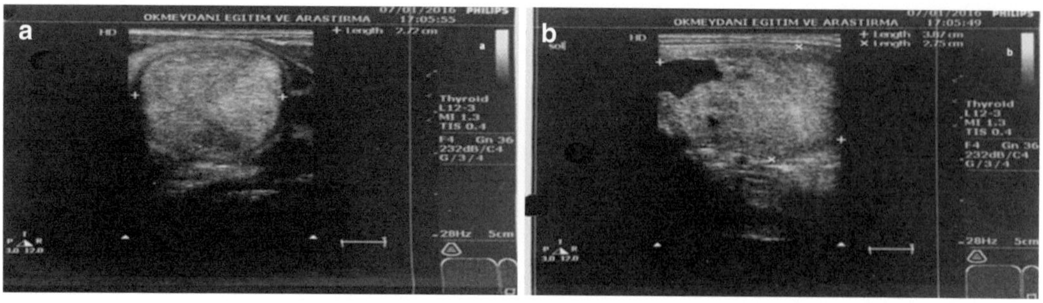

Fig. 19.1 Axial (**a**) and longitudinal (**b**) views of the thyroid nodule on ultrasonography

Pathological findings are as follows: colloid nodule was 4 × 3 cm in size, dimensions of its cross section were 33 × 25 × 21 mm, and it was brownish-creamy in color in some areas and separated from the thyroid tissue with a thick, well-defined fibrotic capsule. In another area, distal to the dominant nodule, another nodule which was 0.1 cm away from the capsule and 6 mm in diameter, with well-defined borders and in yellowish-white color, was found and it was totally sampled. Pathologically result: Papillary microcarsinoma, with encapsulation,without vascular and extrathyroid invasion, HBME-1 (Cell Marque/HBME):1 isthmus and other areas were clean.

19.2 Discussion

19.2.1 Evaluation and Diagnosis

Thyroid nodules are the solid or fluid-filled lumps within the normal thyroid glands. They are usually localized adjacent to the thyroid tissue which gives the patient a sense of a swollen neck and can be recognized easily in slim persons.

It is known that 1 in every 40 young men and 1 in 12–25 young women have thyroid nodules. More than 90% of these are benign, mostly cystic, but sometimes complex in structure and filled mainly with fluid/colloid instead of tissue cells.

The probability of having a nodule in the thyroid gland increases with age. It is well accepted that it is present in almost half of the people aged 50. In our country, iodine depletion is an important etiological factor. Postmortem analyses series conducted in Germany and Central Europe showed that the percentage of nodules with clinical findings is 50% and 5–10% of palpable nodules carry the risk of cancer. Every year in 5 of 100,000 nodules, new thyroid cancer is being detected. These nodules need to be followed up and treated because of the risk of malignancy.

Genetic transmission almost does not exist, but there is a tendency in certain areas and families. Rarely, being single-egg twins and having some other genetic disorders may increase the malignancy risk in people with thyroid nodules. Hormonal change mediators like beta-hCG and IGF-1 may facilitate nodule formation by increasing the TSH levels [1, 2].

In patients with a detected nodule, the decision of following up or suggesting surgical intervention should be based on answers to the following questions: Does the nodule have potential cancer risk? Does it compress on the adjacent organs in the neck? Does it change the functions of the thyroid gland, for example, by excreting too many hormones affecting the metabolism? Is there a cancer case in the family history and has the patient been subject to ionizing radiation in his childhood or adolescence? Are there any lymphadenopathies? Is there a dimensional or structural change of the nodule in time? Also, age (>14 or <70 years) and gender of the patient (more in man than woman) should be taken into consideration while making the decision [1–3].

During the initial visit, a detailed patient history and physical examination are necessary. TSH level measurement and USG evaluation are also vital. Some scoring systems have been developed for the risk evaluation of the patients with a nodule. We prefer to use the definitions of the American Thyroid Association (ATA) guidelines, and precisely indicated FNAB and careful interpretation of the result are very important for the correct approach. According to the latest version of the ATA guidelines published in 2015, low-risk nodules which are smaller than 5 mm can be followed up yearly, and there is no indication of FNAB. For nodules bigger than 5 mm, the following criteria should be considered before performing FNAB: whether the nodules of 5–10 mm in diameter are located subcapsular or paratracheal, the presence of extrathyroidal pathological findings or lymph node enlargement in the neck, and family history of cancer or detection of risk increasing features in the patient history.

If the patient has a moderate or undefined risk, FNAB should be performed in nodes which are 10–20 mm in diameter; if the patient has a high risk, then FNAB should be performed in nodes bigger than 10 mm. If the patient is hyperthyroid and findings are suggesting that the nodule is benign or the patient has lymphocytic thyroiditis, FNAB is not recommended. It should be performed however in nodules >1 cm that are detected incidentally during PET scanning. FNAB results are evaluated according to Bethesda system (the Bethesda System for Reporting Thyroid Cytopathology (TBSRTC)), [3–7] (Table 19.1).

Ultrasonographic (USG) evaluation has a particular value in the identification of the risk. Two major criteria for FNAB decision are the size of the nodule and USG findings [3, 4]. Ultrasonographic evaluation of the thyroid recently described by Horvath (Thyroid Imaging and Reporting Data System (TIRADS)) is also being recommended by the American College of Radiology (ACR). Fine needle aspiration is the most accurate and cost-effective method for the evaluation of thyroid nodules. As false-negative results and underdiagnosis rates will be diminished, it is recommended to be accompanied by USG (ATA Recommendation (R) 9) [1, 6, 7].

Fine needle aspiration indication is consistent with USG findings regarding the structure of the nodule: very low if the nodule is pure cystic and increase a little if the nodule has sponge-like complex cystic/solid structure. It increases significantly if the nodule is solid, and USG shows capsule border irregularity, calcification, lymph node enlargement at the capsule border,

Table 19.1 Risk classification according to US (AACE/ACE/AME)

Category	US findings	Approach
1. Low-risk lesion (<1%) cysts (fluid component >80%)	Mostly cystic nodules with reverberating artifacts and not associated with suspicious US signs Isoechoic spongiform nodules, either confluent or with regular halo "indeterminate"	Follow-up
2. Intermediate-risk thyroid lesion (%1-15	Slightly hypoechoic (vs. thyroid tissue) or isoechoic nodules with ovoid-to-round shape and smooth or ill-defined margins may be present: Intranodular vascularization Elevated stiffness at elastography Macro or continuous rim calcifications Indeterminate hyperechoic spots	Follow-up with FNA
3. High-risk thyroid lesion (50–90%)	Nodules with at least one of the following features: Marked hypoechogenicity (vs. prethyroideal muscles) Spiculated or lobulated margins Microcalcifications Taller-than-wide shape (AP > TR) Extrathyroidal growth Pathologic adenopathy expected risk of malignancy in accordance with the presence of one or more suspicious	Surgery

AACE/ACE/AME American Association of Clinical Endocrinologists/American College of Endocrinology/Associazione Medici Endocrinologi, *AP* anteroposterior or capsizing the capsule border. Each nodule has to be approached individually, changing from low risk to high risk and follow-up to surgical intervention. To decide whether the gray area nodules are candidates for surgery, multidisciplinary but case-specific individual decisions should be based on clinical experience and actual knowledge [3, 7, 8].

If the patient is in the low-risk group, USG every 6 months for 3 years is recommended. According to its results, the patient is reevaluated and follow-up is either continued or discontinued. If FNAB is indicated and it is Bethesda 1 or 2 in the first one, it should be repeated 1 year later; if it is Bethesda 3, it should be repeated at a shorter time interval such as 3 months. If the findings are not explicit, it should be performed even at shorter periods. A case diagnosed with undefined atypical cells subsequently is a candidate for surgery (Table 19.2).

Table 19.2 Comparison of the BRSCT, TI-RADS, and recommended clinical management

Bethesda	TI-RADS	Clinical management
1. Nondiagnostic, cystic fluid only	1. Normal thyroid gland	Repeat FNA with ultrasound guidance
2. Benign	2. Benign lesions	Clinical follow-up
3. AUS/FLUS atypia of undetermined significance or follicular lesion of undetermined significance	3. Probably benign lesions	Repeat FNA
4. Follicular neoplasm or suspicious for follicular neoplasm	4. Suspicious lesions subclassified as 4a, 4b, and later 4c with increasing risk of malignancy (5–10/10–80%)	Surgical lobectomy or thyroidectomy
5. Suspicious for malignancy	5. Probably malignant lesions	Thyroidectomy or surgical lobectomy
6. Malignant	6. Biopsy proven malignancy	Thyroidectomy (+neck dissection)

19.3 Management

A nodule which is radiologically and pathologically benign (TIRADS 2 and Bethesda 2) does not need to be followed up or additional assessment (ATA R11) [1]. For low- to moderate-risk nodules, USG can be repeated every 12 months, for high-risk nodules every 6 months depending on the size of the nodule, USG features, or individual factors even if they are benign (ATA R23–24) [1]. In our case, the patient was risky for the following reasons with the annual USG could be recommended but because of the risk factors in patient's own and family history and individual factors (his grandmother had thyroid carcinoma, he was born in Northern Anatolia in 1986 – Chernobyl nuclear disaster) and pre tracheal placement of the nodule and additionally his mother was a very concerned healthcare worker close follow up or surgical intervention was offered to him. Both choices are discussed in detail regarding the risks and benefits with the subject. The patient chose the surgery option, and total thyroidectomy or hemithyroidectomy was suggested. As the initial diagnosis was not malignant and the necessary conditions for a second surgical intervention were present, surgical lobectomy was planned. The additional blood tests such as thyroid function tests, calcitonin, anti-TPO, and anti-TG which are suggested for subtotal thyroidectomy patients were done (ATA R4, ATA R10c) [1]. All were in the normal range. Left hemithyroidectomy was performed. The initial nodule which was found by the patient himself was diagnosed as a colloid nodule, but incidentally in another area of the same lobe, papillary microcarcinoma (PMC) was detected. Papillary microcarcinoma is an entity with very low metastasis and mortality rates <1%. Similar cases are being seen more often nowadays which brings overdiagnosis and overtreatment concepts into consideration [8, 9]. As even with experienced endocrine surgeons, the morbidity rate is reported to be 1–3%, and it is widely accepted today that total thyroidectomy is not obligatory in this group of patients. It is even being discussed if active follow-up is necessary for them [8–10].

19.4 Follow-Up and Outcome

This case has been discussed at a multidisciplinary endocrine council. Lobectomy was regarded as sufficient and the patient to be followed up [1, 5, 8]. One month after the surgery and from then on every 6 months, the patient has been followed up by TSH level measurements and USG. After 2 years, the follow-up continues with two times TSH level control and 1 USG yearly without problems. The first TSH value was 2.5. Replacement therapy with 75 μgm/day levothyroxine has been initiated. The target TSH value was 0.5–1, and the last measured value was 0.91 for TSH [8–10].

19.4.1 Future

Although there are numerous studies assessing the predictive value of molecular markers and cytogenetic tests, the outcomes and level of the evidence are not satisfactory; they are not included in the current guidelines [10, 11].

For targeted diagnosis and therapy, more studies should be conducted in this area.

What Can We Learn from This Case?

- Thyroid nodules are usually benign and common, and surgery is not suitable or necessary for most of them. When surgical intervention is planned for a diagnosed nodule, surgical morbidity, side effects of hormone replacement therapy, recurrence, redone surgical interventions, their adverse effects on quality of life, and high costs should also be considered carefully. It is also known that in the past many patients had undergone unnecessary surgical interventions.
- The right approach for each patient with a thyroid nodule can be chosen after risk assessment according to the actual guidelines.
- FNAB is the most accurate and cost-effective method in nodule evaluation.
- The size of the nodule and the USG features are the two major factors in FNA decision. It should be accompanied by USG as it reduces the false-negative and underdiagnosis rates (ATA R9).
- The clinical experience of the radiologist and the pathologist (cytologist) is very important.
- The decision regarding the approach toward the nodule differs from the low risk to high risk as follow-up or surgical intervention.
- For the differential diagnosis and surgical intervention decision of the nodules which are in the gray area, patients should be evaluated individually with actual knowledge in a multidisciplinary way.

References

1. Haugen BR, Alexander EK, Bible KC, Doherty GM, Mandel SJ, Nikiforov YE, et al. 2015 American Thyroid Association management guidelines for adult patients with thyroid nodules and differentiated thyroid cancer: the American Thyroid Association guidelines task force on thyroid nodules and differentiated thyroid Cancer. Thyroid. 2016;26:1–133. https://doi.org/10.1089/thy.2015.0020.
2. Horvath E, Majlis S, Rossi R, Franco C, Niedmann JP, Castro A, et al. An ultrasonogram reporting system for thyroid nodules stratifying cancer risk for clinical management. J Clin Endocrinol Metab. 2009;94:1748–51. https://doi.org/10.1210/jc.2008-1724.
3. Gharib H, Papini E, Paschke R, Duick DS, Harrell RM, Hegedüs L, et al. American Association of Clinical Endocrinologists, American College of Endocrinology, and Associazione Medici Endocrinologi medical guidelines for clinical practice for the diagnosis and management of thyroid nodules – 2016 update. Endocr Pract. 2016;22:622–39. https://doi.org/10.4158/EP161208.GL.
4. Kwak JY, Han KH, Yoon JH, Moon HJ, Son EJ, Park SH, et al. Thyroid imaging reporting and data system for US features of nodules: a step in establishing better stratification of cancer risk. Radiology. 2011;260:892–9. https://doi.org/10.1148/radiol.11110206.
5. Xie C, Cox P, Taylor N, LaPorte S. Ultrasonography of thyroid nodules: a pictorial review. Insights

imaging. 2016;7(1):77–86. https://doi.org/10.1007/s13244-015-0446-5.

6. Varshney R, Forest VI, Mascarella MA, et al. The Mcgill thyroid nodule score - does it help with indeterminate thyroid nodules. J Otolaryngol Head Neck Surg. 2015;44:2. https://doi.org/10.1186/s40463-015-0058-6.
7. Renuka V, Saila Bala G, Aparna C, Kumari R, Sumalatha K. The Bethesda system for reporting thyroid cytopathology: interpretation and guidelines in surgical treatment. Indian J Otolaryngol Head Neck Surg. 2012;64:305–11. https://doi.org/10.1007/s12070-011-0289-4.
8. Cibas ES, Ali SZ. The Bethesda system for reporting thyroid cytopathology. Am J Clin Pathol. 2009;132:658–65. https://doi.org/10.1309/AJCPPHLWMI3JV4LA.
9. Leboulleux S, Tuttle RM, Pacini F, Schlumberger M. Papillary thyroid microcarcinoma: time to shift from surgery to active surveillance? Lancet Diabetes Endocrinol. 2016;4:933–42. https://doi.org/10.1016/S2213-8587(16)30180-2. Epub 2016 Aug 20.
10. Nickel B, Brito JP, Barratt A, Jordan S, Moynihan R, McCaffery K. Clinicians views on management and terminology for papillary thyroid microcarcinoma: a qualitative study. Thyroid. 2017;27(5):661–71. https://doi.org/10.1089/thy.2016.0483.
11. Vuong HG, Duong UN, Altibi AM, Ngo HT, Pham TQ, Tran HM, et al. A meta-analysis of prognostic roles of molecular markers in papillary thyroid carcinoma. Endocr Connect. 2017;6:R8–R17. https://doi.org/10.1530/EC-17-0010. Epub 2017 Feb 20. Review.

20 Follow-Up of Nodular-Multinodular Goiter: When Should the Operation Be Performed?

Ali İlker Filiz and Taner Kıvılcım

Abstract

Thyroid nodules are a commonly encountered clinical condition. The follow-up criteria for thyroid nodules principally rest with patient's history, thyroid hormone levels, imaging features, and biopsy results. In this case, a nodular thyroid disease, which was reported as follicular neoplasia, was discussed. Additionally, the management strategy in case the results of fine needle aspiration biopsies are different among several cytology reports as in our case was also discussed. The interesting part of this case was that an incidental malignant nodule was found in the opposite lobe of the thyroid after the operation.

20.1 Case Presentation

A 43-year-old woman presented with a thyroid nodule in the right lobe, which had been found 2 years ago incidentally with a neck ultrasound (USG) examination. She had not experienced any specific symptoms, such as neck pain, dysphagia, hoarseness, or compressive symptoms. There was not any past family or medical history, and she had no history of irradiation to the head or neck. There was no any palpable mass on the neck and the cervical region on physical examination. On laboratory analysis, the serum thyroid-stimulating hormone (TSH) level was within normal range (1.7 mg/dl). Thyroid USG disclosed a well-defined, lobular contoured iso-hypoechoic solid nodule seen with peripheral thin hypoechoic halo sized as 15 × 12 × 27 mm in the right lobe having macrocalcifications. On color Doppler USG, peripheral and central vascularizations were seen. Additionally an irregularly contoured nodule was seen in the left lobe, which sized as 4 × 4.4 mm and showing hypoechoic solid echotexture with microcalcifications. Peripheral blood flow was seen in color Doppler USG (Figs. 20.1 and 20.2). USG also showed a few benign characterized lymph nodes which were smaller than 1 cm. When compared with previous USG report, which had been made 1 year ago, the nodule in the right lobe became larger, but nodule in the left lobe was a new finding. A fine needle aspiration biopsy (FNAB) had been performed from the nodule in the right lobe 2 years ago, and cytological findings were benign. Due to the fact that the nodule in the right lobe became larger and the nodule in the left lobe had the high suspicious characteristics of malignancy, an FNAB was repeated for both nodules. The cytological findings were follicular neoplasia for the nodule in the right

A. İ. Filiz · T. Kıvılcım (✉)
Department of General Surgery, İstanbul Okan University, Faculty of Medicine, Istanbul, Turkey

T. Özülker et al. (eds.), *Thyroid and Parathyroid Diseases*, https://doi.org/10.1007/978-3-319-78476-2_20

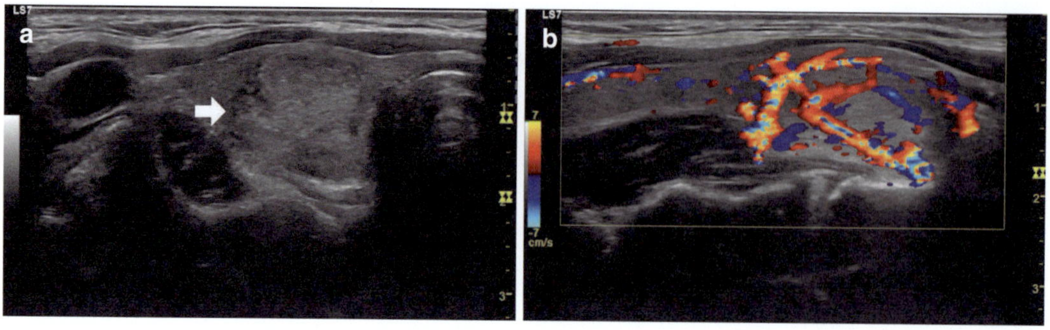

Fig. 20.1 A well-defined, lobular contoured iso-hypoechoic solid thyroid nodule with peripheral thin hypoechoic halo sized as 15 × 12 × 27 mm in the middle posterior part of the right lobe (*arrow*). There are also macrocalcifications within the nodule (**a**). Color Doppler USG shows peripheral and central vascularization (**b**)

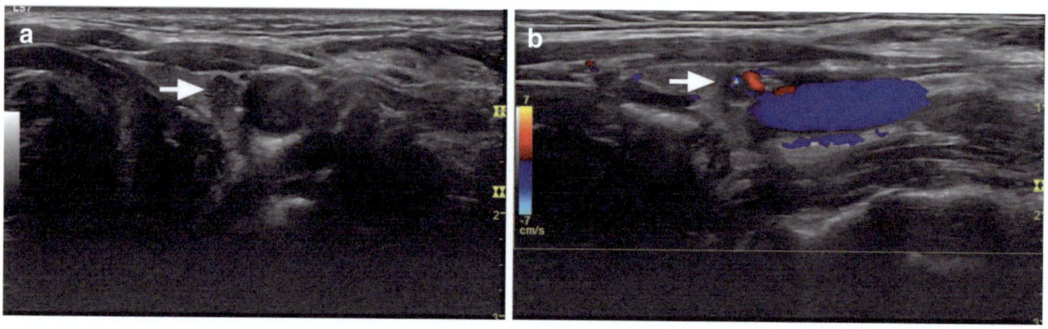

Fig. 20.2 Thyroid nodule in the lower posterior part of the left lobe (*arrows*). Nodule sized as 4 × 4.4 mm shows hypoechoic solid echotexture with microcalcifications and has irregular contours (**a**), peripheral blood flow was seen on color Doppler USG (**b**)

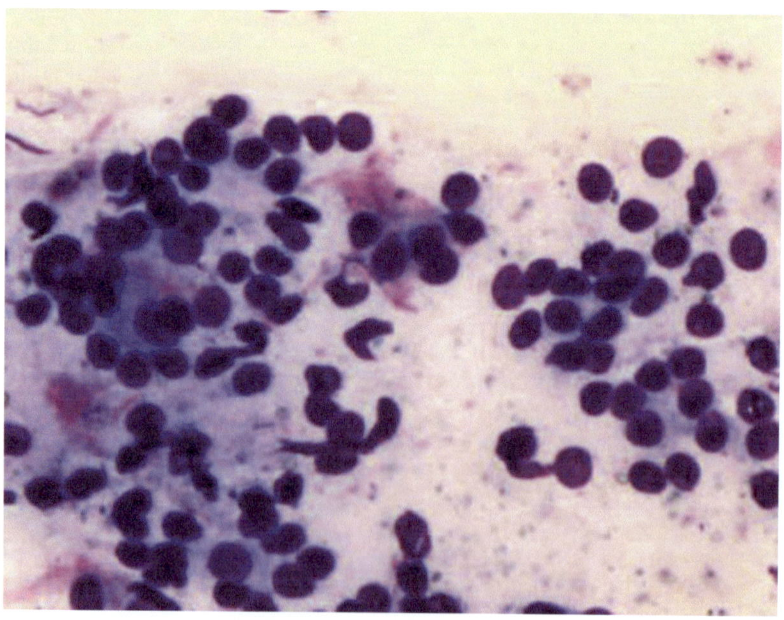

Fig. 20.3 Hypercellular smear with follicular structures compatible with follicular neoplasia (May-Grunwald-Giemsa, 40×)

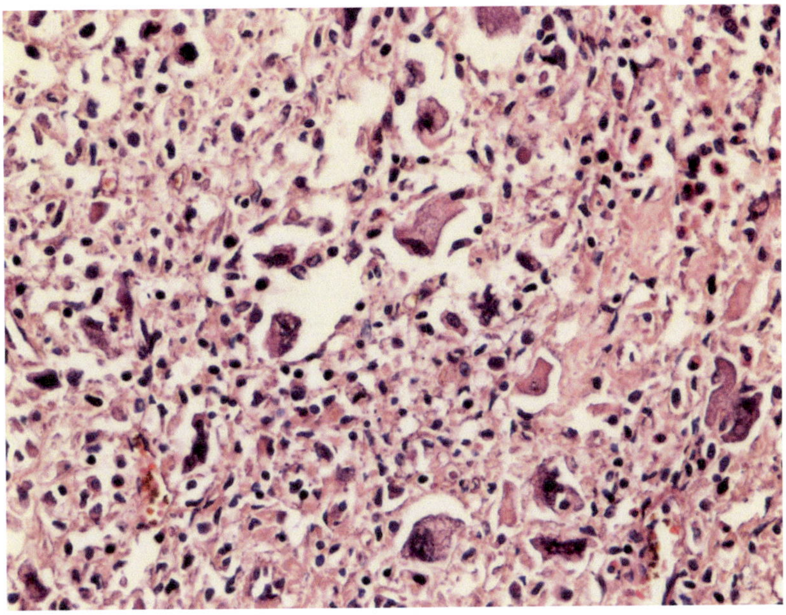

Fig. 20.4 Nodular lesion is showing pleomorphism and multinucleated cells. Compatible with follicular adenoma because there is no capsule or vessel invasion (hematoxylin-eosin, 20×)

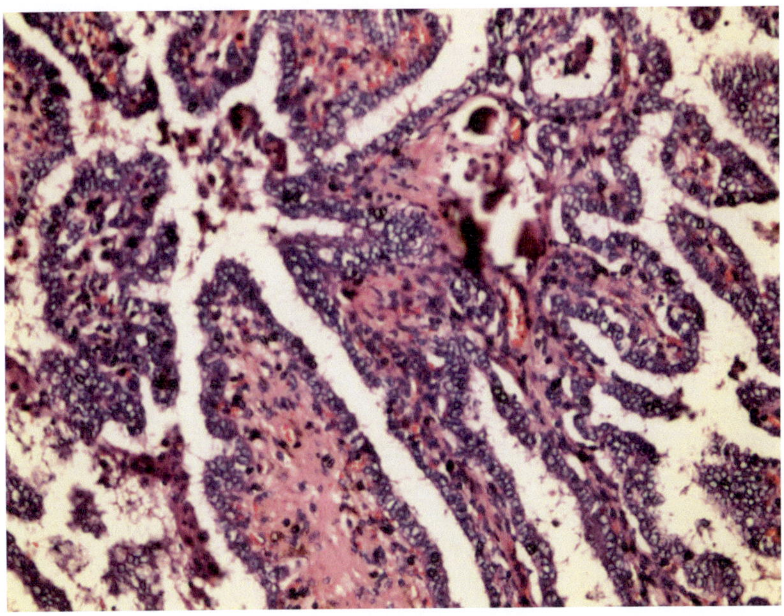

Fig. 20.5 Papillary folding and multinuclear cells, compatible with papillary carcinoma (hematoxylin-eosin, 20×)

lobe (Fig. 20.3) and hypocellular/nondiagnostic for the nodule in the left lobe. According to these results, bilateral total thyroidectomy was performed. The pathological diagnosis was follicular adenoma for right lobe nodule and micropapillary carcinoma for the left lobe nodule (Figs. 20.4 and 20.5).

20.2 Discussion

20.2.1 Evaluation and Diagnosis

Thyroid nodules are a commonly encountered clinical condition. By use of high-resolution USG imaging, the incidence increased to

76% [1]. Over half million people are affected by thyroid cancer in the United States, and thyroid cancer incidence is also increasing worldwide like thyroid nodules [2]. Nevertheless, mortality of thyroid cancer is not increasing [3].

The follow-up criteria for thyroid nodules principally rest with patient's history, thyroid hormone levels, imaging features, and biopsy results.

Radiation history (e.g., childhood head and neck irradiation, total body irradiation for bone marrow transplantation) and family history of thyroid cancer or syndromes associated with thyroid cancer in the first-degree relatives (e.g., PTEN (phosphatase and tensin homolog), hamartoma tumor syndrome (Cowden's disease), familial adenomatous polyposis, Carney complex, multiple endocrine neoplasia [MEN] 2, Werner syndrome/progeria) are situations that require close follow-up [4, 5]. For the initial evaluation of a patient with a thyroid nodule, TSH levels should be measured. For decreased TSH levels, a radionuclide thyroid scan should be performed, and for normal/elevated TSH levels, USG should be performed [5].

The characteristics of the thyroid nodules in USG evaluation are particularly important for the follow-up. The recommendations for USG imaging *in 2015 American Thyroid Association Guideline for Thyroid Nodules* (ATA 2015) are listed in Table 20.1 [5]. In 2009, Horvath et al. reported *Thyroid Imaging Reporting and Data System* (TIRADS) for USG features of thyroid nodules, and Kwak et al. further described it (Table 20.2) [6, 7]. There are different recommendations in various guidelines to consider biopsy according to the diameter of the nodule. As seen at Table 20.1, FNAB is not recommended for nodules below 1 cm even though it comprises highly suspicious features [5]. Additionally, there are many recent publications supporting this approach [7, 8]. On the other hand, in some studies, FNAB is preferred for suspected nodules even if smaller than 1 cm [9, 10].

When FNAB is performed for a nodule, cytology should be reported according to the "Bethesda System for Reporting Thyroid Cytopathology" [5, 11]. In Bethesda System, there are six diagnostic categories (Table 20.3) [11] which declare

Table 20.1 FNAB guidance for thyroid nodules according to USG patterns

Pattern	USG features	Consider FNAB
High suspicion (estimated malignancy risk >70–90%)	• Irregular margins • Microcalcifications • Taller than wide shape • Rim calcifications with small extrusive soft tissue component • Evidence of extrathyroidal extension	>1 cm nodule
Intermediate suspicion (estimated malignancy risk 10–20%)	• Hypoechoic solid nodule with smooth margins	>1 cm nodule
Low suspicion (estimated malignancy risk 5–10%)	• Isoechoic or hyperechoic solid nodule or partially cystic nodule with eccentric solid areas	>1.5 cm nodule
Very low suspicion (estimated malignancy risk <3%)	• Spongiform or partially cystic nodules	>2 cm nodule or observe
Benign (estimated malignancy risk <1%)	• Purely cystic nodules	No biopsy (aspiration may be considered symptomatic cysts)

Table 20.2 TIRADS classification and estimated malignancy risk

TIRADS category		Definition	Estimated malignancy risk (%)
1		Normal	0
2		Benign	0
3		Probably benign	2–2.8
4	a	Low suspicion for malignancy	3.6–12.7
	b	Intermediate suspicion for malignancy	6.8–37.8
	c	Moderate concern but not classic for malignancy	21–91.9
5		Consistent with malignancy	88.7–97.9
6		Malignant	100

Table 20.3 Diagnostic categories according to "Bethesda System for Reporting Thyroid Cytopathology" and risk of malignancy

Diagnostic category	Risk of malignancy (%)
Nondiagnostic or unsatisfactory	1–4
Benign	0–3
Atypia of undetermined significance or follicular lesion of undetermined significance (AUS/FLUS)	5–15
Follicular neoplasm or suspicious for a follicular neoplasm (FN)	15–30
Suspicious for malignancy (SUSP)	60–75
Malignant	97–99

a specific risk of malignancy and recommend the management according to the cytology result.

For nondiagnostic cytology results, ATA 2015 guideline has notified three recommendations. Firstly, FNAB should be performed once more with USG guidance, and, if available, an on-site cytologic evaluation would be better. Secondly, if the nodule demonstrates nondiagnostic cytological result repeatedly, close observation is an option or surgery might be performed for highly suspicious nodules. Thirdly, surgery should be considered for highly suspicious nodules or growing nodules (>20% in two dimensions) or nodules showing malignant clinical features [5]. It is shown that waiting 3 months for the second biopsy is not necessary [12]. On the other hand, Yoon et al. recommend a 6-month interval to repeat FNAB after an initially nondiagnostic thyroid nodule to decrease false positivity [13]. In a survey study with 694 participants for nondiagnostic biopsy results, repeated biopsy was performed to the 13% of the participants at <1 month, 46% in 1–3 months, and 22% at more than 3 months [14].

After the surgical intervention for a nodule with benign cytology, it is shown that the rate of malignancy is 3.2% [15]. Therefore, in ATA 2015 guideline, control USG and USG-guided FNAB are recommended in 12 months for highly suspicious USG pattern nodules and in 12–24 months for low/intermediate suspicious nodules. After two benign FNAB results, the malignancy risk reduces to zero [16]. Thus, follow-up does not seem necessary after two benign FNAB results [5].

When follicular neoplasm or suspicious for follicular neoplasm (FN/SUSP) is encountered as a result of cytology, surgery should be decided. Another way to follow these nodules is using molecular tests, but it is still not the routine approach [5].

20.2.2 Management

The discussed patient had a nodule with low suspicion on follow-up for 2 years. It was seen that the nodule enlarged over 50% in this process. Therefore, a second biopsy was done for this nodule. Additionally, a 4 mm new nodule was found in the contralateral lobe, which was highly suspicious by USG.

The latest guidelines do not recommend an FNAB for <1 cm nodule, even though it has high-risk features [5, 8]. However, because of the two suspicious nodules in different lobes, we preferred to perform FNAB for the nodule, which was 0.4 cm. Cytology result showed us that the bigger nodule in the right lobe was FN, and the smaller one in the left lobe was nondiagnostic. The patient was discussed in the multidisciplinary meeting (MDM), and the risk of malignancy of both nodules was evaluated. The recommendation was total thyroidectomy. After the MDM the patient was informed about the situation, and the surgery was performed with the consensus.

The purpose of MDM is to help the clinician to resolve difficult cases and give advice about the diagnosis, treatment, and care of the disease. All members of this multidisciplinary team are well specialized in their field and settle their judgments according to the current guidelines to make high-quality decision-making and to improve the outcomes of the various diseases. In our center, all patients with thyroid disease are discussed in MDM, and the recommendations are given after evaluation of patient's general health status, disease condition, and guideline advice. Guidelines play an important role in the decision-making process, like a pathfinder.

When cytological examination revealed FN or SUSP of a thyroid nodule, the latest ATA guideline strongly recommends lobectomy. Furthermore, it may be modified according to patient preference or molecular tests [5].

20.2.3 Future

By the standardization of the USG and FNAB reports, it is more clear to plan surgery or follow-up nowadays. Nevertheless, the indeterminate (atypia of undetermined significance/follicular lesion of undetermined significance (AUS/FLUS), FN, SUSP) biopsy results are still a problem leading to unnecessary thyroidectomies. This kind of surgery causes complications (hoarseness, hypocalcemia, etc.) and lifelong medicine dependence. To decrease unnecessary surgeries, molecular tests could play an important role in the future.

What Can We Learn from This Case?

- The follow-up criteria for thyroid nodules principally rest with patient's history, thyroid hormone levels, imaging features and biopsy results.
- After a benign biopsy result, controls should be continued especially for high suspicious nodules. The control biopsy should be done after 12 months.
- When FN/SUSP is encountered as a result of cytology, surgery should be decided. The routine procedure should be lobectomy, but this approach may be modified. For multinodular thyroid disease, to avoid a second surgery, total or near-total thyroidectomy may be decided.
- To decide an initial therapy, multidisciplinary meetings are important. After deciding the therapy, the patient must be informed about the consensus. The final plan should decide after the patients' confirmation.

References

1. Yoon JH, Han K, Kim EK, Moon HJ, Kwak JY. Diagnosis and management of small thyroid nodules: a comparative study with six guidelines for thyroid nodules. Radiology. 2017;283:560–9.
2. Lubitz C, Ali A, Zhan T, Heberle C, White C, Ito Y. The thyroid cancer policy model: a mathematical simulation model of papillary thyroid carcinoma in the U.S. population. PLoS One. 2017;12:e0177068. https://doi.org/10.1371/journal.pone.0177068.
3. SEER. 2015. http://seer.cancer.gov/statfacts/html/thyro.html. Accessed 1 June 2017.
4. RosEs DS. Diagnostic approach to and treatment of thyroid nodules. 2016. https://www.uptodate.com/contents/diagnostic-approach-to-and-treatment-of-thyroid-nodules?source=search_result&search=thyroid%20nodule%20follow%20up&selectedTitle=1~146. Accessed 1 June 2017.
5. Haugen BR, Alexander EK, Bible KC, Doherty GM, Mandel SJ, Nikiforov YE, et al. 2015 American Thyroid Association management guidelines for adult patients with thyroid nodules and differentiated thyroid cancer: the American Thyroid Association guidelines task force on thyroid nodules and differentiated thyroid cancer. Thyroid. 2016;6:1–133. https://doi.org/10.1089/thy.2015.0020.
6. Horvath E, Majlis S, Rossi R, Franco C, Niedmann JP, Castro A, et al. An ultrasonogram reporting system for thyroid nodules stratifying cancer risk for clinical management. J Clin Endocrinol Metab. 2009;90:1748–51.
7. Kwak JY, Han KH, Yoon JH, Moon HJ, Son EJ, Park SH, et al. Thyroid imaging reporting and data system for US features of nodules: a step in establishing better stratification of cancer risk. Radiology. 2011;260:892–9.
8. Haddad RI, Lydiatt WM, Bischoff L, et al. National Comprehensive Cancer Network. NCCN Clinical Practice Guidelines in Oncology (NCCN Guidelines) Thyroid Carcinoma version 1. 2016. www.nccn.org. Accessed 1 June 2017.
9. Yi KH. The revised 2016 Korean thyroid association guidelines for thyroid nodules and cancers: differences from the 2015 American Thyroid Association guidelines. Endocrinol Metab. 2016;31:373–8.
10. Russ G, Royer B, Bigorgne C, Rouxel A, Bienvenu-Perrard M, Leenhardt L. Prospective evaluation of thyroid imaging reporting and data system on 4550 nodules with and without elastography. Eur J Endocrinol. 2013;168:649–55.
11. Cibas ES, Ali SZ. The Bethesda system for reporting thyroid cytopathology. Am J Clin Pathol. 2009;132:658–65.
12. Singh RS, Wang HH. Timing of repeat thyroid fine-needle aspiration in the management of thyroid nodules. Acta Cytol. 2011;55:544–8.
13. Yoon JH, Kim EK, Kwak JY, Moon HJ. Non-diagnostic thyroid nodules after application of

the Bethesda system: a study evaluating the interval for repeat aspiration for non-diagnostic results. Acta Radiol. 2017;0:1–8. https://doi.org/10.1177/0284185117715286.

14. Brito JP, Castro MR, Dean DS, Fatourechi V, Stan M. Survey of current approaches to non-diagnostic fine-needle aspiration from solid thyroid nodules. Endocrine. 2015;49:745–51.
15. Tee YY, Lowe AJ, Brand CA, Judson RT. Fine-needle aspiration may miss a third of all malignancy in palpable thyroid nodules: a comprehensive literature review. Ann Surg. 2007;246:714–20.
16. Kwak JY, Koo H, Youk JH, Kim MJ, Moon HJ, Son EJ, et al. Value of US correlation of a thyroid nodule with initially benign cytologic results. Radiology. 2010;254:292–300.

21 Recurrent Nodular Goiter

Beyza Özçınar and Sibel Özkan Gürdal

Abstract

A 55-year-old man had undergone bilateral subtotal thyroidectomy due to multinodular goiter 30 years ago, and histopathological examination had revealed benign nodular goiter. The patient had been suffering from swelling in the neck and dyspnea for the last 15 years, and the symptoms got worsened by the time. The thyroid ultrasonography revealed a diffusely enlarged thyroid gland, with the right lobe being 11 × 8 × 4 cm, left lobe being 5.5 × 4.5 × 3 cm, and extension to the retrosternal region. He was referred for surgery. The operation was initiated with an enlarged Kocher's incision on the neck. The retrosternal portion of thyroid could not be removed through the neck incision, and thus, partial sternotomy was performed. The definitive treatment of recurrent goiter is primarily surgery. However, adhesions and scar tissue due to previous neck surgery increase the risk of complications during recurrent surgery. The rate of complications increases with the rising number of reoperations. It is essential to find the recurrent laryngeal nerve at the earlier stages of surgery and to give considerable attention to protect it during surgery. Intraoperative nerve monitorization should be used for preservation of recurrent laryngeal nerve. Careful dissection and attentive identification and preservation of parathyroid glands, as well as recurrent laryngeal nerves, should be performed during surgery.

B. Özçınar
Division of Breast and Endocrin Surgery, Istanbul University, Istanbul, Turkey

S. Özkan Gürdal (✉)
Division of Breast and Endocrin Surgery, Tekirdağ Namık Kemal Üniversity, Tekirdağ, Turkey

21.1 Case Presentation

A 55-year-old man had undergone bilateral subtotal thyroidectomy due to multinodular goiter 30 years ago, and histopathological examination had revealed benign nodular goiter. He did not require L-thyroxine replacement therapy after surgery. The patient had been suffering from swelling in the neck and dyspnea for the last 15 years, and the symptoms got worsened by the time (Fig. 21.1). The thyroid ultrasonography (USG) revealed a diffusely enlarged thyroid gland, with the right lobe being 11 × 8 × 4 cm and the left lobe being 5.5 × 4.5 × 3 cm, and extension to the retrosternal region. Cervical and thoracic computed tomography (CT) scan performed afterward revealed the left lobe of the thyroid gland to extend to the ascending aorta level toward mediastinum in the retrosternal region (Fig. 21.2). The tracheal deviation was also detected (Fig. 21.3). Mediastinal thyroid tissue

T. Özülker et al. (eds.), *Thyroid and Parathyroid Diseases*, https://doi.org/10.1007/978-3-319-78476-2_21

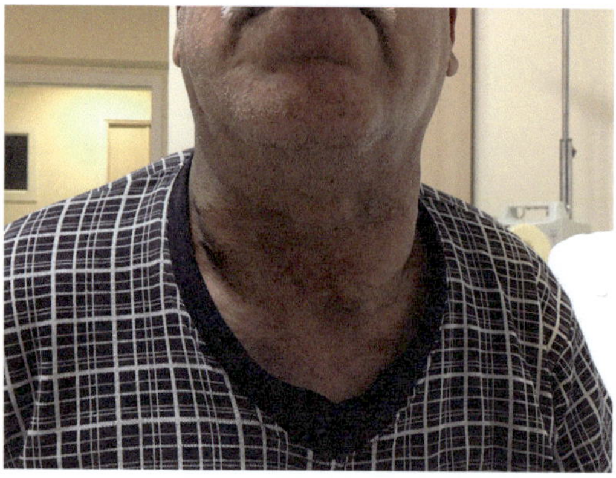

Fig. 21.1 The neck of the patient

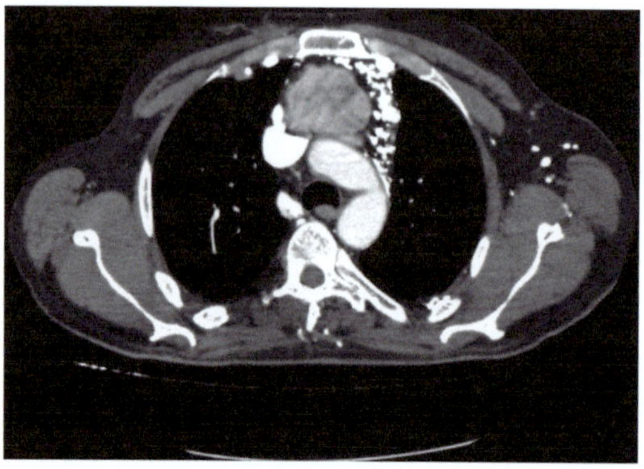

Fig. 21.2 Thoracic CT scan showing thyroid descending to the ascending aorta

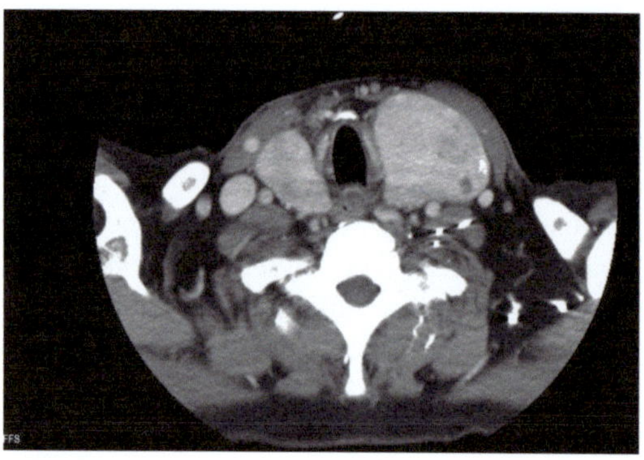

Fig. 21.3 Cervical CT scan showing tracheal deviation to the right

appeared excessively vascular in the CT scan (Fig. 21.4). Therefore, thoracic surgery consultation was requested, and the patient was prepared for partial sternotomy.

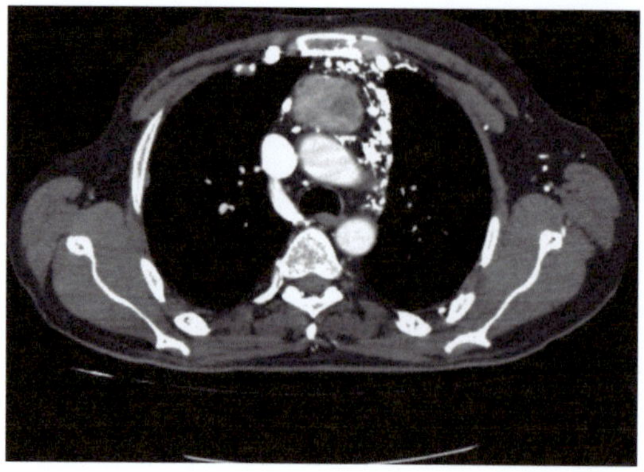

Fig. 21.4 Thoracic CT scan showing high vascularity of retrosternal goiter

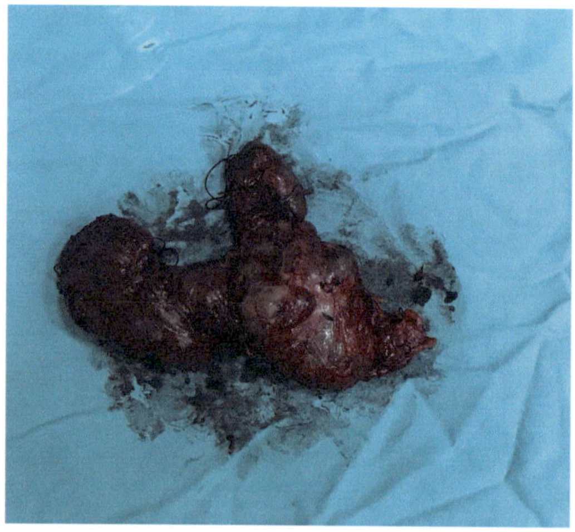

Fig. 21.5 Excised thyroid tissue

The surgery was initiated with an enlarged Kocher's incision on the neck. Both thyroid lobes were extremely large, and a retrosternal portion of the thyroid gland did not come out through neck incision, and partial sternotomy was performed. Mediastinal thyroid tissue was excised in cooperation with thoracic surgery team with precise attention to preserve the recurrent laryngeal nerve (RLN) (Fig. 21.5). Then, the surgery was completed with total thyroidectomy (Fig. 21.6). There was no complication occurred during surgery and no need to open pleura in the mediastinum. The surgery was completed after the insertion of aspiration drainage to thyroidectomy area and to the mediastinum. The patient was taken to the intensive care unit after the surgery

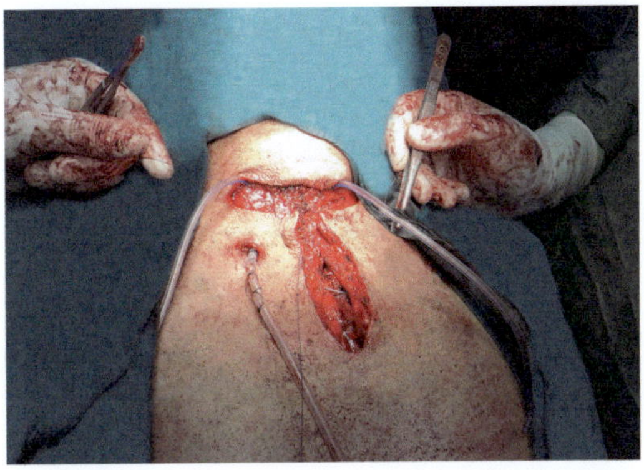

Fig. 21.6 The appearance of the patient before closure of incisions

and was carefully extubated; later he was taken to general surgery service on the first day after surgery. No findings of hoarseness and hypoparathyroidism were detected.

The patient was discharged from hospital on the third day after removal of the drainage. Histopathologic evaluation revealed encapsulated follicular variant thyroid cancer in a dimension of 0.7 cm on the basis of multinodular hyperplasia. No tumoral necrosis and lymphatic or vascular invasion were detected. Surgical borders were observed as negative, and extrathyroidal invasion was not detected. There was no requirement for radioactive iodine treatment, and the patient was taken into routine postoperative follow-up.

21.2 Discussion

21.2.1 Evaluation and Diagnosis

Goiter has been detected in 5–7% of all population worldwide, and researchers anticipated that thyroid nodules would be detected in about 60% of the general population if ultrasonographic screening was performed [1, 2]. Surgical treatment is required in 10–15% of goiter patients. Total thyroidectomy, near-total thyroidectomy, subtotal thyroidectomy, or lobectomy may be the surgery of choice, depending on the case. Recurrence rates reached up to 12% after all thyroid surgeries in the literature [3, 4]. This rate varies between 2.5% and 42% in surgeries where some thyroid tissue is remained, which excludes total thyroidectomy. On the other hand, in the case of total thyroidectomy, the recurrence rate is below 1% [5–8]. The frequency of recurrent cases has declined in the last two decades due to the performance of greater number of total thyroidectomies. Thirty years ago, total thyroidectomy was not performed routinely for multinodular goiter. In this case, the patient also underwent a bilateral subtotal thyroidectomy. As a consequence of rest thyroid tissue, he began to suffer from neck swelling accompanied with dyspnea after 15 years. The most important factor affecting the recurrences after thyroid surgery is the type of initial surgery. Currently, we all performed total thyroidectomy for either benign or malignant thyroid disease in our routine clinical practice [9].

Before deciding on recurrent surgery, the patient's previous reports (surgery reports and ultrasound findings after surgery) should be well-evaluated. The type of first surgery, the remaining amount of thyroid tissue, and any complication during surgery should be investigated. This will allow for clarification of goiter being either a residue or a recurrence. However, surgical indications of both residual and recurrent nodular goiter are the same, and they are similar to the surgical indications of the primary nodular goiter (Appendix).

The rate of cancer incidence is higher in recurrent surgery even when the first surgery is performed due to benign causes. Menegaux et al. [10] reported the cancer rate to be 11.4% in recurrent surgery in their study, while Levin et al. [11] found this rate as 22%. In this recurrent benign nodular goiter case, also we had an encapsulated follicular variant thyroid cancer with the dimension of 0.7 cm in the basis of multinodular hyperplasia. This case should remind us that we should all perform total thyroidectomy even if the case is benign nodular goiter. It is known that performing total thyroidectomy in the first operation decreases the risk of recurrent goiter below to 1% [5–8, 12–14].

The definitive treatment of recurrent goiter is primarily surgery. However, adhesions and scar tissue due to previous neck surgery increase the risk of complications during recurrent surgery.

The rate of complications increases with the rising number of reoperations [15]. In recurrent surgery, the rate of temporary recurrent laryngeal nerve paralysis is 0–22%, the rate of permanent nerve paralysis is 0–13%, the rate of development of temporary hypoparathyroidism is 9–35%, and the rate of permanent hypoparathyroidism is 0–22% [7, 11–14]. Thus, considering the increased risk of complications, the indication of recurrent surgery should be well identified. In this case, the patient had severe dyspnea with tracheal deviation due to huge thyroid and needed surgery to get rid of the obstructive symptoms. In recurrent surgeries, we should give great attention to preserve both parathyroid glands and RLN. The American Thyroid Association (ATA) guideline (2015) strongly suggests that the parathyroid glands and RLN should be completely protected during surgery and also suggests that the external branch of superior laryngeal nerve (EBSLN) should be protected during upper lobe dissection [9]. We gave great attention to protect both RLN and EBSLN during surgery and used intraoperative nerve monitorization (IONM) device. We found the RLN at the beginning of the surgery and preserve during surgery. The ATA (2015) also suggests the use of IONM at a weak recommendation level [9]. Dralle et al. [16] reported an inversely proportional correlation between the effort spent for looking for recurrence nerve and the rate of recurrent nerve injuries in their study. In addition, Sosa et al. [17] demonstrated that as the rate of performing total thyroidectomy increased, complication rates decreased. As we know that the risk of complications during recurrent thyroid surgery is higher [7, 11–14], we suggest that these types of cases should be done in experienced centers to reduce the risk of complications.

21.2.2 Management

Gain and loss balance should be considered thoroughly while deciding for recurrent thyroid surgery, and precautions should be taken against possible complications. Researchers reported that undiagnosed vocal cord paralysis might be detected in 20% of cases after the first surgery [4]. Therefore, bilateral vocal cords should certainly be examined using laryngoscopy before recurrent thyroid surgery. In addition, the presence of both hypothyroidism and hyperthyroidism should be well evaluated, and surgery should be planned when the patient becomes euthyroid after the appropriate treatment. Preoperative measurement of blood calcium and PTH levels is crucial in the detection of coexisting hypoparathyroidism. Preoperative venous thromboembolism prophylaxis and antibiotic prophylaxis should certainly be administered.

Researchers suggest that recurrent surgery may be performed with lateral approach due to adhesions of the first surgery and the increased risk of complications [4, 14]. In addition, identification of recurrent laryngeal nerves in the early stages of surgery and their preservation during surgery have excessive significance [16]. The use of intraoperative nerve monitorization has been recommended during surgery. Barczyński et al. [18] demonstrated in their wide-scaled retrospective series that the use of IONM in recurrent thyroid surgery decreases the rate of recurrent laryngeal nerve injury. The use of IONM is beneficial in better identification of recurrent nerve anatomy and in predicting the rate of postoperative nerve damage. Careful dissection and attentive identification and preservation of parathyroid glands, as well as RLNs, should be performed during surgery.

Complementary total thyroidectomy is recommended in recurrent goiter surgery. In the case of unilateral RLN injury, total thyroidectomy should be performed to the injured side, and a small amount of tissue from the other (healthy) side should be left to prevent the bilateral RLN injury [19]. When malignancy is detected in histopathological examination of the removed thyroid specimen, ablation of the remaining tissue will be possible using radioactive iodine in the postoperative periods [20].

21.3 Follow-Up and Outcome

There was no complication after surgery, and no findings of hoarseness or hypoparathyroidism were detected. The patient was discharged from the hospital in the postoperative third day after the removal of the drainage. Histopathologic evaluation revealed encapsulated follicular variant thyroid cancer in a dimension of 0.7 cm on the basis of multinodular hyperplasia. No tumoral necrosis and lymphatic or vascular invasion were detected. Surgical borders were observed as negative, and extrathyroidal invasion was not detected. There was no requirement for radioactive iodine treatment, and the patient was taken into routine postoperative follow-up.

What Can We Learn from This Case?

- Total thyroidectomy should be preferred in benign nodular goiter to decrease the recurrence risk.
- Permanent and temporary RLN injury and hypoparathyroidism risk are higher than the first surgery in recurrent nodular goiter.
- Indications for surgery in recurrent nodular goiter are similar to the indications of primary nodular goiter.
- Bilateral vocal cord examination should definitely be performed before recurrent surgery.
- Surgery may be initiated with lateral approach to recurrent thyroid surgery.
- Use of IONM is recommended in recurrent thyroid surgery.
- The recommended surgery in recurrent nodular goiter is complementary total thyroidectomy.

Appendix

Surgical indications in recurrent nodular goiter are as follows:

1. Suspicion or presence of malignancy in a nodule or nodules: Fine needle aspiration biopsy (FNAB) is recommended for nodule or nodules in the presence of hypoechogenicity, microcalcifications, interrupted edge calcification, irregular borders, partial or total disappearing of halo sign, increased intranodular blood supply, greater anterior-to-posterior dimension of nodule than the transverse diameter, invasion to anterior neck muscles, or the presence of pathologic cervical lymphadenopathy in thyroid ultrasonography (USG). In addition, FNAB should be performed in the presence of growth in nodule dimension between the two ultrasonographic monitoring (at least 2 mm growth at least in two dimensions or more than 50% increase in volume). Surgery should be performed in patients where FNAB biopsy revealed follicular/Hurthle cell neoplasia or suspicion, suspicion of malignancy, or malignant results.
2. Presence of pressure symptoms (presence of dyspnea, dysphagia, hoarseness, or cough due to pressure).
3. Retrosternal goiter.
4. Accompanying hyperthyroidism.
5. Presence of mutation in RET proto-oncogene.

References

1. Gaitan E, Nelson NC, Poole GV. Endemic goiter and endemic thyroid disorders. World J Surg. 1991;5:205–15.
2. Brander A, Viikinkoski P, Nickels J, Kivisaari L. Thyroid gland: US screening in a random adult population. Radiology. 1991;181:683–7.
3. Kraimps JL, Marechaod R, Gineste D, Fieuzal S, Metaye T, Carretier M, et al. Analysis and prevention of recurrent goiter. Surg Gynecol Obstet. 1993;176:319–22.
4. Seiler CA, Glaser C, Wagner HE. Thyroid gland surgery in an endemic region. World J Surg. 1996;20:593–6.
5. Erbil Y, Barbaros U, Salmaslioglu A, Yanik BT, Bozbora A, Ozarmagan S. The advantage of near total thyroidectomy to avoid postoperative hypoparathyroidism in benign multinodular goiter. Langenbeck's Arch Surg. 2006;391:567–73.
6. Colak T, Akca T, Kanik A, Yapici D, Aydin S. Total versus subtotal thyroidectomy for the management of benign multinodular goiter in an endemic region. ANZ J Surg. 2004;74:974–8.
7. Snook KL, Stalberg PL, Sidhu SB, Sywak MS, Edhouse P, Delbridge L. Recurrence after total thyroidectomy for benign multinodular goiter. World J Surg. 2007;31:593–8.

8. Subbiah S, Collins BJ, Schneider AB. Factors related to the recurrence of thyroid nodules after surgery for benign radiation related nodules. Thyroid. 2007;17:41–7.
9. Haugen BR, Alexander EK, Bible KC, Doherty GM, Mandel SJ, Nikiforov YE, et al. 2015 American Thyroid Association management guidelines for adult patients with thyroid nodules and differentiated thyroid cancer: the American Thyroid Association guidelines task force on thyroid nodules and differentiated thyroid cancer. Thyroid. 2016;26:1–133.
10. Menegaux F, Turpin G, Dahman M, Leenhardt L, Chadarevian R, Aurengo A, et al. Secondary thyroidectomy in patients with prior thyroid surgery for benign disease: a study of 203 cases. Surgery. 1999;125:479–83.
11. Levin KE, Clark AH, Duh QY, Demeure M, Siperstein AE, Clark OH. Reoperative thyroid surgery. Surgery. 1992;111:604–9.
12. Sugrue DD, Drury MI, McEvoy M, Heffernan SJ, O'Malley E. Long term follow-up of hyperthyroid patients treated by subtotal thyroidectomy. Br J Surg. 1983;70:408–11.
13. Erbil Y, Bozbora A, Yanik BT, Ozbey N, Salmaslioglu A, Ozarmagan S. Predictive factors for recurrent non toxic goiter in endemic region. J Laryngol Otol. 2007;121:231–6.
14. Muller PE, Jakoby R, Heinert G, Spelsberg F. Surgery for recurrent goiter: its complications and their risk factors. Eur J Surg. 2001;167:816–21.
15. Reeve TS, Delbridge L, Brady P, Crummer P, Smyth C. Secondary thyroidectomy: a twenty-year experience. World J Surg. 1988;12:449–53.
16. Dralle H, Sekulla C, Haerting J, Timmermann W, Neumann HJ, Kruse E, et al. Risk factors of paralysis and functional outcome after recurrent laryngeal nerve monitoring in thyroid surgery. Surgery. 2004;136:1310–22.
17. Sosa JA, Bowman HM, Tielsch JM, Powe NR, Gordon TA, Udelsman R. The importance of surgeon experience for clinical and economic outcomes from thyroidectomy. Ann Surg. 1998;228:320–30.
18. Barczyński M, Konturek A, Pragacz K, Papier A, Stopa M, Nowak W. Intraoperative nerve monitoring can reduce prevalence of recurrent laryngeal nerve injury in thyroid reoperations: results of a retrospective cohort study. World J Surg. 2014;38:599–606.
19. Seiler CA, Glaser C, Wagner HE. Thyroid gland surgery in an endemic region. World J Surg. 1996;20:593–7.
20. Mitchell AL, Gandhi A, Scott-Coombes D, Perros P. Management of thyroid cancer: United Kingdom national multidisciplinary guidelines. J Laryngol Otol. 2016;130:150–60.

22 Intrathoracic Goiter

Ali Uğur Emre

Abstract

A recurrent intrathoracic goiter and a case of intrathoracic goiter with tracheal narrowing are presented. The symptoms were mainly dyspnea and wheezing, but vascular compression is also a possible severe symptom. The importance of preoperative evaluation regarding the relation of the gland with the surrounding structures such as major vessels and trachea is emphasized. Although ultrasonography is the first step radiologic tool for cervical thyroid pathologies, non-contrast computerized tomography is the preferred method of radiologic evaluation. Valuable information about the extent of gland to the mediastinum and the compressive effect of the gland to the surrounding structures can be evaluated, and operative management can be planned in detail. Intubation of the patient with a tracheal stricture needs to be focused on. The alternatives are discussed on the case with low situated tracheal compression. Most of the intrathoracic goiters can be removed through a cervical incision. Hourglass-shaped goiters or intrathoracic goiters placed in the posterior mediastinum and malignant cases with possible invasions sometimes require a sternotomy or thoracotomy to remove the gland safely thorough vascular structures.

A. U. Emre
Division of Endocrine Surgery, Bülent Ecevit University, Zonguldak, Turkey

22.1 Case 1

A 76-year-old female patient was admitted with dyspnea, dysphagia, and coughing symptoms worsening gradually over the last 3 years. Her medical history revealed a thyroidectomy operation 20 years ago, medical treatment with antiaggregants for coronary arterial stenosis after angiographic evaluation, hypertension for 2 years, and gastritis. She presented the reports of two thyroid fine needle aspiration biopsies (FNAB) that had been nondiagnostic according to Bethesda classification.

In her physical examination, there was a collar incision scar of the previous surgery in the lower neck. The thyroid gland was partially palpated at the jugular notch. The gland was hard in consistency and fixed while swallowing. Her TSH was 1.02 uIU/mL, fT4, 0.90 ng/dl; Ca, 9.6 mg/dl; and P, 4.3 mg/dl. The tracheal air column was deviated to the right in the thoracic inlet. Thyroid ultrasonography demonstrated remnant thyroid tissue of 12.4 × 13 × 23 mm in the right and 27.4 × 39 × 52,4 mm in the left lobe. The left remnant tissue was showing intrathoracic extension and almost entirely solid with minute cystic areas and coarse calcifications. Computerized tomography (CT) imaging of the neck and thorax defined a hypodense, 37 × 27 mm mass lesion on the left of the trachea with an irregular contour and peripheral calcifications that significantly dis-

T. Özülker et al. (eds.), *Thyroid and Parathyroid Diseases*, https://doi.org/10.1007/978-3-319-78476-2_22

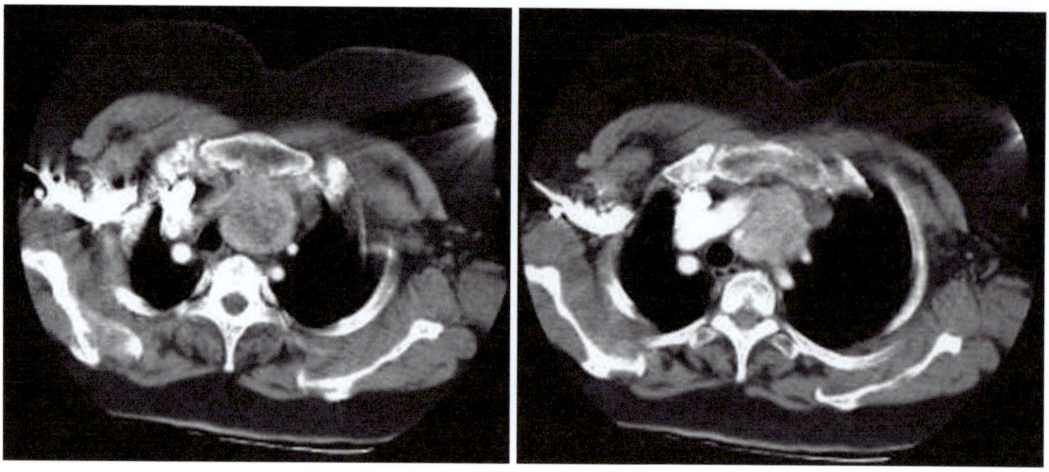

Fig. 22.1 Axial slices CT shows intrathoracic recurrent goiter

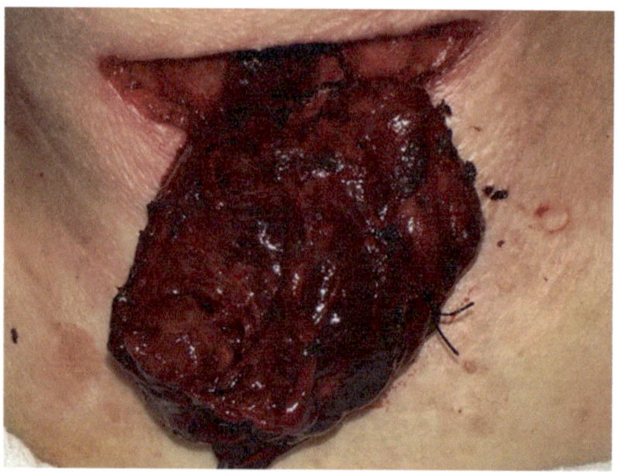

Fig. 22.2 Cervical resection of recurrent goiter

places the trachea to the right (Fig. 22.1). Vocal cords were mobile bilaterally indirect laryngoscopy. After preoperative evaluation for anesthesia, patient was reported as ASA 3 risk group, and thyroid lobectomy was planned for compressive symptoms. A cervical procedure is planned, but the operation room is prepared for a partial sternotomy. A left complementary thyroid lobectomy was performed for the tightly adherent remnant tissue through a cervical incision (Fig. 22.2).

Pathologic findings were a 6 × 5 × 4 cm thyroid lobectomy specimen with a 4 × 4 × 2.9 cm irregular partially calcified and hemorrhagic nodule occupying nearly all of the tissue with a diagnosis of nodular hyperplasia and regressive alterations.

22.2 Case 2

A 64-year-old male patient was admitted to the hospital for painless hematuria. His medical history revealed a myocardial infarction treated with coronary artery stenting 20 years ago. He had a huge grade 4 goiter and hypertension. Cardiologic evaluation for the accompanying dyspnea and palpitation symptoms resulted with ECG findings representing ischemia. Angiographic examination demonstrated 100% and 80% stenosis in the circumflex and right coronary arteries, respectively. Two stents were placed successfully, but the procedure lasted more than 2 h due to the critical localization of the stenosis. Radiological evaluation for the intermittent hematuria continued after that, and two irregular masses, 28 × 10 mm on the right inferior part and 20 × 12 mm on the left, reported as suspicious for bladder carcinoma are defined at the base of the urinary bladder with ultrasonography (USG). Blood tests for the evaluation of the patient for surgery were done. Thyroid hormone profile was TSH, < 0.01 uIU/mL; fT4, 2.4 (0.54–1.24) ng/dl; and fT3, 8.23 (2.00–3.90) pg/mL. Former medical records of the patient were euthyroid, so the hyperthyroid state is diagnosed as Jod-Basedow phenomenon. The thyroid gland was measured as right lobe, 115 × 55 × 42 mm; left lobe, 178 × 62 × 42 mm; and isthmus, 15 mm with many nodules up to 6 cm in diameter, but mediastinal

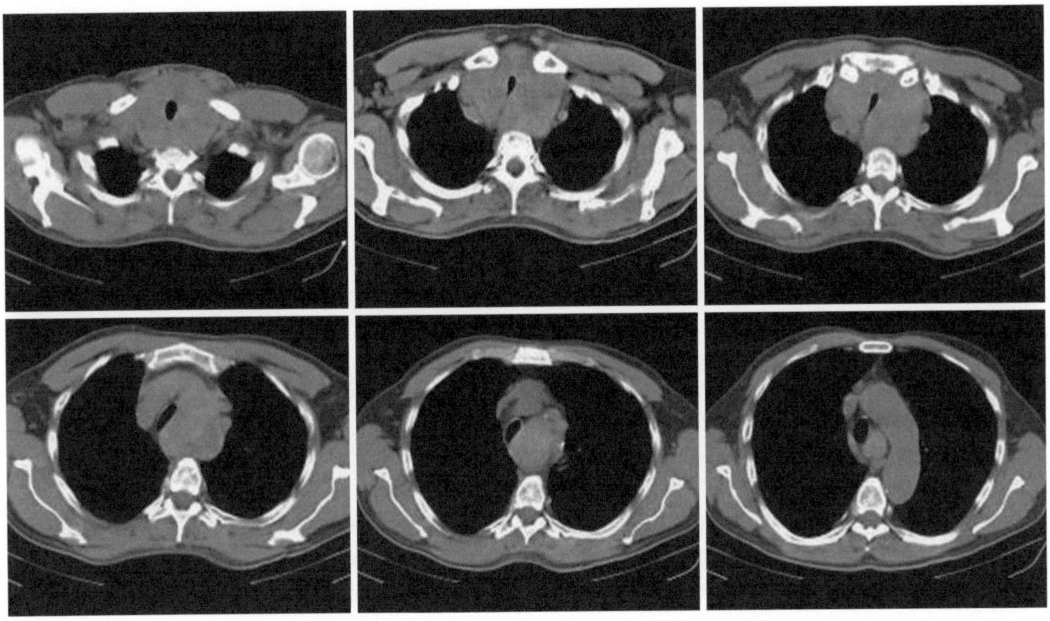

Fig. 22.3 Axial slices CT shows intrathoracic goiter with posterior mediastinal extension and tracheal compression

extensions of the inferior poles could not be interpreted. Non-contrast neck and thorax CT imaging demonstrated a retrosternal goiter extending below the aortic arch to the level of tracheal bifurcation especially on the left side, surrounding the trachea and deviating it to the right. The trachea was constricted to 5 mm luminal width (Fig. 22.3). As strict adherence to dual antiplatelet therapy with aspirin and a thienopyridine is required for drug-eluting coronary artery stents preferably for 1 year but at least for 6 months, it was not suitable to operate the patient immediately. After 6 months of observation period, a thyroidectomy with a possible sternotomy simultaneously with transurethral tumor resection is offered with bronchoscopy-assisted tracheal intubation, but the patient refused thyroidectomy, and after 5 days withdrawal of anticoagulant therapy, he was operated for bladder carcinoma with spinal anesthesia.

22.3 Discussion

22.3.1 Evaluation and Diagnosis

Intrathoracic goiter (ITG), although there are a number of definitions as a gland reaching the level of the aortic arch or a thyroid reaching the level of T4 (on chest x-ray), is widely accepted as the thyroid gland descending below the thoracic inlet or more than 50% of the gland below this point [1, 2]. The terms retrosternal, substernal, or mediastinal goiter are also used to describe this condition. Differences in the criteria of definition cause a variety of incidence from 1% to 20% [3]. About 98% of the intrathoracic goiters are secondary, but there are also rare primary cases which develop in the mediastinum embriologically. Primary mediastinal goiters result from the embryological migration process that is particularly important regarding blood supply to the gland. The variations in the vascular supply as intrathoracic arteries should receive high attention to prevent blood loss and other complications [4]. The majority of the ITG are extensions of cervical thyroid gland through thoracic inlet either on one side or both. The anterior superior mediastinum is the most common site for ITG as the anatomic structures such as the trachea, brachiocephalic veins, and superior vena cava limit the growth to some extent. Posterior mediastinum is rarely occupied by the goiter, but preoperative evaluation is essential in planning of the surgical procedure in such a case.

Intrathoracic goiters can cause symptoms related to compression of surrounding structures. Respiratory complaints such as dyspnea, coughing, and asthma-like syndrome are frequent and followed by dysphagia, hyperthyroidism, dysphonia, and superior vena cava syndrome [5]. Case 1 represents such an asthma-like syndrome with dyspnea that is treated with thyroidectomy.

Diagnostic workup of the patient begins with physical examination of the neck. The inferior border of the gland cannot be palpated when it continues to the mediastinum. Thyroid function tests should be done for hyper- or hypothyroidism beginning with serum TSH testing. The first radiologic evaluation is the USG of the thyroid gland and the neck. USG evaluation of the gland gives information about the dimensions of the gland, the presence of any thyroid nodules, the texture of the nodules in terms of suspicious criteria about malignancy, and the nodules that should be evaluated with FNAB. Unfortunately, most of the intrathoracic goiter cannot be adequately visualized with USG. Tracheal deviation and in some cases tracheal narrowing can be visualized in chest radiograph. CT of the neck and thorax is the preferred and effective way of screening ITG. Patients with obstructive symptoms that are discordant with the cervical goiter must be screened with a non-contrast CT. A contrast agent is only useful for demonstrating vascular supply of the gland especially for suspected primary ITG, but a careful hormonal evaluation, preparation, and observation for clinical or subclinical hyperthyroid patients or patients with a huge mass of thyroid gland must be done to prevent exacerbation of hyperthyroidism as seen in Case 2 that resulted with Jod-Basedow phenomenon. Preconditioning with methimazole can help to manage this complication. In such patients, magnetic resonance imaging is an alternative radiologic tool. These radiological workups give information about the extension of the gland to mediastinum, particularly to the posterior mediastinum and below the aortic arch, and the relation with the surrounding anatomical structures including possible invasive tumors, the extent of tracheal compression, and focal calcifications in the gland [6]. Obstructive symptoms can be seen in patients with a tracheal diameter below 8 mm as exertional dyspnea and when below 5 mm as wheezing and stridor even at resting state as in Case 2 [7]. The compression symptoms include not only of the trachea but the esophagus or vascular structures that can be diagnosed with a Pemberton's maneuver due to increased thoracic inlet pressure and rarely subclavian vein compression and thrombosis.

22.3.2 Management

Surgical removal of the thyroid is the preferred and most effective treatment of ITG. Surgery offers a rapid and permanent relief of symptoms. A total or near-total thyroidectomy should be performed by an experienced surgeon and surgical team in a high-volume center experienced in endocrine surgery with sufficient facilities to prevent recurrence as long as recurrent laryngeal nerves are secured and complications are avoided [8]. Although suppression with exogenous thyroid hormone can achieve some regression in thyroid volume, it is generally insufficient and temporary.

Patients with obstructive symptoms should be managed with great attention and detailed planning. Compression of the trachea is also important throughout the induction of anesthesia, intubation, and extubation procedures. Inability to ventilate the patient is a serious problem, and the airway should be secured carefully. Large volume of the goiter and intrathoracic compression of trachea can be dangerous if the patient cannot be ventilated after induction of anesthesia because emergency tracheotomy will not be useful if the compressed trachea is below this level. Fiber-optic bronchoscopy in a spontaneously breathing patient and correct positioning of endotracheal tube distal to the narrow part of trachea is advised in such patients [9, 10]. Again fiber-optic evaluation of the trachea through the endotracheal tube is effective during the extubation regarding the probability of tracheomalacia. There are conflicting data about the incidence of tracheomalacia from 0% to 10% in the literature, but in terms of safety, it should be carefully evaluated during the surgery [11]. Extubation can be delayed, or immediate surgical interventions can be used in such cases to prevent airway collapse.

Most of the secondary intrathoracic goiters can safely be removed through a cervical incision [12]. Delivering the thyroid through thoracic inlet with careful finger dissection from the mediastinal structures and pulling the inferior pole out and vessel control is generally effective. The decision of the surgical procedure should be planned before surgery. Intrathoracic goiters, those are extending to the posterior mediastinum and descending to the level of the aortic arch, usually require an additional intervention such as manubriotomy and partial or complete sternotomy in addition to the cervical incision and necessitate a thorough preoperative radiologic evaluation [6]. A detailed informed consent is required for these patients as complications are more frequently seen.

In most of the cases, when it is not possible to remove the goiter through a cervical incision, a manubriotomy or partial sternotomy is enough to visualize the mediastinal structures and safely remove the gland with effective control of the vessels [13]. An hourglass-shaped ITG with a narrow thoracic inlet is best treated with such interventions. Primary ITG usually receives their blood supply from mediastinal vasculature and advised to be removed with thoracic approach to obtain a good access to the glands and vascular supply. Dense fibrotic adhesions in recurrent cases and vascular invasions in malignant cases also require thoracic surgery. Posterior mediastinal goiters and mainly ectopic goiters are best resected with a lateral thoracotomy, but it should be kept on mind that transthoracic procedures have significantly higher rates of complications and a lengthened hospital stay [14]. The decision for such cases again should be made preoperatively.

The recurrent laryngeal nerve is at an increased risk for intrathoracic goiters either managed with cervical or thoracic approach when compared with cervical goiters [15]. Neuromonitoring is a valuable tool for identification of recurrent laryngeal nerve and evaluation of paralysis in such cases. A continuous vagal stimulation is preferred.

22.4 Follow-Up and Outcome

Case 1: Immediately after the operation, dyspnea, dysphagia, coughing symptoms, and sleep disturbances are improved. No bleeding, nerve paralysis, or seroma is observed. Thyroid hormone replacement with levothyroxine is initiated after the pathologic diagnosis of a benign condition aiming a serum TSH level around 2 uIU/mL.

Case 2: After the removal of bladder carcinoma, the patient is receiving intraluminal chemo- and immunotherapy. The symptoms of compressive intrathoracic goiter will be followed. A CT scan surveillance will be performed. A tracheal stenting can be offered if tracheal compression increases and patient still refuses thyroidectomy.

What Can We Learn from This Case?

- Intrathoracic goiters can be primary or secondary. Primary goiters deserve a high attention in terms of variations of vascular supply.
- Compression of mediastinal structures especially to the trachea is important. A tracheal diameter below 8 mm results in dyspnea, wheezing, and stridor.
- A thorough preoperative radiologic evaluation is essential.
- Operative management of patients with tracheal compression begins with the planning of intubation and extubation of the patient.
- Intrathoracic goiters extending to the posterior mediastinum, below the aortic arch or infracarinal level, recurrent cases and malignant cases, may require a sternotomy or thoracotomy for a safer surgical removal.

References

1. Rios A, Rodríguez J, Balsalobre M, Tebar F, Parrilla P. The value of various definitions of intrathoracic goiter for predicting intra-operative and postoperative complications. Surgery. 2010;147:233–8. https://doi.org/10.1016/j.surg.2009.06.018.

2. Walz P, Iwenofu O, Essig G. Ectopic mediastinal goiter successfully managed via cervical approach: case report and review of the literature. Head Neck. 2011;35:E94–7. https://doi.org/10.1002/hed.21920.
3. Katlic M, Wang C, Grillo H. Substernal goiter. Ann Thorac Surg. 1985;39:391–9.
4. Foroulis C, Rammos K, Sileli M, Papakonstantinou C. Primary intrathoracic goiter: a rare and potentially serious entity. Thyroid. 2009;19:213–8. https://doi.org/10.1089/thy.2008.0222.
5. Anders H. Compression syndromes caused by substernal goitres. Postgrad Med J. 1998;74:327–9.
6. Qureishi A, Garas G, Tolley N, Palazzo F, Athanasiou T, Zacharakis E. Can pre-operative computed tomography predict the need for a thoracic approach for removal of retrosternal goitre? Int J Surg. 2013;11:203–8. https://doi.org/10.1016/j.ijsu.2013.01.006.
7. Al-Bazzaz F, Grillo H, Kazemi H. Response to exercise in upper airway obstruction. Am Rev Respir Dis. 1975;111(5):631–40. https://doi.org/10.1164/arrd.1975.111.5.631.
8. Nakaya M, Ito A, Mori A, Oka M, Omura S, Kida W, et al. Surgical treatment of substernal goiter: an analysis of 44 cases. Auris Nasus Larynx. 2017;44:111–5. https://doi.org/10.1016/j.anl.2016.02.016.
9. Tan P, Esa N. Anesthesia for massive retrosternal goiter with severe intrathoracic tracheal narrowing: the challenges imposed -a case report. Korean J Anesthesiol. 2012;62:474. https://doi.org/10.4097/kjae.2012.62.5.474.
10. Wong P, Chieh Liew G, Kothandan H. Anaesthesia for goitre surgery: a review. Proc Singap Healthc. 2015;24:165–70. https://doi.org/10.1177/2010105815596095.
11. Huins C, Georgalas C, Mehrzad H, Tolley N. A new classification system for retrosternal goitre based on a systematic review of its complications and management. Int J Surg. 2008;6:71–6. https://doi.org/10.1016/j.ijsu.2007.02.003.
12. Wang L. Surgical management of a substernal goiter. Formosan J Surg. 2012;45:41–4. https://doi.org/10.1016/j.fjs.2012.02.001.
13. Nankee L, Chen H, Schneider D, Sippel R, Elfenbein D. Substernal goiter: when is a sternotomy required? J Surg Res. 2015;199:121–5. https://doi.org/10.1016/j.jss.2015.04.045.
14. Khan M, Goljo E, Owen R, Park R, Yao M, Miles B. Retrosternal Goiter: 30-day morbidity and mortality in the transcervical and transthoracic approaches. Otolaryngol Head Neck Surg. 2016;155:568–74. https://doi.org/10.1177/0194599816649583.
15. Testini M, Gurrado A, Bellantone R, Brazzarola P, Cortese R, De Toma G, et al. Recurrent laryngeal nerve palsy and substernal goiter. An Italian multicenter study. J Visc Surg. 2014;151:183–9. https://doi.org/10.1016/j.jviscsurg.2014.04.006.

23 Persistent Hypothyroidism Despite Levothyroxine Replacement Therapy: Malabsorption or Patient Noncompliance

Dilek Yazıcı

Abstract

The most important reason for being unable to achieve euthyroidism in the treatment of hypothyroidism is noncompliance with treatment. The state of levothyroxine pseudomalabsorption is a factitious disorder where the patients present with noncompliance with L-thyroxine therapy. In order to diagnose levothyroxine pseudomalabsorption, an L-thyroxine absorption test may be performed. There are different protocols for the test, where 1000–2000 mcg L-thyroxine is given to the patient and blood is withdrawn at 2 h intervals, until up to 24 h. If the free thyroid hormone levels increase during the test, then this suggests that there is no malabsorption. The therapy of levothyroxine pseudomalabsorption may be parenteral infusion at the beginning to achieve an initial euthyroid state and giving the medication orally once or twice a day under medical supervision in the follow-up.

A 38-year-old female patient had been followed up with the diagnosis of Graves' disease for 6 years. She had symptoms of nervousness and sweating. She had used propylthiouracil for 4 years and was then given radioactive iodine therapy (RAI). Subsequently, the disease had recurred, and she had undergone near-total thyroidectomy. Following thyroidectomy, she had weakness and loss of her hair, thinning and dryness in her skin, and edema in her feet and hands. She had gained 15 kg in 2 months. She had cold intolerance, numbness in her hands and feet and also numbness in the right part of her head, and headache. She had been amenorrheic for the past 5 years. She consulted a primary care physician with these symptoms, and the laboratory revealed TSH > 100 mU/mL (high); sT3,0.402pg/mL (low); and sT4,0.506 ng/dL (low). The patient was started on 200 mcg L-thyroxine in the morning and 50 mcg L-thyroxine at night. The TSH level 5 weeks later was still >100 mU/mL. The dose of the medication was increased gradually, but TSH did not decrease, and she still was symptomatic. The physician following her also tried different L-thyroxine preparations. When she was first consulted to our outpatient clinic, the dose she was using was 350 mcg/d. Since her TSH was still elevated with this dose, she was evaluated further.

In her past medical history, there were epileptic seizures for two times, nephrolithiasis, and gastrointestinal bleeding. She had been operated for a temporal lobe arachnoid cyst. Her mother had congestive heart failure, father diabetes mellitus and chronic renal failure, and sister colon carcinoma.

D. Yazıcı
Koç University Medical School, Section of Endocrinology and Metabolism, Istanbul, Turkey

T. Özülker et al. (eds.), *Thyroid and Parathyroid Diseases*, https://doi.org/10.1007/978-3-319-78476-2_23

She had been smoking seven packs/year. The medications she was taking other than L-thyroxine were diltiazem 60 mg/day, lansoprazole 30 mg/day, and alverine citrate + simethicone three times a day. The physical examination revealed bilateral exophthalmos, the thyroid gland was nonpalpable, and there was a thyroidectomy scar. Deep tendon reflexes were slow on relaxation. There was no pedal edema but a 2 × 3 cm lesion on the pretibial surface and a 4 × 5 cm lesion on the feet dorsum bilaterally.

23.1 Discussion

Inability to achieve euthyroidism is a common problem in treating hypothyroid patients. The proposed etiological mechanisms for this situation are problems in patient compliance; some physiological (pregnancy, weight), nutritional, or pharmacological conditions of increased or decreased L-thyroxine need; and the presence of malabsorption [1]. The recommended treatment dosage of L-thyroxine is 1.6 mcg/kg body weight a day [2]. Results with this dosage are adequate and reproducible. If greater amounts of L-thyroxine are needed, this may suggest a problem, and further evaluations can be made. Normally L-thyroxine absorption takes place primarily in the jejunum and ileum. Approximately 80% of an orally administered dose is absorbed [2]. L-Thyroxine serum levels peak nearly 2 h after administration of an oral dose [2–4]. However, it has been demonstrated that the intestinal uptake of LT4 is variable even among euthyroid subjects [2, 3].

The most common cause of failure of L-thyroxine therapy seems to be noncompliance with the medication [3, 5]. Pseudomalabsorption is the term used for this situation, and it usually has a psychiatric background. The term pseudomalabsorption of L-thyroxine was first introduced to the literature by Ain et al. in 1991 [2]. They described four patients who could not become euthyroid despite ingesting up to eightfold the mean daily dose of levothyroxine. All patients were found to have normal L-thyroxine absorption when the medication was administered through a nasogastric tube or a double-labeled thyroxine tracer technique was used. They decided that the patients are noncompliant due to psychiatric problems and named this condition as pseudomalabsorption of L-thyroxine [1].

23.1.1 Evaluation and Diagnosis

Malabsorption of L-thyroxine due to adjunctive use of other medications (e.g., laxatives, antacids) and supplements (e.g., calcium, iron) and interference by food should be identified first. Later on malabsorptive conditions (e.g., celiac, pancreatic insufficiency, jejunoileal bypass surgery, lactose intolerance, small intestine bacterial overgrowth, severe hepatic cirrhosis, and congestive heart failure) should be excluded [6–10]. An increased need for oral L-thyroxine has also been identified in gastric disorders (*Helicobacter pylori* infection, chronic gastritis, etc.), indicating a role for the stomach in subsequent intestinal L-thyroxine absorption [11].

Drugs that may interfere with the absorption of L-thyroxine are sucralfate, calcium carbonate, ferrous sulfate, and cholestyramine [6–10]. There is evidence that at least 1 h delay between L-thyroxine tablet ingestion and breakfast may give the best therapeutic result [12]. Drugs like carbamazepine, phenytoin, and phenobarbital increase the metabolism of levothyroxine, leading to higher dose requirements [13].

In our patient, firstly, the dose of L-thyroxine was raised to 600 mcg/day, and TSH did not come down in the follow-up. Meanwhile, alverine citrate + simethicone, proton pump inhibitor, and diltiazem were stopped. Then she had a through laboratory work-up (Table 23.1), which revealed that she did not have anemia, any deficiencies of vitamin B12 or iron. Her liver function tests and amylase were normal. Antigliadin antibody was negative.

After absorption problems and drug interactions are eliminated, L-thyroxine absorption test is performed to evaluate L-thyroxine pseudomalabsorption. The test is performed after an overnight fast, and the patient is not allowed to ingest anything except fluids during the test. The test is

Table 23.1 Laboratory values of the patient

	Value	Normals
FBG (mg/dL)	82	<100
BUN (mg/dL)	11	3–20
Creatinine (mg/dL)	0.78	0.4–1.1
T protein (mg/dL)	7.7	6.3–7.9
Albumin (mg/dL)	4.16	3.5–5.0
AST (U/L)	13	8–43
ALT (U/L)	11	7–45
ALP (U/L)	64	37–98
GT (U/L)	12	6–29
Na (mEq/L)	141	135–145
K (mEq/L)	4.46	3.6–5.2
Calcium (mg/dL)	8.7	8.9–10.2
Phosphorus (mg/dL)	4.10	2.5–4.5
T cholesterol (mg/dL)	183	<200
Triglycerides (mg/dL)	144	<150
HDL (mg/dL)	47	>45
LDL (mg/dL)	107	<100
Creatinine phosphokinase (U/L)	630	38–176
WBC (103/uL)	4600	3500–10,500
PNL (%)	49.5	
Hb (g/dL)	11.3	12.0–15.5
HCT (%)	33	34.9–44.5
MCV (FL)	90.3	80–100
PLT (103/uL)	226,000	150,000–450,000
Iron (μg/dL)	72	35–145
Total iron-binding capacity (μg/dL)	377	250–400
Ferritin (ng/mL)	74.13	11–307
Folic acid (ng/mL)	8.03	>4
Vitamin B12 (pg/mL)	567.8	180–914
Antigliadin IgG	<20EU/mL	
TSH (mU/mL)	>100	0.5–4.0
Free T4 (ng/dL)	0.08	0.9–1.7
Anti-TPO (μIU/mL)	124.8	<35
Atg (μIU/mL)	431	<20
FSH (mIU/mL)	4.29	2.5–10.2
LH (mIU/mL)	3.38	1.9–12.5
E2 (pg/mL)	45.6	39–375
Prolactin (ng/mL)	26.3	3–30

performed in the fasting state because L-thyroxine absorption is greater while fasting [14]. Blood samples are obtained at the baseline and 2, 4, and 6 h following the ingestion of L-thyroxine orally. Proper ingestion and possible surreptitious regurgitation should be checked by the attending physician or the nurse during the test [2, 15]. Multiple protocols for clinical L-thyroxine absorption test have been published. These involve oral administration of 1000–2000 mcg of L-thyroxine, and the duration of the test can vary from 4 to 24 h [2, 3]. A rapid (2 h long) test was suggested by a group of authors. This group also informed the patients 3 weeks prior to the test, so the patients had already started to ingest the medication properly before the test, and therefore all three patients started the test with high free T3 and free T4 levels, which increased even further during the test [16]. They commented that the plan of an L-thyroxine absorption test had motivated the patients already. If the free T4 levels increase throughout the test, then this excludes the presence of malabsorption. Some authors suggest performing the test even before doing all kinds of troublesome investigations for malabsorption [14].

Lastly thinking of L-thyroxine pseudomalabsorption, our patient was hospitalized to perform the L-thyroxine loading test. During the test, 2000 mcg of L-thyroxine was given to the patient in the fasting state. Free T3 and TSH levels were determined every 2 h for 6 h. An increase in free T3 and decrease in TSH were observed (Fig. 23.1). This suggested L-thyroxine pseudomalabsorption since the patient was able to absorb the medication orally.

Dermatology consultation for the lesions on the pretibial region and the dorsum of the feet suggested lichen chronicus simplex. This lesion resulted from scratching the skin continuously and was suggested to have psychogenic etiology.

23.1.2 Management

There are different approaches to the treatment of L-thyroxine pseudomalabsorption. Since this is a psychiatric problem, originally the underlying psychiatric condition should be solved. The psychiatric problems are usually due to a depressive state, which is a common manifestation of hypothyroidism; however, some patients may present with some other psychotic problems [2, 13, 15]. The usual approach is giving the patient parenteral infusion initially to ensure euthyroidism. The problem with parenteral infusion is

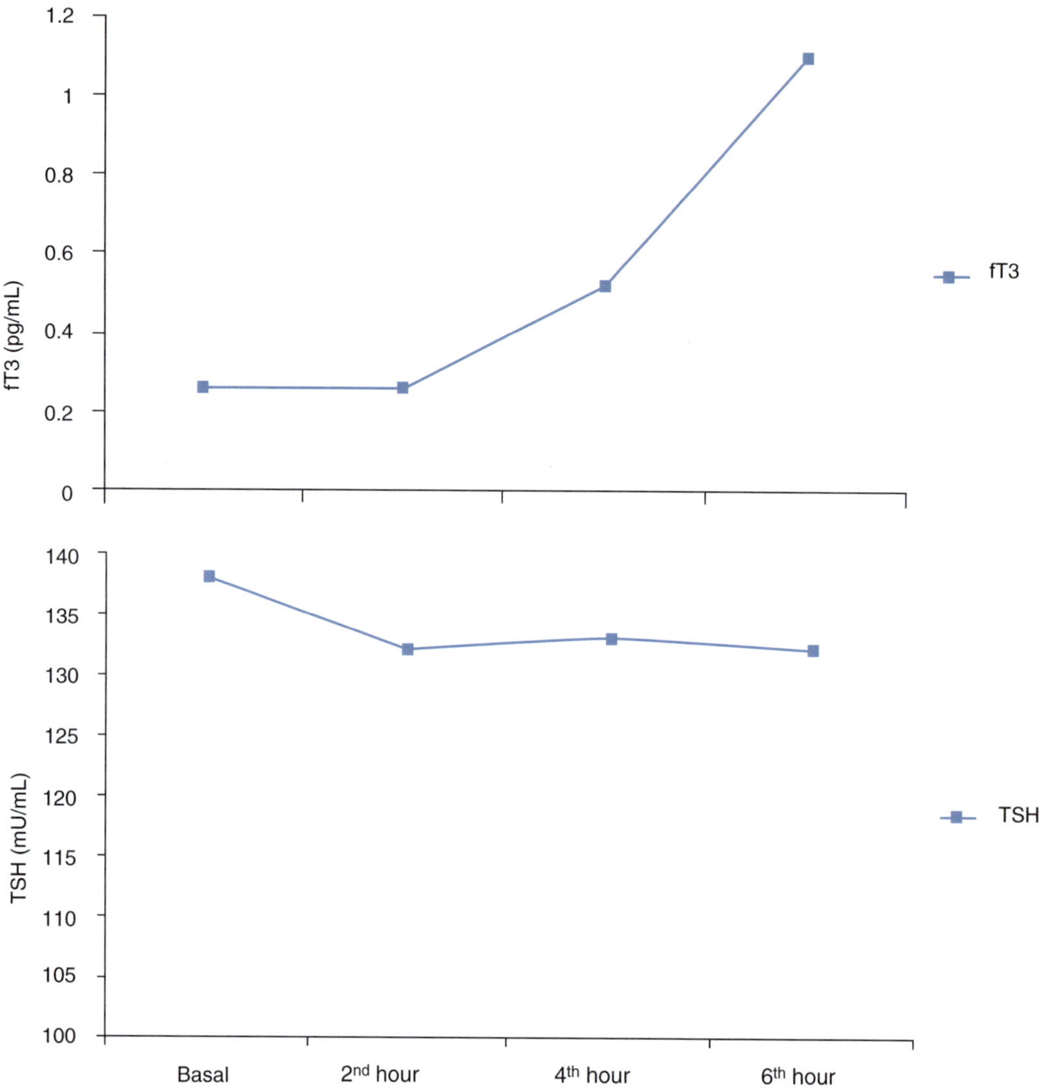

Fig. 23.1 Diagram showing increase in free T3 and decrease in TSH during L-thyroxine loading test

that it is not available in some countries and can only be applied for short periods. Following this, oral therapy can be continued in different ways. Thus, one of the groups used the method of giving the patient oral L-thyroxine under medical supervision within the hospital. The authors claim that by this way the patient was not confronted with the problem, and the physicians did not show their judgment to the patient, and the patient continued to be the "patient" that she desires to be all the time [17]. Patients tend to drop out when they are told of their noncompliance by physicians. Confronting the patient with the possibility of noncompliance may affect the patient negatively and worsen the situation. The patients should be handled with very much care.

23.2 Follow-Up and Outcome

Our patient was externalized with a dose of 1600 mcg/day L-thyroxine. In the follow-up, her TSH level went down to 0.3 mU/mL. She continued with the same dose, and the TSH went up to 38 mU/mL and later 100 mU/mL in a few months' time, despite her claiming to take the medication.

She was living in another city, so we could not offer her to come a few days a week to take the medication. Besides, intravenous form of the medication is not available in our country.

Inability to achieve euthyroidism is a common problem in hypothyroidism. Malabsorption is a common problem, and for that different formulations have been designed, such as soft gel formulation [18]. For pseudomalabsorption, literature search shows that giving the medication weekly or twice weekly under medical supervision is helpful. One group tried to use the L-thyroxine absorption test as a therapeutic means, and they informed the patients 3 weeks prior to the test. It turned out that the patients were more keen on using the medication and the free hormone levels went up at the beginning of the test. The demonstration of continued interest in the patients' "disease states" seems to be of help for the patients' psychology.

What Can We Learn from This Case?

- The most important reason for not being able to achieve euthyroidism is noncompliance with treatment.
- When this has a psychological background, this state is called L-thyroxine pseudomalabsorption.
- The way to diagnose levothyroxine pseudomalabsorption is to perform an L-thyroxine absorption test, where 1000–2000 mcg L-thyroxine is given to the patient and blood is withdrawn at 2 h intervals, until up to 24 h, in different protocols.
- The therapy of levothyroxine pseudomalabsorption may be parenteral infusion at the beginning to achieve the euthyroid state and afterward giving the medication orally once or twice a week, preferentially at the hospital, under supervision.

References

1. Centanni M. Thyroxine treatment: absorption, malabsorption, and novel therapeutic approaches. Endocrine. 2013;43:8–9.
2. Ain KB, Refetoff S, Fein HG, Weintraub BD. Pseudomalabsorption of levothyroxine. JAMA. 1991;266:2118–20.
3. Lips DJ, van Reisen MT, Voigt V, Venekamp W. Diagnosis and treatment of levothyroxine pseudomalabsorption. Neth J Med. 2004;62:114–8.
4. Hays MT. Localization of human thyroxine absorption. Thyroid. 1991;1:241–8.
5. Mandel SJ, Brent GA, Larsen PR. Levothyroxine therapy in patients with thyroid disease. Ann Intern Med. 1993;119:492–502.
6. Bevan JS, Munro JF. Thyroxine malabsorption following intestinal bypass surgery. Int J Obes. 1986; 10:245–6.
7. Mandel SJ, Larsen PR, Seely EW, Brent GA. Increased need for thyroxine during pregnancy in women with primary hypothyroidism. N Engl J Med. 1990;323:91–6.
8. Harmon SM, Seifert CF. Levothyroxine-cholestyramine interaction reemphasized. Ann Intern Med. 1991;115:658–9.
9. Leger CS, Ooi TC. Ferrous fumarate-induced malabsorption of thyroxine. Endocrinologist. 1999;9:493–5.
10. Singh N, Singh PN, Hershman JM. Effect of calcium carbonate on the absorption of levothyroxine. JAMA. 2000;283:2822–5.
11. Centanni M, Gargano L, Canettieri G, Viceconti N, Franchi A, Delle Fave G, et al. Thyroxine in goiter, *Helicobacter pylori* infection, and chronic gastritis. N Engl J Med. 2006;354:1787–95.
12. Bach-Huynh TG, Nayak B, Loh J, Soldin S, Jonklaas J. Timing of levothyroxine administration affects serum thyrotropin concentration. J Clin Endocrinol Metab. 2009;94:3905–12.
13. Surks MI, Sievert R. Drugs and thyroid function. N Engl J Med. 1995;333:1688–94.
14. Ogawa D, Otsuka F, Mimura Y, Ueno A, Hashimoto H, Kishida M, et al. Pseudomalabsorption of levothyroxine: a case report. Endocr J. 2000;47:45–50.
15. Payer J, Sladekova K, Kinova S, Cesnakova Z, Killinger Z, Krizko M, et al. Autoimmune thyroiditis with severe hypothyroidism resistant to the treatment with high peroral doses of thyroxine: case report. Endocr Regul. 2000;34:189–93.
16. Balla M, Jhingan RM, Rubin DJ. Rapid levothyroxine absorption testing: a case series of nonadherent patients. Int J Endocrinol Metab. 2015;13:e31051.
17. Jauk B, Mikosch P, Gallowitsch HJ, Kresnik E, Molnar M, Gomez I, et al. Unusual malabsorption of levothyroxine. Thyroid. 2000;10:93–5.
18. Santaguida MG, Virili C, Del Duca SC, Cellini M, Gatto I, Brusca N, et al. Thyroxine soft gel capsule in patients with gastric-related T4 malabsorption. Endocrine. 2015;49:51–7.

Malpractise and Ethical Violations in Thyroid Surgery

24

Tamer Akça and Nursel Gamsız Bilgin

Abstract

In this article we aimed to give information about the legal process, to reveal the troubles encountered, to inform the physicians, and to attract attention when an unexpected condition occurs in the thyroid surgery and is referred to the judiciary. For this purpose, based on the cases referred and finalized in the Turkish jurisdiction, short information on the subject of ethical, medical, and legal responsibilities, informed consent, discrimination of complication from malpractice, the concept of expertise and expertise institutions, and criminal and compensation cases of the physicians is provided.

24.1 Case 1: Complication

24.1.1 Case Presentation [1]

A patient was diagnosed with papillary carcinoma of the thyroid, based on fine needle aspiration cytology (FNAC) of a nodule located within the right lobe of the gland. The patient was scheduled for total thyroidectomy. The patient provided an informed consent for thyroid surgery and anesthesia procedures and underwent an operation on the same day. The surgical report stated that hematoma was present in relation to the FNAC site, predominantly in the right lobe; the right recurrent laryngeal nerve was identified and preserved after a difficult dissection; parathyroid glands were identified and preserved, and a mini-drain was inserted. In the postoperative period, the patient suffered from hoarseness and shortness of breath and was diagnosed with vocal cord and laryngeal paralysis. Follow-up examinations were recommended, but the complaints significantly worsened within a year, for which the patient received voice therapy. Vocal cord paralysis persisted 18 months after the initial surgery, and it was stated that medialization laryngoplasty could be considered if there was no improvement in the voice quality.

24.1.2 Discussion

Although there are many definitions of medical interventions in legal parlance, they generally refer to procedures performed by licensed professionals in compliance with medical principles and techniques, with the aim of protecting the physical and/or mental integrity of the patient

T. Akça (✉)
Division of Breast and Endocrin Surgery, University of Mersin, Mersin, Turkey

Department of Medical History and Ethics, Mersin University, Mersin, Turkey

N. Gamsız Bilgin
Division of Forensic Medicine, University of Mersin, Mersin, Turkey

T. Özülker et al. (eds.), *Thyroid and Parathyroid Diseases*, https://doi.org/10.1007/978-3-319-78476-2_24

regarding the diagnosis, treatment, and prevention with the informed consent of the patient. In a precedent decree by the 4th Civil Chamber of Supreme Court, the legal terms for medical interventions were identified as follows:

1. The physician has to be authorized by law to practice medicine.
2. The patient has to provide an informed consent for the procedure.
3. The medical act has to be conducted within objective and subjective boundaries of medical science (4th Civil Chamber of Supreme Court E.1976/6297, K.1977/2541, T. 7.3.1977) [2, 3].

For medical interventions to have legal grounds, the physician has contractual obligations. These include diagnosis and treatment, provision of related information, loyalty and care, recording of clinical information, and confidentiality. Contract breaches, negligence, malpractice, and causal relation are infractions to hold the physician responsible for criminal liability [2–6].

Complications can be defined as adverse outcomes beyond acceptable risks without any case of negligence. In terms of practice of health legislation, it is important to differentiate between malpractice and complication. In medical practice, treatment of severe cases may require making quick decisions and taking risks. This particular case of medical practice may also result in controversies regarding the legal approach. Medical interventions are performed in patients with different characteristics and findings, and the outcomes may not be similar in every case. Therefore, medical interventions are performed on the basis of data derived from generalizations and scientific studies instead of individual-specific outcomes. A physician cannot be held liable for certain outcomes associated with the treatment, provided that medical interventions are performed in compliance with the risks and deviations considered normal in medical practice. If inevitability or unpredictability is present in terms of outcomes, the case is considered a complication and not negligence. For a physician to avoid legal responsibility, he/she should inform the patients of the complications, have their informed consent, and fulfill the conditions of a medical intervention [2, 4, 7–9].

If an unwanted outcome is unpredicted or if no precautions are taken by the average physician in terms of prediction and prevention of anticipated risks or mitigation of unwanted outcomes, then the outcome cannot be considered as a complication even without the physician's will. In this case, the conduct of the physician is considered negligence, and the physician is held liable. Predictable and preventable unwanted outcomes are considered a case of medical malpractice [8, 10, 11].

Predictability is defined as foreseeing the unwanted outcomes that may arise from medical interventions beforehand, and it is determined according to the subjective criteria established by the physician conducting the medical intervention. According to Turkish Criminal Law decree number 5237, "In negligent offenses, the offender should be in a condition to predict and act in compliance with objective duty of care depending on his/her own skills, has the ability of perception, knowledge, and circumstances" [2, 5, 8, 10, 11].

The decision by the General Assembly of the Supreme Court for Criminal Matters dated November 05, 2014, stated there is no negligence "when the characteristics of the offender (age, experience, occupation, etc.) should be taken into consideration to determine whether the outcome is predictable by the offender." In case prediction is not possible, accident and coincidence must be considered rather than negligence (YCGK 11.05.2005 T, 2004/2-97E, 2004/115K) [2].

24.1.3 Follow-Up and Outcome

A lawsuit was filed upon the defendant's complaint. Information, documents, and findings in the case file were reviewed by the Supreme Council of Health. After the trial, tests performed before surgery and the decision to operate were judged to be justifiable.

It was concluded that the patient's problems after surgery were a case of complication, practice of the respondent physician was in accordance with medical principles, the case was not of medical negligence, and the physician could not be held liable.

What Can We Learn from This Case?

- Predictable but unavoidable conditions are considered to be complications, whereas predictable and avoidable conditions are considered medical interventions.
- Predictability is foreseeing the unwanted outcomes that may arise in advance.
- The condition is considered a complication if an average physician has taken measures to predict and prevent anticipated risks or to mitigate/eliminate the unwanted outcomes.
- The physician cannot be held liable for outcomes arising from complication.

24.2 Case 2: Malpractice, Liability of Private Hospitals [12]

24.2.1 Case Presentation

A lawsuit has been filed against the doctors and hospital by the spouse of a patient who died after goiter surgery at a private hospital. In the case file, the operating surgeon was accused of gross negligence for not informing the patient regarding treatment options and choosing a hospital with insufficient equipment for the surgery. It was alleged that responsible manager and owner of the hospital was liable in allowing such surgical intervention in a facility that did not conform to the requirements of a hospital and did not possess the necessary equipment. It was also claimed that no doctor on call was present to intervene any unwanted outcomes that might arise after surgery.

24.2.2 Discussion

Criminal law states that there is no crime if there is no negligence. Wrongful intention is the highest degree of fault. The Turkish Penal Code article 21 states that the existence of a criminal offense depends upon the presence of intent. Intent is defined as "knowingly and willingly conducting the elements in the legal definition of an offense." In Turkish Penal Code article 22/2, negligence is defined as "conducting an act without foreseeing the results as stated in the legal definition of the offense, because of failure to discharge duty of care and attention" [4–6].

The Turkish Medical Association Ethical Principles of Healthcare item 13 defines medical intervention as "harm to the patient as a result of lack of knowledge, inexperience, or inattention." In the announcement titled "Medical Malpractice" published at the 44th General Assembly of the World Medical Association in 1992, medical malpractice was defined as "the physician's failure to conform to the standard of care for the treatment of patient's condition, or lack of a skill, or negligence in providing care" [2, 5, 6].

Medical malpractice may be caused by reasons such as failure to diagnose, failure to perform the required tests or leave them incomplete, failure to intervene, administering wrong treatment techniques, retaining foreign objects, not having control and surveillance, confusing patients, operating on the wrong body part, failure to notice complications, incorrect surgical technique, failure to conform to infection and hygiene principles, insufficiency in the use of technical instruments, and failure to refer or consult a specialist, or a delayed consultation [5, 6, 8, 10, 11, 13–15].

In 2016, Karakaya et al. published an article titled "Evaluation of expert reports provided by the Institution of Forensic Medicine for recurrent laryngeal nerve paralysis during thyroidectomy" in Turkish Journal of Surgery [16]. Thirty-eight files evaluated by the Third Specialization Board of the Institution of Forensic Medicine were retrospectively reviewed with respect to age, gender, diagnosis, vocal cord compression before surgery, identification of nerves during surgery, use of intraoperative nerve monitoring, recognition of the injury during surgery and attempts at rehabilitation, and type of nerve injury. Nineteen bilateral and 19 unilateral nerve injuries were identified, and all cases of bilateral injury were considered malpractice cases by the Institution of Forensic Medicine. Cases where there was not a situation complicating the identification of the nerve in terms of imaging methods and pathology reports were considered to be malpractice. It was concluded that if the physician ensures preservation of the nerve in one side after meticulous nerve dissection before proceeding to the other lobe, malpractice lawsuits could be avoided.

24.2.3 Follow-Up and Outcome

The physician, who is also the responsible manager of the hospital, and the operating surgeon were convicted of causing the death of the patient and sentenced to imprisonment and punitive fine.

The Ministry of Health was also condemned to pay compensation because of "failure to audit."

The cases where imaging methods and pathology reports cannot demonstrate the presence of a condition complicating the identification of the nerve are considered to be malpractice by the Institution of Forensic Medicine.

What Can We Learn from This Case?

- Injuries caused by physician's failure to perform medical standards during treatment and injuries caused by lack of skills and failure to provide treatment are considered as malpractice.
- Failure of the surgeon to inform the patient of treatment methods is considered as malpractice.
- Injuries caused by the insufficiency of personnel, medical equipment, etc., both in public or private hospitals, are considered as malpractice.
- Turkish Penal Code judges the malpractice cases based on the articles on wrongful intent and negligence.

24.3 Case 3: Assignment of New Experts [1]

24.3.1 Case Presentation

A patient underwent goiter surgery by the defendant general surgeon for multinodular goiter. The patient started oral intake during the postoperative hospitalization period; however, because of postoperative vomiting from the tube inserted, the defendant physician referred the patient to the university hospital. Surgical intervention in the university hospital revealed that both the trachea and esophagus were dissected during initial surgery.

Defendant physician asserted that the intubation process was difficult because of the anatomic features of the patient and the intubation was successful only after the third attempt and that esophageal perforation developed as a complication of multiple attempts at intubation. The defendant physician further claimed that tracheal perforation did not occur during or after surgery and there was no evidence of tracheal perforation during surgery.

The report issued by the Institution of Forensic Medicine concluded: "It is evident from the medical documents of the patient and various statements that the intubation of the patient was complicated, that esophageal intubation and associated esophageal perforation could occur in cases of difficult intubation and tracheal perforation might develop as a result of surgery." It was claimed that esophageal and tracheal perforations should be considered as complications. It was also stated that all necessary measures were taken after the initiation of oral intake in the first day after surgery because of suspicion of esophageal perforation and that the patient was referred to an advanced healthcare facility. The institution came to the conclusion that "the complications caused by the incidence were not mild to be eliminated by simple medical treatment, and diagnosis of the physician and complications that arose as a result of the surgery were in accordance with medical principles."

On the other hand, it was also noted that the report of the Institution of Forensic Medicine was not binding but that it should be considered as an evidence to be considered together with other evidence. Upon the assessment of patient's claims, defense of the doctor, and all medical information and documents, it was ruled that an expert opinion from specialist doctors in the university must be obtained to detect the causes of the two injuries above suspicion.

24.3.2 Discussion

Expert opinion. The legal doctrine requires consulting a specialist or an expert opinion in cases beyond legal knowledge and experience where special and technical knowledge is the absolute source required for the revelation of truth and conclusion of a lawsuit. The regulations on expertise are mentioned in respective articles of the Code of Criminal Procedure, which states that "where a special or technical knowledge for the solution of some cases is required, it may be decided to obtain the vote of an expert…."

The decision to appoint an expert is left to the court. The Institution of Forensic Medicine (IFM), Supreme Council of Health (SCH), universities, and medical chambers are authorized institutions of expertise in Turkish Republic.

IFM was founded in 1982 in affiliation with the Ministry of Justice. It houses specialization boards (SB) and specialization departments. Along with providing routine forensic medicine services in forensic cases, it provides scientific and technical opinions on subjects upon the demands of judges and prosecutors, and it also conducts studies on forensic medicine and forensic sciences and provides training programs.

SCH functions as an official panel of experts in malpractice offenses in accordance with the decree number 1219. It was founded within the body of the Ministry to present expert opinion to courts on forensic cases in reference to practice of healthcare professionals and to compile a list of experts to be assigned for administrative investigations and the commissions of conciliation. The decisions rendered by the Supreme Council of Health are not binding for criminal courts.

According to the Code of Criminal Procedure, the Department of Forensic Medicine and other related branches in universities are considered as official experts for the resolution of forensic cases and other forensic issues in accordance with Institution of Forensic Medicine decree number 2659 article 31.

Furthermore, a patient who is harmed or claims to be harmed by malpractice or the patient's relative or a legal representative has the right to file a petition to the medical chambers. The executive board and discipline committee of the medical chambers are in charge of such matters.

Experts and panel of experts are obliged to be unprejudiced and professionally competent. The Code of Civil Procedure takes precautions against prejudices by having the experts to take an oath: "I will perform my duty of expertise impartially and objectively with loyalty and care in accordance with science" [5, 11, 15–18].

In a study conducted by Erkol et al. that retrospectively reviewed expert reports issued by the Third SB of the Institution of Forensic Medicine on unwanted outcomes associated with thyroid surgery between 2006 and 2009, 28 cases were identified, and 10 of them were hypoparathyroidism, 7 were unilateral vocal cord paralysis, 5 were bilateral vocal cord paralysis, 3 were hematoma, and 1 was hematoma plus bilateral vocal cord paralysis plus esophageal injury. In all of the cases, informed consents of the patients were obtained. Three cases were detected to be death from hematoma plus respiratory difficulty. When the expert reports were reviewed, analyses (thyroid function tests, thyroid ultrasonography, thyroid scintigraphy, FNAC), outcomes, and histopathological diagnoses following the surgery were evaluated to investigate whether indications to perform surgery were accurate, and expert decision ruled that six cases were of malpractice [17].

24.3.3 Follow-Up and Outcome

Although judicial decision is final in lawsuits of medical issues, expert reports based on scientific and evidence-based investigations are of prime importance in court decision. Since differentiation between complications and malpractice is only possible through a complete expert investigation, accurate and objective expertise by physicians specialized in their fields make a significant contribution to the administration of justice.

According to the law of the Turkish Republic, reports issued by the Institution of Forensic Medicine are not considered to be binding; rather they are taken as an evidence to be investigated.

At this case, it was ruled that a panel of experts composed of specialist physicians in the university were to issue an expert report to determine if there is any case of negligence or malpractice, and if the case involves negligence, the causal relation should be established.

What Can We Learn from This Case?

- Appealing to expert opinion is required in conditions where resolution of the case necessitates special or technical knowledge.
- Appealing to expert opinion in medical issues is an obligation according to the law and judicial decisions.
- Differentiation between complications and malpractice is only possible through a thorough expert investigation.
- The Third SB of the Institution of Forensic Medicine, Supreme Council of Health, Departments of Forensic Medicine and General Surgery in the universities, and medical chambers are authorized bodies of expertise in Turkey.

24.4 Case 4: Missing Informed Consent

24.4.1 Case Presentation [13]

A patient who underwent goiter surgery filed a lawsuit against the physician and claimed material and moral indemnities because of permanent vocal damage after surgery for which the patient's consent was taken with a simple consent form. As a result of expert investigation, physician was not found negligent for the damage, and the outcome was considered a complication.

Nevertheless, forensic medicine specialist investigating the case found the physician negligent for providing the patient with insufficient information regarding the surgery, even though the physician might not be regarded negligent in terms of medical intervention.

24.4.2 Discussion

Informed consent, which is one of the code of conducts of good medical practice, represents patients' acceptance or rejection of medical or surgical intervention with his/her free will and without enforcement [19]. Informed consent, defined in the documents of universal medical ethics, is protected by the Constitution of the Republic of Turkey (article 17), Turkish Penal Code (articles 86 and 89), Turkish Civil Code (articles 23 and 24), Turkish Code of Obligations (articles 41, 45–47), and various articles of the regulations on Patient Rights of the Ministry of Health as well as international legal documents such as Universal Declaration of Human Rights and European Convention on Human Rights. Through this right, the individual has the authority to make decisions regarding his/her own body [4, 5, 13].

Informed consent is a process of communication based on trust between the physician and the patient in terms of its dynamics and principles rather than a spontaneous occurrence [9, 20]. As one of the four basic principles of biomedical ethics, this right arises with respect to "autonomy," and it primarily requires that the patient should have the capacity to comprehend the given information. For the patient to make a completely autonomous decision, he/she must be informed of all treatment methods with pros and cons with a plain language, and the patient must be provided with sufficient time to think. Furthermore, mental capacities of the patient should also be adequate to reason, process, and make decisions. The fulfillment of these principles is under direct and/or indirect responsibility of the physician [21]. In this regard, there is a misconception in Turkey that general consent form signed by the patient upon admission to the hospital would be sufficient. However, open consent requires that the patient is informed of "each and every medical intervention."

Main prerequisites of informed consent include disclosure of information to the patient, ability of the patient to understand the information provided, voluntariness, ability of the patient to provide consent, and supervision of the patient's competency by the information provider and giving authorization. Information that should be disclosed to the patient include health status and diagnosis of the patient, type of recommended treatment, likelihood of treatment success and its duration, potential risks of the treatment to the patient's health, use of prescribed medications and possible side effects, possible outcomes in case the patient refuses the proposed treatment, and alternative treatment options and their risks [9].

Any consent obtained before fulfillment of physician's responsibility to disclose and subsequent medical intervention would be considered as a violation of the patient's rights to self-determination for which the physician is held liable. There are other decisions by the Supreme Court and Council of State in which physicians were convicted to indemnity because of their failure to fulfill their responsibility to provide information. Such decisions even date back to 1977 [3–6, 13].

Negligence. According to Turkish Code of Obligations, an agency contract exists between patient and physician. Articles 386–390 of the Turkish Code of Obligations establish that the agent is responsible for his/her inadequate efforts to reach the intended result. The objective responsibility of the physician to fulfill the duty of care involves standard precautions and attention applicable to the health conditions of the country. The duty of loyalty and care obliges the physician to protect the well-being of the patient and avoid practices that might be hazardous to the patient. It also implies that the physician should possess and practice the generally acclaimed and standardized principles and take all necessary precautions. In other words, it requires the physician to hold the patient's interest over his/her own interests [3–7, 9, 13].

24.4.3 Follow-Up and Outcome

The physician was found not to be negligent although the lawsuit was filed against physician's negligence; however, the violation of disclosure by the physician became a matter of dispute, printed informed consent form was not regarded as sufficient, and it was ruled that the burden of proof of disclosure was the physician's responsibility and that informed consent form did not necessarily imply disclosure.

Supreme Court ruled that "The physician as an agent is responsible for all acts of negligence even if minor based on the civil liability of the physician, and burden of accuracy. The physician is obliged to fulfill all professional provisions to avoid any hazard to the patient, promptly ascertain the medical condition of the patient, take complete precautions necessitated by the case and administer the adequate treatment methods."

During the course of the trial, the physician claimed to obtain the written informed consent from the patient and verbally informed the patient regarding the surgery; the court deemed the defense invalid and claimed that disclosure principle was not fulfilled because of the absence of written consent. The 13th Civil Chamber of the Supreme Court affirmed the indemnity verdict given by the district court because of failure to fulfill the principles of disclosure.

The court decision indicated the failure to provide sufficient information regarding the potential complications during and after surgery.

The patient's lawyer claimed compensation through the guidance of the medical examiner, and the court sentenced the physician to pay compensation for his failure to fulfill his responsibility to disclosure.

What Can We Learn from This Case?

- It is the physician's primary responsibility to provide information to the patient regarding the disease and appropriate treatment options.
- Disclosure is a different notion from providing information. A didactic interview with the patient using technical terms will only provide superficial information to the patient.
- Ensuring that the patient understands the provided information and mentally participates in the process and obtaining written document only thereafter will support patient-physician relationship and protect the physician against legal issues.

24.5 Case 5: Statute of Limitations [22]

24.5.1 Case Presentation

The patient suffering from vocal cord paralysis 2 years after goiter surgery sued the physician for delaying necessary treatment after surgery, claiming that no information was provided regarding the consequences, that multiple interventions were made to the surgical site, and that finally he/she had to have a microphone inserted because of vocal cord paralysis. The patient claimed material and moral indemnities from the surgeon.

The defendants filed a motion to dismiss claiming the physician was not negligent and the statute of limitation was expired. The court dismissed the case on the grounds that statute of limitation expired; and the plaintiffs appealed the decision.

The lawsuit was refiled for compensation against negligence by the hospital and the physician during the surgery and treatment process, and the accusation was based on the failure to fulfill duty of care arising from agency contract.

The court ruled the verdict with the following justification: "The plaintiff patient underwent emergency surgery at a training and research hospital 18 months after goiter surgery and was discharged after tracheostomy." The patient discovered 18 months after initial surgery that he/she suffered hazard. Therefore, the plaintiff was entitled to file a lawsuit at the time of discovery of the hazard, and the statute of limitation began before the time of discovering the hazard, and that discovery of the hazard was sufficient for the statute of limitation to begin.

24.5.2 Discussion

Claims for damage are filed for the compensation of hazards arising from the injury by the person liable for the loss. In case of voluntary malpractice or negligence resulting in harm to the patient, the physician liable for the injury is obliged to pay compensations. The following conditions must be met before filing claim for hazards: a wrongful act should be committed, medical interventions must result in an injury, and the injury must be related to negligence [1, 5, 6, 13]. If there is no harm, claim for hazards is invalid.

According to Turkish Code of Obligations number 6098 article 72, statute of limitation in claims for compensations expires after 2 years the plaintiff ascertains the hazard and 10 years after the date the liable party performs the deed that causes the hazard. The expiration of the statute begins upon recognition of the deed which is against the contract. However, expiration of the statute begins at the time of actual injury if there are any visible and detectable injuries such as falling into a vegetative state and loss of limbs/organs [2, 5, 6].

The insurance coverage protecting the professionals against claims for injuries caused by medical interventions occurring during provision of medical services is called professional liability insurance. In 2004, the Prime Ministry Undersecretariat of Treasury General Directorate of Insurance authorized to regulate general requirements of the policyholders in Turkey established professional liability insurance. Expert Committee also covers physicians. The committee outlined the general requirements, published in the Official Gazette Number 26110 in January 16, 2006. Medical Professionals Liability Insurance became valid in September 21, 2006. From 2006 onward, physicians started being insured by the insurance companies through policies designed according to various risk levels. Depending on the insurance coverage, the risk is considered actual simultaneously as the policyholder discovers the claim for compensation or as the damaged party directly appeals to the insurance company [2, 5, 6, 18].

24.5.3 Follow-Up and Outcome

The patient sued the physician for delaying necessary treatment after surgery, claiming that no information was provided regarding the consequences, multiple interventions were made to the surgical site, and finally he/she had to have a microphone inserted because of vocal cord paralysis.

The patient filed a lawsuit and claimed material and moral indemnities because of negligence of the hospital and the physician during surgery and treatment.

The accusation was based on the failure to fulfill duty of care arising from the agency contract. In this concrete incidence, the statute of limitations began to expire after the discovery of the problem by the patient, which is 18 months after surgery. The relation between the two parties is based on the agency contract. Claims related to the agency contract are subject to 5-year statute of limitations. It was ruled that dismissal of charges because of statute of limitations is non-procedural and against the law and requires dismissal.

What Can We Learn from This Case?

- A physician can be held liable by private law for negligence while practicing medicine.
- Medical interventions and lawsuits are filed for the compensation of hazards arising from the injury by the person liable for the loss.
- The physician liable for the injury is obliged to pay compensations in case the patient is injured by voluntary malpractice or negligence.
- The statute of limitation begins to expire when the patient discovered the problem.
- If there is no harm, claim for hazards is invalid. The insurance coverage protecting the professionals against claims for injuries caused by medical interventions occurring during provision of medical services is called professional liability insurance.

References

1. Erdem Ü. Yargıtay 12. Ceza dairesi (2014–2016) kararlarında hekimin sorumluluğu (Physician's liability in decisions by 12th civil chamber of supreme court), Hukuk Kitapları Serisi. 1st ed. İstanbul: Legal Yayıncılık; 2016. p.109–10, 293–5, 328–9.
2. Savaş H. Yargıya yansıyan tıbbi müdahale hataları. tıbbi malpraktis-tıbbi davaların seyri ve sonuçları (Medical errors. Medical malpractice – the course and outcome of medical lawsuits). 3rd ed. Ankara: Seçkin Yayıncılık; 2013. p. 25–70, 181–228.
3. Oral T. Hekimin aydınlatma ve hastanın rızasını alma yükümü. http://www.ankarabarosu.org.tr/siteler/ankarabarosu/tekmakale/2011-2/2011-2-8.pdf. Accessed 20 Apr 2017.
4. Çakmut ÖY. Sağlık hukukunun temel esasları ve özellikle aydınlatılmış onam. Tıbbi müdahaleden kaynaklanan hukuki sorumluluk. Sempozyum Bildiri Kitabı [Physician's liability to disclosure and receive patient's consent]. Ankara: Mersin Barosu; 2009. p. 1–40.
5. Doğan M. Hekimin hukuki sorumluluğu. Tıbbi müdahaleden kaynaklanan hukuki sorumluluk. Sempozyum Bildiri Kitabı [Civil liabilities of the

physician. Liabilities arising from medical interventions]. Ankara: Mersin Barosu; 2009. p. 41–60.
6. Hakeri H. Tıp Hukuku (medical jurisprudance). Ankara: Seçkin Yayıncılık; 2007. p. 93–185, 289–388.
7. TC. Yargıtay 13. Hukuk Dairesi Esas No:2013/23012 Karar No:2014/22561. http://www.hukukmedeniyeti.org/ictihatyazdir.asp?id=612. Accessed 20 Apr 2017.
8. World Medical Association. Statement on medical malpractice. Santiago: WMA; 2005. http://www.wma.net/en/30publications/10policies/20archives/m2/index.html. Accessed 20 Apr 2017.
9. Türk Tabipleri Birliği. Aydınlatılmış Onam Kılavuzu (Turkish Medical Association. Informed consent manual). Madde 26. 2013. http://www.ttb.org.tr/mevzuat/index.php?option=com_content&view=article&id=983:onam&Itemid=65. Accessed 18 Apr 2017.
10. Buzzacchi L, Scellato G, Ughetto E. Frequency of medical malpractice claims: the effects of volumes and specialties. Soc Sci Med. 2016;170:152–60. https://doi.org/10.1016/j.socscimed.2016.10.021.
11. Üzün İ, Özdemir E, Melez İE, Melez DO, Akçakaya A. Evaluation of medical malpractice in emergency and elective general surgery cases resulting in death. Ulus Travma Acil Cerrahi Derg. 2016;22:365–73. https://doi.org/10.5505/tjtes.2015.26543.
12. http://www.medimagazin.com.tr/ana-sayfa/kategorisiz/tr-guatr-ameliyati-sonrasi-olum-davasi-1-666-3460.html. Accessed 18 Apr 2017.
13. Hakeri H. Yargıtayın Aydınlatma Konusundaki Son Kararı ve Bu Kararın Sonuçları (Final decision by the Supreme Court on disclosure and its outcomes). http://www.medimagazin.com.tr/authors/hakan-hakeri/tr-yargitayin-aydinlatma-konusundaki-son-karari-ve-bu-kararin-sonuclari-72-64-1815.html. Accessed 05 Jan 2017.
14. Dralle H, Schneider R, Lorenz K, Phuong NT, Sekulla C, Machens A. Vocal cord paralysis after thyroid surgery: current medicolegal aspects of intraoperative neuromonitorin. Chirurg. 2015;86:698–706. https://doi.org/10.1007/s00104-015-0033-9.
15. Singer MC, Iverson KC, Terris DJ. Thyroidectomy-related malpractice claims. Otolaryngol Head Neck Surg. 2012;146(3):358–61. https://doi.org/10.1177/0194599811430898.
16. Karakaya MA, Koç O, Ekiz F, Ağaçhan AF, Göret NE. İstanbul Adli Tıp Kurumu tarafından 2008-21012 yılları arasında tiroidektomi sırasında gelişen rekürren laringeal sinir yaralanmaları nedeni ile verilen bilirkişi kararlarının irdelenmesi (Evaluation of expert reports provided by the Institution of Forensic Medicine (IFM) for recurrent laryngeal nerve paralysis during thyroidectomy between 2008-2012). Ulus Cerrahi Derg. 2016;32:43–6.
17. Erkol Z, Ertan A, Gökdoğan C, Kadıoğlu P, Yavuz N, Erkol H, et al. İstenmeyen Sonuçlar Gelişmesi Nedeniyle Dava Konusu Olan Tiroidektomi Olgularının Retrospektif Değerlendirilmesi (retrospective evaluation of thyroidectomy incidences in dispute due to unwanted outcomes). Türkiye Klinikleri J Med. 2012;32:130–8.
18. Tümer AR. Tıp mensupları için hukuki yönleri ile adli bilirkişilik (Forensic expertise for medical proffesionals). İstanbul: Matsis Matbaa; 2013. p. 13–6, 93–104.
19. Hanson M, Pitt D. Informed consent for surgery: risk discussion and documentation. Can J Surg. 2017;60(1):69–70.
20. Childress JF, Beauchamp TL. The concept of autonomy and the principle of respect of autonomy. In: Childress JF, Beauchamp TL, editors. Principles of biomedical ethics. 7th ed. New York: Oxford; 2013. p. 101–14.
21. Childress JF, Beauchamp TL. The capacity of autonomous choice. In: Childress JF, Beauchamp TL, editors. Principles of biomedical ethics. 7th ed. New York: Oxford; 2013. p. 114–20.
22. http://hastahukuku.com/yargitayk.php?recordID. Accessed 05 Jan 2017.

25 Application of Ultrasound by the Surgeon in Thyroid-Parathyroid Surgery

Güldeniz Karadeniz Çakmak

Abstract

In general ultrasound (USG) serves as the first-line imaging modality for diseases of the thyroid and parathyroid gland. Currently, in the hands of a surgeon, USG not only provides invaluable data about nodular thyroid disease and parathyroid adenomas but plays a crucial role in the preoperative and intraoperative setting to design minimal-sized incisions for the best cosmetic effect and to guide invasive procedures with higher diagnostic accuracy. Moreover, routine use of USG after positioning results in designing the most appropriate incision for focused parathyroidectomy. The confirmatory USG scanning of the neck region by the surgeon after removal of the predicted lesion is of paramount importance acting as an insurance policy for the surgeon. Beyond the initial diagnosis, in recurrent malignant cases, the surgeon-performed intraoperative USG is a safe way to detect and visualize nonpalpable, subcentimeter lymph nodes in an adequate fashion which is otherwise a great dilemma for the surgeon. As for the issue of recurrence in a previously dissected compartment, surgeon-performed intraoperative USG directed focused dissection is one of the best approaches warranted. The most critical point to be emphasized is that surgeon-performed thyroid, and parathyroid USG requires training, validation, experience, and establishment of competency.

G. K. Çakmak
Division of Breast and Endocrin Surgery, Bülent Ecevit Üniversity, Zonguldak, Turkey

25.1 Case Presentations

Case 1

A 50-year-old female with a history of thyroidectomy 27 years ago was referred to the endocrine department for the evaluation of hypercalcemia of unclear etiology. Her medical history revealed weakness, joint pain, vague abdominal pain, easy fatigability, and depression and was notable for recurrent nephrolithiasis since the age of 25. Physical examination was proven to be unremarkable, and she was not under any medication. A complete laboratory scan was performed, which demonstrated increased albumin-adjusted serum calcium level (11.3 mg/dl) with elevated parathormone (PTH) (137.7 pg/mL) indicating the diagnosis of primary hyperparathyroidism (PHPT). The rest of her biochemistry results were insignificant. Her neck ultrasound (USG) revealed a normal-sized thyroid gland and a 4.2 × 10.1 × 12 mm hypoechoic mass located on the right lower side of her cervical region suspicious for a parathyroid adenoma (Fig. 25.1). Further examination with 99m Tc-MIBI parathyroid scintigraphy depicted nothing significant.

T. Özülker et al. (eds.), *Thyroid and Parathyroid Diseases*, https://doi.org/10.1007/978-3-319-78476-2_25

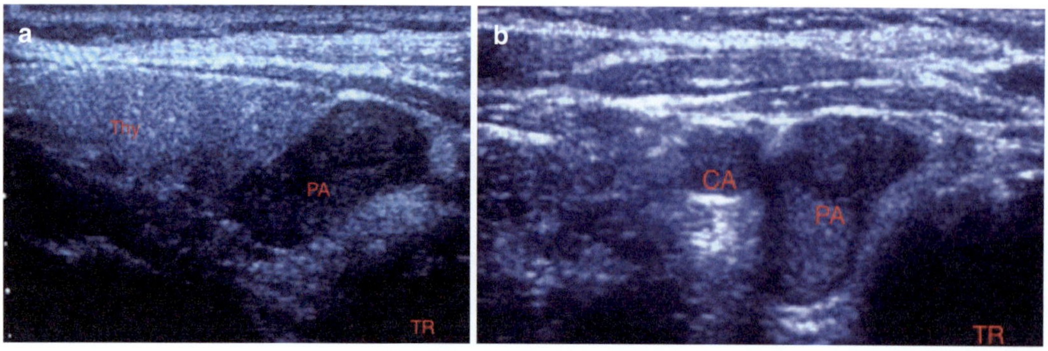

Fig. 25.1 Longitudinal sonographic view of parathyroid adenoma (**a**), transverse sonographic view of parathyroid adenoma (**b**). *PA* parathyroid adenoma, *Thy* thyroid gland, *CA* carotid artery

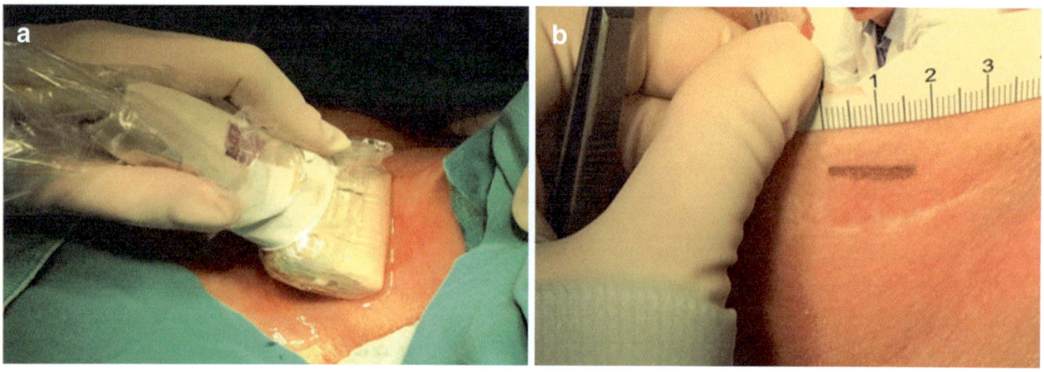

Fig. 25.2 Surgeon-performed pre-incision ultrasound after positioning (**a**), marking best position for a minimally invasive parathyroidectomy incision (**b**)

Preoperatively, the surgeon-performed ultrasound-guided fine needle aspiration (FNA) washout was performed, and elevated PTH level (>3384.4 mg/dl) confirmed the diagnosis. She was discussed in endocrine board and scheduled for focused parathyroidectomy without intraoperative PTH (IOPTH) monitoring which was unavailable. In theater, after positioning, a surgeon-performed pre-incision USG to locate the best position for a minimally invasive parathyroidectomy incision was performed (Fig. 25.2). The parathyroid adenoma was successfully removed, and intraoperative sonography of the area confirmed excision. Following surgery, PTH was normalized (39.4 pg/ml), hypocalcemia developed (7.8 mg/dl), and treatment with calcium and calcitriol was started to stabilize normocalcemia. The pathologic diagnosis was reported to be parathyroid adenoma. The follow-up period was uneventful without recurrence within 2 years.

Case 2

A 55-year-old female with a history of thyroidectomy 20 years ago presented to her primary care physician with progressive neck swelling and referred to our clinic for evaluation. She suffered no associated symptoms such as voice changes, hoarseness, and systemic-type symptoms. The patient was without any history of radiation exposure or family history of thyroid cancer. At physical examination, thyroid was enlarged, with an irregular surface and multiple discrete nodules in the right and left lobes with the greatest dimension of 1 cm. No cervical lymphadenopathy was clinically noted. The remaining of the physical examination was unremarkable. An ultrasound of the neck revealed bilateral residual thyroid gland

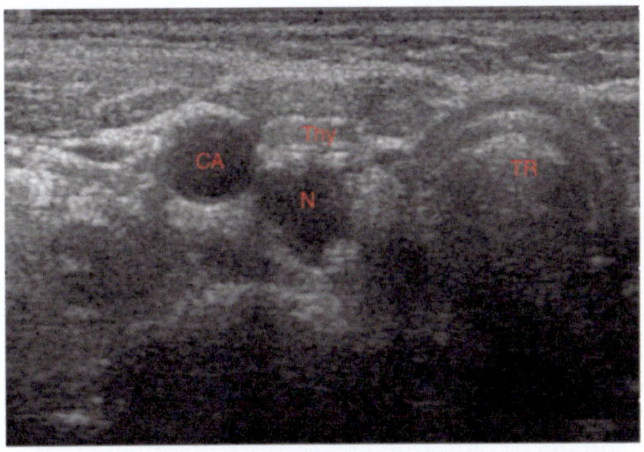

Fig. 25.3 A hypoechoic nodule with irregular lobulated margins located in the lower right lobe. *CA* carotid artery, *Thy* thyroid gland, *N* nodule, *TR* trachea

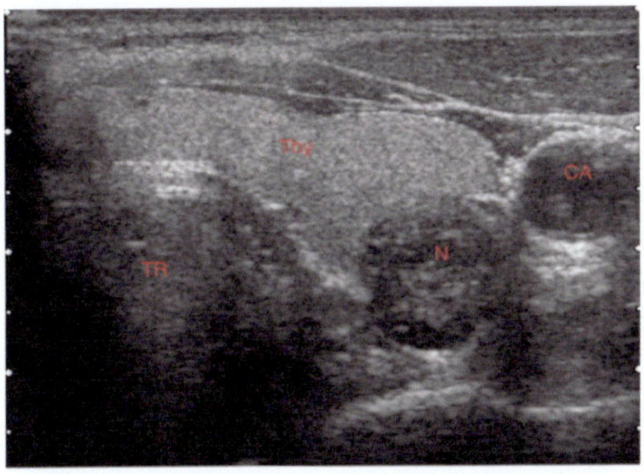

Fig. 25.4 A hypoechoic heterogeneous nodule with lobulated margins and central microcalcifications together with peripheral patchy rim calcifications located in the lower pole of the left lobe. *CA* carotid artery, *Thy* thyroid gland, *N* nodule, *TR* trachea

with a size of 21 × 18 × 18 mm on the right and 20 × 11 × 17 mm on the left side with enlarging nodules possessing calcifications. Two heterogeneous solid nodules were determined in the right lobe, the largest of which is located in the lower pole measured 12 × 10 × 8 mm with lobulated margins and hypoechogenicity (Fig. 25.3). The second nodule was located in the mid-pole measured <1 cm in size without worrisome sonographic features. The left lobe contained a third hypoechoic nodule with a size of 15 × 12 × 10 mm, was located in the lower pole, and had lobulated margins with central microcalcifications and peripheral patchy rim calcifications (Fig. 25.4). No pathologic lymph node was noted in the neck. The surgeon-performed USG-guided FNA of these nodules revealed adenomatoid nodule in the right lobe and highly suspicious features for papillary carcinoma in the left lobe. She was subsequently offered total thyroidectomy. In the theater, after positioning, surgeon-performed USG of the neck was performed, and suspicious nodules were marked to design incision according to real-time sonographic data of the diseased gland (Fig. 25.5). Completion thyroidectomy was followed by sonographic evaluation of operative field to confirm no residual disease had been left behind. The histopathologic evaluation confirmed the diagnosis of papillary cancer at the left-sided nodule with the largest diameter of 15 mm without extrathyroidal extension. She proceeded to receive radioactive iodine ablation therapy under rhTSH stimulation and was administered suppressive doses of levothyroxine to maintain a TSH of <0.01 mIU/L. Her post-therapy whole-body 131-I scan noted no radioiodine uptake in the thyroid bed. Her stimulated thyroglobulin was 2.0 ng/mL, and thyroglobulin antibody was <20 IU/mL. Two years

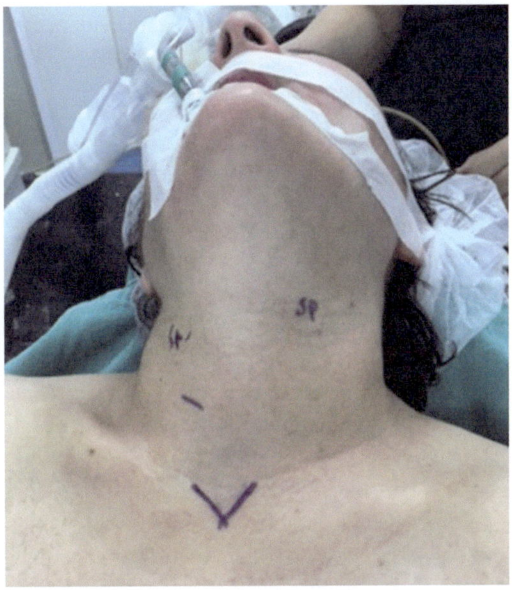

Fig. 25.5 Surgeon-performed USG of the neck after positioning to mark suspicious nodules to design the most appropriate incision according to real-time sonographic data of the diseased gland and peripheral anatomic landmarks

after initial surgery, she showed no evidence of local recurrence or distant metastases. Neck USG was also unremarkable.

25.2 Discussion

USG is accepted as the first-line imaging modality for diseases of thyroid and parathyroid gland by radiologists [1]. As technological improvement made it possible to achieve higher-resolution devices with low costs, USG has gained an important role in clinical management of the neck in the hands of nonradiologists, particularly surgeons. In the routine examination, USG not only provides invaluable data about nodular thyroid disease, parathyroid adenomas, cervical lymph nodes, head and neck masses outside of the central compartment, or residual disease but serves as a beneficial preoperative and intraoperative tool to design minimal-sized incisions for the best cosmetic effect and to guide invasive procedures with higher diagnostic accuracy [2]. The clinical features of parathyroid adenoma are primarily due to hypercalcemia, and therefore the challenge to the clinician is to make diagnosis and the surgeon is to accurately predict the location to allow minimally invasive surgery. More than 85% of cases of primary hyperparathyroidism are caused by a single adenoma, and less frequently, it can be caused by double adenomas, multigland hyperplasia, or rarely parathyroid carcinoma [3]. In the past, the conventional operation for primary hyperparathyroidism was a bilateral neck exploration (BNE), with improvement in preoperative localizing studies such as USG, technetium-99m-sestamibi with single-photon computed tomography (SPECT), and four-dimensional computed tomography, along with the use of intraoperative parathyroid hormone monitoring and minimally invasive interventions like focused parathyroidectomy, emerged as an acceptable alternative to the standard BNE with shorter operative time and reduced surgical morbidity [4, 5]. The accuracy of USG is similar or superior to that of sestamibi-SPECT, particularly when performed by surgeon, at 70–87% [6, 7]. Concomitant thyroid pathology, including thyroid cancer and benign nodules, is identified on USG in 30–50% of patients with primary hyperparathyroidism [8], and USG-guided FNA also may be used to aspirate suspected adenomas for confirmation. Series demonstrate that concordant sestamibi-SPECT and USG have operative cure rates up to 99%, suggesting that this may be an alternative to IOPTH monitoring [9]. Currently, office-based or theater portable ultrasound without exposing patients to radiation and costing less than nuclear medicine or multidimensional studies is the primary diagnostic and localizing tool to guide surgeons for focused operation [10]. Preoperative USG-directed FNA biopsy of parathyroid lesions is highly specific but can have undesirable consequences [11]. Therefore, this technique should be reserved for selected cases. One of the other advantages of surgeon-performed USG is to allow sampling in case of equivocal sonographic findings and sestamibi scan, either in recurrent disease or to make distinction between thyroid and parathyroid pathologies following previous neck surgery. In the first case that we presented, we performed USG-guided FNA to confirm the lesion was a parathyroid adenoma, since parathyroid scintigraphy depicted nothing significant and IOPTH measurement was not available. However, it should be emphasized that FNA should be avoided regarding any suspicion of malignant disease.

Analogously, surgeon-performed USG serves as an invaluable tool for thyroid disease. After the discovery of a thyroid nodule, evaluation for malignancy is necessary to determine appropriate management recommendations. FNA is the gold standard method to make diagnosis. The malignancy risk in nondiagnostic or unsatisfactory samples is 1–4%. Repeated aspiration of the nodule with USG guidance should lead to a diagnostic result in 50–88% of cases [12]. The surgeon-performed USG guidance increases the accuracy of FNA of thyroid nodules [2]. Moreover, there is a great enthusiasm on performing thyroidectomies through minimal-sized incisions for the best cosmetic outcome. The preoperative real-time localization of thyroid gland can aid in designing minimal-sized incisions by means of predicting technical issues before operation. In the operative setting, after positioning, pre-incision ultrasound is useful to real-time locate the best position for thyroid and parathyroid exploration. Routine use of USG after patients are positioned on the operating table also results in designing the most appropriate incision for focused parathyroidectomy. The confirmatory scanning of the neck region by surgeon after removal of the predicted lesion is of paramount importance. Since parathyroid adenomas are very tiny lesions with fatty appearance, surgeon should be secure by means of sonographic visualization of the area demonstrating that the adenoma is successfully removed. Another advantage of surgeon-performed USG is that it can frequently identify an intrathyroidal parathyroid gland not easily detected by other modalities (Fig. 25.6) and provide opportunity to perform FNA at the same time without multiple hospital visits or appointments [10]. In thyroid surgery, sonographic scanning demonstrates the location of superior and inferior poles with respect to anatomic landmarks, including cricoid and thyroid cartilages, hyoid bone, and the clavicles for technically the most comfortable incision to be placed [1]. The extension of the neck can be evaluated and modified based on real-time objective, individualized position of the lobes to improve access to superior extension of the gland.

Another critical issue to be emphasized is the lymph node status of the neck. Routine preoperative sonographic imaging of the cervical nodal basins changes the extent of surgery up to 40% of patients in case of malignancy [13]. The surgeon-performed USG of neck compartments is very crucial to determine pathologic lymph node presence regarding the malignant disease. A definitive diagnosis of malignancy in a cervical lymph node is best obtained by ultrasound-guided FNA biopsy [14]. In theater, pre-incision USG of the neck compartments for metastatic lymph node localization can also be very beneficial to the operating surgeon. Moreover, intraoperative USG after the completion of neck dissection to determine residual disease or to confirm the absence of metastatic lymph nodes possesses great value for the surgeon, as an adjunct [15]. One of the most crucial contributions of USG in the operative setting is in case of recurrence in a previously dissected compartment. Surgeon-performed intraoperative USG guidance is the best way to plan and direct the approach and extend the dissection for recurrent disease [16, 17]. Surgical anatomy of the neck is complex. USG becomes increasingly effective when performed by the operating surgeon, owing to the familiarity of the surgical anatomy. The real-time images that can be taken in multiple planes and compared with surrounding anatomy allow a more comprehensive and detailed assessment of structures to discriminate thyroid nodules from parathyroid adenoma or a metastatic lymph node. Recurrent and persistent primary hyperparathyroidism has been called the bête noir of the endocrine surgeon. In case of recurrence after minimally invasive parathyroidectomy, surgeon-performed USG of the neck and FNA of any suspicious structure for localization may predict the initial landmark area to begin

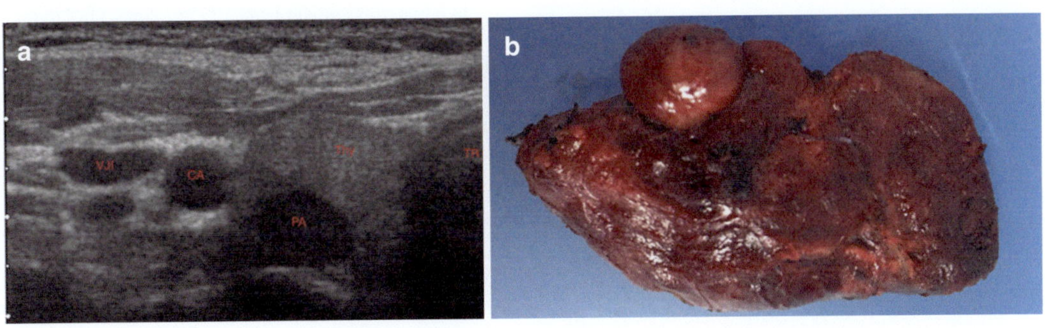

Fig. 25.6 Sonographic view of an intrathyroidal parathyroid gland (**a**), specimen view of intrathyroidal parathyroid adenoma (**b**). *CA* carotid artery, *Thy* thyroid gland, *TR* trachea, *PA* parathyroid adenoma, *VJI* vena jugularis inferior

neck exploration. Moreover, surgeon-performed USG-guided FNA with higher reported rates of accuracy is another advantage of the procedure [2]. After thyroid surgery for malignant disease, the sonographic evaluation of the neck by surgeon allows the imaging and localization to be performed by the same individual who has performed the surgery. Unfortunately, neck recurrence is a common scenario in papillary thyroid cancer. Beyond the initial diagnosis, the usefulness of surgeon-performed USG for surgical planning just before incision after positioning in recurrent cases is of paramount importance. Properly removing nonpalpable, subcentimeter lymph nodes based on only macroscopic visual features adequately is a dilemma for the surgeon. Therefore, in the course of surveillance for papillary thyroid cancer, sonographically suspicious lymph nodes should be interrogated with FNA biopsy. The aspirate may be assayed for thyroglobulin to increase the sensitivity and specificity for metastatic disease. When a nodal recurrence is found in a previously dissected central or lateral neck field, the reoperation should focus on the areas where recurrence is demonstrated [15]. As for the issue of recurrence in a previously dissected compartment, surgeon-performed intraoperative USG directed focused dissection is the best approach warranted [17].

What Can We Learn from This Case?

- The surgeon-performed USG is a specific tool for defining and determining thyroid and parathyroid disease.
- For the operative surgeon, USG has a significant role to play in the operating room providing accurate, informative, and more comprehensive evaluation of thyroid, parathyroid, and lymph node diseases.
- Thyroid and parathyroid USG require training, validation, experience, and establishment of competency.
- The surgeon-performed USG is an invaluable tool to explore the neck for thyroid and parathyroid pathology, to serve as a guide for FNA, to design incision after positioning for either benign or malignant thyroid disease, to determine pathologic lymph nodes that are clinically not evident, to determine residual disease after compartmental dissection with the aim of N0 neck, to act as a guide in minimally invasive parathyroidectomy, to localize parathyroid adenoma, and to confirm the resection after intervention.
- The surgeon-performed USG in the preoperative, operative, and postoperative setting is nothing more than a stethoscope of a clinician, which clarifies anatomic boundaries in a real-time fashion and valuable adjunct to benign and malignant endocrine surgical practice.
- The surgeon-performed neck USG benefits patient care and impacts surgical decisions.

References

1. Coltera MD. Clinician-performed thyroid ultrasound. Otolaryngol Clin N Am. 2014;47:491–507. https://doi.org/10.1016/j.otc.2014.04.001.
2. Karadeniz Cakmak G, Emre AU, Tascilar O, Gultekin FA, Ozdamar SO, Comert M. Diagnostic adequacy of surgeon-performed ultrasound-guided fine needle aspiration biopsy of thyroid nodules. J Surg Oncol. 2013;107:206–10. https://doi.org/10.1002/jso.23212.
3. Ruda JM, Hollenbeak CS, Stack BC. A systematic review of the diagnosis and treatment of primary hyperparathyroidism from 1995 to 2003. Otolaryngol Head Neck Surg. 2005;132:359–72.
4. Udelsman R, Lin Z, Donovan P. The superiority of minimally invasive parathyroidectomy based on 1650 consecutive patients with primary hyperparathyroidism. Ann Surg. 2011;253:585–91.
5. Laird AM, Libutti SK. Minimally invasive parathyroidectomy versus bilateral neck exploration for primary hyperparathyroidism. Surg Oncol Clin N Am. 2016;25:103–18.
6. Untch BR, Adam MA, Scheri RP, Bennett KM, Dixit D, Webb C, et al. Surgeon-performed ultrasound is superior to 99Tc-sestamibi scanning to localize parathyroid adenomas in patients with primary hyperparathyroidism: results in 516 patients over 10 years. J

Am Coll Surg. 2011;212:522–9. discussion 529–31. https://doi.org/10.1016/j.jamcollsurg.2010.12.038.
7. Solorzano CC, Carneiro-Pla DM, Irvin GL 3rd. Surgeon-performed ultrasonography as the initial and only localizing study in sporadic primary hyperparathyroidism. J Am Coll Surg. 2006;202:18–24.
8. Morita SY, Somervell H, Umbricht CB, Dackiw AP, Zeiger MA. Evaluation for concomitant thyroid nodules and primary hyperparathyroidism in patients undergoing parathyroidectomy or thyroidectomy. Surgery. 2008;144:862–6. [discussion: 866–8].
9. Suliburk JW, Sywak MS, Sidhu SB, Delbridge LW. 1000 minimally invasive parathyroidectomies without intra-operative parathyroid hormone measurement: lessons learned. ANZ J Surg. 2011;81:362–5.
10. Solorzano CC, Carneiro-Pla D. Minimizing cost and maximizing success in the preoperative localization strategy for primary hyperparathyroidism. Surg Clin North Am. 2014;94:587–605.
11. Wilhelm SM, Wang TS, Ruan DT, Lee JA, Asa SL, Duh QY, et al. The American Association of Endocrine Surgeons guidelines for definitive management of primary hyperparathyroidism. JAMA Surg. 2016;151:959–68. https://doi.org/10.1001/jamasurg.2016.2310.
12. Cibas ES, Ali SZ. The Bethesda system for reporting thyroid cytopathology. Am J Clin Pathol. 2009;132:658–65.
13. Stulak JM, Grant CS, Farley DR, Thompson GB, van Heerden JA, Hay ID. Value of preoperative ultrasonography in the surgical management of initial and reoperative papillary thyroid cancer. Arch Surg. 2006;141:489–94. [discussion: 494–6].
14. Sturgeon C, Yang A, Elaraj D. Surgical management of lymph node compartments in papillary thyroid cancer. Surg Oncol Clin N Am. 2016;25:17–40. https://doi.org/10.1016/j.soc.2015.08.013.
15. Agcaoglu O, Aliyev S, Taskin HE, Aksoy E, Siperstein A, Berber E. The utility of intraoperative ultrasound in modified radical neck dissection: a pilot study. Surg Innov. 2014;21:166–9.
16. McCoy KL, Yim JH, Tublin ME, Burmeister LA, Ogilvie JB, Carty SE. Same-day ultrasound guidance in reoperation for locally recurrent papillary thyroid cancer. Surgery. 2007;142:965–72.
17. Yoo JY, Stang MT. Current guidelines for postoperative treatment and follow-up of well-differentiated thyroid cancer. Surg Oncol Clin N Am. 2016;25:41–59. https://doi.org/10.1016/j.soc.2015.08.002.

Intraoperative Nerve Monitorization 26

Günay Gürleyik and Emin Gürleyik

Abstract

The anatomical integrity of the recurrent laryngeal nerve (RLN) is generally preserved by visual identification, and its exposure is mandatory during thyroid surgery. Intraoperative nerve monitoring (IONM) is used as an adjunct to visual identification to confirm the motor activity of both the RLN and the external branch of the superior laryngeal nerve (EBSLN).

We performed total thyroidectomy for the treatment of hyperthyroidism using IONM for both these nerves. The procedure was started from the dominant left lobe. Pre-dissection stimulation (V1) of the left vagus nerve showed normal function of the intrinsic laryngeal muscles. We could not visually, but could functionally, identify the left EBSLN by IONM. EBSLN stimulation generating cricothyroid muscle (CTM) contraction also induced vocal cord action recorded by nerve monitoring. We identified an extralaryngeal terminal bifurcation of the left RLN. Analysis of sound signal and wave amplitude after predissection (R1) stimulation showed normal motor activity on the anterior branch and sensory function on the posterior branch. Stimulation of the left RLN also induced CTM twitches. At the end of the surgery, postdissection (R2) and (V2) stimulations confirmed proper motor function of the RLN. EBSLN stimulation generated cricothyroid muscle (CTM) contraction revealing the normal function of this branch. The right lobe was also dissected under the guidance of IONM. All stages of monitoring were the same as on the left side, which showed proper function of the nerves at the end of the surgery.

IONM contributes to the identification of the EBSLN and establishes its proper motor function by observation of CTM contraction. It assesses the function of the RLN at the beginning, during, and the end of the surgery, with vocal cord mobility being received by surface electrodes creating a sound signal while recording the waveform amplitude. Based on recordable amplitudes after stimulation of EBSLN and induction of CTM twitches by stimulation of the left RLN, IONM establishes real-time motor interconnections between EBSLN and RLN via laryngeal anastomosis.

G. Gürleyik
Department of Surgery, Haydarpaşa Numune Training and Research Hospital, Istanbul, Turkey

E. Gürleyik (✉)
Department of Surgery, Düzce University, Düzce, Turkey

26.1 Introduction

Intrinsic and extrinsic laryngeal muscles, which are responsible for vocal cord (VCs) movements, are innervated by superior and inferior laryngeal

T. Özülker et al. (eds.), *Thyroid and Parathyroid Diseases*, https://doi.org/10.1007/978-3-319-78476-2_26

nerves. During thyroid surgery, proper function of the laryngeal musculature is the key to avoid any complication that depends on the functional integrity of both the recurrent laryngeal nerve (RLN) and external branch of the superior laryngeal nerve (EBSLN). Their anatomical integrity is generally preserved by visual identification and exposure of the nerves using good surgical technique by experienced surgeons. However, the anatomical integrity of nerve branches does not necessarily guarantee preserved motor function. Intraoperative nerve monitoring (IONM) is used as an adjunct to visual identification to confirm motor activity of the nerves. Electrophysiological stimulation of EBSLN and RLN produced contraction of the laryngeal musculature that establishes the functional integrity of the nerve during thyroid surgery [1–4]. The present case is an example of various steps of IONM and monitoring motor relations between superior and inferior laryngeal nerves.

26.2 Case Presentation

A 64-year-old woman presented to our clinic with symptoms of hyperthyroidism. Blood biochemical analysis showed reduced serum thyroid-stimulating hormone and high free thyroid hormone (FT4 and FT3) levels. Ultrasound and a nuclear scan of the thyroid gland revealed large, solid, hot, and hyperactive nodules in both lobes. Of the two lobes, higher voluminous glandular tissue and more hyperactive nodules were located in the left lobe. Based on these findings, a diagnosis of toxic multinodular goiter was made. We first prescribed methimazole (30 mg/day) as preoperative thyrostatic treatment. Later, the dose was increased to 100 mg/day for normalizing serum hormone levels. We planned on performing total thyroidectomy as the appropriate surgical procedure with the use of IONM for both nerves. IONM was performed using a nerve integrity monitor (NIM-Response 3.0 System; Medtronic Xomed, Jacksonville, FL, USA). The device was used in the following settings: stimulation intensity of 1 mA and amplitude threshold of 100 μV. The nerve integrity monitor was connected to surface electrodes integrated with an endotracheal tube 7.0 which was inserted between VCs under direct vision during intubation.

The procedure was started from the dominant left lobe. After medial traction of the lobe, we incised the neurovascular sheet and identified the vagus nerve (VN) posterior to the common carotid artery and jugular vein. The stimulator probe was directly applied (V1) on VN, and the sound signal was obtained from the device while recording the wave amplitude and latency. After dissection of the inferior pole, we dissected the superior pole of the left lobe under monitoring EBSLN. After lateral and caudal retraction of the upper pole of the thyroid, the upper thyroid vessels were ligated closer to the glandular tissue under nerve monitoring. However, we could not visually identify the left EBSLN. The nerve tract on the constrictor muscle was stimulated (S1) indirectly with an intensity of 1 mA without observation of the physiological response. The intensity was increased to 2 mA, and the nerve tract was restimulated (S1). We macroscopically observed the physiological contraction of the cricothyroid muscle (CTM) while recording its first amplitude. After completing upper pole dissection, final stimulation (S2) was applied on the nerve tract, and the amplitude was recorded while macroscopically observing CTM contraction. After medial mobilization of the left lobe, RLN was identified using the conventional lateral approach. Once RLN was visually identified, it was directly stimulated (R1). The left RLN was then fully isolated and completely exposed, and extralaryngeal terminal bifurcation was observed as an anatomical variation. Later, post-dissection final stimulation (R2) was applied to the main trunk and anterior and posterior branches of RLN (Fig. 26.1). Based on IONM data, the anterior branch was identified as the motor with a positive signal, and the posterior branch was identified as the sensory with no signal. In addition to VC movement, the stimulation (R2) of the left RLN also induced CTM twitches. The left VN was reidentified and restimulated (V2) at the end of surgery. After V1, S1, R1, S2, R2, and V2 stimulations, waveform amplitudes and latencies were recorded separately (Table 26.1).

Dissection of the right lobe: After VN stimulation (V1) and dissection of the inferior pole, we

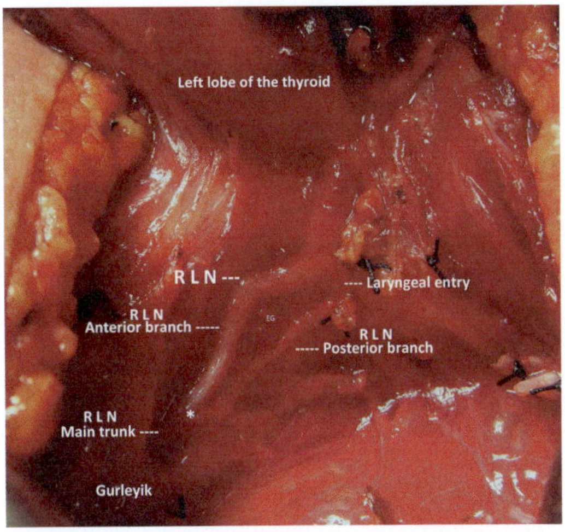

Fig. 26.1 The left recurrent laryngeal nerve (RLN) has extralaryngeal terminal bifurcation. Main trunk is divided at bifurcation point (*): anterior and thinner posterior branches that enter separately into the larynx

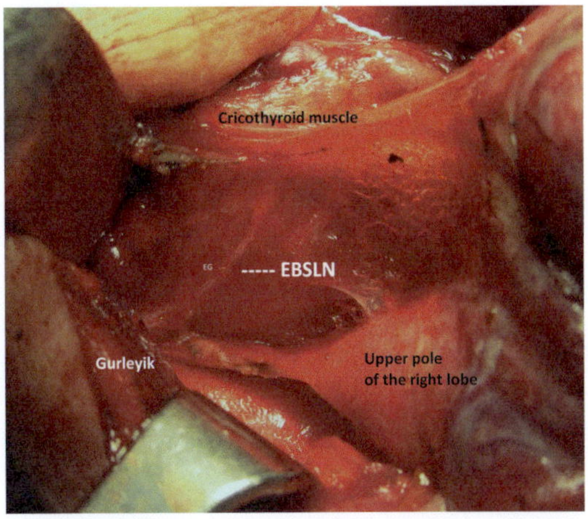

Fig. 26.2 The right external branch of superior laryngeal nerve (EBSLN). Distal part of the nerve branch running on the constrictor muscle is visually identified and fully exposed (Friedmann type 1)

Table 26.1 Results of IONM

Definition	Steps of IONM	Right side		Left side	
		Amplitude (μV)	Latency (mS)	Amplitude (μV)	Latency (mS)
Pre-dissection VN stimulation	V1	746	6.0	593	9.38
Pre-dissection EBSLN stimulation	S1	215	4.63	313	4.38
Pre-dissection RLN stimulation	R1	2044	4.38	1362	4.0
Post-dissection EBSLN stimulation	S2	279	2.88	547	3.63
Post-dissection RLN stimulation	R2	1316	3.5	1759	4.13
Post-dissection VN stimulation	V2	515	6.25	870	9.6

Table 26.2 Anatomical and physiological identification of laryngeal nerves

Anatomical identification and nerve monitoring	Right side	Left side
EBSLN: visual identification	Yes	No
EBSLN: functional identification with CTM contraction by IONM	Yes	Yes
EBSLN: stimulation creating recordable amplitude	Yes	Yes
RLN: visual identification	Yes	Yes
RLN: functional identification with VC movement by IONM	Yes	Yes
RLN: stimulation creating CTM twitch	No	Yes

EBSLN external branch of superior laryngeal nerve, *RLN* recurrent laryngeal nerve

visually identified the right EBSLN (Fig. 26.2) during dissection of the superior pole which was stimulated (S1) directly with an intensity of 1 mA. At the end of pole dissection, EBSLN was restimulated (S2), and we observed contraction of the right CTM. After complete exposure of the right RLN, we observed an uncommon course of the nerve on the lateral surface of the right lobe (Fig. 26.3). All steps of IONM (V1, S1, R1, S2, R2, and V2) were performed similarly on the right side, and waveform amplitudes and latencies were recorded (Table 26.1).

Normal VC action was determined by postoperative video laryngoscopy. At both sides, we performed anatomical identification of the laryngeal nerves (except left EBSLN) by surgical dissection and physiological identification with contraction of the laryngeal musculature using IONM (Table 26.2).

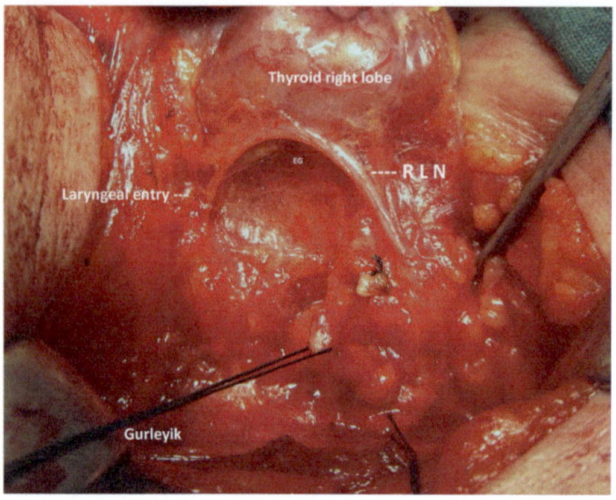

Fig. 26.3 Cervical part of the right recurrent laryngeal nerve is identified and completely exposed; the nerve has a superficial course and is adherent on the lateral surface of the right lobe

26.3 Discussion

In this toxic multinodular goiter case, total thyroidectomy was performed under the guidance of IONM. First, we attempted the dissection of the left lobe that was identified as the dominant lobe after clinical and radiological evaluation. After checking functional integrity by IONM at the left side, we completed total resection uneventfully. The first rule of nerve monitoring is to start the surgery on the dominant lobe that harbors the main pathology. At the end of first lobe dissection, the surgeon checks the functional integrity of RLN by nerve monitoring and proceeds to dissect the contralateral lobe. In case of loss of signal and amplitude (an indicator of VCs palsy) during dissection of the first lobe, surgery of the second lobe may be delayed or postponed [5, 6]. Consequences of bilateral RLN injuries are more severe and catastrophic than unilateral ones. One of the main advantages of IONM is the prevention of bilateral injuries to RLN.

The first step of IONM is pre-dissection monitoring (V1) of VN. In our case, V1 of both sides showed functional neural integrity. Electrophysiological V1 stimulation confirms the proper function of the inferior neural system of the larynx at the beginning of the surgery. We think that right V1 stimulation is slightly more important than left V1 as signals from the right VN (V1) are rarely negative at a distal standard contact point of the stimulator probe despite proper function of VCs. The absence of the V1 signal is a pathognomonic determinant of a non-recurrent course of the nerve indicating a rare anatomical variation of RLN. The V1 signal was negative if the stimulator probe contact point was located distal to the non-RLN separation and positive if it was located proximal to the separation [7]. Early detection of a risky anatomical variation of RLN appears to be an advantage of IONM.

The nerve monitoring begins with the visual identification of laryngeal nerves followed by functional identification by electrophysiological stimulation. We could visually identify the right EBSLN but not the left one. Visualization of EBSLN is not always possible because of the deep course of the nerve through the muscle fibers. Approximately, 15–20% of the nerve branches run distally through the pharyngeal constrictor muscle and are not visualized with standard dissection [8, 9]. EBSLN innervates CTM which plays an important role in maintaining the tension and length of VCs. Adequate tension and length are essential for vibration frequency of VCs to ensure optimal voice quality [1, 2, 9]. IONM directly checks the functional integrity of the visualized nerve with the observation of CTM twitches as done during the dissection of right lobe in our case. On the other hand, observation of CTM contraction after stimulation of the nerve tract with 2 mA intensity confirms the contribution of nerve monitoring to the identification of non-visualized nerves as observed during the dissection of the left lobe in our case. At the end of each pole dissection, final stimulation (S2) of EBSLN and detection of CTM twitches is required to establish the motor integrity of the nerve branch. Thus, IONM has a clear advantage in the anatomical identification and establishing the functional integrity of non-visualized nerves.

RLN has many anatomical variations. We discovered extralaryngeal terminal bifurcation of the left RLN and superficial course of the right RLN on the lateral surface of the thyroid gland.

Terminal bifurcation is a common variation with approximately 30% of incidence [10, 11]. Visual misidentification of the posterior branch as a single nerve trunk may increase the risk of the inadvertent division of the anterior motor branch. This can result in postoperative VC palsy, even though the surgeon believes to have preserved the integrity of the nerve. In case of a bifid nerve, IONM is a good adjunct to visual nerve identification because it can help the surgeon to clearly identify the motor function of the main trunk and both branches. In the present case, nerve monitoring established the functional integrity of the nerve branches: anterior (motor) and posterior (sensory). We can comment that in the case of anatomical variation, nerve monitoring may be a good guide for determining the functional integrity of nerves and for preventing inadvertent nerve injury. The anterior branch of RLN always provides motor function, while the posterior branch only rarely has motor fibers and is usually sensory [12].

The superficial course of RLN adherent on the lateral surface of the gland and lateral to Zuckerkandl's tubercle is another uncommon variation, with the incidence being less than 10% [13]. The thyroid surgeon must be familiar with the surgical anatomy of RLN including all anatomical variations. At the end of surgery, stimulation (R2) of RLN checks the motor integrity of the distal part of the nerve, and stimulation (V2) of VN establishes the motor integrity of the inferior laryngeal motor nerves. Sometimes, a proximal injury may be missed if nerve monitoring checks the distal cervical part of the nerve. V2 stimulation confirms the integrity of the inferior motor neural system of the larynx. IONM helps in identifying motor nerves with anatomical variations and may decrease injury risk in uncommon situations.

At the end of surgery, final stimulation (S2) of both EBSLNs resulted in recordable amplitude (right, 278 μV; left, 547 μV) due to contraction of intrinsic laryngeal musculature. RLN innervates these muscles and induces movements of VCs which are also determined by IONM. Thus, recordable amplitudes, due to the laryngeal muscle movements after stimulation of EBSLN, led us to think about motor communications between two nerves. Microdissection of 90 larynges obtained from necropsies established some form of anastomoses between the laryngeal nerves. An anastomosis between the EBSLNs and RLNs was present in 68% of cases as a connecting branch throughout CTM [14], while human communicating nerve has been reported to be present in 70% of humans [15]. On the other hand, induction of CTM twitches by stimulation (R2) of the left RLN is another confirmation of these relations in the present case. In the study by Miyauchi et al. [16], following stimulation of the 51 (73%) ipsilateral RLNs, CTM contractions were observed providing further confirmation of motor communication between the superior and the inferior laryngeal systems. Martin-Oviedo et al. [17] observed response in CTM in 7 of 13 (53.8%) patients after RLN stimulation. Recently, Liddy et al. [18] have described target and nontarget muscles for RLN and EBSLN after their monitoring. Based on available data, we can argue that CTM is the target muscle for EBSLN and nontarget muscle for RLN, while all intrinsic laryngeal muscles are target for RLN and nontarget for EBSLN.

Conclusion

Visual identification of neural structures based on good surgical skill and full anatomical knowledge including variations of laryngeal nerves is the gold standard in thyroid surgery. IONM has gained widespread acceptance as an adjunct to the gold standard of anatomical identification.

Thyroid surgeon can use IONM in all cases of thyroid surgery as an adjunct to surgical dissection. Besides visual integrity of the nerves after their full exposure, IONM detects motor integrity of laryngeal nerves during and at the end of the surgery. IONM is a reliable way to identify motor nerves and their motor integrity. In our opinion, IONM should be in the armamentarium of thyroid surgeons.

The surgeon must keep in mind that IONM cannot always prevent injury to RLN. Surgeon's skill and full anatomical knowledge are still the key, essential, and main factor for safe thyroid surgery. An experienced surgeon can perform thyroidectomy with a low complication incidence, but not with nil complication rate. We need a technology which can prevent intraoperative VC palsy secondary to nerve injury especially under complicated conditions.

What Can We Learn from This Case?

- Total thyroidectomy is a procedure of choice for patients with bilateral surgical pathology of the thyroid gland.
- Starting dissection from the dominant lobe harboring the main pathology is the first rule of total thyroidectomy with nerve monitoring.
- The surgeon can visually identify and expose EBSLN. It is impossible to expose some branches running deep through the constrictor muscle. IONM contributes by electrophysiological identification of non-visualized nerve and establishing motor integrity of EBSLN with observation of CTM contraction.
- IONM verifies motor integrity of RLNs of which anatomical identification and total exposure are mandatory during thyroid surgery.
- IONM is a good adjunct to anatomic exposure, especially for RLN with anatomical variations like extralaryngeal bifid nerve, and premature and early bifurcation of the nerve prior to laryngeal entry.
- Uncommon and superficial course of the nerve on the lateral surface of the lobe may increase injury risk that IONM may assist identification and gentle dissection of the nerve from underlying tissue.
- IONM may establish motor communication between laryngeal nerves. Electrophysiological stimulation of both EBSLNs created recordable amplitude secondary to movement of intrinsic laryngeal muscles received by surface electrodes integrated on endotracheal tube. Additionally, stimulation of the left RLN induced CTM twitches. These findings reveal motor interconnection between superior and inferior laryngeal nerves.
- Many anatomical variations of laryngeal nerves have been described previously. Nerves with variations increase the importance of nerve integrity monitor in thyroid surgery. It is generally impossible to discover anatomical variations preoperatively; therefore, the use of IONM seems advisable during thyroid surgery.

References

1. Tewari A, Samy RN, Castle J, Frye TM, Habeych ME, Mohamed M. Intraoperative neurophysiological monitoring of the laryngeal nerves during anterior neck surgery: a review. Ann Otol Rhinol Laryngol. 2017;126:67–72.
2. Wojtczak B, Barczyński M. Intermittent neural monitoring of the recurrent laryngeal nerve in surgery for recurrent goiter. Gland Surg. 2016;5:481–9.
3. Lee J, Fraser S, Glover A, et al. Prospective evaluation of the utility of routine neuromonitoring for an established thyroid surgical practice. ANZ J Surg. 2016;87:E138–42. https://doi.org/10.1111/ans.13606.
4. Wong KP, Mak KL, Wong CK, Lang BH. Systematic review and meta-analysis on intra-operative neuromonitoring in high-risk thyroidectomy. Int J Surg. 2017;38:21–30.
5. Randolph GW, Kamani D. Intraoperative electrophysiologic monitoring of the recurrent laryngeal nerve during thyroid and parathyroid surgery: experience with 1,381 nerves at risk. Laryngoscope. 2017;127:280–6.
6. Stopa M, Barczyński M. Prognostic value of intraoperative neural monitoring of the recurrent laryngeal nerve in thyroid surgery. Langenbeck's Arch Surg. 2016;402:957–64.
7. Gurleyik E, Gurleyik G. Nonrecurrent laryngeal nerve in the era of intraoperative nerve monitoring. Adv Med. 2016;2016:1606029.

8. Lennquist S, Cahlin C, Smeds S. The superior laryngeal nerve in thyroid surgery. Surgery. 1987;102:999–1008.
9. Friedman M, LoSavio P, Ibrahim H. Superior laryngeal nerve identification and preservation in thyroidectomy. Arch Otolaryngol Head Neck Surg. 2002;128:296–303.
10. Gurleyik E. Extralaryngeal terminal division of the inferior laryngeal nerve: anatomical classification by a surgical point of view. J Thyroid Res. 2013;2013:731250. https://doi.org/10.1155/2013/731250.
11. Gurleyik E. Surgical anatomy of bilateral extralaryngeal bifurcation of the recurrent laryngeal nerve: similarities and differences between both sides. N Am J Med Sci. 2014;6:445–9.
12. Gurleyik E. Location of motor fibers within branches of the recurrent laryngeal nerve with extralaryngeal terminal bifurcation; functional identification by intraoperative neuromonitoring. Surgery. 2015;158:1339–44.
13. Gurleyik E, Gurleyik G. Incidence and surgical importance of Zuckerkandl's tubercle of the thyroid and its relations with recurrent laryngeal nerve. ISRN Surg. 2012;2012:450589. https://doi.org/10.5402/2012/450589.
14. Sanudo JR, Maranillo E, León X, et al. An anatomical study of anastomoses between the laryngeal nerves. Laryngoscope. 1999;109:983–7.
15. Randolph GW. Surgical anatomy and monitoring of the recurrent laryngeal nerve, SLN monitoring. In: Randolph GW, editor. Surgery of the thyroid and parathyroid glands. 2nd ed. Philadelphia: Elsevier; 2013. p. 338–40.
16. Miyauchi A, Masuoka H, Nakayama A, Higashiyama T. Innervation of the cricothyroid muscle by extralaryngeal branches of the recurrent laryngeal nerve. Laryngoscope. 2016;126:1157–62.
17. Martin-Oviedo C, Maranillo E, Lowy-Benoliel A, Pascual-Font A, et al. Functional role of human laryngeal nerve connections. Laryngoscope. 2011;121:2338–43.
18. Liddy W, Barber SR, Cinquepalmi M, et al. The electrophysiology of thyroid surgery: electrophysiologic and muscular responses with stimulation of the vagus nerve, recurrent laryngeal nerve, and external branch of the superior laryngeal nerve. Laryngoscope. 2017;127:764–71.

Recurrent Laryngeal Nerve Injury in Thyroid Surgery with Intraoperative Nerve Monitoring

27

Emin Gürleyik and Günay Gürleyik

Abstract

IONM assesses the motor function of the recurrent laryngeal nerve (RLN) while exposing the anatomical integrity, which does not always ensure the normal function. However, despite its advantages, IONM cannot always prevent injury to the nerve. Nevertheless, nerve monitoring can still play an important role in case of an inadvertent nerve injury. We present a case of an RLN injury in thyroid surgery performed under the guidance of IONM.

We planned for total thyroidectomy for the surgical treatment of papillary cancer under the guidance of IONM. We first dissected the right lobe harboring the malignant solid nodule. Pre-dissection sound signals (V1 and R1) after vagus nerve (VN) and RLN stimulations were obtained from the device while recording the wave amplitude. The right RLN was isolated and completely exposed. In the end, post-dissection stimulation (R2) of the anatomically intact RLN determined the loss of signal (LOS) without a recordable waveform amplitude. Post-dissection stimulation of the right VN confirmed the LOS, revealing the transient or permanent injury to the nerve. Electrophysiological monitoring of the RLN detected a segmental (type 1) injury. The resection of the left lobe was abandoned after right hemithyroidectomy. Postoperative laryngoscopy showed unilateral right VC palsy. The final pathological diagnosis was papillary thyroid cancer in the right lobe. The normal function of the right VC was recovered in the third postoperative month. Completion left lobe excision was performed under the guidance of IONM as a delayed procedure after 4 months of primary surgery. Postoperative laryngoscopy confirmed the normal function of both VCs.

IONM assesses and confirms the functional integrity of the laryngeal nerves. Intraoperative LOS indicates an injury to the nerve and the presence of palsy. In case of unfavorable complications, IONM detects the type of injury to the RLN. IONM establishes the outcome of the neural palsy, affects the surgical decision-making, and prevents the risk of bilateral palsy.

E. Gürleyik
Department of Surgery, Düzce University, Düzce, Turkey

G. Gürleyik (✉)
Department of Surgery, Haydarpaşa Numune Training and Research Hospital, Istanbul, Turkey

27.1 Introduction

During thyroid surgery, anatomical identification and complete exposure of the cervical part of the recurrent laryngeal nerve (RLN) are mandatory.

T. Özülker et al. (eds.), *Thyroid and Parathyroid Diseases*, https://doi.org/10.1007/978-3-319-78476-2_27

The anatomical integrity of the nerve is the first key to a safe surgery. Protection of the structural integrity is primarily based on a complete anatomical knowledge including the variations and the surgical skill. Thyroid surgery performed by an experienced surgeon will have a very low complication rate. In addition to anatomical integrity, the motor integrity of the nerve has paramount importance for a complication-free thyroidectomy. Intraoperative nerve monitoring (IONM) has now become an adjunct to anatomical identification and integrity of the RLN. IONM assesses the motor function of the nerve while exposing the anatomical integrity, which does not always ensure the normal function. The medical literature presents some reports demonstrating that IONM can reduce the incidence of vocal cord (VC) palsy [1–6]. However, despite its advantages, IONM cannot always prevent injury to the nerve. In this situation, it is necessary to assess the intraoperative utility of nerve monitoring in the case of an inadvertent RLN injury. We hypothesize that nerve monitoring still has an important role during thyroid surgery even in the case of a nerve injury.

We present a case of RLN injury in thyroid surgery performed under the guidance of IONM.

27.2 Case Presentation

A 60-year-old woman presented to our clinic with an anterior cervical mass. Biochemical analysis of her blood sample showed a euthyroid state. Thyroid ultrasound revealed a hypoechoic nodule measuring 23 × 33 × 39 mm with a cystic component in the right lobe and an isoechoic nodule measuring 4 × 5 × 8 mm with regular borders in the left lobe. After a fine needle aspiration biopsy of the larger nodule, a cytological diagnosis of papillary cancer was suspected. We planned for a total thyroidectomy under the guidance of IONM that was performed using a nerve integrity monitor (NIM-Response 3.0 System; Medtronic Xomed, Jacksonville, FL, USA). The setup of the device included a stimulation intensity of 1 mA and an amplitude threshold of 100 μV. The nerve integrity monitor was connected to the surface electrodes integrated with an endotracheal tube 7.0 ID (NIM®EMG standard reinforced endotracheal tube; Medtronic Xomed, Jacksonville, FL, USA), which was inserted between the VCs under direct vision during intubation. We first dissected the right lobe harboring the larger solid nodule with a suspicious cytology. After medial traction of the lateral lobe, we incised the neurovascular sheet and then identified the vagus nerve (VN) posterior to the common carotid artery and the jugular vein. The stimulator probe was directly applied on the VN, and the pre-dissection sound signal (V1) was obtained from the device while recording the wave amplitude. After dissecting the inferior pole, we dissected the superior pole of the right lobe and ligated the upper thyroid vessels closer to the glandular tissue under the guidance of nerve monitoring. After medial mobilization of the lobe, the RLN was identified using a conventional lateral approach. When first identified under direct vision, the RLN was directly stimulated, and the pre-dissection sound signal (R1) was obtained from the device while recording the wave amplitude. The RLN was isolated until the ligament of Berry with observation of the disappearance of the nerve in the ligament layers. At the end of lobe dissection, a final post-dissection stimulation (R2) was applied on anatomically intact RLN. We determined the loss of signal (LOS) without a recordable waveform amplitude. The right VN was reidentified and restimulated (V2), which confirmed the LOS, revealing the transient or permanent injury to the nerve. Surgical exploration of the cervical part of the RLN showed an anatomically intact nerve. Electrophysiological monitoring of the RLN detected a segmental (type 1) injury at approximately 15 mm to the laryngeal entry. The IONM created a sound signal on the distal 15 mm of the nerve and revealed the LOS on the proximal part. We waited for 30 min for the return of the motor function and the physiological signal and amplitude. However, the motor function of the RLN was not recovered during the waiting period. We abandoned the resection of the left lobe and performed right hemithyroidectomy, including the larger nodule with a suspicious cytological diagnosis of papillary cancer. Postoperative laryngoscopy showed unilateral right VC palsy. The final histopathological diagnosis was papillary thyroid cancer (encapsulated follicular variant) with a tumor size of 30 × 25 mm. The tumor was intrathyroidal without lymphovascular invasion. Follow-up monthly laryngoscopic examinations showed that the normal function of the right VC was recovered in the third postoperative month. Completion left lobe excision was performed as a delayed procedure after 4 months of primary surgery. All stages of nerve monitoring showed functional integrity of the left laryngeal nerves. Postoperative laryngoscopy confirmed the normal function of both VCs. The pathological diagnosis in the left lobe was a benign nodular goiter. A suppressive dose of L-thyroxin was prescribed postoperatively. The follow-up period was uneventful in the third year.

27.3 Discussion

The identification and complete exposure of the RLN are the gold standard during thyroidectomy. IONM has been accepted as a good adjunct to anatomical identification. Despite some advantages of monitoring, injury to the nerve uncommonly occurs during thyroid surgery under the guidance of IONM. Even in the case of an injury, IONM may still have an important role in the surgical procedure. The present case of thyroid surgery is an example of injury to an anatomically intact nerve detected by IONM, which may affect the intraoperative surgical decision, the intended preoperative plan, and the outcome of the surgical procedure.

27.3.1 IONM Assesses and Confirms the Functional Integrity of Laryngeal Nerves

During thyroid surgery, nerve monitoring determines the integrity of motor function of the nerve, and IONM has been demonstrated to have not only a very high sensitivity and a negative predictive value but also good specificity and positive predictive value [7]. Meta-analyses have shown that IONM is associated with a reduction in overall and permanent RLN palsy during thyroid reoperations and also reduces the rate of injury [1–3]. IONM could be an effective method to increase the rate of RLN identification and reduce the temporary phonation alteration after thyroid surgery. The use of IONM significantly decreases the occurrence of RLN injuries [4–6]. On the other hand, there are contradictory reports that the use of IONM does not prevent permanent nerve palsy; no significant benefit of IONM compared with visualization alone in reducing the rate of RLN injuries could be proven [8, 9]. Monitoring the RLN and the VN at the end of the surgery has been especially accepted as a good determinant for the prognostication of normal neural function. In our present case, predissection stimulation of the VN and the RLN confirmed the normal function of both nerves. However, post-dissection retesting by IONM showed unexpected unfavorable findings despite the anatomical integrity of the RLN. Randolph and Kamani [10] reported that intraoperative monitoring of the RLN during thyroid and other neck surgeries could aid in nerve mapping, nerve identification, and prognostication of postoperative VC function. Our finding in the present case confirmed that visual integrity of the RLN trunk does not always ensure the normal motor function of the nerve. In the case of an anatomically intact nerve without monitoring, we believe that a complication-free surgery has been performed, but the results of IONM indicated loss of motor integrity despite visual integrity. Therefore, the surgeon can miss neural palsy without the assistance of electrophysiological monitoring.

27.3.2 IONM Detects Injury, Neural Palsy, and Intraoperative Loss of Motor Function

In the present case, the identification, isolation, and exposure of the right RLN were uneventful. The nerve was anatomically intact at the end of right lobe dissection. Therefore, we believe that the procedure was uncomplicated before rechecking the functions of the RLN and the VN by IONM. Both right R2 and V2 stimulation showed LOS and a nonrecordable wave amplitude that revealed the injury to the nerve. Postoperative laryngoscopy confirmed ipsilateral VC palsy. Recognizable intraoperative nerve damage was almost 100% by IONM [11]. The LOS was successfully diagnosed in a series of 500 total thyroidectomies, including 20 temporary and 5 permanent nerve lesions, that allows for optimizing the predictive values of IONM in the prognostication of postoperative RLN function [12]. We can comment that our finding of post-dissection LOS is an important advantage of nerve monitoring as it can detect the presence of an intraoperative nerve injury. In the case of an intraoperative RLN injury, IONM provides reliable and appropriate feedback on the functional status of the RLN on the side of the initial dissection during a total thyroidectomy [13]. The LOS on the RLN reveals a deterioration of motor integrity, and in such a situation, expert surgeons advise a waiting period of 20–30 min for the return of motor function in the case of a transient palsy. Sitges-Serra et al. [14] reported that the majority of initially silent nerves recovered an electromyographic signal at retesting. The mean time to recovery was 20.2 (range: 10–35) min. After the LOS on the RLN dissected initially, there is a high probability of intraoperative signal recovery. In this setting, judicious bilateral thyroidectomy can be performed without the risk of bilateral recurrent nerve paresis [14]. Sometimes, the motor function of the nerve is recovered intraoperatively and allows the completion of the procedure. Otherwise, we recommend discontinuation of the procedure and consideration of a delayed or staged surgery. In the present case, the absence of motor function recovery during the waiting period prompted us to change the surgical plan of the intended total thyroidectomy. Therefore, nerve monitoring was found to be useful also for the early detection of nerve palsy, which affects the ongoing procedure and the surgical plan. Anuwong et al. [11] reported that the standardized technique of nerve monitoring allows to cumulate stage procedures and reset bilateral RLN palsy.

27.3.3 IONM Detects the Type of Injury and Injury Mechanism of the RLN

The mechanism of injury to the RLN has been categorized into traction, mechanical compression, ligation, heat damage, and transection. The types of an RLN injury include segmental (type 1) and global (type 2). If an inadvertent neural injury occurs during surgery, IONM can clarify the type of injury as segmental or global. In our case, a positive signal on the distal segment and no signal on the proximal part of the nerve confirmed the presence of type 1 injury. After the segmental loss of motor function in the anatomically intact RLN, we believed that the mechanism of injury to the nerve could be traction, compression, or thermal damage. These findings based on the results of nerve monitoring and anatomical observations increased the probability of a transient palsy and the expectation of functional recovery. The functional outcome after an RLN palsy may depend on the type of nerve injury [15]. There are two possible intramural injuries to a macroscopically intact nerve, disruption of axons (axonotmesis) and conduction block affecting Schwann cells and nodes of Ranvier. An intact axon with a surrounding myelin injury presents a conduction block on electromyography. Myelin and axonal injuries resulting in Wallerian degeneration present as a conduction block and denervation on electromyography [15]. For prognostication of recovery in cases of laryngeal dysfunction and voice changes after thyroid surgery, the surgeon would first need to define the presence, location, and type of nerve injury [16]. Intramural damage inside an anatomically intact nerve is caused due to traction, pressure, or heating. Neurapraxia affects the surrounding Schwann cells, despite maintaining the integrity of the axon. The LOS during surgery indicates a discontinuity in the electrical propagation of the nerve. The surgeon can pinpoint the exact location of the injury using the stimulator probe along the course of the nerve [16]. In our case, the important advantages of nerve monitoring were the detection of the functional loss, the exact location of the injury line on the anatomically intact nerve, defining the injury type, and the observation of the intraoperative outcome of nerve palsy. We can state that the IONM has a beneficial and predictive role in thyroid surgery even in the case of RLN palsy.

27.3.4 IONM Establishes the Outcome of Neural Palsy and Affects Surgical Decision-Making

Certain mild traction and compression injuries cause neurapraxia and are sometimes reversible within 20–30 min if the traction or compression is relaxed. If the IONM indicates an early functional recovery, the surgeon can continue and complete the surgery. In our case, the normal motor function was not recovered during the intraoperative waiting period, which increased the suspicion of a moderate or severe injury. In this situation, excision of the left lobe was abandoned to prevent the probability of bilateral palsy. Henry et al. [17] presented five meta-analyses demonstrating a nonsignificant reduction in RLN injury using IONM versus nerve visualization alone. On the other hand, the concept of a staged thyroidectomy in the case of LOS on the first side to prevent bilateral RLN injury may provide additional benefits [17]. Ten (4.9%) of 206 procedures were staged based on unfavorable signal changes. The IONM results accurately indicated postoperative ipsilateral VC dysfunction with high reliability [13]. Therefore, we can comment that the IONM is a reliable tool that can be used for staging thyroid surgery. An important rule of nerve monitoring is to start the surgery by dissecting the lobe harboring the primary, dominant pathology to prevent bilateral palsy in the case of unilateral loss of motor integrity. Nerve monitoring has been found to be useful also for the intraoperative decision of continuation or postponement of surgery based on the motor function of laryngeal nerves. Bergenfelz et al. [18] reported that bilateral RLN injury did not occur during thyroid surgery with IONM. Randolph and Kamani [10] reported that IONM aids in the prognostication of postoperative VC function, which in turn can influence the surgeon's decision to proceed to bilateral surgery. Because an abnormal intraoperative electromyogram indicates a high risk for early postoperative VC palsy, the initial plan of bilateral surgery needs to be critically reviewed after the occurrence of LOS on the first side of resection. Since the majority of affected nerves will fully recover after the operation, a staged completion thyroidectomy is recommended [19]. In the present case, the RLN injury determined by IONM and the right VC palsy identified by postoperative laryngoscopy supported the current decision of interrupting the surgical procedure. Another rule of nerve monitoring is the staged surgery implying delaying or postponing the excision of the contralateral lobe in the case of LOS on the side of the initial dissection. An important advantage of IONM is the protection of the patient from the risk of bilateral VC palsy. With proper use of nerve monitoring, there would be no incidence of bilateral RLN injury.

In the present case, the cytological diagnosis indicated total thyroidectomy as surgical treatment. We first delayed the surgery after observing the intraoperative LOS and the nonrecordable wave amplitude on electromyography. Right VC palsy established by postoperative laryngoscopy confirmed the intraoperative result. The pathological diagnosis of papillary carcinoma in the excised right lobe revealed the indication of completion surgery for the remaining left lobe. Recovery of the normal VC function in the postoperative third month indicated that the injury to the right RLN was transient. Normal VC activity detected by the third month of laryngoscopy allowed us to perform completion thyroidectomy. Surgical treatment of the papillary cancer was completed with delayed resection of the remaining lobe. Total thyroidectomy is a procedure of choice for patients with papillary thyroid cancer, but in the case of LOS on the first side after excision of the primary pathology, staged surgery is a good and widely accepted alternative for preventing the probability of bilateral VC palsy. The decision of a staged surgery after the recovery of VC activity provides motor integrity to both RLNs or at least protects the unilateral motor integrity of the nerve against catastrophic bilateral injuries. If the VC function is not recovered, discontinuation of resection of the contralateral lobe should be considered.

Anatomical identification of the RLN is the gold standard during thyroidectomy, and IONM can be a valuable adjunct to visual identification. Even in the case of nerve palsy, IONM has an important role in defining the presence, cause, and type of injury and in the surgical decision-making and outcome of the ongoing procedure.

27.4 Follow-Up and Outcome

In the present case, the initial surgical plan was total thyroidectomy. At the end of excision of the first lobe, the IONM results showed that unilateral loss of motor integrity of the RLN affected the outcome of the procedure. Excision of the contralateral lobe was abandoned to prevent the probability of bilateral nerve palsy. The surgical treatment of papillary thyroid cancer was completed with a two-stage surgery after the detection of normal VC function by the third month of laryngoscopy. The IONM results during the second surgery and those of the laryngoscopy after completion thyroidectomy revealed the motor integrity of both nerves and the normal function of VCs. Unfavorable events were not detected at the third year of follow-up.

IONM assesses and establishes the functional integrity of laryngeal nerves. Its role is more apparent and significant especially in an anatomically intact nerve that does not always ensure a normal function. In the case of a visually intact but functionally injured nerve, IONM can also be used to detect the deterioration of motor integrity, define the type of injury, assess the early outcome of nerve palsy, change the initial surgical plan, and affect the surgical decision-making. In addition to RLN identification, it plays an important role in the case of nerve injury. Therefore, as a useful adjunct to surgical skill and anatomical dissection, IONM should be included in the armamentarium of the surgeon.

What Can We Learn from This Case?

- Visual identification, exposure of the RLN, and protection of its anatomical integrity are the gold standard of thyroid surgery. IONM is a valuable adjunct to anatomical exposure of the nerve.
- Anatomical integrity does not always ensure normal motor function, and IONM can be used to assess the functional integrity.
- Nerve monitoring may also have an important role in the case of injury to the laryngeal nerves. IONM with LOS and a nonrecordable waveform amplitude aids in the early detection of injury to the RLN.
- IONM may define the type, cause, and mechanism of injury, which is important for the prognostication and outcome of VC palsy.
- In the case of a transient injury, IONM is beneficial to determine the intraoperative recovery of a transient nerve palsy that allows continuation of the surgical procedure.
- In the case of an injury detected by nerve monitoring, IONM has an important role in surgical decision-making. Loss of signal and amplitude during dissection on the first side changes the intended surgical plan so that the excision of the contralateral side is postponed.
- The decision of a staged completion surgery based on the results of IONM appears to be a good alternative for preventing the probability of bilateral palsy. The standard use of IONM prevents bilateral injury to the RLN.

References

1. Sun W, Liu J, Zhang H, Zhang P, Wang Z, Dong W, et al. Meta-analysis of intraoperative neuromonitoring of recurrent laryngeal nerve palsy during thyroid reoperations. Clin Endocrinol. 2017;87(5):572–80. https://doi.org/10.1111/cen.13379.

2. Yang S, Zhou L, Lu Z, Ma B, Ji Q, Wang Y. Systematic review with meta-analysis of intraoperative neuromonitoring during thyroidectomy. Int J Surg. 2017;39:104–13.
3. Wong KP, Mak KL, Wong CK, Lang BH. Systematic review and meta-analysis on intra-operative neuromonitoring in high-risk thyroidectomy. Int J Surg. 2017;38:21–30.
4. Baek SK, Lee K, Oh D, Kang SH, Kwon SY, Woo JS, et al. Efficiency of intraoperative neuromonitoringon voice outcomes after thyroid surgery. Auris Nasus Larynx. 2017;44:583–9.
5. Vasileiadis I, Karatzas T, Charitoudis G, Karakostas E, Tseleni-Balafouta S, Kouraklis G. Association of intraoperative neuromonitoring with reduced recurrent laryngeal nerve injury in patients undergoing total thyroidectomy. JAMA Otolaryngol Head Neck Surg. 2016;142:994–1001.
6. Wojtczak B, Sutkowski K, Kaliszewski K, Głód M, Barczyński M. Experience with intraoperative neuromonitoring of the recurrent laryngeal nerve improves surgical skills and outcomes of non-monitored thyroidectomy. Langenbeck's Arch Surg. 2017;402:709–17.
7. Calò PG, Medas F, Conzo G, Podda F, Canu GL, Gambardella C, et al. Intraoperative neuromonitoring in thyroid surgery: is the two-staged thyroidectomy justified? Int J Surg. 2017;41(Suppl 1):S13–20.
8. Lombardi CP, Carnassale G, Damiani G, Acampora A, Raffaelli M, De Crea C, et al. "The final countdown": is intraoperative, intermittent neuromonitoring really useful in preventing permanent nerve palsy? Evidence from a meta-analysis. Surgery. 2016;160:1693–706.
9. Brajcich BC, McHenry CR. The utility of intraoperative nerve monitoring during thyroid surgery. J Surg Res. 2016;204:29–33.
10. Randolph GW, Kamani D. Intraoperative electrophysiologic monitoring of the recurrent laryngeal nerve during thyroid and parathyroid surgery: experience with 1,381 nerves at risk. Laryngoscope. 2017;127:280–6.
11. Anuwong A, Lavazza M, Kim HY, Wu CW, Rausei S, Pappalardo V, et al. Recurrent laryngeal nerve management in thyroid surgery: consequences of routine visualization, application of intermittent, standardized and continuous nerve monitoring. Updat Surg. 2016;68:331–41.
12. Stopa M, Barczyński M. Prognostic value of intraoperative neural monitoring of the recurrent laryngeal nerve in thyroid surgery. Langenbeck's Arch Surg. 2016;402:957–64. https://doi.org/10.1007/s00423-016-1441-0.
13. Fontenot TE, Randolph GW, Setton TE, Alsaleh N, Kandil E. Does intraoperative nerve monitoring reliably aid in staging of total thyroidectomies? Laryngoscope. 2015;125:2232–5.
14. Sitges-Serra A, Fontané J, Dueñas JP, Duque CS, Lorente L, Trillo L, et al. Prospective study on loss of signal on the first side during neuromonitoring of the recurrent laryngeal nerve in total thyroidectomy. Br J Surg. 2013;100:662–6.
15. Hydman J, Björck G, Persson JK, Zedenius J, Mattsson P. Diagnosis and prognosis of iatrogenic injury of the recurrent laryngeal nerve. Ann Otol Rhinol Laryngol. 2009;118:506–11.
16. Mattsson P, Hydman J, Svensson M. Recovery of laryngeal function after intraoperative injury to the recurrent laryngeal nerve. Gland Surg. 2015;4:27–35.
17. Henry BM, Graves MJ, Vikse J, Sanna B, Pękala PA, Walocha JA, et al. The current state of intermittent intraoperative neural monitoring for prevention of recurrent laryngeal nerve injury during thyroidectomy: a PRISMA-compliant systematic review of overlapping meta-analyses. Langenbeck's Arch Surg. 2017;402:663–73.
18. Bergenfelz A, Salem AF, Jacobsson H, Nordenström E, Almquist M, Steering Committee for the Scandinavian Quality Register for Thyroid, Parathyroid and Adrenal Surgery (SQRTPA). Risk of recurrent laryngeal nerve palsy in patients undergoing thyroidectomy with and without intraoperative nerve monitoring. Br J Surg. 2016;103:1828–38.
19. Schneider R, Lorenz K, Sekulla C, Machens A, Nguyen-Thanh P, Dralle H. Surgical strategy during intended total thyroidectomy after loss of EMG signal on the first side of resection. Chirurg. 2015;86:154–63.

Part II

Thyroid Cancer

28 Preoperative Cervical USG Mapping in a Patient Undergoing Thyroidectomy for Malignant Cytological Findings

Seyfettin Ilgan

Abstract

Papillary thyroid carcinoma has a propensity for early spread to regional lymph nodes but a low incidence of distance metastases. Cervical lymph nodes are involved in 20–60% of patients in most series using standard pathologic techniques. Although lymph node metastases are more common with increased tumor size and extrathyroidal extension, it may be present with small, intrathyroidal tumors. Since the lymph node metastases are the most common independent risk factor for persistent and recurrent disease, identification and removal of the locoregional disease remains an essential component of initial surgical treatment. Hence, optimal management of thyroid cancer is highly dependent on accurate staging of the extent of disease before surgery. It is known that preoperative physical examination is inadequate for the detection of cervical lymph node metastases in both lateral and central compartments and preoperative staging and follow-up should depend on better diagnostic tools in patients with thyroid cancer. Neck ultrasound is generally considered to be the most sensitive imaging modality to assess the primary tumor and identify lymph node metastases. Though sonography is becoming widely accepted as the technique of choice for staging papillary thyroid carcinoma, assessment of lymph nodes is more challenging compared to thyroid nodule evaluation. While missed findings on preoperative USG may lead to understaging and inadequate surgical management, excessively skeptical reporting of nodal findings may result in submission of the majority of patients to fine needle aspiration biopsy, causing anxiety and extended preoperative workup with many unnecessary biopsies.

S. Ilgan
Department of Nuclear Medicine, Güven Hospital, Ankara, Turkey

28.1 Case Presentation

A 46-year-old man presented to our hospital for consideration of treatment for newly diagnosed papillary thyroid carcinoma. A suspicious palpable nodule had been found on physical examination and neck sonography ordered for further evaluation in a local hospital. Neck sonography had confirmed that palpable nodule was a solitary solid hypoechoic nodule in the right thyroid lobe sized 11 mm in largest diameter. No abnormal lymph node had been appreciated on the nodal survey, and fine needle aspiration biopsy of nodule had been recommended which was turned out to be papillary thyroid carcinoma later on. He was euthyroid and had no history of radiation exposure or family history of thyroid disease.

T. Özülker et al. (eds.), *Thyroid and Parathyroid Diseases*, https://doi.org/10.1007/978-3-319-78476-2_28

The patient was seen by a local general surgeon, who offered a near-total thyroidectomy to him. He came to our center to discuss over whether active surveillance and lobectomy also could be suitable alternatives for him. Given the cytological and ultrasonographic (USG) findings, he was a candidate for lobectomy with intraoperative node assessment according to our institutional approach of multidisciplinary endocrine tumor board.

A comprehensive USG of the neck was performed by an experienced neck sonographer of the multidisciplinary team as a routine part of our preoperative workup. A 12 mm single, solid hypoechoic nodule with irregular margins and several internal punctate echogenic foci possibly representing microcalcifications (psammoma bodies) was found in the inferior and medial part of the right thyroid lobe highly suggestive of primary thyroid malignancy (Fig. 28.1). Though nodule was close to thyroid capsule on the tracheal face, a thin intervening normal thyroid tissue was appreciated between the nodule and thyroid capsule excluding gross extrathyroidal extension (ETE). Thyroid echo was slightly decreased with linear echogenic bands suggesting chronic thyroiditis. In addition, a 27 × 9 mm enlarged lymph node containing microcalcifications and showing chaotic vascularity on color Doppler imaging was seen at the level of right carotid bifurcation (Fig. 28.2). Although not as typical as this one, a 10 × 7 mm ill-defined lymph node, showing a few punctate echogenic foci and increased vascularity, was detected behind the internal jugular vein in the level IV (Fig. 28.3). Both lymph nodes were highly suggestive of nodal metastases. On further surveillance, a 9 × 6 mm hypervascular lymph node, which is

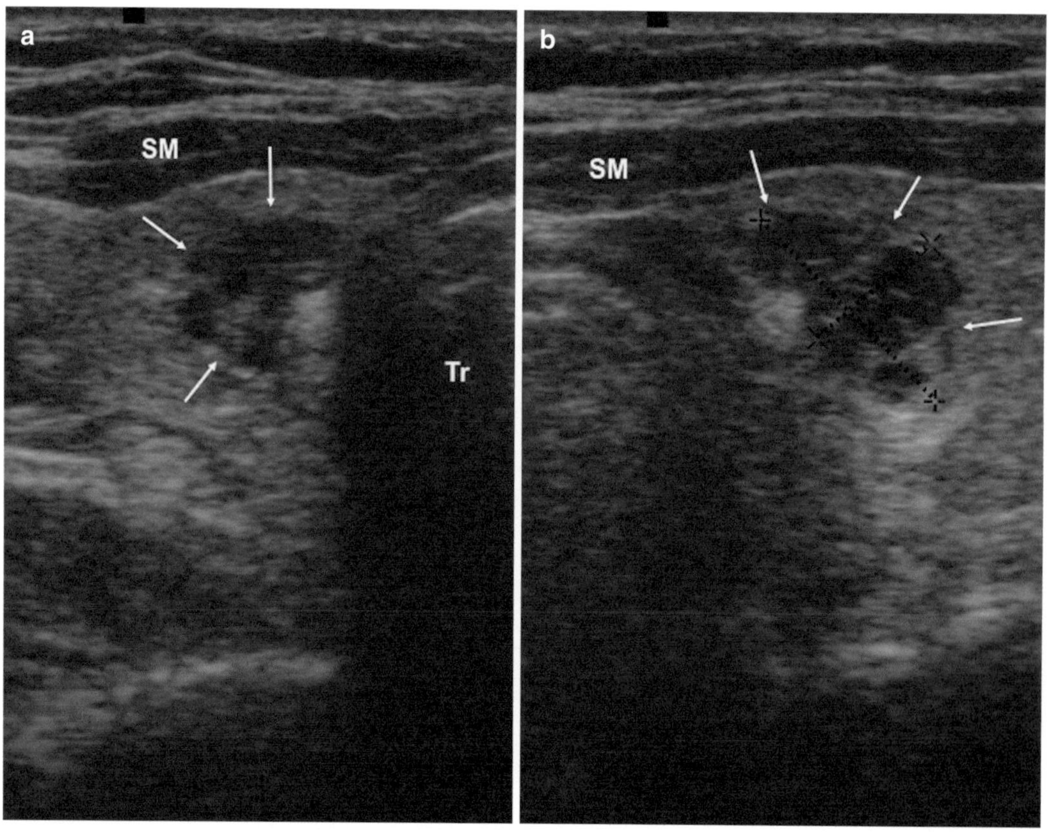

Fig. 28.1 Axial (**a**) and longitudinal (**b**) sonograms of the right thyroid lobe show hypoechoic solid nodule with irregular margins (arrows). *SM* strap muscles, *Tr* trachea

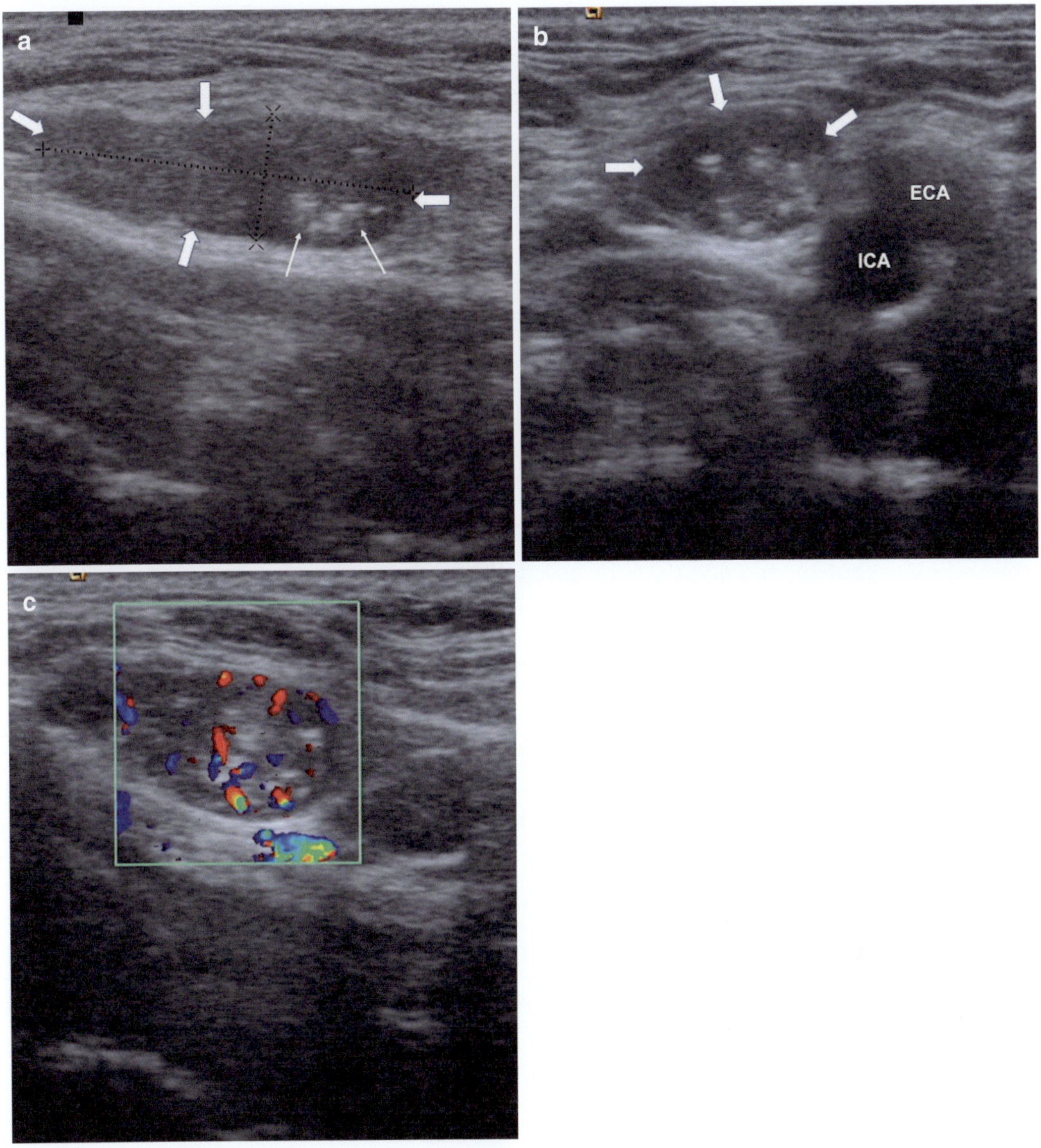

Fig. 28.2 Longitudinal (**a**) and axial (**b**) images of level II lymph node (thick arrows) containing microcalcification (thin arrows). On color Doppler image (**c**), lymph node shows peripheral and chaotic vascularization. Metastatic nature of lymph node confirmed by FNAB and Tg washout. *ICA* internal carotid artery, *ECA* external carotid artery

hardly noticeable among the central fatty tissue, was also seen in the deep pretracheal area while neck hyperextended (Fig. 28.4). None of these lymph nodes were respected during the first neck USG which has been done before cytological diagnosis. Cytological findings and Tg washout of the dominant suspicious lymph node in right segment II confirmed papillary carcinoma metastasis. Under the light of these new findings, he was scheduled for total thyroidectomy with right functional neck dissection and bilateral therapeutic central compartment dissection. Lateral and central neck dissection was carried out as a comprehensive compartment dissection including right levels II, III, and IV and central neck (level VI).

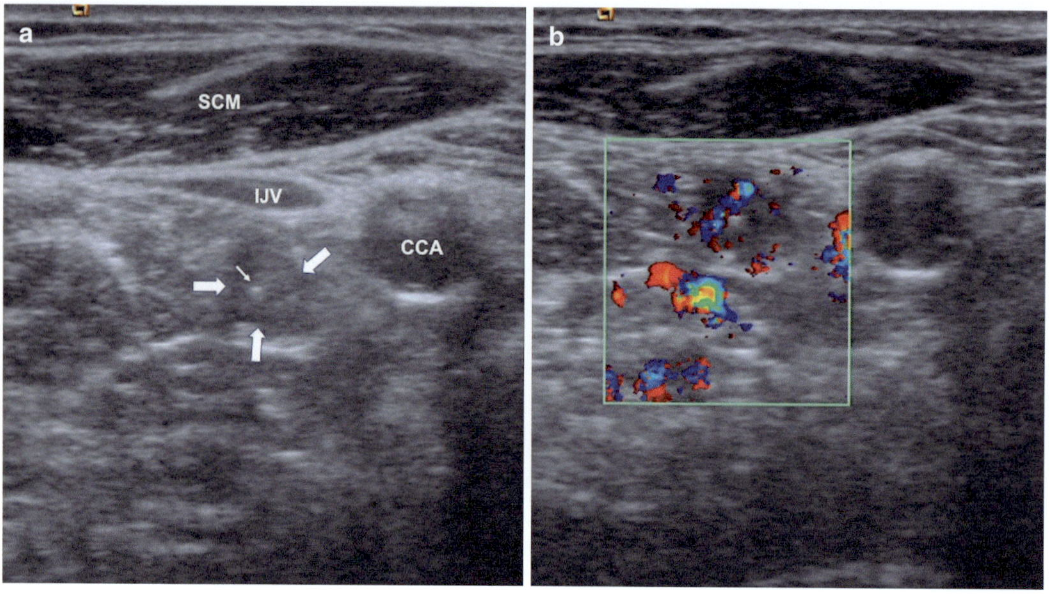

Fig. 28.3 (**a**) Axial USG image of level IV lymph node (thick arrows) behind the internal jugular vein image showing a few microcalcification (thin arrows). (**b**) Lymph node shows chaotic and peripheral vascularization on color Doppler image. *SCM* sternocleidomastoid muscle, *IJV* internal jugular vein, *CCA* common carotid artery

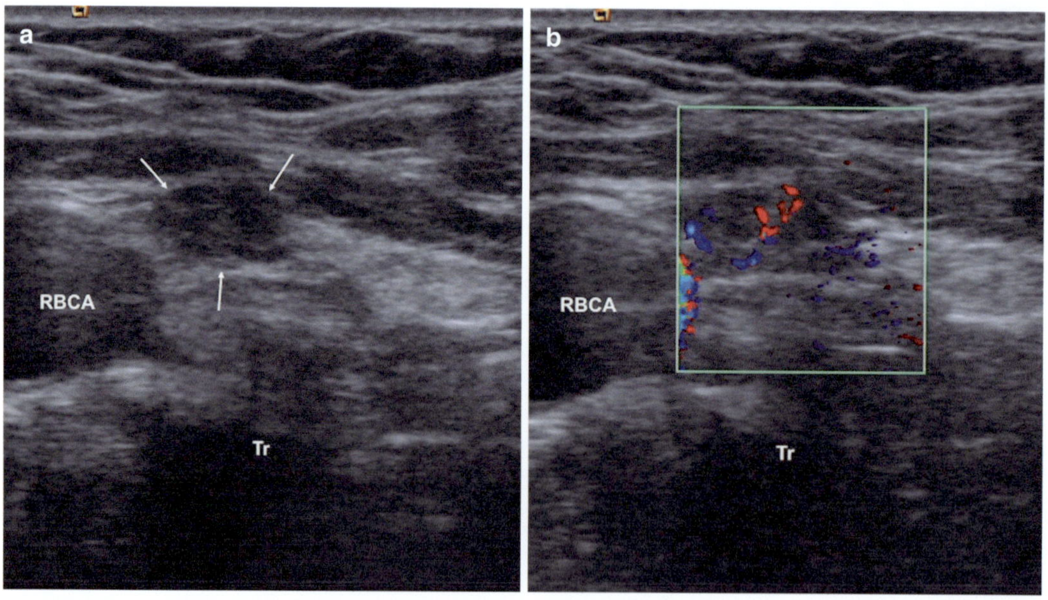

Fig. 28.4 (**a**) Axial sonogram of the central lymph node located in the pretracheal soft tissue (arrows). (**b**) Despite small size lymph node shows pathologic vascularization. *RBCA* right brachiocephalic artery, *Tr* trachea

The final pathology report presented a 1.2 cm classical variant of papillary thyroid carcinoma (PTC) with lymphovascular invasion in the right lobe (Fig. 28.5). There was no evidence of ETE. Background lymphocytic thyroiditis was present. Lateral cervical dissection revealed 4 metastatic nodes out of 20 resected, largest being biopsied one and having a size of 2.5 cm. There were three out of seven lymph node metastases in central compartment dissection material also,

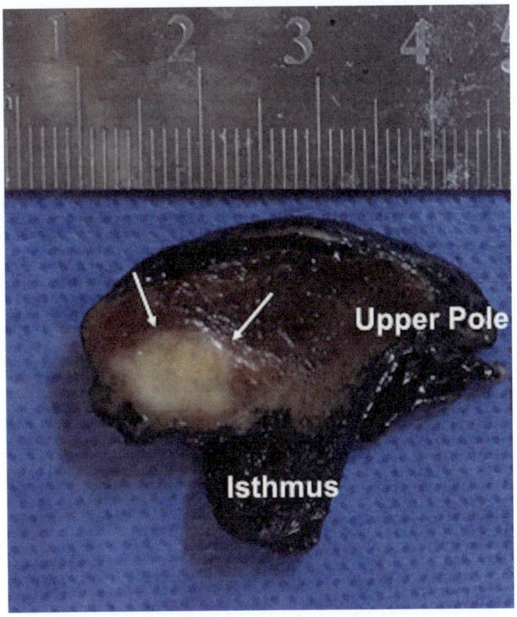

Fig. 28.5 Surgical specimen of the same patient containing white, solid, firm tumor (arrows) with irregular margins sized 1.2 cm in greatest diameter in the right lobe

largest size 0.7 cm. None of the metastatic lymph nodes showed extranodal extension. The clinicopathologic stage of disease in our case was interpreted as follows:

- T1aN1bMx (Stage I) per the AJCC/TNM VIII system [1] (it was Stage IVa previously [2])
- American Thyroid Association (ATA 2015) intermediate risk of recurrence [3]

28.2 Discussion

PTC has a propensity for early spread to regional lymph nodes but a low incidence of distance metastases. Cervical lymph nodes are involved in 20–60% of patients in most series using standard pathologic techniques [4–6]. Although lymph node metastases are more common with increased tumor size and extrathyroidal extension, it may be present with small, intrathyroidal tumors [7]. Since the lymph node metastases are the most common independent risk factor for persistent and recurrent disease, identification and removal of the locoregional disease remains an essential component of initial surgical treatment. Hence, optimal management of thyroid cancer is highly dependent on accurate staging of the extent of disease before surgery.

28.2.1 Evaluation and Diagnosis

It is known that preoperative physical examination is inadequate for the detection of cervical lymph node metastases in both lateral and central compartments, and preoperative staging and follow-up should depend on better diagnostic tools in patients with thyroid cancer. Neck USG is generally considered to be the most sensitive imaging modality to assess the primary tumor and identify lymph node metastases [8]. Though sonography is becoming widely accepted as the technique of choice for staging papillary thyroid carcinoma, assessment of lymph nodes is more challenging compared to thyroid nodule evaluation. While missed findings on preoperative USG may lead to understaging and inadequate surgical management, excessively skeptical reporting of nodal findings may result in submission of the majority of patients to FNAB, causing anxiety and extended preoperative workup with many unnecessary biopsies.

The accuracy of preoperative USG for the assessment of lateral compartment node metastases is well documented. Preoperative ultrasound has a reported sensitivity of 70–94% and specificity of 80–84% for the detection of lateral cervical lymph node metastases [9, 10]. However, its role in the identification of central compartment node metastases is more limited. The existence of thyroid gland, multinodular goiter, patients with short neck and limited extension, and poor ultrasound penetration due to obesity could be counted among the reasons why most false-negative USG results occurred in the central neck compartment. The existence of chronic lymphocytic thyroiditis could also affect the evaluation of central compartment since it is frequently associated with lymph node enlargement in the central compartment. However, preoperative USG may still play a role in the assessment of central compartment with high specificity (95%) and acceptable sensitivity (52%) [11].

The overall USG appearance of metastatic lymph nodes is usually abnormal, though micrometastases cannot be excluded in a sonographically normal lymph node. Normal and reactive lymph nodes have an echogenic hilus and tend to be hypoechoic compared with surrounding muscles and oval in shape. On color/power Doppler imaging, normal cervical nodes show either hilar vascularity or appear avascular, and reactive nodes predominantly show hilar vascularity. USG criteria used for differential diagnosis of metastatic lymph nodes include location, size, shape and border, echogenicity, loss of echogenic hilus, cystic changes, the presence of punctate calcification, and peripheral or mixed vascularity [12]. Each criterion is explained below briefly:

28.2.1.1 Location

Lymphatic flow is not a random process and follows certain patterns. Therefore, the location of the lymph nodes may also be useful for management. Most commonly first nodal metastases will be in the pre- and paratracheal region (level VI) followed by in levels III and IV, ipsilaterally [13]. Exceptionally, tumors arising in the upper pole of the thyroid have a higher tendency to demonstrate skip metastases to levels III and II [14].

28.2.1.2 Size

In general, larger nodes tend to have a higher incidence of malignancy, although reactive nodes can be as large as metastatic ones [15]. Different cutoffs of the nodal size have been proposed to differentiate reactive and metastatic nodes between 5 and 10 mm. Selecting lower cutoff value results in increased diagnostic sensitivity but decreased specificity and vice versa. Size criteria for cervical lymph node metastasis have yet to be determined. However, increasing nodal size on serial examinations in a patient with a history of thyroid carcinoma could be more important.

28.2.1.3 Shape and Borders

Metastatic nodes tend to be round in shape (short-axis to long-axis ratio >0.5), while normal or reactive lymph nodes are elliptical. Since the normal submandibular and parotid lymph nodes are round in shape, it should not be used as the sole criterion of nodal evaluation. Regardless of size, eccentric cortical thickening of lymph nodes, which is thought to be focal tumoral infiltration, should be alerting sign for metastases [16]. Metastatic lymph nodes generally have well-defined borders but may demonstrate ill-defined borders also. The nodal border itself is therefore not a reliable sign in the differential diagnosis. However, the presence of unclear margins and perinodal edema in a lymph node with suspicious USG findings strongly suggests extracapsular extension [16].

28.2.1.4 Echogenicity

Metastatic lymph nodes from papillary thyroid carcinoma may show increased echogenicity resembling thyroid echo, which is related to intranodal deposition of thyroglobulin. This USG feature is highly specific for thyroid origin of metastasis if it exists. On the contrary, most of the metastatic nodes are predominantly hypoechoic, irrespective of the primary origin of malignancy [15].

28.2.1.5 Loss of Echogenic Hilus

Most of the normal or reactive lymph nodes with a maximum transverse diameter larger than 5 mm will show a hilus, which is a linear, echogenic, non-shadowing structure containing nodal vessels. Metastatic nodes usually do not show an echogenic hilus. Despite high sensitivity, the presence or absence of echogenic hilus cannot be used as the single criterion in the differential diagnosis of cervical lymph nodes.

28.2.1.6 Cystic Changes

Cystic changes in a lymph node represent intranodal necrosis (cystic necrosis or coagulation necrosis) and should be regarded pathologic regardless of nodal size [15]. The existence of intranodal necrosis is highly suggestive of metastasis, although it could be found in tuberculosis nodes as well.

28.2.1.7 Punctate Calcification

Punctate calcifications are one of the most valuable signs of PTC representing psammomatous microcalcifications. Studies show that majority of such foci are found in benign nodules and represent sonographic artifacts at the back walls of microcystic areas or colloid crystals [17]. Metastatic lymph nodes from papillary thyroid carcinoma may also show microcalcifications, though it is quite uncommon for normal or reactive lymph nodes. Like the increased echo, the existence of microcalcification within lymph node is considered highly suggestive of metastases from papillary thyroid carcinoma [12]. Although the incidence is substantially lower than papillary carcinoma, metastatic lymph nodes from medullary thyroid carcinoma may also contain micro- or macrocalcifications [15].

28.2.1.8 Peripheral or Mixed Vascularity

On Doppler USG, most of the normal lymph nodes with a maximum transverse diameter larger than 5 mm will show either hilar vascularity or appear as avascular [15]. On the other hand, peripheral or mixed (both hilar and peripheral) vascularity, which is believed to be related to tumor infiltration, is considered pathologic.

Sonographic classification of cervical lymph nodes is straightforward in patients with known or suspected malignancy, if lymph nodes show highly specific USG features like cystic changes, microcalcification, increased echo, or pathologic vascularization. Unfortunately, these USG features are not sensitive enough, and most of the suspicious lymph nodes will show weak criteria like loss of echogenic hilus or increased size. Therefore, USG evaluation of cervical lymph nodes is not just an imaging study and should be done in light of all available laboratory and clinical data. Clinical risk factors for lymph node metastases such as tumor size, multifocality, thyroid capsule invasion, ETE, poor prognostic histopathologic type, male gender, or pediatric age should also be used for decisionmaking [15].

Cervical lymph nodes with a suspicious sonographic feature warrant further workup with FNAB and Tg in needle washout. Though there is no standardization of Tg washout procedures including diluent type and volume, Tg values in needle washout are generally found unquestionably high compared with the serum levels. The method is particularly valuable when the lymph nodes are cystic, aspirate is nondiagnostic or cytological, and sonographic findings are conflicting. Contrary to serum Tg measurements, FNA measurement of Tg is not prone to interference from anti-Tg autoantibodies, which commonly cause falsely low serum Tg measurements. Tg washout technique is not generally recommended in the central compartment when the thyroid gland is present due to possible contamination from thyroid gland [3].

28.2.2 Management

According to our postoperative risk stratification and RAI decision protocol, T4 suppression started after operation for 3 weeks and stopped for another 3 weeks to check stimulated thyroglobulin (Tg) levels. At 6-week follow-up, TSH was 66 μIU/mL, and Tg level was 0.156 ng/mL without Tg antibodies. Neck USG was unremarkable. Based on the excellent response to initial therapy, follow-up without RAI ablation was recommended to him by our endocrine tumor board.

The use of adjuvant RAI therapy in ATA intermediate-risk patients is not the standard approach, and selective use is recommended according to individual risk assessment [3]. Postoperative Tg values could be one of the most useful prognostic tools along with the neck USG that can be used to guide decisionmaking. Postoperative Tg values are expected to reach its nadir 3–4 weeks after the operation [18]. It has been reported that a nonstimulated postoperative Tg < 1 ng/mL was associated with excellent clinical outcomes and recurrence rates $<1\%$ in ATA low- and intermediate-risk patients that did not receive RAI remnant ablation [19]. Therefore, postoperative serum Tg combined with neck USG could provide critical information to decide on adjuvant RAI treatment.

28.3 Follow-Up and Outcome

Six months after the surgery, serum Tg was undetectable under suppression therapy, and USG of the neck did not show any suspicious lymph node in central and lateral neck, compatible with clinical remission. He has been scheduled for annual Tg and neck USG.

What Can We Learn from This Case?

- USG evaluation of patients with known or suspected malignancy should always include bilateral cervical lymph node compartments (levels I–VI) to guide a complete resection of the primary tumor and affected lymph nodes.
- Preoperative USG evaluation should be done in light of all available data including laboratory and pathology results with a clinical perspective.
- Cystic changes, microcalcification, increased echo, and peripheral or mixed vascularity are highly predictive of lymph node metastasis in patients with known or suspected thyroid malignancy.
- Lateral cervical lymph nodes with a suspicious sonographic feature warrant further workup with FNAB and Tg measurement in needle washout.
- Adjuvant RAI therapy would not be necessary for ATA intermediate-risk patients with excellent response to initial therapy. Follow-up without RAI ablation could be an acceptable alternative in patients with low Tg values and normal neck USG.

References

1. Amin MB, Edge SB, Greene FL, Compton CC, Gershenwald JE, Brookland RK, et al., editors. AJCC cancer staging manual. 8th ed. New York: Springer; 2017.
2. Edge SB, Byrd DR, Compton CC, Fritz AG, Greene FL, Trotti A, editors. AJCC cancer staging manual. 7th ed. New York: Springer; 2010.
3. Haugen BR, Alexander EK, Bible KC, Doherty GM, Mandel SJ, Nikiforov YE, et al. 2015 American Thyroid Association management guidelines for adult patients with thyroid nodules and differentiated thyroid cancer: the American Thyroid Association guidelines task force on thyroid nodules and differentiated thyroid cancer. Thyroid. 2016;26:1–133. https://doi.org/10.1089/thy.2015.0020.
4. Scheumann G, Gimm O, Wegener G, Hundeshagen H, Dralle H. Prognostic significance and surgical management of locoregional lymph node metastases in papillary thyroid cancer. World J Surg. 1994;18:559–67; discussion 567–8.
5. Ito Y, Uruno T, Nakano K, Takamura Y, Miya A, Kobayashi K, et al. An observation trial without surgical treatment in patients with papillary microcarcinoma of the thyroid. Thyroid. 2003;13:381–7.
6. Chow S, Law S, Chan J, Au S, Yau S, Lau W. Papillary microcarcinoma of the thyroid – prognostic significance of lymph node metastasis and multifocality. Cancer. 2003;98:31–40.
7. Hay ID, Grant CS, van Heerden JA, Goellner JR, Ebersold JR, Bergstralh EJ. Papillary thyroid microcarcinoma: a study of 535 cases observed in a 50-year period. Surgery. 1992;112:1139–46; discussion 1146–7.
8. Morita S, Mizoguchi K, Suzuki M, Iizuka K. The accuracy of (18)[F]-fluoro-2-deoxy-D-glucose-positron emission tomography/computed tomography, ultrasonography, and enhanced computed tomography alone in the preoperative diagnosis of cervical lymph node metastasis in patients with papillary thyroid carcinoma. World J Surg. 2010;34:2564–9. https://doi.org/10.1007/s00268-010-0733-8.
9. Hwang H, Orloff L. Efficacy of preoperative neck ultrasound in the detection of cervical lymph node metastasis form thyroid cancer. Laryngoscope. 2011;121:487–91. https://doi.org/10.1002/lary.21227.
10. Lee D, Ji Y, Sung E, Park JS, Lee YJ, Park DW, et al. Roles of ultrasonography and computed tomography in the surgical management of cervical lymph node metastases in papillary thyroid carcinoma. Eur J Surg Oncol. 2013;39:191–6. https://doi.org/10.1006/j.ejso.2012.07.119.
11. Kouvaraki MA, Shapiro SE, Fornage BD, Edeiken-Monro BS, Sherman SI, Vassilopoulou-Sellin R, et al. Role of preoperative ultrasonography in the surgical management of patients with thyroid cancer. Surgery. 2003;134:946–54; discussion 954–5.
12. Leboulleux S, Girard E, Rose M, Travagli JP, Sabbah N, Caillou B, et al. Ultrasound criteria of malignancy for cervical lymph nodes in patients followed up for differentiated thyroid cancer. J Clin Endocrinol Metab. 2007;92:3590–4.
13. Machens A, Hinze R, Thomusch O, Dralle H. Pattern of nodal metastasis for primary and reoperative thyroid cancer. World J Surg. 2002;26:22–8.
14. Park JH, Lee YS, Kim BW, Chang HS, Park CS. Skip lateral neck node metastases in papillary thyroid carcinoma. World J Surg. 2012;36:743–7. https://doi.org/10.1007/s00268-012-1476-5.
15. Ahuja AT, Ying M, Ho SY, Antonio G, Lee YP, King AD, et al. Ultrasound of malignant cervical lymph nodes. Cancer Imaging. 2008;8:48–56. https://doi.org/10.1102/1470-7330.2008.0006.

16. Qualliotine JR, Coquia SF, Hamper UM, Fakhry C. Association of ultrasound characteristics with extranodal extension in metastatic papillary thyroid carcinoma. JAMA Otolaryngol Head Neck Surg. 2016;142:263–9. https://doi.org/10.1001/jamaoto.2015.3558.
17. Malhi H, Beland MD, Cen SY, Allgood E, Daley K, Martin SE, et al. Echogenic foci in thyroid nodules: significance of posterior acoustic artifacts. AJR Am J Roentgenol. 2014;203:1310–6. https://doi.org/10.2214/AJR-13.11934.
18. Giovanella L, Ceriani L, Maffioli M. Postsurgery serum thyroglobulin disappearance kinetic in patients with differentiated thyroid carcinoma. Head Neck. 2010;32:568–71. https://doi.org/10.1002/hed.21214.
19. Ibrahimpasic T, Nixon IJ, Palmer FL, Whitcher MM, Tuttle RM, Shaha A, et al. Undetectable thyroglobulin after total thyroidectomy in patients with low- and intermediate-risk papillary thyroid cancer—is there a need for radioactive iodine therapy? Surgery. 2012;152:1096–105. https://doi.org/10.1016/j.surg.2012.08.034.

Papillary Thyroid Carcinoma and Microcarcinoma

29

Ülkem Yararbaş and Zehra Özcan

Abstract

Papillary thyroid carcinoma (PTC) is the most common thyroid cancer subtype and constitutes 80% of all thyroid malignancies. PTC lesions that are 1 cm or less in size are defined as "papillary thyroid microcarcinoma" (PTMC). The incidence of occult PTC cases detected on autopsy series is very high, ranging from 10 to 35%. With the increased use of diagnostic imaging modalities, the detection rate of thyroid cancer is increasing worldwide. Both PTC and PTMC have good prognosis. Due to indolent nature of the disease, especially in PTMC cases, both the extent of the initial surgery and the need for RAI treatment remain controversial.

In this section, two cases are presented. One of them is a PTC with lymph node metastases, and the other is a PTMC case with multifocal disease.

Ü. Yararbaş (✉) · Z. Özcan
Department of Nuclear Medicine, Ege University School of Medicine, Izmir, Turkey

29.1 Case Presentation

29.1.1 Case 1

A 62-year-old female patient with known Hashimoto thyroiditis and a 3 cm thyroid nodule with benign cytology underwent a routine neck thyroid ultrasonography (USG) in 2012. Besides heterogeneous echotexture related to Hashimoto's disease and the known benign nodule in the right thyroid lobe, a new, 10 × 8 mm, hypoechoic nodular lesion with microcalcifications and lobulated margins was observed in left thyroid lobe. The nodule had peripheral and internal vascular flow on Doppler evaluation. Additionally, an 8 × 5 mm lymph node located on the medial border of the internal jugular vein was also detected. Both the thyroid nodule in the left lobe and the lymph node were reported as highly suspicious for malignancy. The patient underwent total thyroidectomy and central lymph node dissection. Histopathological analysis of the nodule revealed a 1.2 cm thyroid papillary carcinoma, classical variant with intrathyroidal infiltrations. The tumor was located near the thyroid capsule, but there was no sign of capsular or vascular invasion. Among seven lymph nodes dissected, four of them were found to be metastatic. Three of four metastatic nodes were micrometastasis (tumor deposit <2 mm). According to AJCC 7th Edition/TNM Classification System Differentiated Thyroid

T. Özülker et al. (eds.), *Thyroid and Parathyroid Diseases*, https://doi.org/10.1007/978-3-319-78476-2_29

Carcinoma, the patient was classified as stage III (T1aN1aM0, patient age ≥45).

Four weeks after surgery, without starting thyroxine (T4) replacement, laboratory tests and thyroid scan with Tc99m pertechnetate were performed. Thyroid-stimulating hormone (TSH) level was 124 μIU/mL (normal range, 0.35–5.50 μIU/mL), and thyroglobulin (Tg) level was 1.24 ng/dL. Anti-Tg antibody was <20 IU/mL. Thyroid scan showed residual thyroid tissue at pyramidal lobe location. The patient underwent high dose (150 mCi) radioactive iodine (RAI) therapy. Whole-body images obtained at the tenth day of the RAI treatment were in concordance with Tc99m pertechnetate scintigraphy and showed a small residual thyroid tissue in pyramidal lobe location. No additional focus suggesting metastatic involvement was detected. Since the patient had metastatic disease, thyroxine replacement was started at TSH suppression dose (TSH level < 0.1 μIU/mL).

29.1.2 Case 2

A 32-year-old female patient underwent total thyroidectomy due to multinodular goiter in 2002. Histopathological analysis showed three incidental foci of papillary microcarcinoma, classical variant. Lesions were 2, 3, and 5 mm in diameter. There was no sign of capsular or lymphovascular invasions. According to the AJCC 7th Edition/TNM Classification System Differentiated Thyroid Carcinoma, the patient was classified as stage I (T1N0M0, patient age < 45). Postoperative laboratory data obtained 4 weeks after the surgery was as follows: TSH, 120 μIU/mL, and Tg, 1.1 g/dL. Anti-Tg antibody was <20 IU/mL. Since histopathological characteristics of the tumor were favorable, and the patient was at the childbearing age, tumor board decision was in favor of follow-up instead of RAI therapy. Thyroxine replacement was started at a dose targeting TSH level below normal limits (TSH level < 0.1 μIU/mL).

29.2 Discussion

Papillary thyroid carcinoma (PTC) is the most common thyroid cancer subtype and constitutes 80% of all thyroid malignancies [1]. Among environmental, genetic, and hormonal etiological factors, radiation exposure is the best-defined factor for the development of PTC [2]. Although thyroid cancers account for less than 1% of all cancers, the incidence of occult PTC cases detected on autopsy series is very high, ranging from 10 to 35% [3]. The incidence of PTC is known to increase worldwide [3]. A significant proportion of this increase is due to the rise in the detection rate of these occult and relatively small lesions. Incidental lesions which are diagnosed histopathologically in a patient operated for benign thyroid disease are much more common when compared with patients having symptomatic thyroid cancer. Most of the PTC have excellent prognosis [4]. Patient age exceeding 45 years, the presence of lymph node metastasis, significant extrathyroidal extension, and aggressive histological features are indicators of relatively poor outcome [5–7].

According to the World Health Organization (WHO) histologic classification, "papillary thyroid microcarcinoma" (PTMC) is described as a lesion 1 cm or less in size. PTMC is more frequent in females and young people (<45 years old). Multifocal disease and regional lymph node metastasis are common [8]. PTMC is known to have a very good prognosis with disease-specific mortality rate lower than 1% [9].

The general approach in the management differentiated thyroid cancers consists of adequate surgery that may be followed by RAI treatment and TSH suppression as adjuvant therapies. However, due to indolent nature of the disease especially in PTMC cases, both the extent of the initial surgery and the need of RAI treatment remain controversial. In the light of cumulative data, recommendations of guidelines and expert opinions evolve to a more conservative approach. One of the studies justifying the use of conservative approach is performed by Ito et al. The study is conducted on 1235 patients having PTMC lesions which are not accompanied by sign of lymph node metastasis on ultrasonography, located far from trachea and recurrent laryngeal nerve, and not having progressive signs on follow-up showed that most of the patients will not need surgery since only a small proportion developed lymph node metastasis (1.7% in 5 years and 3.8% in 10 years follow-up) or tumor size progression exceeding 3 mm (5% in 5 years and 10% in 10 years) [10].

The 2009 American Thyroid Association (ATA) risk stratification system that is predicting recurrent and/or persistent disease risk has been modified in 2015 regarding the definition of low risk to include small-volume lymph node metastases (clinical N0 or ≤5 pathologic N1 micrometastases, <0.2 cm in largest dimension), intrathyroidal well-differentiated follicular cancer with capsular or minor vascular invasion (<4 vessels involved), and intrathyroidal papillary microcarcinomas having BRAF wild-type or BRAF mutations [9, 11]. In the modified version of the guideline, intermediate risk is defined as clinical N1 or >5 pathologic N1 with all involved lymph nodes <3 cm in largest dimension.

Primary tumor characteristics of Case 1 presented in this section remain in low-risk group both before and after modification since the lesion is intrathyroidal without vascular invasion. However, when lymph node status is considered, our case which was classified as intermediate risk in 2009 ATA risk stratification system shifts to a place between low- and intermediate-risk group. Although for patients with ATA intermediate- or low-risk DTC, RAI therapy is not considered as necessary, the impact of RAI treatment in improving patient outcome especially in older age, unfavorable histological subtypes, and lymph node metastasis particularly when located in outside of central neck should be considered.

As seen in Case 2, multifocality of PTMC is a frequent finding [12]. Although some earlier reports support the benefit of radioiodine therapy in PTMC especially in multifocal lesions, currently, in American Thyroid Association (ATA) guideline, both unifocal and multifocal PTMC are included in low-risk group even in the presence of $BRAF^{V600E}$ mutation [9, 13, 14]. The ATA guideline summarizes molecular characteristics that cause a less favorable prognosis in PTMC patients as the coexistence of BRAF mutations with other oncogenic mutations like PIK3CA, AKT1, and also the presence of TERT promoter, TP53 mutations [9]. Tumor characteristics that cause risk group modification toward intermediate risk are aggressive histology including tall cell variant, hobnail variant and columnar cell carcinoma, and multifocal papillary microcarcinoma with extrathyroidal extension.

Hashimoto's thyroiditis (HT) is a common autoimmune disease leading to hypothyroidism and therefore elevated TSH levels. As in Case 1, co-occurrence of HT and PTC is frequently seen. Although the effect of HT on PTC development is still unclear, there are studies showing significantly increased PTC incidence in HT patients with elevated TSH levels [15].

Another point with the coexisting HT in a PTC patient is the fact that Anti-Tg antibodies existing in HT patients may interfere and diminish the reliability of Tg measurements [16].

29.3 Follow-Up and Clinical Course

29.3.1 Case 1

After 8 months following RAI therapy, a radioiodine scan was performed with thyroxine (T4) withdrawal. No residual functioning thyroid tissue was detected on I-131 whole-body scan. Currently, the patient is in her sixth year of follow-up. Yearly performed neck USGs did not show any sign of recurrence. Tg levels measured every 6 months while on thyroxine replacement are <0.9 ng/dL. Starting from fourth year of the diagnosis, thyroxine dosage was gradually decreased targeting TSH level within low reference range (0.5–2 μIU/mL).

29.3.2 Case 2

Currently, the patient is in her fifteenth year of follow-up. Neck USGs performed yearly, and non-stimulated Tg measurements show no evidence of recurrence. Starting from the second year of the diagnosis, thyroxine dosage has been set to target TSH level between 0.5 and 2 μIU/mL.

What Can We Learn from This Case?

- Lymph node metastasis is frequently seen in PTC even in patients with small tumors. However, life expectancy is still very high in this group of patients.
- Even in the presence of metastatic lymph nodes in central neck area, PTC cases bear low risk for recurrent or persistent diseases.
- Multifocality is frequently seen in PTMCs. Patients with multifocal disease are still considered in the low-risk group for development or persistence of disease following surgery.
- Coexistence of Hashimoto's thyroiditis and PTC is high. In patients having elevated Anti-Tg antibodies, the reliability of Tg measurements can be diminished.

References

1. Sadler GP, Clark OH. Schwartz's principles of surgery, vol. 36. 7th ed. New York: McGraw-Hill; 1999. p. 1661–87.
2. Lloyd RV, Buehler D, Khanafshar E. Papillary thyroid carcinoma variants. Head Neck Pathol. 2011;5:51–6. https://doi.org/10.1007/s12105-010-0236-9.
3. Shah JP. Thyroid carcinoma: epidemiology, histology, and diagnosis. Clin Adv Hematol Oncol. 2015;13(4 Suppl 4):3–6.
4. Ito Y, Masuoka H, Fukushima M, Inoue H, Kihara M, Tomoda C, et al. Excellent prognosis of patients with solitary T1N0M0 papillary thyroid carcinoma who underwent thyroidectomy and elective lymph node dissection without radioiodine therapy. World J Surg. 2010;34:1285–90. https://doi.org/10.1007/s00268-009-0356-0.
5. Zaydfudim V, Feurer ID, Griffin MR, Phay JE. The impact of lymph node involvement on survival in patients with papillary and follicular thyroid carcinoma. Surgery. 2008;144:1070–7. https://doi.org/10.1016/j.surg.2008.08.034.
6. Gilliland FD, Hunt WC, Morris DM, Key CR. Prognostic factors for thyroid carcinoma. A population-based study of 15,698 cases from the Surveillance, Epidemiology and End Results (SEER) program 1973-1991. Cancer. 1997;79:564–73.
7. Ito Y, Kudo T, Kobayashi K, Miya A, Ichihara K, Miyauchi A. Prognostic factors for recurrence of papillary thyroid carcinoma in the lymph nodes, lung, and bone: analysis of 5,768 patients with average 10-year follow-up. World J Surg. 2012;36:1274–8. https://doi.org/10.1007/s00268-012-1423-5.
8. Xu Y, Xu L, Wang J. Clinical predictors of lymph node metastasis and survival rate in papillary thyroid microcarcinoma: analysis of 3607 patients at a single institution. J Surg Res. 2018;221:128–34. https://doi.org/10.1016/j.jss.2017.08.007.
9. Haugen BR, Alexander EK, Bible KC, Doherty GM, Mandel SJ, Nikiforov YE, et al. 2015 American Thyroid Association management guidelines for adult patients with thyroid nodules and differentiated thyroid cancer: the American Thyroid Association guidelines task force on thyroid nodules and differentiated thyroid cancer. Thyroid. 2016;26:1–133. https://doi.org/10.1089/thy.2015.0020.
10. Ito Y, Miyauchi A, Inoue H, Fukushima M, Kihara M, Higashiyama T, et al. An observational trial for papillary thyroid microcarcinoma in Japanese patients. World J Surg. 2010;34:28. https://doi.org/10.1007/s00268-009-0303-0.
11. Fabián P, Fernando J, Carolina U, Angélica S, Erika A, Fernanda B, et al. Implementing the modified 2009 American Thyroid Association risk stratification system in thyroid cancer patients with low and intermediate risk of recurrence. Thyroid. 2015;25:1235–42. https://doi.org/10.1089/thy.2015.0121.
12. Hay ID, Grant CS, van Heerden JA, Goellner JR, Ebersold JR, Bergstralh EJ. Papillary thyroid microcarcinoma: a study of 535 cases observed in a 50-year period. Surgery. 1992;112:1139–46.
13. Dietlein M, Luyken WA, Schicha H, Larena-Avellaneda A. Incidental multifocal papillary microcarcinomas of the thyroid: is subtotal thyroidectomy combined with radioiodine ablation enough? Nucl Med Commun. 2005;26:3–8.
14. Küçük NO, Tari P, Tokmak E, Aras G. Treatment for microcarcinoma of the thyroid—clinical experience. Clin Nucl Med. 2007;32:279–81.
15. Lun Y, Wu X, Xia Q, Han Y, Zhang X, Liu Z, et al. Hashimoto's thyroiditis as a risk factor of papillary thyroid cancer may improve cancer prognosis. Otolaryngol Head Neck Surg. 2013;148:396–402. https://doi.org/10.1177/0194599812472426.
16. Spencer C, Petrovic I, Fatemi S. Current thyroglobulin autoantibody (TgAb) assays often fail to detect interfering TgAb that can result in the reporting of falsely low/undetectable serum Tg IMA values for patients with differentiated thyroid cancer. J Clin Endocrinol Metab. 2011;96:1283–91. https://doi.org/10.1210/jc.2010-2762.

30 A Patient Presented with Extensive Lung Metastases of Papillary Thyroid Carcinoma Without Any Primary Focus Detected on Total Thyroidectomy

Tevfik Fikret Çermik and Nurhan Ergül

Abstract

The most common metastatic sites of differentiated thyroid cancer (DTC) are the lung and bone after lymph nodes. A newly defined type of occult DTC is consistent with metastatic disease without an identified primary malignancy in the thyroid gland after total resection. We present a patient with multiple lung metastases of occult DTC showing mild ^{18}F-fluorodeoxyglucose (FDG) uptake and intense radioiodine uptake without a primary lesion in the thyroid gland.

30.1 Case Presentation

A 68-year-old woman presented with cough and chest pain. Thorax computerized tomography (CT) examination revealed multiple non-calcified nodular lesions suspected of metastases. The patient underwent ^{18}F-fluorodeoxyglucose positron emission tomography/computerized tomography (FDG PET/CT) for metabolic characterization of nodules and localization of a possible primary malignancy (Fig. 30.1). Mild FDG uptake was observed in lung nodules (SUVmax = 1.9) and reported as nonspecific/inflammatory lesions. There was a peripherally calcified nodular lesion in the posterior region of the right thyroid lobe approximately 2 cm in diameter having FDG uptake at background levels. A wedge resection from the lung demonstrated metastasis of follicular variant of papillary thyroid carcinoma. Bilateral total thyroidectomy operation was performed upon this finding. The histopathological examination showed adenomatous hyperplasia in both thyroid lobes and no finding of malignancy. The patient was treated with 200 mCi I-131 for lung metastases. The whole-body scan after therapy showed intense radioiodine uptake in lung nodules and mediastinum (Fig. 30.2). The thyroglobulin (Tg) level was 2462 ng/mL before radioiodine therapy. Three months after the therapy, Tg level decreased to 17.6 ng/mL. The patient was under L-thyroxine therapy with suppressed TSH levels. A control ^{18}F-FDG PET/CT scan was performed after 9 months of therapy (Fig. 30.3). Most of the lung nodules that were detected in first PET/CT study were regressed both in size and FDG uptake, and some of them were not visualized anymore. At this time, Tg level was 2.56 ng/mL, and second cure of radioiodine therapy was administered. The whole-body scan after 200 mCi I-131 administration did not show any pathologic uptake in the thyroid region, lungs, and other parts of the body, and the patient was ablated (Fig. 30.4). After 2 months of radioiodine therapy, Tg level was 0.06 ng/mL under TSH suppression.

T. F. Çermik · N. Ergül (✉)
University of Health Sciences, İstanbul Training and Research Hospital, Clinic of Nuclear Medicine, Istanbul, Turkey

T. Özülker et al. (eds.), *Thyroid and Parathyroid Diseases*, https://doi.org/10.1007/978-3-319-78476-2_30

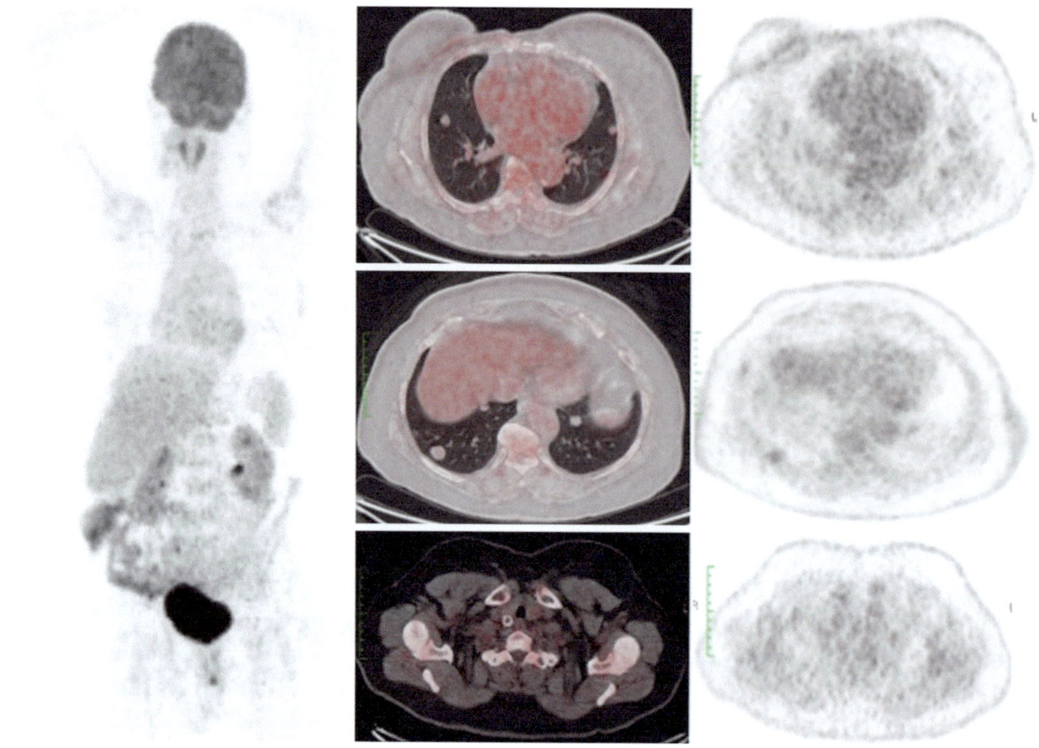

Fig. 30.1 Mild FDG uptake in lung nodules and no pathological uptake in the thyroid nodule in the right lobe

30.2 Discussion

Differentiated thyroid cancer (DTC) referring to papillary and follicular carcinoma is usually characterized by good prognosis. The incidence of the distant metastatic disease has been reported to be 7–23% after initial treatment and 1–9% at first presentation before any treatment [1]. The lung and bone are the most common metastatic sites of DTC after lymph nodes [2]. A retrospective study with 49 patients having distant metastases at the presentation of thyroid carcinoma revealed 3-year and 5-year survival rates of 69% and 50%, respectively. The 3-year survival rates were better for patients aged ≤45, with lung-only versus bone-only metastasis, having papillary versus follicular carcinoma and iodine-avid disease versus non-avid [1].

Occult thyroid carcinoma (OTC) is usually considered as similar to papillary microcarcinoma. The tumor is either detected incidentally after total thyroidectomy for benign disease or at autopsy. In some cases, the patient is presented with apparent metastases of thyroid carcinoma, and the malign lesion is detected in the pathological examination of total thyroidectomy material. Liu et al. have defined a new group of OTC that presented with metastases of thyroid carcinoma at cervical lymph nodes or distant sites; however, the primary malign lesion is not detected in total thyroidectomy specimen. They reported a patient with lymph node metastasis of thyroid carcinoma and no malignity found in the thyroid gland after total thyroidectomy [3]. Our patient seems to be belonging to this group with lung metastases of thyroid carcinoma having no primary at thyroid gland. Borsò et al. also reported a case with disseminating bone metastases of DTC; however, primary malign focus was not detected in thyroidectomy [4]. Xu et al. have recently reported seven cases with this phenomenon having cervical lymph node metastases from thyroid cancer without an identifiable malign lesion in the thyroid gland. A papillary carcinoma phenotype was found in all cases, and most of them were BRAFV600E-positive tumors [5].

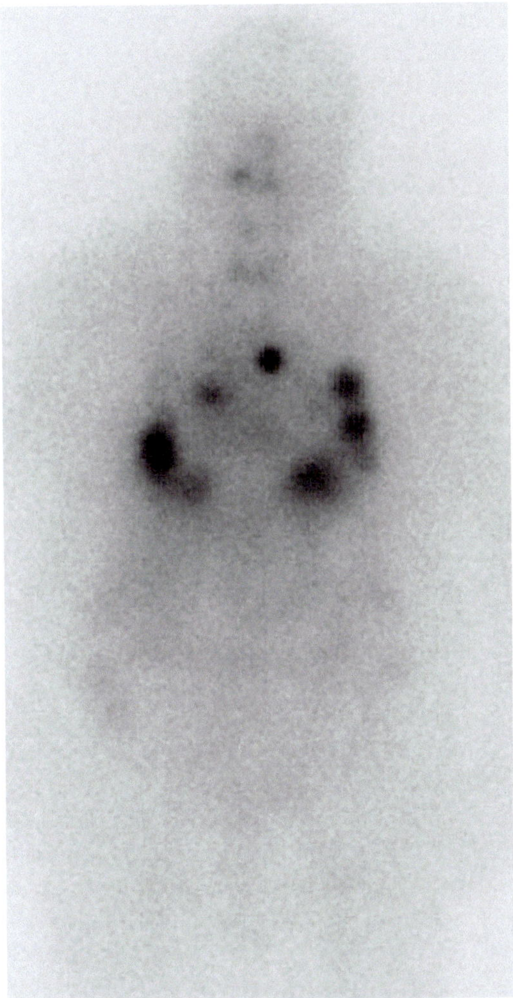

Fig. 30.2 Whole-body scan after 200 mCi radioiodine therapy; intense uptake in lung nodules and mediastinum

The lung is a common organ for metastasis from various tumor types. Pulmonary metastases of thyroid carcinoma are often seen as micronodular or miliary spread throughout both lungs. However, solitary nodular metastasis from thyroid cancer is also reported [6]. In a retrospective study with 75 patients having pulmonary metastases from DTC in different patterns like nodular, diffuse, or combined, it was reported that the treatment responses were not significantly different between patients with varying types of metastasis. However, there was a significant difference between patients with different types of tumor, papillary versus follicular thyroid carcinoma [7]. The initial size of the lung metastasis was also reported to be a significant prognostic factor revealing that patients having macronodular metastases (≥1 cm) had significantly poor treatment responses and disease progression irrespective of radioiodine avidity [8].

The first-line therapy for patients having pulmonary metastases from DTC should be I-131 therapy, as long as the metastases are iodine-avid [9–11]. Song et al. reported the therapy responses and prognostic factors in 372 patients with pulmonary metastases from DTC that received radioiodine therapy. Among patients with iodine-avid pulmonary metastases (68.8%), 60.9% showed a significant decrease in serum Tg levels after I-131 therapy and 60.3% showed a reduction in the size of pulmonary metastases on CT. In only 24.2% of patients, a complete cure

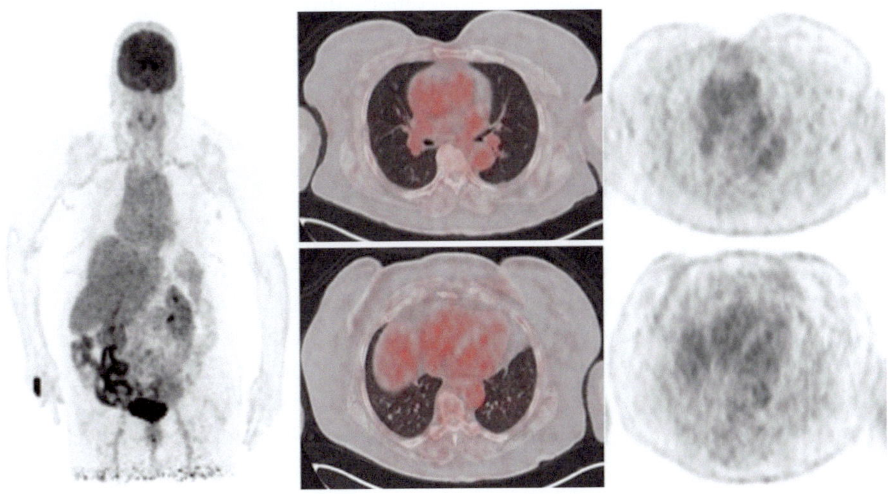

Fig. 30.3 FDG PET/CT after radioiodine therapy; lung nodules are regressed; some of them are not visualized

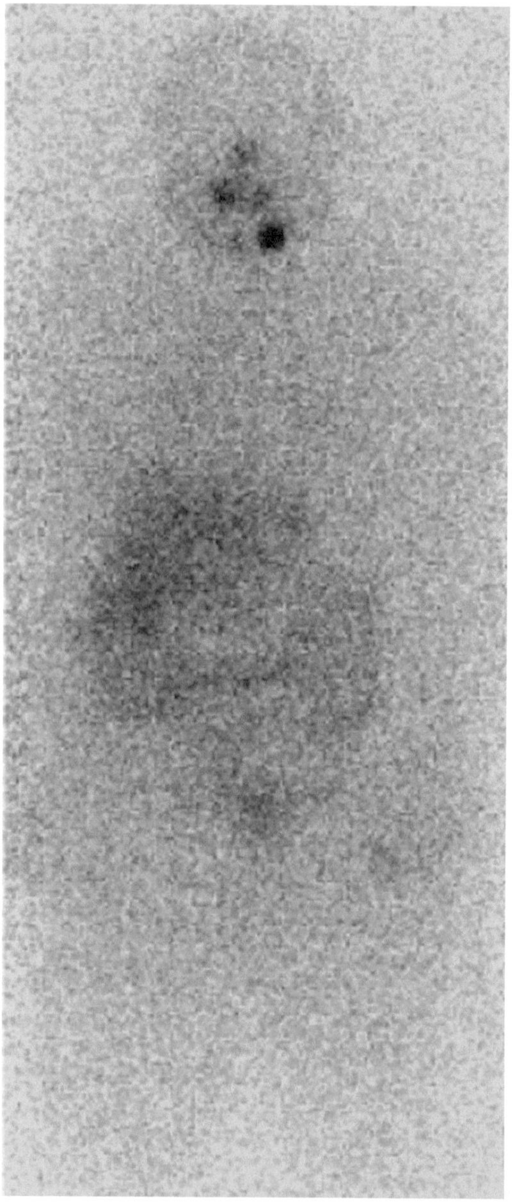

Fig. 30.4 Whole-body scan after the second cure of 200 mCi radioiodine therapy; no uptake in lung nodules and mediastinum

was achieved. The significant independent variables between the groups of iodine-avid and non-avid groups were age, the presence of multiple distant metastases, and pulmonary metastatic nodule size; the patients under 40 years old with lung-only metastatic disease and micronodular or miliary metastases seemed to have favorable outcomes [9]. In another recent study with eight patients, the overall effective rate of radioiodine therapy for lung metastases of DTC was 72.5%. This study showed that gender, pulmonary nodule size, the absence or presence of extrapulmonary distant metastases, age, and Tg level at diagnosis were significantly associated with I-131 therapy efficacy; older patients with higher Tg levels at diagnosis and extrapulmonary distant metastases more likely showed poor prognosis. The optimal cutoffs for age and Tg level to predict therapy efficacy were reported to be 46 years old and 55.50 ng/mL, respectively [10].

The contribution of PET/CT with different radiolabelled agents to staging and follow-up of thyroid cancer has been reported in many studies up-to-date. ^{18}F-FDG PET/CT is routinely used in patients of DTC presenting with high Tg levels and negative iodine scintigraphy (TENIS), and in medullary thyroid carcinoma with elevated tumor markers (calcitonin and carcinoembryonic antigen) detected after thyroidectomy. Another application of PET/CT in thyroid cancer is the use of somatostatin analogs labeled with ^{68}Ga-DOTA compounds for evaluation of peptide receptor radionuclide therapy for patients having non-iodine-avid metastatic disease or considering the heterogeneous behavior of metastatic lesions. PET/CT with iodine-124 has also been reported to be used for dosimetric studies to achieve an individualized therapy [12]. As in many other tumor types, intense uptake of ^{18}F-FDG in primary lesion or metastases of DTC indicates a rapidly dividing and dedifferentiated tumor and poor prognosis [13]. In a study comparing the efficacy of ^{18}F-FDG PET/CT and PET/MRI in patients with dedifferentiated thyroid cancer, PET/CT was found to be superior to PET/MRI to detect the pulmonary metastases, while for cervical status, they were equal when PET/CT is performed with contrast enhancement [14]. The pathologic uptake in the thyroid gland or metastases associated with thyroid carcinoma may be found incidentally in a ^{18}F-FDG PET/CT scan made for another known malignancy in other parts of the body [15]. In our patient, the pulmonary metastatic nodules had shown mild ^{18}F-FDG uptake not reaching levels of malignancy, however, intense radioiodine uptake revealing the good differentiation of the tumor and a favorable outcome after radioiodine therapy.

What Can We Learn from This Case?

- Occult thyroid carcinoma may present with distant metastases without a primary lesion detected on total thyroidectomy.
- Well-differentiated thyroid cancer metastases may show low ^{18}F-FDG uptake while they are intensely iodine-avid.
- I-131 therapy is the preferred therapy for metastatic DTC as long as the metastases show iodine uptake.

References

1. Sampson E, Brierley JD, Le LW, Rotstein L, Tsang RW. Clinical management and outcome of papillary and follicular (differentiated) thyroid cancer presenting with distant metastasis at diagnosis. Cancer. 2007;110:1451–6.
2. Kalra R, Pawar R, Hasija S, Chandna A, Sankla M, Malhotra C. Frontal bone metastasis from an occult follicular thyroid carcinoma: diagnosed by FNAC. J Cytol. 2017;34:59–61.
3. Liu H, Lv L, Yang K. Occult thyroid carcinoma: a rare case report and review of literature. Int J Clin Exp Pathol. 2014;7:5210–4.
4. Borsò E, Boni G, Mazzarri S, Cocciaro A, Gambacciani C, Traino AC, et al. Disseminated bone metastases from occult thyroid cancer effectively treated with debulking surgery and a single dosimetry-guided administration of radioiodine. Rev Esp Med Nucl Imagen Mol. 2015;34:111–5.
5. Xu B, Scognamiglio T, Cohen PR, Prasad ML, Hasanovic A, Michael Tuttle R, et al. Metastatic thyroid carcinoma without identifiable primary tumor within the thyroid gland: a retrospective study of a rare phenomenon. Hum Pathol. 2017;65:133–9.
6. Kaseda K, Watanabe K, Sakamaki H, Kazama A. Solitary pulmonary metastasis from occult papillary thyroid carcinoma. Thorac Cancer. 2016;7:261–3.
7. Qutbi M, Shafeie B, Amoui M, Tabeie F, Azizmohammadi Z, Mahmoud-Pashazadeh A, et al. Evaluation of prognostic factors associated with differentiated thyroid carcinoma with pulmonary metastasis. Clin Nucl Med. 2016;41:917–21.
8. Kim M, Kim WG, Park S, Kwon H, Jeon MJ, Lee JJ, et al. Initial size of metastatic lesions is best prognostic factor in patients with metastatic differentiated thyroid carcinoma confined to the lung. Thyroid. 2017;27:49–58.
9. Song HJ, Qiu ZL, Shen CT, Wei WJ, Luo QY. Pulmonary metastases in differentiated thyroid cancer: efficacy of radioiodine therapy and prognostic factors. Eur J Endocrinol. 2015;173:399–408.
10. Wang R, Zhang Y, Tan J, Zhang G, Zhang R, Zheng W, et al. Analysis of radioiodine therapy and prognostic factors of differentiated thyroid cancer patients with pulmonary metastasis: an 8-year retrospective study. Medicine (Baltimore). 2017;96:e6809. https://doi.org/10.1097/MD.0000000000006809.
11. Biko J, Reiners C, Kreissl MC, Verburg FA, Demidchik Y, Drozd V. Favourable course of disease after incomplete remission on (131)I therapy in children with pulmonary metastases of papillary thyroid carcinoma: 10 years follow-up. Eur J Nucl Med Mol Imaging. 2011;38:651–5.
12. Basu S, Parghane RV. Designing and developing PET-based precision model in thyroid carcinoma: the potential avenues for a personalized clinical care. PET Clin. 2017;12:27–37.
13. Giraudet AL, Taïeb D. PET imaging for thyroid cancers: current status and future directions. Ann Endocrinol. 2017;78:38–42.
14. Vrachimis A, Burg MC, Wenning C, Allkemper T, Weckesser M, Schäfers M. [(18)F]FDG PET/CT outperforms [(18)F]FDG PET/MRI in differentiated thyroid cancer. Eur J Nucl Med Mol Imaging. 2016;43:212–20.
15. Kim MS, Sim YS, Lee SY, Jeon DG. Occult thyroid carcinoma detected by FDG-PET scan in elderly osteosarcoma patients: report of two cases. Ann Nucl Med. 2007;21:529–32.

31 Thyrotoxicosis Caused by Functioning Metastases of Differentiated Thyroid Cancer

Gülin Uçmak and Burcu Esen Akkaş

Abstract

Differentiated thyroid cancer is a malignant disease with favorable prognosis. The rate of distant metastases is rare. In general, metastases of well-differentiated thyroid cancer carry the main biological features of the thyroid cells such as Na-I symporter gene expression and thyroglobulin synthesis, since the cell does not transfer to an undifferentiated form. However, thyroid hormone synthesis by distant metastasis is uncommon. However, rarely hyperfunctioning distant metastases from DTC after total thyroidectomy can be seen and may result in hyperthyroidism or euthyroidism. In this chapter, the clinical management of a patient presenting with thyrotoxicosis due to hyperfunctioning bone metastases of thyroid cancer is discussed.

G. Uçmak (✉) · B. E. Akkaş
Department of Nuclear Medicine, University of Health Sciences (SBÜ) Dr. Abdurrahman Yurtaslan Ankara Oncology Training and Research Hospital, Ankara, Turkey

31.1 Case Presentation

A 54-year-old female patient was referred to our Nuclear Medicine Department with a diagnosis of bone metastases secondary to papillary thyroid cancer for clinical management and the evaluation of radioiodine treatment. Two months ago, she had undergone total hip replacement surgery following femoral head fracture. On surgical exploration, the fracture was recognized to be a pathological fracture, and histopathological examination revealed the metastases of papillary thyroid cancer. On her past medical history, we learned that she had undergone total thyroidectomy 10 years ago for multinodular goiter with a missing pathology report.

On neck ultrasound, small foci of residual thyroid tissue were observed on thyroid bed, 1 cm in size in the left lobe bed and 2 cm in the right lobe bed. In addition, enlarged cervical and supraclavicular lymph nodes were detected. On thyroid scan performed after the IV administration of 5 mCi Tc-99m pertechnetate, minimal uptake was seen reflecting normal functioning residual thyroid tissue. The patient was not receiving any thyroid replacement medication. Her thyroid function test results were as follows: free triiodothyronine (fT3) level of 8.4 pg/mL (reference range, 2.50–4.30 pg/mL), free thyroxine (fT4) level of 4.2 ng/dL (reference range, 0.90–1.70 ng/dL), and thyroid-stimulating hormone (TSH) level of 0.08 μIU/mL (reference range,

T. Özülker et al. (eds.), *Thyroid and Parathyroid Diseases*, https://doi.org/10.1007/978-3-319-78476-2_31

0.35–5.00 μIU/mL). Serum thyroglobulin (Tg) level was significantly elevated and measured as 19,000 ng/mL. Anti-thyroglobulin antibodies (TgAb) were within normal ranges. Liver function tests (LFT) and complete blood counts (CBC) were within normal ranges.

Antithyroid medication with propylthiouracil (PTU), four times 50 mg/day, was administrated to control thyrotoxicosis. Beta-blockers were also given to better control symptoms.

To evaluate disease extent, computed tomography (CT) of the thorax, magnetic resonance imaging (MRI) for the brain, bone scintigraphy, and radioiodine whole-body scan (WBS) with 2 mCi of I-131 were performed. On WBS performed 48 h after the oral administration of I-131, multiple sites of pathological uptake consistent with bone metastases in the calvarium, ribs, vertebral colon, pelvic bones, hips, and bilateral femurs were observed in addition to uptake in residual thyroid tissue (Fig. 31.1). Increased osteoblastic activity was detected on bone scintigraphy at the sites of iodine uptake on postsurgery radioiodine WBS. MRI was negative for brain metastases. A pulmonary nodule was detected on the right lung base on thorax CT. The dose of PTU was increased to six times 50 mg/day since TSH level was still low and FT3 was still elevated. No abnormality was seen in serum aspartate aminotransferase (AST) and alanine aminotransferase (ALT) levels on laboratory follow-up. External beam radiation therapy (EBRT) was given to the left femur and lumbar spine to palliate bone pain.

Then, the patient underwent completion thyroidectomy and bilateral neck dissection. Histopathology was consistent with lymph node metastases of papillary thyroid cancer.

Following surgery, I-131 treatment was planned with a dose of 200 mCi when the patient was still on antithyroid medication with PTU. After hospitalization for I-131 treatment, a careful physical examination and a detailed laboratory check including CBC, LFT, FT3, FT4, serum TSH, Tg, and TgAb levels were performed. CBC and LFT were normal. Serum Tg was elevated at 19700 ng/mL; TSH level was 0.37 μIU/mL despite high doses of PTU. Premedication with oral corticosteroids and beta-blockers was given starting a few days before iodine treatment. Antithyroid medication was stopped the day before the treatment. On the day of I-131 administration, short-acting steroids were administrated intravenously to prevent a possible thyroid storm resulting from the sudden release of preformed hormones from destructed metastatic deposits. In addition, antiemetics were administrated, and careful hydration was performed. A dose of 200 mCi of I-131 was administrated orally. Following treatment, the patient was kept in an isolated room specially designed for radionuclide therapy in our Nuclear Medicine Department. No complication was seen during the hospitalization period. On post-therapy WBS performed 4 days after therapy, intense uptake was seen at the same sites detected on postsurgery WBS performed with low-dose I-131 (Fig. 31.2).

The patient was examined 15 days after the administration of iodine. CBC, LFT, and thyroid function tests were checked. Serum TSH level was elevated at 15 μIU/mL; Tg level was 12,800 ng/mL. PTU dose decreased to three times 50 mg daily, and steroid treatment was stopped following gradual decrease of daily administered dose. We planned the second control of the patient 1 month after radioiodine treatment. On her control visit, PTU was stopped since TSH level increased to 28 μIU/mL. Serum LFTs and CBC were within normal range. L-thyroxin replacement was planned to be administered depending on serum TSH level on follow-up.

A second dose of 250 mCi was administered 9 months after the initial I-131 treatment dose. On laboratory examinations, serum TSH, Tg, FT3, and FT4 levels were 1.5 μIU/mL, 6065 ng/mL, 2.98 pg/mL, and 0.97 ng/mL, respectively. CBC was normal. The patient was not receiving antithyroid medication, but serum TSH level was within normal ranges due to hyperfunctioning metastases. On patient preparation, corticosteroids, oral hydration, and antiemetics were given. Recombinant human TSH (rhTSH) was not administered to elevate serum TSH levels to prevent possible thyroid storm due to sudden efflux of preformed thyroid hormone. On posttreatment

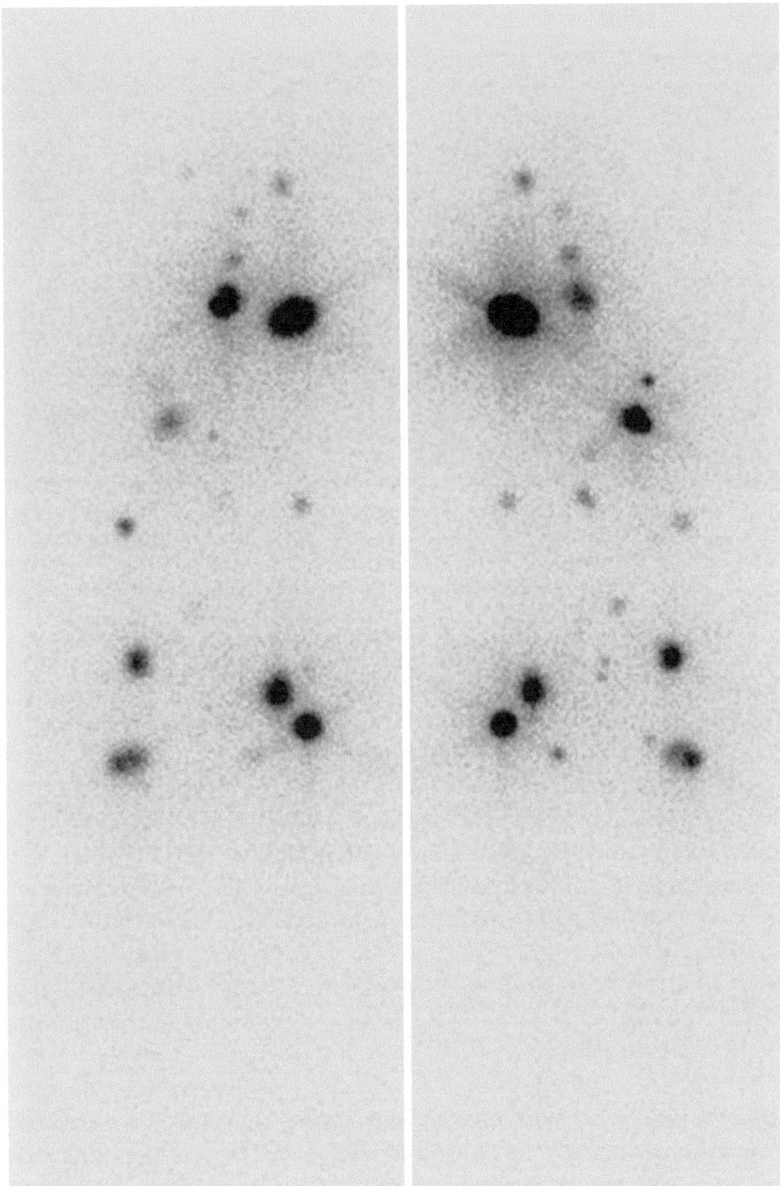

Fig. 31.1 I-131 DxWBS after administration of 2 mCi radioiodine. Anterior (left) and posterior (right) whole-body scan images acquired 48 h after the oral administration of 2 mCi I-131 demonstrate multiple sites of pathological uptake consistent with bone metastases in the calvarium, ribs, vertebral colon, pelvic bones, hips, and bilateral femurs were observed in addition to uptake in residual thyroid tissue

scan, multiple sites of intense iodine uptake were observed at the same sites seen on the posttreatment scan following the initial treatment. However, the intensity was slightly lower compared to the initial uptake on some of the lesions (Fig. 31.2).

On follow-up, serum TSH was within normal ranges despite the considerable amount of radioiodine given. Serum Tg level was decreased to 1700 ng/mL. Radiological imaging demonstrated partial response to treatment according to RECIST criteria. Nine months after the second radioiodine treatment, the third radioiodine treatment was given with 300 mCi. Serum TSH and Tg were 10 μIU/mL and 1650 ng/mL, respectively. On posttreatment WBS, we observed a significant decrease in the intensity, size, and number of metastatic sites parallel to the decrease in Tg levels (Fig. 31.2).

The fourth radioiodine treatment was administered 1 year after the last treatment following a careful physical and laboratory examination

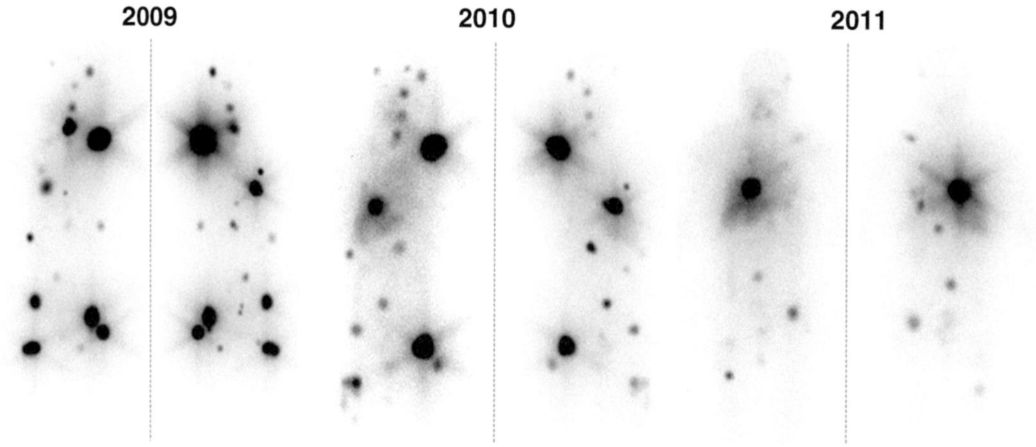

Fig. 31.2 I-131 RxWBS after administration of successive doses of high dose radioiodine. Figure demonstrates the post-therapy whole-body scan images of sequential radioiodine treatments in years 2009, 2010, and 2011. On the left column, post-therapy WBS after the initial radioiodine treatment with 200 mCi I-131 (serum TSH, 0.37 μIU/mL; Tg, 19700 ng/mL) in the year 2009 is shown. Multiple sites of intense and pathological uptakes are observed on the bone metastases similar to the diagnostic WBS. On the posttreatment WBS on the year 2010 (middle column, 250 mCi) and 2011 (right column, 300 mCi), significant decrease on the intensity, size, and number of metastatic sites can be seen clearly. Serum Tg levels gradually decreased from 19,700 ng/mL to 6065 ng/mL in the year 2010 and finally to 1650 ng/mL in the year 2011. Serum TSH levels gradually increased from 0.37 μIU/mL under PTU treatment to 1.6 μIU/mL and finally to 15 μIU/mL without antithyroid medication. Both the elevation in TSH and decline in serum Tg demonstrate the appropriate treatment response to consecutive radioiodine therapies

including CBC, full blood biochemistry, and thyroid function tests. On posttreatment WBS, we observed the same sites of radioiodine uptake with the same intensity with the previous posttreatment scan.

31.2 Discussion

Differentiated thyroid cancer is a malignant disease with excellent disease-specific survival, and the 10-year overall relative survival rate is 90% [1]. Thyroid cancer generally remains localized to the thyroid gland. The rate of distant metastases is rare within a range of 4–15% [2]. The most common site of distant metastases is the lung, followed by the bone [2]. In general, metastases of well-differentiated thyroid cancer carry the main biological features of the thyroid cells such as Na-I symporter gene expression and thyroglobulin synthesis, since the cell does not transfer to an undifferentiated form. However, in general, DTC metastases differ from thyrocytes in thyroid hormone synthesis. Serum thyroid hormone levels remain significantly low in thyroidectomized patients and need to be replaced by exogenous hormone therapies.

Thyrotoxicosis resulting from excessive hormone production by thyroid cancer is extremely rare. Fewer than 100 case reports have been published since its first description in 1946 by Leiter et al. presenting a patient with hyperthyroidism due to metastatic thyroid cancer [3]. Most of the reported cases involve metastatic follicular cancer resulting from excessive hormone production by thyroid cancer cells [4]. The lesions causing thyrotoxicosis are usually bulky, and the bulk of tumor mass is believed to be responsible for thyrotoxicosis rather than an endogenous increased hormonal activity [5].

Papillary thyroid cancer (PTC) is very rarely associated with thyrotoxicosis. Basaria and Salvatori reported thyrotoxicosis due to metastatic papillary thyroid cancer in a patient with Graves' disease, and they considered that the presence of thyroid-stimulating immunoglobulins (TSIs) was responsible for the increased hormonal synthesis and secretion by the metastases [5].

The pathogenesis of hormone production with resulting hyperthyroidism from metastatic thyroid cancer remains largely unknown. Several possible mechanisms have been proposed including endogenous TSH stimulation, iodine deficiency, and environmental causes [5]. Yoshimura Noh et al. reported that one possible mechanism was the activation of receptors on the cancer cells with high level of TSH-binding inhibitor immunoglobulin and thyroid-stimulating antibody in the absence of thyroid tissue that occurred in metastatic site after the completion of radioiodine treatment for many years [6]. Miyauchi et al. reported increased peripheral conversion of fT4 to fT3 causing fT3 toxicosis in patients with massive metastatic follicular thyroid carcinoma [7]. Others suggested that thyroid-stimulating immunoglobulins, which could stimulate and increase the thyrotropin receptors (TSHR), may promote the growth of DTC cells and allow metastatic deposits to synthesize thyroid hormones autonomously [8, 9].

Most functional thyroid cancer metastases produce predominantly T3 toxicosis with normal fT4 serum levels. The possible mechanisms of this effect could be either preferential T3 production or accelerated peripheral conversion of fT4 to fT3 [7, 10]. Another possibility could also include "defect" in the structure of intra-tumoral Tg with rapid removal of the molecule from the iodination site [11]. Although both fT3 and fT4 levels were high in our patient, we observed T3 toxicosis predominantly.

The clinical management of patients with DTC associated with hyperfunctioning distant metastases represents a challenge for the lack of definitive clinical data. Most published studies have been either individual case reports or small case series of patients with hyperthyroidism or euthyroidism [12]. In patients with thyrotoxicosis caused by DTC metastases, I-131 treatment may cause complications due to intralesional edema and hemorrhage, may induce thyrotoxic storm, and may even result in lethal outcome [13]. Thus, it may seem advisable to use combination therapies of antithyroid drugs and glucocorticoids as premedication to reduce the size of metastasis, decrease thyroid hormone levels, and make radioiodine treatment less hazardous and more effective. Antithyroid drugs inhibit iodination of tyrosyl residues in thyroglobulin driven by thyroid peroxidase, thereby inhibiting the synthesis of thyroid hormones. PTU may also act in the peripheral tissues by inhibiting the conversion of thyroxine to triiodothyronine.

Achievement of euthyroidism with antithyroid drugs before I-131 therapy helps to prevent thyroid storm, probably by reducing the amount of stored thyroid hormones in the metastases [5].

Glucocorticoids have proven to have strong anti-inflammatory effects that may be crucial to prevent complications caused by radiation-related inflammation after iodine therapy. Also, high-dose glucocorticoids have long been known to affect serum TSH levels in humans [14]. High doses of glucocorticoids can lower serum TSH levels and decrease TSH secretion and thyroid hormone production through direct effects on TRH in the hypothalamus [14]. Another beneficial role of glucocorticoids is their ability to block peripheral conversion of fT4 to fT3. The use of glucocorticoids has proven to increase survival in case of thyroid storm. In our case, we used dexamethasone 5 mg/day starting 3 days before iodine therapy and 30 mg prednisolone on the day of treatment. To prevent gastric side effects, proton pump inhibitors were also administered. We did not observe any side effects related to steroid use. We would like to remind that absolute and relative contraindications for glucocorticoids, such as diabetes mellitus, gastric or duodenal ulcers, or electrolyte disorders, must be taken into account when considering the use of steroids.

For patients with hyperfunctioning metastases, a high TSH level of >30 ng/mL which is essential to achieve maximal iodine uptake in the remnant tissue or metastatic deposits cannot be reached. Recombinant human TSH has been developed to meet the need for safe, adequate exogenous TSH stimulation in patients with papillary and follicular thyroid carcinoma. The use of rhTSH may be considered to elevate serum TSH levels; however, the necessity of rhTSH injection is questionable since the metastases significantly accumulate radioiodine and use iodine in hormone synthesis and may not require additional intervention to accentuate iodine uptake. Besides, we consider that augmentation of serum TSH levels may induce complications by stimulating the hyperfunctioning metastatic lesions and may cause intralesional edema, hemorrhage, and compression and may carry a potential risk for thyroid storm. Rotman-Pikielny et al. reported that rhTSH could be potentially used to increase TSH to an optimal level and maximize the iodine uptake by the metastatic tumors before radioiodine therapy in patients with hypersecretory metastatic thyroid cancer [11]. However, in the American Thyroid Association guideline published in 2015, the use of rhTSH is not recommended due to insufficient evidence in patients with high-risk DTC with attendant higher risks of disease-related mortality and morbidity. The authors report that more controlled data from long-term outcome studies are needed before rTSH preparation for RAI adjuvant treatment can be recommended in this patient group [15]. We consider that patients with hyperfunctioning metastases must be accepted as high-risk DTC with high risk of disease-related mortality and morbidity not only for the metastatic spread but also for the risk of thyroid storm that may be seen following sudden efflux of thyroid hormones after iodine administration.

Due to the lack of a randomized clinical control study, the effect of radioiodine treatment of metastases in patients with hyperfunctioning metastases in comparison with nonfunctioning metastases remains unclear. However, as a general rule of thumb for thyroid cancer, radioiodine avidity is a characteristic behavior of well-differentiated tumors and predicts a favorable prognosis. Previously published studies report favorable prognosis in patients with hyperfunctioning metastases. In a group of patients with hyperfunctioning metastases limited to the lung, Qiu et al. reported the 10-year cause-specific survival was 92.9% which was higher than the common expectation in this patient group [16]. In general, disease-specific survival is lower in patients with distant metastases [8]. Haq et al. reported cause-specific survival at 10 years as 59% in patients with functioning metastases vs. 55% with nonfunctioning metastases [4]. As bone metastases indicate poorer prognosis and worse survival compared to disease limited to the lung, we considered the higher survival rate reported by Qiu et al. might arise from their patient group of lung-limited metastases.

Hindié et al. reported that radioiodine therapy has a beneficial impact on functioning metastases from thyroid cancer [17]. Also, as observed in our case, authors report excellent avidity for I-131 in functioning metastases that would provide improved overall survival to patients with hyperfunctioning metastases compared to their counterparts.

Another important point in the clinical care of patients with functioning metastases is the fact that hyperfunctioning metastases may retain radioiodine for a longer period than nonfunctioning metastases. This retention of radioactivity may impart harmful levels of radiation to the bone marrow. On this basis, many authors have advocated the value of dosimetry in these patients [18]. If dosimetric calculations are not applicable, the reduction of the appropriate I-131 doses can be discussed. For this case, we were unable to apply dosimetric calculations. However, radioiodine treatments were not administered closer than 9-month period, and we closely monitored bone marrow reserve and did not observe any decrease in complete blood counts.

The management of bone metastases must include a multidisciplinary approach with a combination therapy. Such patients are susceptible to morbid complications of inflammatory tumor expansion and compression to surrounding tissues such as the spinal cord. Resection surgery was proven to improve overall survival in patients with bone metastases [19, 20]. In patients with multiple organ involvements, the role of metastasectomy is less well understood. Even the involvement of multiple bones may preclude curative resection of bony disease. Palliative surgery with partial removal of bone metastases or complete resection of the bone tumor but leaving residual tumor in other organs helps to deliver higher radioiodine dose to the residual tumor and provide maximal benefit from radioiodine therapy by reducing tumor burden. Due to widespread bony metastases, surgeons considered that our patient was not a suitable candidate for resection of metastatic deposits. We planned completion thyroidectomy and bilateral neck dissection for reduction of tumor burden and removal of the non-tumoral gland to provide sufficient radioiodine dose to metastatic deposits.

External beam radiation therapy (EBRT) should be considered in the management of painful bone metastases or of metastases in critical locations likely to result in fractures or neurological or compressive symptoms, if these lesions are not amenable to surgery [21]. EBRT may provide lesion shrinkage and helps palliate pain and reduce the risk of inflammatory tumor expansion or tumor growth. Also, as EBRT delivers lower radiation doses to metastases compared to radioiodine therapy, it may be reasonable to administer EBRT with coadministration of steroids before iodine therapy to avoid sudden efflux of preformed thyroid hormones from the metastatic deposits. In our case, EBRT provided a significant palliation of her bone pain.

The development of osseous metastases from thyroid carcinoma is associated with poorer patient survival and prognosis. Patients with multiple bone metastases have poorer survival than those with solitary bone metastases. Clinical situation is more complicated when metastases function and secrete excess amount of thyroid hormone to the peripheral circulation. The management of DTC patients with hyperfunctioning metastases needs special care and clinical awareness of complications that may increase disease-related mortality and morbidity.

31.3 Follow-Up and Outcome

After the final radioiodine therapy, we observed that serum Tg level was significantly decreased to 260 ng/mL and TSH level rose to 66 μIU/mL on follow-up. L-thyroxine replacement was started. During clinical follow-up, we observed a gradual decrease in serum Tg. Serum Tg levels ranged between 1.5 and 2 ng/mL following the final radioiodine treatment on L-thyroxine replacement therapy. The patient is still alive with a stable and limited disease for 7 years. All blood counts and blood chemistry are within normal ranges. And the patient is free of bone pain. The presented case is a unique example of a successfully treated patient with hyperfunctioning metastases without any complications.

What Can We Learn from This Case?

- Thyrotoxicosis resulting from excessive hormone production by thyroid cancer is extremely rare and needs careful clinical management.
- In patients with hyperfunctioning metastasis, I-131 treatment may cause severe complications due to radiation-caused inflammation, edema, and hemorrhage and may even induce thyrotoxic storm. Therefore, careful patient preparation and premedication for symptomatic control of hyperthyroidism and to avoid thyroid storm are crucial.
- The use of rhTSH in hyperfunctioning metastasis may not be necessary, may even exacerbate symptoms of hyperthyroidism, and must be carefully considered on an individualized patient base.

References

1. Sipos JA, Mazzaferri EL. Thyroid cancer epidemiology and prognostic variables. Clin Oncol. 2010;22:395–404. https://doi.org/10.1016/j.clon.2010.05.00.
2. Schlumberger M, Challeton C, De Vathaire F, Travagli JP, Gardet P, Lumbroso JD, et al. Radioactive iodine treatment and external radiotherapy for lung and bone metastases from thyroid carcinoma. J Nucl Med. 1996;37:598–605.
3. Leiter L, Seidlin SM, Marinelli LD. Adenocarcinoma of the thyroid with hyperthyroidism and functional metastases. J Clin Endocrinol Metab. 1946;6:247–51.
4. Haq M, Hyer S, Flux G, Cook G, Harmer C. Differentiated thyroid cancer presenting with thyrotoxicosis due to functioning metastases. Br J Radiol. 2007;80:38–43.
5. Basaria S, Salvatori RJ. Thyrotoxicosis due to metastatic papillary thyroid cancer in a patient with Graves' disease. J Endocrinol Invest. 2002;25:639–42.
6. Yoshimura Noh J, Mimura T, Kawano M, Hamada N, Ito K. Appearance of TSH receptor antibody

and hyperthyroidism associated with metastatic thyroid cancer after total thyroidectomy. Endocr J. 1997;44:855–9.

7. Miyauchi A, Takamura Y, Ito Y, Miya A, Kobayashi K, Matsuzuka F, et al. 3,5,3′-Triiodothyronine thyrotoxicosis due to increased conversion of administered levothyroxine in patients with massive metastatic follicular thyroid carcinoma. J Clin Endocrinol Metab. 2008;93:2239–42. https://doi.org/10.1210/jc.2007-2282.
8. Salvatori M, Saletnich I, Rufini V, Dottorini ME, Corsello SM, Troncone L, et al. Severe thyrotoxicosis due to functioning pulmonary metastases of well-differentiated thyroid cancer. J Nucl Med. 1998;39:1202–7.
9. Nishihara E, Amino N, Miyauchi A. Fractionated radioiodine therapy for hyperthyroidism caused by wide spread metastatic follicular thyroid carcinoma. Thyroid. 2010;20:569–70. https://doi.org/10.1089/thy.2009.0460.
10. Paul SJ, Sisson JC. Thyrotoxicosis caused by thyroid cancer. Endocrinol Metab Clin N Am. 1990;19:593–612.
11. Rotman-Pikielny P, Reynolds JC, Barker WC, Yen PM, Skarulis MC, Sarlis NJ. Recombinant human thyrotropin for the diagnosis and treatment of a highly functional metastatic struma ovarii. J Clin Endocrinol Metab. 2000;85:237–44.
12. Lee JI, Chung YJ, Park SJ, Ryu HS, Cho BY. Euthyroid status after total thyroidectomy due to functioning lung metastases from a clear cell variant of papillary thyroid carcinoma. Thyroid. 2012;22:1084–7. https://doi.org/10.1089/thy.2011.0437.
13. Cerletty JM, Listwan WJ. Hyperthyroidism due to functioning metastatic thyroid carcinoma. Precipitation of thyroid storm with therapeutic radioactive iodine. JAMA. 1979;242:269–70.
14. Wilber JF, Utiger RD. The effect of glucocorticoids on thyrotropin secretion. J Clin Invest. 1969;48:2096–103.
15. Haugen BR, Alexander EK, Bible KC, Doherty GM, Mandel SJ, Nikiforov YE, et al. 2015 American Thyroid Association management guidelines for adult patients with thyroid nodules and differentiated thyroid Cancer: the American Thyroid Association guidelines task force on thyroid nodules and differentiated thyroid cancer. Thyroid. 2016;26:1–133. https://doi.org/10.1089/thy.2015.0020.
16. Qiu ZL, Shen CT, Luo QY. Clinical management and outcomes in patients with hyperfunctioning distant metastases from differentiated thyroid cancer after total thyroidectomy and radioactive iodine therapy. Thyroid. 2015;25:229–37. https://doi.org/10.1089/thy.2014.0233.
17. Hindié E, Mellière D, Lange F, Hallaj I, de Labriolle-Vaylet C, Jeanguillaume C, et al. Functioning pulmonary metastases of thyroid cancer: does radioiodine influence the prognosis? Eur J Nucl Med Mol Imaging. 2003;30:974–81.
18. Sisson JC. Practical dosimetry of 131I in patients with thyroid carcinoma. Cancer Biother Radiopharm. 2002;17:101–5.
19. Wexler JA. Approach to the thyroid cancer patient with bone metastases. J Clin Endocrinol Metab. 2011;96:2296–307. https://doi.org/10.1210/jc.2010-1996.
20. Satcher RL, Lin P, Harun N, Feng L, Moon BS, Lewis VO. Surgical management of appendicular skeletal metastases in thyroid carcinoma. Int J Surg Oncol. 2012;2012:417086. https://doi.org/10.1155/2012/417086.
21. Luster M, Clarke SE, Dietlein M, Lassmann M, Lind P, Oyen WJ, European Association of Nuclear Medicine (EANM), et al. Guidelines for radioiodine therapy of differentiated thyroid cancer. Eur J Nucl Med Mol Imaging. 2008;35:1941–59. https://doi.org/10.1007/s00259-008-0883-1.

32 Papillary Thyroid Carcinoma

Yasemin Giles Şenyürek and İsmail Cem Sormaz

Abstract

Although most thyroid nodules are a result of a benign disease process (>90%), the possibility of thyroid cancer is always a consideration. Ultrasonography can help for differential diagnosis of thyroid nodules. Fine needle aspiration biopsy is the traditional diagnostic test to determine malignancy in thyroid nodules. We present a 58-year-old female patient with low-risk papillary thyroid carcinoma (PTC) who was treated by total thyroidectomy. Although the recent ATA guideline recommends that the extent of initial surgery can be a total or near-total thyroidectomy or lobectomy in low-risk unilateral PTC >1 cm and <4 cm, the extent of thyroidectomy in such patients should be decided according to the judgment of the treatment team and postoperative histopathological findings. In low-risk PTC patients, a suppressed or stimulated Tg <1 ng/mL by 3–4 weeks postoperatively and no evidence of disease by imaging further confirm classification of these patients as being at low risk. RAI (radioactive iodine) remnant ablation is not routinely recommended after thyroidectomy for ATA low-risk PTC patients.

Y. G. Şenyürek · İ. C. Sormaz (✉)
Division of Endocrine Surgery, Istanbul University, Istanbul Medical Faculty, Istanbul, Turkey

32.1 Case Presentation

A 58-year-old female patient applied to our outpatient clinic in March 2014. Her history revealed that she had been diagnosed with Hashimoto thyroiditis (HT) in 2004 and has been using thyroxine supplementation since then. She had no family history of thyroid cancer or history of head and neck irradiation. Neck ultrasonography (USG) which had been performed in 2004 showed an iso-hyperechoic nodule that was 6.3 × 4.8 mm in the right upper lobe of the thyroid gland and a hypoechoic nodule in the middle left lobe which was measured as 1.7 × 1.8 mm. No additional USG imaging had been performed between the years 2004 and 2014.

Her initial physical examination at the time of reference revealed one dominant nodule in each thyroid lobe which was estimated as 1.5 cm by palpation. Serum levels of thyroid-stimulating hormone (TSH), antithyroid peroxidase (anti-TPO) antibody, and anti-thyroglobulin (anti-Tg) antibody were found as 3.2 mU/L (0.27–4.2 mU/L), 460 IU/mL (0–34 IU/mL), and 235 IU/mL (0–115 IU/mL), respectively. Neck USG showed an iso-hyperechoic solid nodule that was 8.6 × 8.6 × 11.7 mm in size and a subcentimetric (3.8 mm) hypoechoic nodule in the right lobe and a predominantly cystic nodule that was measured as 8.9 × 9.8 × 13.6 mm in the left lobe (Fig. 32.1). Although these nodules seemed to increase in size during the last 10 years, they

T. Özülker et al. (eds.), *Thyroid and Parathyroid Diseases*, https://doi.org/10.1007/978-3-319-78476-2_32

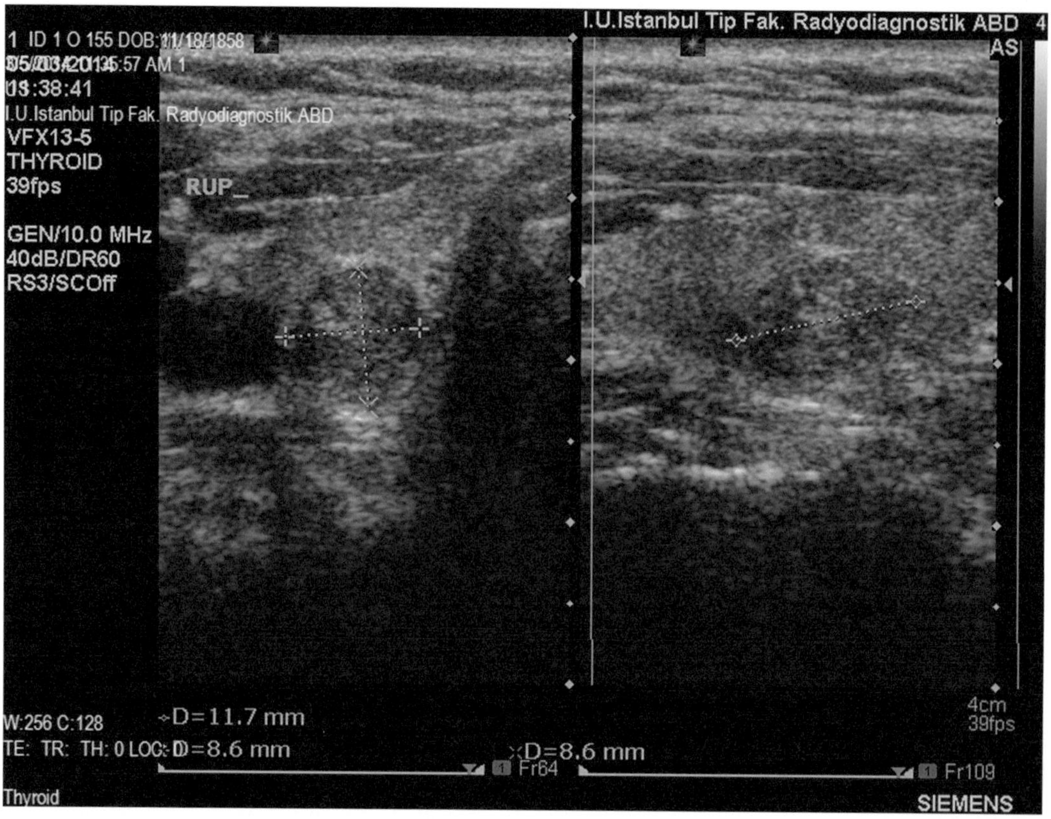

Fig. 32.1 Sonographic image of the dominant thyroid nodule in the right lobe showing iso-hyperechoic nodule with regular borders

exhibited low-suspicion category findings by USG and were smaller than 1.5 cm. We decided annual USG surveillance for these nodules. Repeat neck USG that was performed 1 year later revealed that the size of the dominant nodule in the right lobe increased by 1.5 and 2.0 mm in two dimensions. Although this nodule was observed as being iso-hyperechoic on the former USG, it appeared mildly hypoechoic on repeat USG (Fig. 32.2). The size of the predominantly cystic nodule in the left lobe was slightly increased as well (1 and 0.6 mm increase in two dimensions). USG revealed multiple subcentimetric lymph nodes in bilateral cervicolateral compartments. These lymph nodes appeared to be oval shaped and had echogenic hilum which were common sonographic characteristics of benign lymph nodes (Figs. 32.3 and 32.4). No suspicious cervical lymph nodes were detected by neck USG. As the nodule in the right lobe increased in size and turned in a hypoechogenic state, fine needle aspiration biopsy (FNAB) was performed to this nodule. FNAB cytology was reported as suspicious for papillary thyroid carcinoma (PTC). Total thyroidectomy was performed with intraoperative nerve monitoring. No lymph nodes suspicious of malignancy were observed in the central compartment during the operation. There were no postoperative complications. Histopathological examination revealed nonencapsulated PTC of 1.3 cm in the right lobe. The microscopic variant was oncocytic follicular subtype of PTC. Lymph-vascular invasion, extrathyroidal extension (ETE), and multifocality were not observed. There were no postoperative complications.

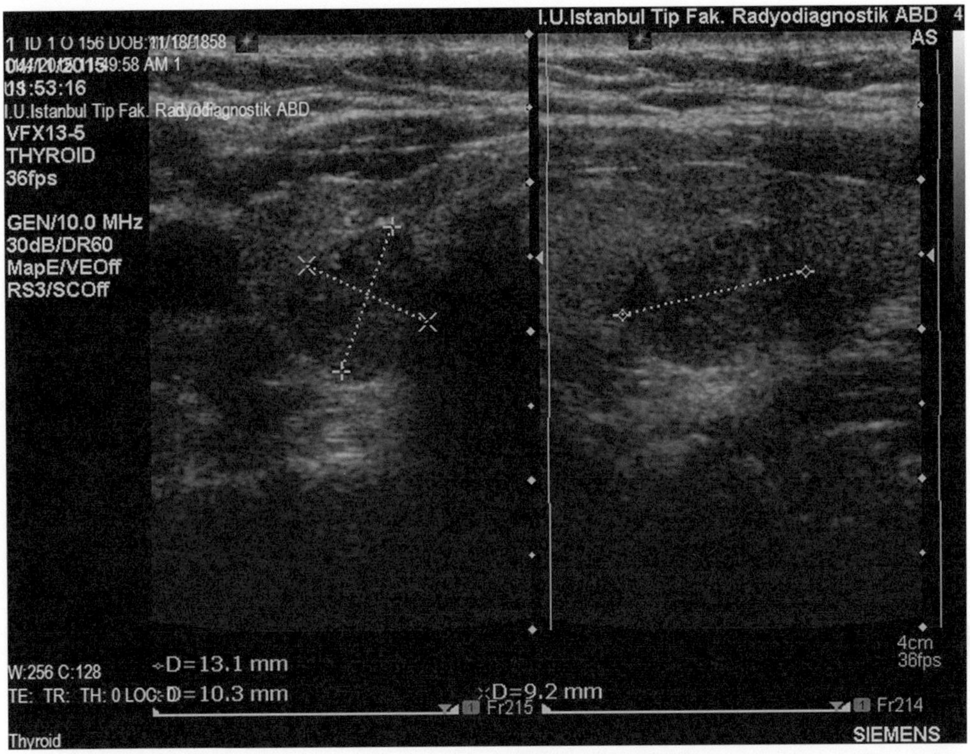

Fig. 32.2 The image on repeat USG shows that the dominant nodule in the right lobe increased in size and echogenic structure changed from iso-hyperechogenicity to mild hypoechogenicity

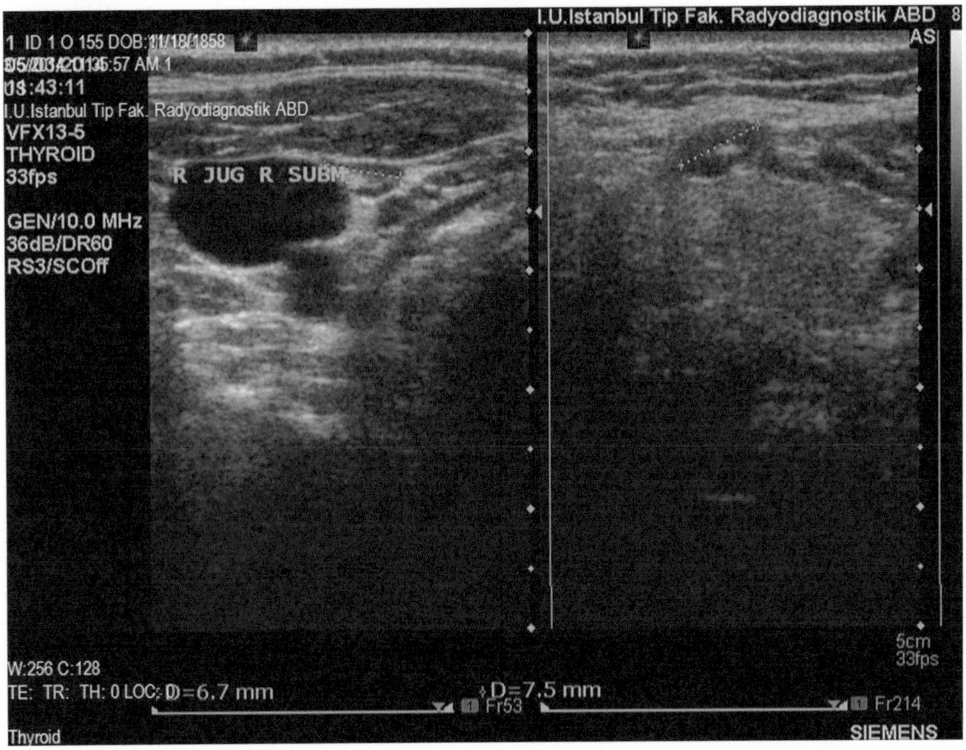

Fig. 32.3 Subcentimetric cervicolateral lymph nodes with echogenic hilum which is a USG feature associated with benign cervical lymph nodes

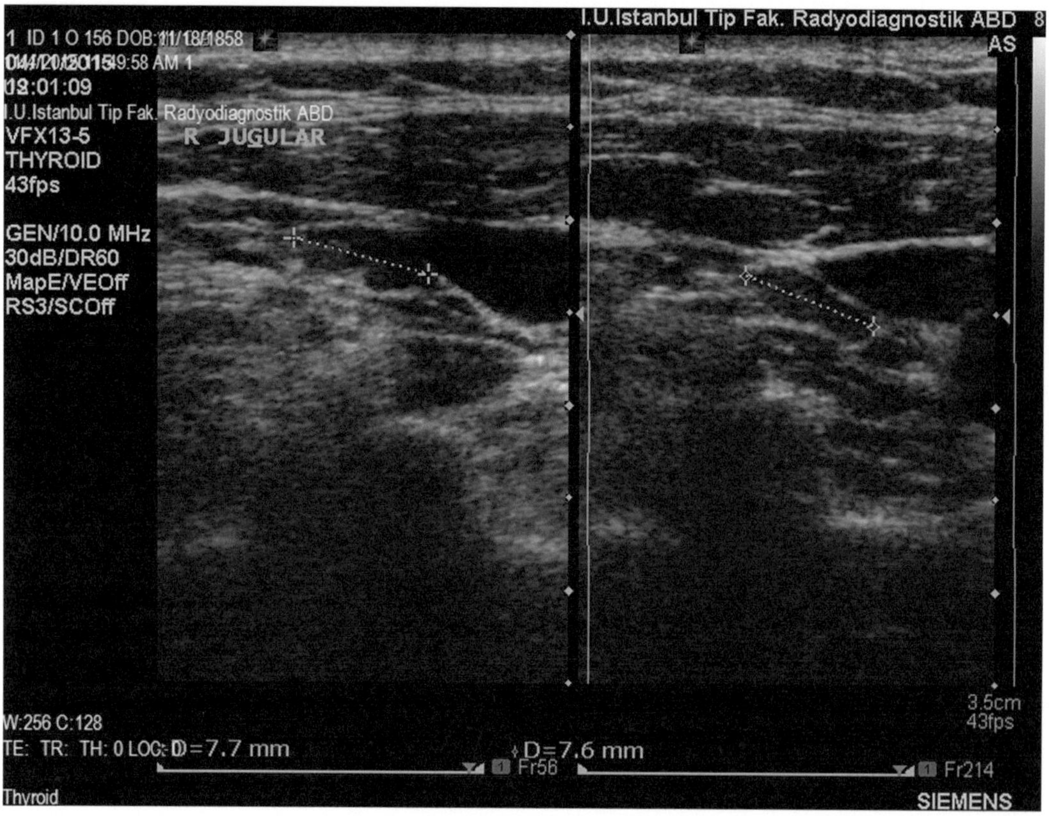

Fig. 32.4 Sonographic image of subcentimetric oval-shaped cervicolateral lymph nodes. A marked difference between the short-axis and long-axis diameter with long-axis diameter longer than short-axis diameter is a common sonographic feature in benign cervical lymph nodes

32.2 Discussion

32.2.1 Evaluation and Diagnosis

Although most thyroid nodules are a result of benign disease process (>90%), the possibility of thyroid cancer is always a consideration [1]. History of childhood head/neck irradiation; family history of PTC, MTC, or multiple endocrine neoplasia type 2 (MEN2); age <20 or >70 years; male sex; enlarging nodule; abnormal cervical adenopathy; fixed nodule; and vocal cord paralysis are features that are associated with increased risk of cancer in patients with thyroid nodules [1].

There has long been a controversy in the literature about a possible link between HT and PTC. Population-based FNAB studies did not find a statistically significant correlation between HT and PTC, whereas a recent meta-analysis showed that PTC was significantly associated with pathologically confirmed HT [2]. PTCs with coexisting HT were found to be significantly related to female patients, multifocal involvement, no extrathyroidal extension, and no lymph node metastasis. Moreover, PTCs with HT were significantly associated with long recurrence-free survival [3].

Serum TSH should be measured during the initial evaluation of a patient with a thyroid nodule [4]. In the patients with high TSH values or who are suspected to have HT, the laboratory diagnosis of HT is established with the assay of serologic markers, including serum levels of anti-TPO and anti-Tg antibodies [5]. Circulating anti-TPO antibodies are now considered the best serological marker to establish a diagnosis of HT. The presence of positive anti-Tg antibodies is less sensitive and specific than anti-TPO antibodies to diagnose HT [5]. A recent systematic review of the literature showed that USG features that suggested malignancy in a thyroid nodule included a blurred or ill-defined margin, irregular shape, solid echo structure, hypoechogenicity, absent halo, fine calcifications, and intranodular vascular pattern [6]. Most of the malignant nodules had more than two USG features characteristic of malignancy [6]. Kwak et al. documented that the probability of malignancy was found relatively higher in thyroid nodules with microcalcifications alone and in those with microlobulated margins alone compared to other suspicious USG features [7]. The authors also reported that the risk of malignancy in a nodule increased as the number of suspicious USG features increased [7]. Microcalcification, marked hypoechogenicity, irregular border, and taller-than-wide features were reported to be individual sonographic criteria for malignant nodules with high specificity and accuracy [8]. The recent ATA guideline classifies the nodules as highly suspicious if they have a combination of such highly suspicious USG features or associated suspicious cervicolateral lymph nodes [4]. A nodule that is observed to be hypoechoic nodule with regular border on USG is defined as intermediate risk [4]. Hyperechoic or isoechoic nodules are defined as low-suspicion category. FNAB is recommended for nodules ≥1 cm which has high or intermediate suspicious findings by USG and for nodules ≥1.5 cm with low suspicion of malignancy according to sonographic pattern [4].

Although enlarging thyroid nodules has been previously reported to be a definite risk factor for thyroid cancer, recent studies suggested that the malignancy rate of growing thyroid nodules was not very high [6, 9, 10]. Nakamura et al. found that nodule growth was a predictor of malignancy in the nodules with follicular neoplasm cytology, whereas enlarged thyroid nodules with benign cytology had a malignancy rate of 1% [10]. Although there are conflicting results related to risk of malignancy associated with nodule growth, repeat USG at 12–24-month intervals are recommended to follow up low-suspicion thyroid nodules [4]. FNAB is recommended if the USG findings show nodule growth (20% increase in at least two nodule dimensions with a minimal increase of 2 mm or more than a 50% change in volume) or development of new suspicious sonographic features [4]. In our patient, FNAB was performed to the dominant nodule as this nodule showed size enlargement and developed hypoechogenicity during sonographic surveillance. FNAB cytology was reported as suspicious for papillary thyroid carcinoma (PTC). The risk of malignancy ranges between 60 and 75% in FNAB results reported as suspicious for PTC [11]. If the cytology is reported as suspicious for papillary carcinoma, surgical management should be similar to that of malignant cytology, depending on clinical risk factors, sonographic features, patient preference, and possibly results of mutational testing [4].

Fine needle aspiration cytology might present some potential sources of error when performed in glands harboring autoimmune thyroiditis. The similarity of epithelial cell nuclear atypia in HT and cellular neoplasm may cause false-positive results. On the other hand, pleomorphic Hürthle cells may be present in aspirates from Hürthle cell neoplasms and underdiagnosed as HT, especially when they are associated with a few lymphocytes, resulting in false negatives [12, 13].

In HT patients, hyperplastic lymph nodes are commonly detected by neck USG [14]. Ultrasonographic features such as round shape (short-axis/long-axis ratio <0.60), absence of hilar echo, sharp nodal borders, hypoechoic internal echogenicity, and presence of intranodal necrosis were determined to be highly suggestive of metastatic cervical lymph nodes [15]. Brancato et al. reported that an increased number of benign hyperplastic neck nodes (oval shaped and with echogenic hilum), especially in levels II, III, and IV, were a characteristic sonographic finding associated with HT [14].

32.2.2 Management

Papillary thyroid cancer is defined as low risk when there is no local or distant metastasis, no macroscopic or microscopic local invasion, no aggressive histology, no vascular invasion, and no lymph node metastasis or ≤5 are micrometastasis [4]. In the former revised ATA Management Guidelines for Patients with Thyroid Nodules and Differentiated Thyroid Cancer (2009), total or near-total thyroidectomy was recommended for PTC >1 cm [16]. This recommendation was based on the results of an analysis of 52.173 PTC patients who were treated either by total thyroidectomy or lobectomy. This analysis demonstrated a slightly higher 10-year relative overall survival and slightly lower 10-year recurrence rate for total thyroidectomy as opposed to thyroid lobectomy [17]. A recently updated analysis of a similar population including 61.775 PTC patients demonstrated that the slight overall survival advantage was seen for patients with 1–4 cm PTC who underwent total thyroidectomy disappeared when further adjustment was made for additional variables such as clinicopathological features and severity of illness [18]. The recent ATA guideline (2015) recommends that the extent of initial surgery can be a total or near-total thyroidectomy or lobectomy in low-risk PTC >1 cm and <4 cm [4]. However, there is still an ongoing debate on the extent of thyroidectomy in PTC >1 cm. Proponents of total thyroidectomy argue that multifocality is a well-known feature of PTC and that total thyroidectomy decreases the risk of recurrence and risk of reoperations that are associated with high morbidity, improves survival, enables detection and elimination of persistent and/or metastatic disease by radioiodine, and enhances follow-up with serum Tg levels, and the operation has low morbidity in experienced hands [19]. The main argument against total thyroidectomy is high rate of complications of the procedure with no proven potential benefit on recurrence and survival. Opponents for total thyroidectomy argue that occult tumor foci have no implications on disease outcome, RAI therapy has no proven benefit in low-risk patients, and adequate follow-up can be achieved after lobectomy with Tg measurements and neck USG [19]. They further argue that the majority of the reoperations after lobectomy involve the contralateral lobe which can be removed with no increased morbidity compared to primary lobectomy. It is important to emphasize that the surgeon should take account of pre-, intra-, and postoperative prognostic features as well as risk group to decide on the extent of thyroidectomy [19]. Total thyroidectomy is the treatment of choice for all patients with PTC if further therapy such as RAI is being considered and the operation can be done safely [20]. Lobectomy can be performed in low-risk PTC patients with unilateral tumor according to the judgment of the treatment team if postoperative histopathological findings do not necessitate RAI therapy [4]. We preferred to perform total thyroidectomy in our patient because there were nodules in both thyroid lobes and these nodules showed size enlargement during the follow-up.

The postoperative Tg value is an important prognostic factor that can be used to guide clinical management. In low-risk PTC patients, a suppressed or stimulated Tg <1 ng/mL by 3–4 weeks postoperatively and no evidence of disease by imaging further confirm classification of these patients as being at low risk [4]. RAI remnant ablation is not routinely recommended after thyroidectomy for ATA low-risk DTC patients [4]. In low-risk patients who underwent a total thyroidectomy without postoperative RAI therapy, the recommended strategy of follow-up is based on serum Tg determination on thyroxine and neck USG at 9–12 months.

32.3 Follow-Up and Outcome

The patient was classified as low risk according to the ATA 2009 Risk Stratification System with Proposed Modifications [4]. Serum level of stimulated thyroglobulin (sTg) was found as 0.4 ng/mL (in the absence of anti-Tg antibodies) on postoperative third week when TSH level was 56 mIU/L. Radioactive iodine (RAI) therapy was not considered in our case as the patient was classified as low-risk PTC according to the clinicopathological features and detection of very low level of sTg on postoperative third week. Thyroxine treatment was started to maintain TSH values as 0.1–0.5 mIU/L. The follow-up included TSH, Tg, and anti-TG assay at 6-month intervals and neck USG annually. There was no evidence of recurrence during the follow-up period of 36 months.

32.3.1 The Future

Current knowledge assures that lobectomy is sufficient treatment for small, unifocal, intrathyroidal papillary microcarcinomas in the absence of prior head and neck radiation, familial thyroid carcinoma, or clinically detectable cervical nodal metastases. It is still controversial if lobectomy is a sufficient treatment in low-risk PTC >1 cm. Future studies related to the impact of molecular markers on the outcome of PTC may be helpful to achieve a more definite risk stratification of PTC preoperatively. In PTC >1 cm, preoperative risk assessment with the evaluation of molecular markers along with clinicopathological features would help proper selection of patients for whom lobectomy is a sufficient treatment or those for whom total thyroidectomy is indicated.

What Can We Learn from This Case?

- Although there is no clear evidence to support the correlation between HT and PTC, thyroidectomy studies reported a positive correlation. Patients with HT need to be carefully monitored for the development of PTC.
- FNAB should be considered in thyroid nodules if the USG findings show nodule growth (20% increase in at least two nodule dimensions with a minimal increase of 2 mm or more than a 50% change in volume) or development of new suspicious sonographic features during USG surveillance.
- A definitive correlation between the extent of thyroid resection and long-term survival has not yet been established. The decision-making regarding lobectomy or total thyroidectomy in PTC > 1 cm should be based on pre-, intra-, and postoperative prognostic features in low-risk patients.
- Total thyroidectomy is the treatment of choice for PTC if postoperative RAI therapy is being considered and the operation can be done with low morbidity.
- Routine RAI ablation is not recommended for low-risk PTC patients. Postoperative sTg assay and imaging findings are helpful in postoperative RAI therapy decision-making. Postoperative sTg <1 ng/mL and negative imaging confirm the low-risk state of the patient, and these patients can be safely managed without postoperative RAI therapy.

References

1. Gharib H, Papini E. Thyroid nodules: clinical importance, assessment, and treatment. Endocrinol Metab Clin N Am. 2007;36:707–35. https://doi.org/10.1016/j.ecl.2007.04.009.
2. Jankovic B, Le KT, Hershman JM. Clinical Review: Hashimoto's thyroiditis and papillary thyroid carcinoma: is there a correlation? J Clin Endocrinol Metab. 2009;98:474–82. https://doi.org/10.1210/jc.2012-2978.
3. Lee JH, Kim Y, Choi JW, Kim YS. The association between papillary thyroid carcinoma and histologically proven Hashimoto's thyroiditis: a meta-analysis. Eur J Endocrinol. 2013;168:343–9. https://doi.org/10.1530/EJE-12-0903.
4. Haugen BR, Alexander EK, Bible KC, Doherty GM, Mandel SJ, Nikiforov YE, et al. American Thyroid Association management guidelines for adult patients with thyroid nodules and differentiated thyroid cancer: the American Thyroid Association guidelines task force on thyroid nodules and differentiated thyroid cancer. Thyroid. 2016;26:1–133. https://doi.org/10.1089/thy.2015.0020.
5. Caturegli P, De Remigis A, Rose NR. Hashimoto thyroiditis: clinical and diagnostic criteria. Autoimmun Rev. 2014;13:391–7. https://doi.org/10.1016/j.autrev.2014.01.007.
6. Morris LF, Ragavendra N, Yeh MW. Evidence-based assessment of the role of ultrasonography in the management of benign thyroid nodules. World J Surg. 2008;32:1253–63. https://doi.org/10.1007/s00268-008-9494-z.

7. Kwak JY, Han KH, Yoon JH, Moon HJ, Son EJ, Park SH, et al. Thyroid imaging reporting and data system for US features of nodules: a step in establishing better stratification of cancer risk. Radiology. 2011;260:892–9. https://doi.org/10.1148/radiol.11110206.
8. Kim EK, Park CS, Chung WY, Oh KK, Kim DI, Lee JT, et al. New sonographic criteria for recommending fine-needle aspiration biopsy of nonpalpable solid nodules of the thyroid. AJR Am J Roentgenol. 2002;178:687–91. https://doi.org/10.2214/ajr.178.3.1780687.
9. Kuma K, Matsuzuka F, Kobayashi A, Hirai K, Morita S, Miyauchi A, et al. Outcome of long standing solitary thyroid nodules. World J Surg. 1992;16:583–8.
10. Nakamura H, Hirokawa M, Ota H, Kihara M, Miya A, Miyauchi A. Is an increase in thyroid nodule volume a risk factor for malignancy? Thyroid. 2015;25:804–11. https://doi.org/10.1089/thy.2014.0567.
11. Cibas ES, Ali SZ. The Bethesda system for reporting thyroid cytopathology. Thyroid. 2009;19:1159–65. https://doi.org/10.1089/thy.2009.0274.
12. Kini SR, Miller JM, Hamburger JI. Problems in the cytologic diagnosis of the "cold" thyroid nodule in patients with lymphocytic thyroiditis. Acta Cytol. 1981;25:506–12.
13. MacDonald L, Yazdi HM. Fine needle aspiration biopsy of Hashimoto's thyroiditis. Sources of diagnostic error. Acta Cytol. 1999;43:400–6.
14. Brancato D, Citarrella R, Richiusa P, Amato MC, Vetro C, Galluzzo CG. Neck lymph nodes in chronic autoimmune thyroiditis: the sonographic pattern. Thyroid. 2013;3:173–7. https://doi.org/10.1089/thy.2012.0375.
15. Raja Lakshmi C, Sudhakara Rao M, Ravikiran A, Sathish S, Bhavana SM. Evaluation of reliability of ultrasonographic parameters in differentiating benign and metastatic cervical group of lymph nodes. ISRN Otolaryngol. 2014;2014:238740. https://doi.org/10.1155/2014/238740.
16. Cooper DS, Doherty GM, Haugen BR, Kloos RT, Lee SL, Mandel SJ, et al. Revised American Thyroid Association management guidelines for patients with thyroid nodules and differentiated thyroid cancer. Thyroid. 2009;19:1167–214. https://doi.org/10.1089/thy.2009.0110.
17. Bilimoria KY, Bentrem DJ, Ko CY, Stewart AK, Winchester DP, Talamonti MS, et al. Extent of surgery affects survival for papillary thyroid cancer. Ann Surg. 2007;246:375–84. https://doi.org/10.1097/SLA.0b013e31814697d9.
18. Adam MA, Pura J, Gu L, Dinan MA, Tyler DS, Reed SD, et al. Extent of surgery for papillary thyroid cancer is not associated with survival: an analysis of 61,775 patients. Ann Surg. 2014;260:601–5. https://doi.org/10.1097/SLA.0000000000000925.
19. Miccoli P, Bakkar S. Surgical management of papillary thyroid carcinoma: an overview. Updat Surg. 2017;69(2):145–50. https://doi.org/10.1007/s13304-017-0449-5. [Epub ahead of print].
20. Robbins J, Merino MJ, Boice JD Jr, Ron E, Ain KB, Alexander HR, et al. Thyroid cancer: a lethal endocrine neoplasm. Ann Intern Med. 1991;115:133–47.

33

Papillary Thyroid Carcinoma with Central Lymph Node Metastases

Yasemin Giles Şenyürek and İsmail Cem Sormaz

Abstract

Lymph nodal involvement in papillary thyroid carcinoma (PTC) is very common. Preoperative neck ultrasonography (USG) allows for the early detection of nonpalpable cervical lymph node metastasis prior to thyroidectomy in patients with FNAB-proven or suspected thyroid cancer. In patients with clinically involved central nodes, therapeutic central compartment (level VI) neck dissection should be performed. Lateral neck dissection performed for macroscopic PTC metastases should be the selective neck dissection of levels IIa, III, IV, and Vb. We present a 38-year-old female patient of unilateral PTC with central and ipsilateral lateral lymph node metastasis who underwent total thyroidectomy and bilateral central and ipsilateral lateral lymph node dissection followed by radioactive iodine ablation (RAI) treatment. Postoperative RAI adjuvant therapy should be considered in ATA intermediate-/high-risk level patients. In PTC patients, no biochemical, clinical, or radiological evidence of tumor during the follow-up after total thyroidectomy and RAI treatment is defined as excellent response to treatment. The rate of recurrence ranges between 1 and 4% in patients with excellent response. In intermediate-risk patients who are subsequently reclassified into excellent response category, non-stimulated thyroglobulin assays and neck USG at 12–24-month intervals are considered to be appropriate in the follow-up.

33.1 Case Presentation

A 38-year-old female patient was referred to our institution for thyroidectomy in January 2016. She has been suffering from a gradually enlarging neck lump for 3 years. She had undergone neck ultrasonography (USG) previously at another institution, and fine needle aspiration biopsy (FNAB) had been performed for a large thyroid nodule located in the left thyroid lobe. The cytologic features of FNAB specimen have been reported as a highly cellular specimen with enlarged, oval, and irregular nucleus and intranuclear grooves. The findings were consistent with papillary thyroid carcinoma (PTC) (Bethesda 6). She had no family history of thyroid cancer or history of radiation to the head and neck. Physical examination revealed a large thyroid nodule sized approximately 4 cm in the left thyroid lobe. Serum thyrotropin (TSH) level was 2.5 mIU/L. The patient was scheduled for surgery. In our institution, routine preoperative

Y. G. Şenyürek (✉) · İ. C. Sormaz
Division of Endocrine Surgery, Istanbul University Istanbul Medical Faculty, Istanbul, Turkey

T. Özülker et al. (eds.), *Thyroid and Parathyroid Diseases*, https://doi.org/10.1007/978-3-319-78476-2_33

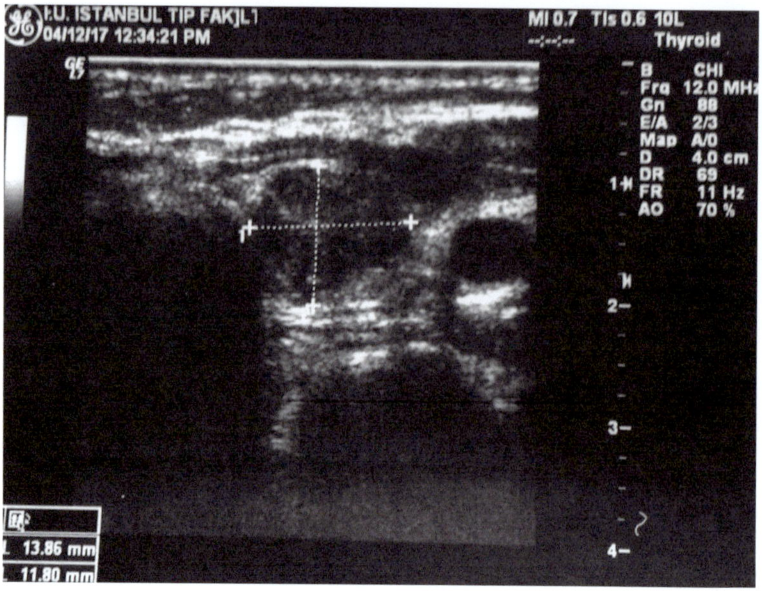

Fig. 33.1 Ultrasonographic image of enlarged central lymph node with hypoechogenicity, rounded shape, and irregular borders

neck USG is performed in patients with a diagnosis of PTC in order to detect central or lateral suspicious lymph nodes, if any, which might have been missed during previous imaging studies. Preoperative neck USG showed a heterogenous, hypoechoic thyroid nodule with ill-defined borders in the left thyroid lobe. The transverse and longitudinal diameters of the nodule were measured as 39 and 20 mm, respectively. There were no nodules detected by USG in the right lobe. Preoperative neck USG also revealed an enlarged and hypoechoic lymph node with a rounded shape and irregular borders located at the inferior border of the left thyroid lobe (central lymph node) and suspicious subcentimetric lymph nodes at level IV at the left lateral compartment. The largest diameter of the central lymph node was measured as 13.9 mm (Fig. 33.1). The size of the largest lymph node at the left lateral compartment was measured as 9 mm. Thyroglobulin (Tg) measurement of fine needle aspiration (FNA-Tg) from the central and lateral lymph nodes was found as 355 ng/mL and 780 ng/mL, respectively. Macroscopic central lymph nodes in the left paratracheal compartment were observed intraoperatively (Fig. 33.2). The patient underwent total thyroidectomy, bilateral central lymph node dissection, and left lateral lymph node dissection with continuous nerve monitoring. Lateral lymph node dissection included levels III and IV. At the left side, macroscopic paratracheal central lymph nodes were found to show dense adherence to the recurrent laryngeal nerve. The postoperative histopathological diagnosis revealed classical variant PTC with a maximum diameter of

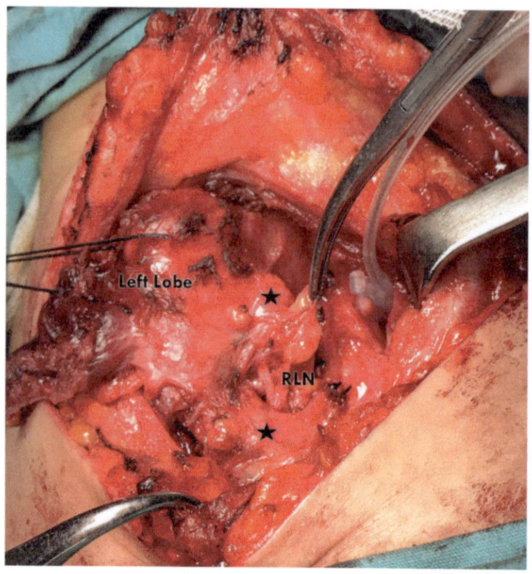

Fig. 33.2 Intraoperative image of macroscopic central lymph nodes (★)

3.8 cm located in the left lobe. The tumor showed microscopic extrathyroidal extension (ETE) and lymphatic invasion. No vascular invasion was recorded. Of 12 lymph nodes dissected from the central compartment, ipsilateral metastasis was found in 5. Of 14 lymph nodes dissected from the left lateral compartment, metastasis was detected in 6. Two of the metastatic lateral lymph nodes showed extranodal extension. Postoperative stimulated Tg (sTg) value was 5.6 ng/mL in the absence of anti-thyroglobulin (Anti-Tg) antibodies. Transient hypoparathyroidism developed postoperatively which was managed by oral calcium and vitamin D supplementation for 2 weeks following surgery. The stage of the PTC was defined as stage I according to the AJCC/UICC TNM system and ATA intermediate risk according to the ATA 2009 Risk Stratification System with Proposed Modifications [1].

33.2 Discussion

33.2.1 Evaluation and Diagnosis

The clinical importance of thyroid nodules, besides local compressive symptoms or thyroid dysfunction, is primarily the possibility of thyroid cancer which occurs in about 5% of thyroid nodules [2]. Thyroid nodules should be evaluated primarily to rule out thyroid malignancy. USG is the most reliable diagnostic modality to detect thyroid nodules, and USG-guided FNAB is the gold standard method to determine the malignant potential of the thyroid nodules [3, 4]. Several ultrasonographic thyroid nodule characteristics have been found to correlate highly with malignancy, including irregular borders, microcalcifications, height greater than width, hypoechogenicity, and increased vascularity [3, 4]. Combination of these suspicious sonographic features, especially of hypoechogenicity, irregular borders, and microcalcifications, is strongly associated with an increased risk for differentiated thyroid cancer [4]. USG-guided FNAB is strongly recommended in nodules ≥1 cm with highly suspicious findings [1]. Lymph nodal involvement in PTC is very common, and in up to 90% of cases, lymph node micrometastases are observed [5, 6]. In PTC patients with lymph node metastasis, the nodal metastasis predominates in the ipsilateral central and ipsilateral cervicolateral compartments [7, 8]. The extent of initial thyroidectomy should be total or near total thyroidectomy in patients with clinical evidence of metastatic lymph nodes [1]. Preoperative neck USG for cervical lymph nodes is recommended for all patients undergoing thyroidectomy for malignant or suspicious for malignancy cytologic findings [1]. Preoperative neck USG allows for the early detection of nonpalpable cervical lymph node metastasis prior to thyroidectomy in patients with FNAB-proven or suspected thyroid cancer that otherwise might have been missed intraoperatively, thereby minimizing the risk for persistent disease [9, 10]. Preoperative USG can identify suspicious cervical lymphadenopathy, thereby potentially altering the extent of and overall surgical approach in 1/3 of these PTC patients [9, 10]. The sonographic features which are associated with metastatic lymph nodes include hypoechogenicity, rounded appearance, irregular borders, macro- or microcalcifications, loss of the fatty hilus, cystic appearance, and increased size [3]. The sensitivity of USG to detect central compartment metastatic lymph nodes is low prior to primary thyroidectomy when the thyroid gland is in situ. Kouvaraki et al. reported the sensitivity of preoperative USG to detect metastatic lymph nodes in the central and ipsilateral compartments as 52% and 77%, respectively [9]. The authors documented that most false-negative USG results occurred in the central neck compartment, especially in patients whose thyroid gland was still in situ. Confirmation of malignancy in lymph nodes with a suspicious sonographic appearance is achieved by USG-guided FNA for cytology and/or measurement of Tg in the needle washout [3]. Although the cutoff values for the FNA-Tg have not been standardized, preoperative values of >32.04 ng/mL and postoperative values of >0.9 ng/mL are recommended for identifying neck LN metastasis [11]. Several studies reported that tumor size >2 cm, male sex, age <45 years, lymphatic invasion, ETE, multifocality, BRAF mutation, and the presence of lateral cervical lymph node metastasis were significant predictive factors for central lymph node metastasis in PTC [12–17].

33.2.2 Management

In patients with clinically involved central nodes, therapeutic central compartment (level VI) neck dissection should be performed [1]. At a minimum, central compartment neck dissection should include the prelaryngeal, pretracheal, and at least one paratracheal lymph node basin [18]. The presence of ipsilateral central or lateral cervical lymph node metastasis is a strong predictor of contralateral central lymph node metastasis in PTC [19, 20]. Skip metastasis to the lateral neck sparing the central compartment is uncommon but may be found up to 21.8% of the patients with upper pole tumors [21]. In patients who present with clinically evident disease involving cervical lymph nodes, the standard of care is to perform a therapeutic neck dissection, which entails the systematic removal of the lymph nodes in the central compartment [1]. Lateral neck dissection performed for macroscopic PTC metastases should be the selective neck dissection of levels IIa, III, IV, and Vb [1]. However, the patients with image-based, isolated lateral level IV involvement and no macroscopic extranodal extension might be potential candidates for limited levels III–IV dissection [22].

Because the AJCC/TNM risk of mortality staging system does not adequately predict the risk of recurrence in PTC, ATA thyroid cancer guidelines proposed a postoperative risk stratification system that classified patients as having low, intermediate, or high risk of recurrence according to clinicopathological and imaging findings [1]. Our patient was classified as intermediate risk due to the presence of microscopic ETE and >5 pathologic N1 with all involved lymph nodes <3 cm in the largest dimension. Of the patients who are classified as intermediate risk, approximately 60% have been reported to show excellent response to total thyroidectomy and RAI ablation treatment [1]. However, 20–30% of such patients may have persistent disease or develop locoregional or distant metastasis. Large tumor size (>4 cm), macroscopic lymph node in more than five nodes or metastatic nodes larger than >3 cm, extranodal invasion, gross extrathyroidal invasion, vascular invasion, and detection of certain molecular markers, such as BRAF, TERT, or TP53 mutations, were found to be associated with increased risk of recurrence in PTC [1]. Recently, the percentage of positive lymph nodes among the total number of nodes removed (lymph node ratio(LNR)) has been used to predict the risk of recurrence in PTC. A LNR >0.3 in the central, lateral, or both compartments has been reported to present a strong prognostic factor for recurrence [23]. In PTC patients, postoperative disease status can be determined by means of serum Tg levels, neck USG, and diagnostic whole-body scan (WBS) [1]. Postoperative Tg is expected to reach its nadir by 3–4 weeks after surgery. Postoperative sTg level <1–2 ng/mL (in the absence of Anti-Tg antibodies) and no evidence of disease by radiological evaluation are strong predictors of remission [1]. Low postoperative serum Tg (<1 ng/mL) levels in low-risk patients confirm the classification of such patients as being low risk and might alter the decision of RAI ablation therapy [1]. Postoperative RAI adjuvant therapy should be considered in ATA intermediate-/high-risk level patients. In intermediate-risk level PTC patients, thyroid hormone treatment at suppressive doses is recommended for TSH suppression to 0.1–0.5 mU/L. In patients who underwent total thyroidectomy and RAI treatment, the criteria for disease-free status include all of the following findings: (1) no clinical evidence of tumor, (2) no imaging evidence of tumor (WBS or neck US), and (3) serum Tg levels <0.2 ng/mL under TSH suppressive therapy or sTg <1 ng/mL following stimulation. The follow-up of the intermediate-risk level PTC patients includes serum Tg assay and neck USG at 6–12-month intervals following surgery and RAI ablation therapy. In intermediate-risk PTC patients who have clinical features associated with increased risk of recurrent or persistent disease, diagnostic WBS 6–12 months after RAI treatment is recommended [1]. Routine diagnostic WBS 6–12 months after RAI treatment is not recommended in intermediate-risk patients without high-risk factors and undetectable levels of serum Tg (in the absence of Anti-Tg antibodies) on thyroid hormone and negative US [1]. The adjustment of risk stratification in PTC patients during the course of further follow-up is important to provide an individualized therapeutic approach. After thyroidectomy and RAI treatment, biochemical and radiological findings during the first 2 years can be used to determine the individual response to initial treatment and reclassify the patients (dynamic risk assessment) [1]. The response to initial treatment is defined as excellent, biochemical incomplete, structural incomplete, and indeterminate response according to the serum Tg and/or Anti-Tg levels and radiological or clinical evidence of recurrent or persistent disease [1]. Excellent response to treatment is defined as no biochemical, clinical, or radiological evidence of tumor. The patients with negative or nonspecific imaging findings but abnormal Tg and Anti-Tg levels are reclassified as biochemical incomplete or indeterminate response. The patients with structural and functional evidence of tumor despite appropriate initial treatment are redefined as structural incomplete response. The rate of recurrence ranges between 1 and 4% in patients with excellent response, whereas it is 20% in patients with biochemical incomplete or indeterminate response. In patients with structural incomplete response, disease-specific death rate might be as high as 11%. Appropriate reclassification of intermediate-risk patients into the excellent response category with its very low risk of recurrence should lead to reevaluation of intensity of diagnostic surveillance procedures and treatment [1]). In intermediate-risk patients who are subsequently reclassified into excellent response category, the recommended TSH goal is 0.5–2 mU/L. Non-stimulated Tg assays and neck US at 12–24-month intervals are considered to be appropriate in the follow-up of such patients [1].

33.3 Follow-Up and Outcome

The patient received 150 mCi adjuvant radioactive iodine (RAI) therapy. There were no RAI-avid metastatic foci outside the thyroid bed on the first posttreatment WBS. After RAI therapy, the patient received thyroxine therapy to maintain TSH levels between 0.1 and 0.5 mU/L. Measurement of serum Tg values on thyroxine therapy and neck USG was performed at 6-month intervals during the first year after RAI treatment. The diagnostic WBS with thyroid hormone withdrawal which was done 12 months after RAI showed no uptake in the neck and distant sites. The sTg level at the time of diagnostic WBS was found 0.04 ng/mL. Further follow-up of the patient was planned as Tg measurement at 6-month intervals and neck USG annually.

33.3.1 The Future

Future research related to the identification of gene mutations which are associated with aggressive tumor behavior and the impact of such mutations on the clinical course of the disease would guide the therapeutic decision-making in PTC patients.

What Can We Learn from This Case?

- Cervical lymph nodes should be evaluated by preoperative neck USG in all patients undergoing thyroidectomy for malignant or suspicious for malignancy cytologic findings.
- Preoperative neck USG allows for the detection of nonpalpable cervical lymph node metastasis prior to thyroidectomy. When the thyroid gland is in situ, the sensitivity of USG to detect central compartment metastatic lymph nodes is lower compared to lateral metastatic lymph nodes.
- In patients with clinically involved central nodes, therapeutic central compartment (level VI) neck dissection should

be performed. At a minimum, central compartment neck dissection should include the prelaryngeal, pretracheal, and at least one paratracheal lymph node basin.

- The presence of ipsilateral central or lateral cervical lymph node metastasis is a strong predictor of contralateral central lymph node metastasis in PTC. In patients who present with clinically evident disease involving cervical lymph nodes, the standard of care is to perform a therapeutic neck dissection, which entails the systematic removal of the lymph nodes in the central compartment.
- The PTC patients with more than five metastatic lymph nodes with all involved lymph nodes <3 cm in the largest dimension are defined as ATA intermediate risk. Postoperative RAI adjuvant treatment should be considered in ATA intermediate-risk patients.

References

1. Haugen BR, Alexander EK, Bible KC, Doherty GM, Mandel SJ, Nikiforov YE, et al. American Thyroid Association management guidelines for adult patients with thyroid nodules and differentiated thyroid cancer: the American Thyroid Association guidelines task force on thyroid nodules and differentiated thyroid cancer. Thyroid. 2016;26:1–133. https://doi.org/10.1089/thy.2015.0020.
2. Gharib H, Papini E. Thyroid nodules: clinical importance, assessment, and treatment. Endocrinol Metab Clin N Am. 2007;36:707–35. https://doi.org/10.1016/j.ecl.2007.04.009.
3. Lew IJ, Solorzano CC. Use of ultrasound in the management of thyroid cancer. Oncologist. 2010;15:253–8. https://doi.org/10.1634/theoncologist.2009-0324.
4. Jabiev AA, Ikeda MH, Reis IM, Solorzano CC, Lew JI. Surgeon-performed ultrasound can predict differentiated thyroid cancer in patients with solitary thyroid nodules. Ann Surg Oncol. 2009;16:3140–5. https://doi.org/10.1245/s10434-009-0652-9.
5. Sherman SI. Thyroid carcinoma. Lancet. 2003;361:501–11.
6. Trimboli P, Ulisse S, Graziano FM, Marzullo A, Ruggieri M, Calvanese A, et al. Trend in thyroid carcinoma size, age at diagnosis and histology in a retrospective study of 500 cases diagnosed over 20 years. Thyroid. 2006;16:1151–5. https://doi.org/10.1089/thy.2006.16.1151.
7. Mirallié E, Visset J, Sagan C, Hamy A, Le Bodic MF, Paineau J. Localization of cervical node metastasis of papillary thyroid carcinoma. World J Surg. 1999;23:970–4.
8. Machens A, Hinze R, Thomusch O, Dralle H. Pattern of nodal metastasis for primary and reoperative thyroid cancer. World J Surg. 2002;26:22–8. https://doi.org/10.1007/s00268-001-0176-3.
9. Kouvaraki MA, Shapiro SE, Fornage BD, Edeiken-Monro BS, Sherman SI, Vassilopoulou-Sellin R, et al. Role of preoperative ultrasonography in the surgical management of patients with thyroid cancer. Surgery. 2003;134:946–55. https://doi.org/10.1016/S0039-6060(03)00424-0.
10. Stulak JM, Grant CS, Farley DR, Thompson GB, van Heerden JA, Hay ID, et al. Value of preoperative ultrasonography in the surgical management of initial and reoperative papillary thyroid cancer. Arch Surg. 2006;141:489–96. https://doi.org/10.1001/archsurg.141.5.489.
11. Pak K, Suh S, Hong H, Kim SJ, Kim IJ, Kim EE, et al. Diagnostic values of thyroglobulin measurement in fine-needle aspiration of lymph nodes in patients with thyroid cancer. Endocrine. 2015;49:70–7. https://doi.org/10.1007/s12020-014-0410-z.
12. Lee KE, Chung Y, Kang E, Koo do H, Kim KH, Kim SW, et al. Ipsilateral and contralateral central lymph node metastasis in papillary thyroid cancer: patterns and predictive factors of nodal metastasis. Head Neck. 2013;35:672–6. https://doi.org/10.1002/hed.23016.
13. Roh JL, Kim JM, Park CI. Central lymph node metastasis of unilateral papillary thyroid carcinoma: patterns and factors predictive of nodal metastasis, morbidity, and recurrence. Ann Surg Oncol. 2011;18:2245–50. https://doi.org/10.1245/s10434-011-1600-z.
14. Ito Y, Fukushima M, Higashiyama H, Kihara M, Takamura Y, Kobayashi K, et al. Tumor size is the strongest predictor of microscopic lymph node metastasis and lymph node recurrence of N0 papillary thyroid carcinoma. Endocr J. 2013;60:113–7.
15. Roh JL, Kim JM, Park CI. Lateral cervical lymph node metastases from papillary thyroid carcinoma: pattern of nodal metastases and optimal strategy for neck dissection. Ann Surg Oncol. 2008;15:1177–82. https://doi.org/10.1245/s10434-008-9813-5.
16. Zhao Q, Ming J, Liu C, Shi L, Xu X, Nie X, et al. Multifocality and total tumor diameter predict central neck lymph node metastases in papillary thyroid microcarcinoma. Ann Surg Oncol. 2013;20:746–52. https://doi.org/10.1245/s10434-012-2654-2.
17. So YK, Son YI, Park JY, Baek CH, Jeong HS, Chung MK. Preoperative BRAF mutation has different predictive values for lymph node metastasis according to tumor size. Otolaryngol Head Neck Surg. 2011;145:422–7. https://doi.org/10.1177/0194599811404649.

18. Carty SE, Cooper DS, Doherty GM, Duh QY, Kloos RT, Mandel SJ, American Thyroid Association Surgery Working Group, American Association of Endocrine Surgeons, American Academy of Otolaryngology-Head and Neck Surgery, American Head and Neck Society, et al. Consensus statement on the terminology and classification of central neck dissection for thyroid cancer. Thyroid. 2009;19:1153–8. https://doi.org/10.1089/thy.2009.0159.
19. Koo BS, Choi EC, Yoon YH, Kim DH, Kim EH, Lim YC. Predictive factors for ipsilateral or contralateral central lymph node metastasis in unilateral papillary thyroid carcinoma. Ann Surg. 2009;249:840–4. https://doi.org/10.1097/SLA.0b013e3181a40919.
20. Koo BS, Choi EC, Park YH, Kim EH, Lim YC. Occult contralateral central lymph node metastases in papillary thyroid carcinoma with unilateral lymph node metastasis in the lateral neck. J Am Coll Surg. 2010;210:895–900. https://doi.org/10.1016/j.jamcollsurg.2010.01.037.
21. Park JH, Lee YS, Kim BW, Chang HS, Park CS. Skip lateral neck node metastases in papillary thyroid carcinoma. World J Surg. 2012;36:743–7. https://doi.org/10.1007/s00268-012-1476-5.
22. Kang BC, Roh JL, Lee JH, Cho KJ, Gong G, Choi SH, et al. Candidates for limited lateral neck dissection among patients with metastatic papillary thyroid carcinoma. World J Surg. 2014;38:863–71. https://doi.org/10.1007/s00268-013-2361-6.
23. Chereau N, Buffet C, Tresallet C, Tissier F, Leenhardt L, Menegaux F. Recurrence of papillary thyroid carcinoma with lateral cervical node metastases: predictive factors and operative management. Surgery. 2016;159:755–62. https://doi.org/10.1016/j.surg.2015.08.033.

34

A Case of Papillary Carcinoma of the Thyroid with Minimal Extrathyroidal Extension

Banu Bilezikçi and Seyfettin Ilgan

Abstract

Authors present a case with papillary thyroid carcinoma showing minimal extrathyroidal extension (ETE). The ETE, which is defined as tumor extension beyond the thyroid gland in surrounding tissues, is one of the major determinants of accurate staging. Though it is considered as a prognostic parameter in all guidelines, the evaluation and interpretation of microscopic ETE remain problematic due to the thyroid gland's anatomical features. By TNM classification (seventh edition), differentiated thyroid carcinoma with ETE is designated by T3 (minimal invasion, invasion into the sternothyroid muscle or perithyroid tissues), T4a (extended invasion), or T4b (more extensive unresectable invasion) according to the degree of tumor involvement. Though outcomes from gross ETE are worse than those from microscopic ETE, both are recognized as risk factors on prognosis and recurrence rate.

B. Bilezikçi
Department of Pathology, Güven Hospital, Ankara, Turkey

S. Ilgan (✉)
Department of Nuclear Medicine, Güven Hospital, Ankara, Turkey

34.1 Case Presentation

A 49-year-old woman presented for routine screening of thyroid gland due to newly diagnosed papillary thyroid carcinoma in her daughter. The patient was euthyroid and asymptomatic. Physical examination was unremarkable except a palpable firm nodule on the right lobe. Thyroid ultrasonography (USG) revealed 10 × 8 mm markedly hypoechoic solid solitary nodule with microlobulated margins and increased anteroposterior diameter on the upper pole of the right lobe showing bulging into the adjacent structures on the anterior face (Fig. 34.1). The thyroid gland was slightly heterogeneous suggesting autoimmune thyroiditis. The contralateral lobe was normal, and no abnormal lymph nodes were visualized in the central compartment and lateral neck.

USG-guided fine needle aspiration (FNA) cytology of the nodule showed a "malignant/ papillary thyroid carcinoma" (Bethesda class VI). Total thyroidectomy and prophylactic central lymph node dissection were recommended to her by multidisciplinary team mainly because of suspicious sonographic findings for extrathyroidal extension (ETE). On gross examination, the cut surface of the tumor in the upper pole of the right lobe was gray-white and hard with infiltration into the adjacent thyroid parenchyma measuring 1.2 × 0.8 × 0.8 cm.

T. Özülker et al. (eds.), *Thyroid and Parathyroid Diseases*, https://doi.org/10.1007/978-3-319-78476-2_34

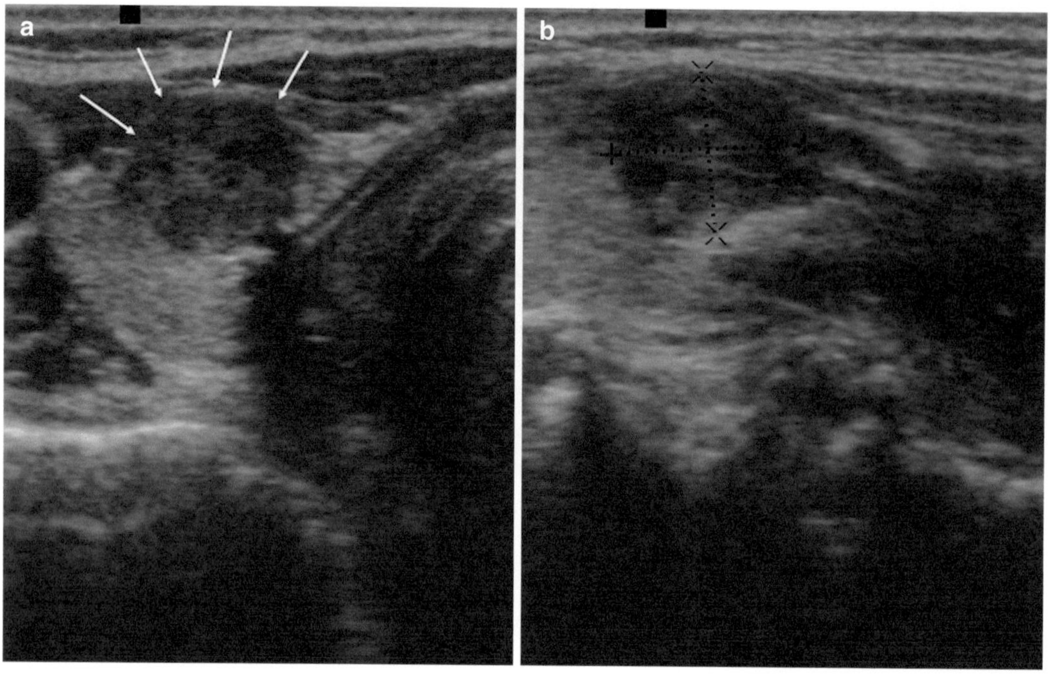

Fig. 34.1 Axial (**a**) and longitudinal (**b**) sonograms of the right thyroid lobe show markedly hypoechoic solid nodule with microlobulated margins which proved to be a papillary thyroid carcinoma. The tumor shows anterior protrusion (arrows) with disruption of thyroid capsule in some areas suggesting extrathyroidal extension. Skeletal muscle invasion is confirmed at the final pathology

Central lymph node dissection material was also sent along with thyroid specimen measured 2 × 2 × 0.6 cm. Materials were fixed in 10% formalin and embedded in paraffin, and deparaffinized sections were stained with hematoxylin-eosin. The histopathologic findings were consistent with follicular variant of papillary thyroid carcinoma without tumor capsule [1]. The tumor showed microscopic ETE, including infiltration of the skeletal muscle (Fig. 34.2), and the outer surface of the specimen (inked edge) was positive. The remainder of the thyroid parenchyma showed Hashimoto's thyroiditis. The tumor was staged as T3b using the eighth edition of the *American Joint Committee on Cancer/Union for International Cancer Control* manual [2]. There was no lymphovascular invasion at the periphery of the tumor. Seven lymph nodes in the central compartment were examined; none of them presented metastatic deposits of thyroid carcinoma. The patient was stage III according to the AJCC/UICC TNM system and in intermediate-risk group according to the *2015 American Thyroid Association Management Guidelines for Adult Patients with Thyroid Nodules and Differentiated Thyroid Cancer* [3].

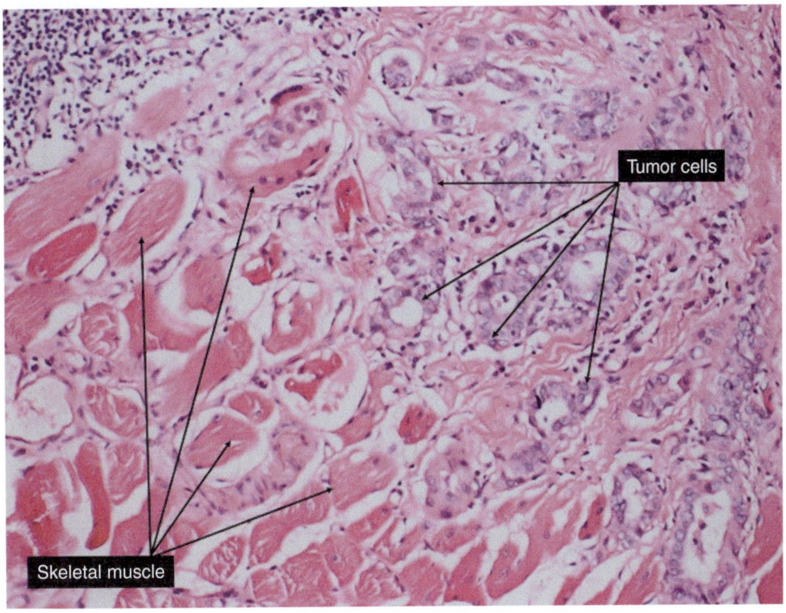

Fig. 34.2 Neoplastic cells are arranged in a follicular pattern of growth. Skeletal muscle invasion is visible at the periphery of the tumor (arrows) (hematoxylin and eosin staining, magnification 20×)

34.2 Discussion

One of the most important determinants of treatment and prognosis in patients with malignancy is the stage of cancer. In papillary thyroid carcinomas, the ETE, which is defined as tumor extension beyond the thyroid gland in surrounding tissues, is one of the main determinants of accurate staging. Therefore, the exact diagnosis of ETE is crucial for both therapy and management [4, 5].

Identifying the stage of the disease (stage III or IV) depends on the evaluation of ETE. In spite of the fact that it is considered as a prognostic parameter in all guidelines, the evaluation and interpretation of microscopic ETE remain problematic due to the thyroid gland's anatomical features [4].

On macroscopic examination, the capsule may appear complete. However, Komorowski et al. [6] showed that the thyroid capsule might be focally incomplete or absent; thyroid follicles may be found in the capsule or outside the gland during the microscopic examination in a majority of thyroid glands evaluated at the autopsy. Moreover, extension into perithyroidal adipose tissue is not a criterion for ETE because adipose tissue can appear in the thyroid gland under normal conditions or various thyroid diseases [4, 7].

Thyroid tumor within adipose tissue and capsule invasion cannot be accepted as a standard of ETE or as a thyroid carcinoma particularly in minimal extension (pT3). For this reason, skeletal muscle's invasion is a more exact diagnostic finding of ETE. Similar to adipose tissue in the thyroid, skeletal muscle may be seen in the thyroid gland under normal conditions, especially in relation to the isthmus portion of the thyroid gland. It may be seen in a variety of pathologic conditions as well. In this situation, if present, a desmoplastic response may be considered as evidence of ETE [4, 7].

Similarly, pathology reports should give the data of surgical margin status just as in other organs. The outer surface of the thyroid gland and/or the inked edge of the specimen are described as the "margin" [4, 7]. In contrast to other cancers, the role of margin status in differentiated papillary thyroid carcinoma is not well-known. Recently, Wang et al. [8] reported that positive microscopic margins in differentiated thyroid carcinoma are not an independent predictor of local failure.

By TNM classification (seventh edition), differentiated thyroid carcinoma with ETE is designated by T3 (minimal invasion, invasion into the sternothyroid muscle or perithyroid tissues), T4a (extended invasion), or T4b (more extensive unresectable invasion) according to the degree of tumor involvement [9].

Depending on the applied pathologic criteria, nearly 10–15% of thyroid cancers present with ETE, with the most common structures involved including the strap muscle, RLN, trachea, esophagus, and larynx [10, 11]. Minimal ETE is common, with a reported prevalence between 11 and 44%. However, it must be distinguished from the major extrathyroidal extension, which implies more advanced disease and worse prognosis [12]. Recently, Youngwirth et al. [5] reported that compared with patients without ETE, patients with minimal and extensive ETE were more likely to have larger tumors (1.4 cm vs. 1.8 cm and 2.0 cm, respectively), lymphovascular invasion (8.6% vs. 28.0% and 35.1%, respectively), positive margins after thyroidectomy (6.1% vs. 35.2% and 45.9%, respectively), and regional lymph node metastases (32.5% vs. 67.0% and 74.6%, respectively; all $p < 0.01$). It has also been shown in a large group of patients that differentiated thyroid cancer patients with no ETE had improved overall survival compared with those with minimal and extensive ETE. Other studies concluded that though outcomes from gross ETE are worse than those from microscopic ETE, both are recognized risk factors on prognosis and recurrence rate [13].

Furthermore, according to the ATA, minimal ETE is associated with intermediate risk, and extensive ETE is associated with high risk for differentiated thyroid cancer [3, 5]. The definition of T3 has been revised for papillary carcinoma in the eighth edition of AJCC. If the tumor is more than 4 cm in greatest diameter and is limited to the thyroid, it is reclassified as a T3a. Tumors renamed as a T3b are defined by tumors of any size with gross extrathyroidal extension invading only strap muscles (sternohyoid, sternothyroid, or omohyoid) [2]. The new version of AJCC accepts the invasion of the skeletal muscle as the identifier for microscopic ETE. Therefore, it seems necessary to adapt the new classification to other guides (ATA, cap protocol, etc.).

Although thyroid lobectomy alone is seen as sufficient treatment for small low-risk tumors (unifocal, intrathyroidal carcinomas in the absence of prior head and neck radiation, familial thyroid carcinoma, or clinically detectable cervical nodal metastases), bilateral surgical procedure and prophylactic central lymph node dissection would be preferred in tumors with ETE to allow for the possible use of RAI remnant ablation and facilitate detection of recurrent/persistent disease during follow-up [3, 14].

34.2.1 Evaluation and Diagnosis

High-resolution sonography has become an essential tool for preoperative evaluation of known or suspected thyroid cancer. In fact, surgical planning mostly depends on sonographic findings such as tumor size, multifocality, ETE, and lymph node metastasis. Defining ETE during preoperative imaging has significant importance in surgical planning and decision process. There have been several studies evaluating the value of preoperative sonography in the prediction of ETE. The sensitivity and specificity of sonography in the evaluation of ETE were reported between 62.9–85.3% and 68.9–97.6%, respectively [15, 16].

Diagnostic performance of preoperative USG in the preoperative evaluation of primary tumors and cervical lymph nodes in patients with papillary thyroid carcinoma has been compared with computerized tomography (CT) by Choi et al. [17]. In a series of 299 patients with PTC who underwent preoperative CT and USG, USG was more accurate than CT in predicting ETE and multifocal bilobar disease. The accuracy of staging was better overall with USG, and USG had greater sensitivity than CT at predicting lateral compartment metastases. USG also compared with magnetic resonance imaging (MRI) in preoperative prediction of the ETE and showed higher sensitivity (80% vs. 64.7%) and lower specificity (70.4% vs. 84.9%) than MRI for predicting minimal ETE of PTC [4, 7]. Although the diagnostic performance of USG was comparable with MRI in the assessment of extensive ETE ($p > 0.05$), USG had a significantly higher sensitivity (100%), NPV (100%), and accuracy (92.6%) than MRI in the prediction of overall ETE ($p < 0.001$).

There have been only a few studies defining sonographic risk factors in the prediction of the ETE. The existence of intervening normal thyroid tissue between the malignant nodule and the thyroid capsule practically rules out gross ETE with high accuracy. However, microscopic ETE could not be excluded with this finding [18]. On the other hand, (1) direct contact of the malignant nodule with thyroid capsule (abutment), (2) disruption of the perithyroidal echogenic line (thyroid capsule), and (3) protrusion of tumor directly into the adjacent structures were suggested as sonographic risk factors for ETE [15–22]. A capsular protrusion is defined as the bulging of the tumor into the adjacent structures, while capsular abutment is defined as the lack of intervening tissue between the malignant nodule and the thyroid capsule. The relationships between tumor and thyroid capsule are further categorized according to the degree of the capsular abutment (<25%, 25–50%, and >50%) since higher scores reflect a higher possibility of ETE [15, 20].

Shimamoto et al. reported that protrusion of malignant nodule into the surrounding tissue with loss of normal tissue boundaries was an equivocal finding for ETE, but protrusion with loss of mobility during vending was a definite sonographic evidence of T4 tumor [15]. Lee et al. found that protrusion was a statistically significantly better predictive factor than abutment [22]. In addition, an increasing perimeter ratio was also reported as a statistically significant predictive factor of ETE. On the other hand, the location of tumor (anterior vs. posterior) and echotexture of thyroid gland (heterogeneous vs. homogenous) were not statistically significant factors for prediction of ETE [22].

34.2.2 Management

The ETE by primary tumors and lymph node metastasis are previously reported as independent risk factors of recurrence [23]. Moreover, a larger tumor size and a higher lymph node stage have been found as the best predictors of ETE in sonographically suspected patients [21]. Though both are recognized risk factors for prognosis and recurrence rate [5, 13], there is a clear prognostic difference between gross and microscopic ETE. While patients with only microscopic ETE had an overall excellent prognosis, gross ETE had markedly impaired prognosis [24]. This distinction is reflected in modern TNM staging system and guidelines also.

Since the microscopic ETE someway suggests slightly more aggressive tumor biology, groups may elect total thyroidectomy as initial surgical treatment in patients with suspicious preoperative sonographic findings for ETE, as we did. However, lobectomy would also be preferred in carefully selected patient groups.

Though no nodal metastases were detected in central compartment dissection material in our case, skip lateral nodal metastasis should be expected with primary tumors of the upper pole [25]. So, we decided to use stimulated Tg levels to rule out occult lateral nodal metastases and for decision of RAI use. According to our postoperative risk stratification and RAI decision protocol, T4 suppression started after operation for 3 weeks and stopped for another 3 weeks to check stimulated thyroglobulin (Tg) levels. At 6-week follow-up, TSH was 73 μIU/mL, and Tg level was <0.1 ng/mL without Tg antibodies. Based on excellent response to initial therapy, patient was reclassified as low risk, and follow-up without RAI ablation, using neck USG and serum Tg, is recommended to her. At the 12-month follow-up,

USG of the neck did not show any pathologic lymph nodes in the central and lateral neck, and serum Tg levels were undetectable with negative Tg antibodies.

ATA 2015 intermediate-risk category includes microscopic ETE, cervical lymph node metastases, RAI-avid disease in the neck outside the thyroid bed, vascular invasion, or aggressive tumor histology [3]. Though postsurgical RAI was generally favored based on the risk of recurrent disease, to help guide this decision, local factors such as the quality of preoperative and postoperative USG evaluations, availability of stimulated/suppressed Tg measurements, experience of the surgical team, and follow-up conditions should also be taken into consideration in postoperative RAI use. Still, we need high-quality evidence to understand the therapeutic efficacy of the adjuvant use of RAI in various subgroups of patients in the ATA intermediate-risk category. In our case, adjuvant RAI was not indicated for her management.

What Can We Learn from This Case?

- Ultrasound could supply critical information about preoperative prediction of ETE and alter preferred initial surgical strategy in patients with known or suspected thyroid malignancy.
- Existence and degree of capsular abutment, disruption of perithyroidal echogenic line (thyroid capsule), and protrusion of tumor directly into the adjacent structures are recognized sonographic risk factors for ETE.
- Though outcomes from gross ETE are worse than those from microscopic ETE, both are recognized risk factors for prognosis and recurrence rate. Currently, there is no consensus on the use of adjuvant RAI treatment in patients with microscopic ETE. Use of RAI therapy in this setting (either for remnant ablation to make follow-up easier or as an adjuvant therapy) would depend on many factors such as clinicopathological details, postoperative Tg levels, USG finding, and experience of the center.
- Unlike macroscopic ETE of papillary carcinoma, microscopic diagnosis of minimal gross extrathyroidal extension is quite problematic.
- Safe diagnostic finding of ETE is skeletal muscle invasion.
- Microscopic ETE should be presented on final pathology reports.
- We hope that the new revision (eighth edition) of AJCC staging criteria will lead to more efficient and standard diagnosis of ETE.

References

1. Lloyd R, De Lellis RPH. World Health Organization classification of tumours: pathology and genetics of tumours of the endocrine organs. 3rd ed. Lyon: IARC Press International Agency for Research on Cancer; 2004.
2. Amin MB, Edge SB, Greene FL, Compton CC, Gershenwald JE, Brookland RK, et al., editors. AJCC cancer staging manual. 8th ed. New York: Springer; 2017.
3. Haugen BR, Alexander EK, Bible KC, Doherty GM, Mandel SJ, Nikiforov YE, et al. 2015 American Thyroid Association management guidelines for adult patients with thyroid nodules and differentiated thyroid cancer: the American Thyroid Association guidelines task force on thyroid nodules and differentiated thyroid cancer. Thyroid. 2016;26:1–133. https://doi.org/10.1089/thy.2015.0020.
4. Mete O, Rotstein L, Asa SL. Controversies in thyroid pathology: thyroid capsule invasion and extrathyroidal extension. Ann Surg Oncol. 2010;17:386–91. https://doi.org/10.1245/s10434-009-0832-7.
5. Youngwirth LM, Adam MA, Scheri RP, Roman SA, Sosa JA. Extrathyroidal extension is associated with compromised survival in patients with thyroid cancer. Thyroid. 2017;27:626–31. https://doi.org/10.1089/thy.2016.0132.
6. Komorowski RA, Hanson GA. Occult thyroid pathology in the young adult: an autopsy study of 138 patients without clinical thyroid disease. Hum Pathol. 1988;19:689–96.
7. Seethala RR, Asa SL, Carty SE, Hodak SP, McHugh JB, Richardson MS, et al. Protocol for the examina-

tion of specimens from patients with carcinomas of the thyroid gland. Northfield: College of American Pathologists; 2016. p. 1–22.

8. Wang LY, Ghossein R, Palmer FL, Nixon IJ, Tuttle RM, Shaha AR, et al. Microscopic positive margins in differentiated thyroid cancer is not an independent predictor of local failure. Thyroid. 2015;25:993–8. https://doi.org/10.1089/thy.2015.0141.
9. Edge SB, Byrd DR, Carducci MA, Compton CC, editors. AJCC cancer staging manual. 7th ed. New York: Springer; 2009.
10. Dralle H, Sekulla C, Haerting J, Timmermann W, Neumann HJ, Kruse E, et al. Risk factors of paralysis and functional outcome after recurrent laryngeal nerve monitoring in thyroid surgery. Surgery. 2004;136:1310–22.
11. Shindo ML, Caruana S, Kandil E, McCaffrey JC, Orloff LA, Porterfield JR, et al. Management of invasive well-differentiated thyroid cancer an American Head and Neck Society consensus statement. Head Neck. 2014;36:1379–90. https://doi.org/10.1002/hed.23619.
12. Yin DT, Yu K, Lu RQ, Li X, Xu J, Lei M. Prognostic impact of minimal extrathyroidal extension in papillary thyroid carcinoma. Medicine (Baltimore). 2016;95:e5794. https://doi.org/10.1097/MD.0000000000005794.
13. Radowsky JS, Howard RS, Burch HB, Stojadinovic A. Impact of degree of extrathyroidal extension of disease on papillary thyroid cancer outcome. Thyroid. 2014;24:241–4. https://doi.org/10.1089/thy.2012.0567.
14. Kim KJ, Hong SW, Lee YS, Kim BW, Lee SC, Chang HS, et al. Tumor margin histology predicts tumor aggressiveness in papillary thyroid carcinoma: a study of 514 consecutive patients. J Korean Med Sci. 2011;26:346–51. https://doi.org/10.3346/jkms.2011.26.3.346.
15. Shimamoto K, Satake H, Sawaki A, Ishigaki T, Funahashi H, Imai T. Preoperative staging of thyroid papillary carcinoma with ultrasonography. Eur J Radiol. 1998;29:4–10.
16. Park JS, Son KR, Na DG, Kim E, Kim S. Performance of preoperative sonographic staging of papillary thyroid carcinoma based on the sixth edition of the AJCC/UICC TNM classification system. AJR Am J Roentgenol. 2009;192:66–72. https://doi.org/10.2214/AJR.07.3731.
17. Choi JS, Kim J, Kwak JY, Kim MJ, Chang HS, Kim EK. Preoperative staging of papillary thyroid carcinoma: comparison of ultrasound imaging and CT. AJR Am J Roentgenol. 2009;193:871–8. https://doi.org/10.2214/AJR.09.2386.
18. Kim H. Preoperative prediction of the extrathyroidal extension of papillary thyroid carcinoma with ultrasonography versus MRI: a retrospective cohort study. Int J Surg. 2014;12:544–8. https://doi.org/10.1016/j.ijsu.2014.03.003.
19. Rim JH, Chong S, Ryu HS, Chung BM, Ahn HS. Feasibility study of ultrasonographic criteria for microscopic and macroscopic extra-thyroidal extension based on thyroid capsular continuity and tumor contour in patients with papillary thyroid carcinomas. Ultrasound Med Biol. 2016;42:2391–400. https://doi.org/10.1016/j.ultrasmedbio.2016.06.014.
20. Kim SS, Lee BJ, Lee JC, Kim SJ, Lee SH, Jeon YK, et al. Preoperative ultrasonographic tumor characteristics as a predictive factor of tumor stage in papillary thyroid carcinoma. Head Neck. 2011;33:1719–26. https://doi.org/10.1002/hed.21658.
21. Kwak JY, Kim EK, Youk JH, Kim MJ, Son EJ, Choi SH, et al. Extrathyroid extension of well-differentiated papillary thyroid microcarcinoma on US. Thyroid. 2008;18:609–14. https://doi.org/10.1089/thy.2007.0345.
22. Lee CY, Kim SJ, Ko KR, Chung KW, Lee JH. Predictive factors for extrathyroidal extension of papillary thyroid carcinoma based on preoperative sonography. J Ultrasound Med. 2014;33:231–8. https://doi.org/10.7863/ultra.33.2.231.
23. Hay ID, Bergstralh EJ, Goellner JR, Ebersold JR, Grant CS. Predicting outcome in papillary thyroid carcinoma: development of a reliable prognostic scoring system in a cohort of 1779 patients surgically treated at one institution during 1940 through 1989. Surgery. 1993;114:1050–7; discussion 1057–1058.
24. Hotomi M, Sugitani I, Toda K, Kawabata K, Fujimoto Y. A novel definition of extrathyroidal invasion for patients with papillary thyroid carcinoma for predicting prognosis. World J Surg. 2012;36:1231–40. https://doi.org/10.1007/s00268-012-1518-z.
25. Park JH, Lee YS, Kim BW, Chang HS, Park CS. Skip lateral neck node metastases in papillary thyroid carcinoma. World J Surg. 2012;36:743–7. https://doi.org/10.1007/s00268-012-1476-5.

Therapeutic Neck Dissection for Differentiated Thyroid Cancer, to Whom and to What Extent?

35

Betül Bozkurt

Abstract

Bilateral total thyroidectomy is the standard surgical procedure for metastatic thyroid cancers. In this section, the definition and the extent of neck dissection will be discussed for thyroid cancer patients with lateral neck metastases. Since the first description of the radical neck dissection by George Crile almost a century ago, the surgical management of thyroid cancer patients with metastatic regional lymph nodes continues to be a challenge. The level of regional lymphatic spread in thyroid cancer is independent of tumor size and its location in the thyroid. In treatment, cervical lymphatic dissection has a place only in clinically proven metastatic disease. In clinically proven cases of nodal disease with preoperative USG and fine needle aspiration cytology (FNAC) or thyroglobulin (Tg) measurements, lymph node dissection during surgery may reduce the risk of relapses and possible mortality. In proven cervical metastatic disease, compartmental lymph node dissection is effective and adequate for treatment and which is also the recommendations of the guidelines.

B. Bozkurt
Division of Endocrine and Breast Surgery, Hitit University Medical Faculty General Surgery Department, Çorum, Turkey

35.1 Case Presentation

A 59-year-old male patient presented with thyroid nodules and cervical lymphadenopathy. He stated that he had a mass on his neck for a long while and that it had started growing recently. Thus, he was revisiting his doctor. On physical examination of the neck, the thyroid gland was palpated as heterogeneous, multinodular, and enlarged. There was a subclavicular extension on the right lobe. Cervical lymphadenopathy could not be found on the neck examination. His general physical examination was normal. Thyroid ultrasonography (USG) that was performed at the Endocrinology Department revealed a 26 × 42 × 43 mm nodule with mixed echogenicity. This nodule covered the left lobe and harbored cystic components with border calcifications. On the right lobe, there was a nodule of 21 × 37 × 43 mm with cystic components; the nodule filled the middle and lower posterior parts of this lobe. Numerous nodules were observed within the parenchyma, and the sizes of the largest ones were provided (Fig. 35.1).

On the neck USG, in right level III, there was a hypoechoic lymph node of 13.0 × 10.0 × 5.4 mm with cystic components; its hilus could not be visualized. Neighboring this node, there was another one measuring 9.2 × 7.0 × 4.3 mm. In right level IV, lymph nodes (LN) of 7.2 × 6 × 3.1 mm and 7 × 5.4 × 4.8 mm were

T. Özülker et al. (eds.), *Thyroid and Parathyroid Diseases*, https://doi.org/10.1007/978-3-319-78476-2_35

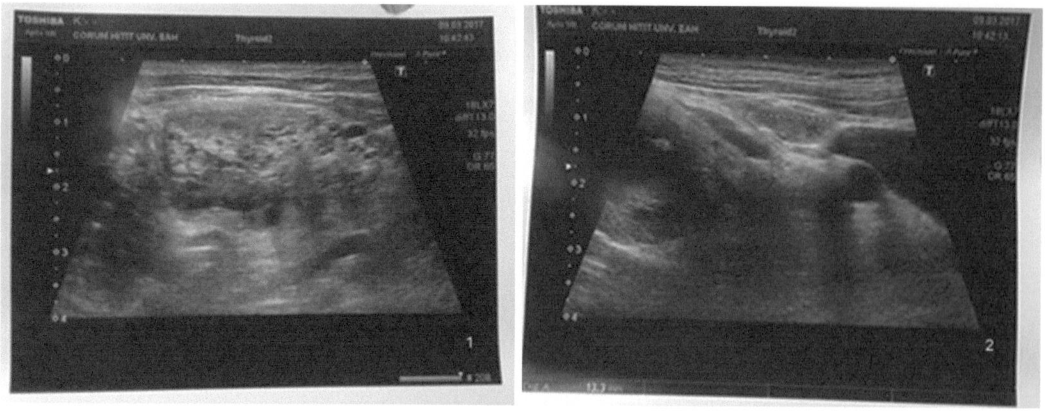

Fig. 35.1 Thyroid and neck USG

observed; their hili could not be visualized either (Fig. 35.1).

We mostly prefer to use the definitions of the American Thyroid Association (ATA) guidelines in our clinical practice. The latest revised ATA guideline for thyroid cancer was published in 2016 [1]. With these findings, a fine needle aspiration biopsy (FNAB) was performed from the right lobe of the thyroid gland.

The pathology report was as follows: On a ground laid with colloid poor blood cells, there were stratified thyroid follicular epithelial cells in layers together with several Hürthle cells either in solitude or small groups. There were histiocytes in between, as well as spindle-like atypical cellular groups that were not very rare and that might be associated with cyst lining epithelium. There was no increase in the lymphoid cells (atypia of undetermined significance (AUS) right middle thyroid FNAB [2]). The described cytological findings may represent Hürthle cell hyperplasia in a patient with multiple nodules. However, Hürthle cell neoplasia cannot be ruled out.

This case was reported as "clinical correlation is recommended." FNAB from the LN in level III on the right was reported as malignant cytological findings compatible with papillary carcinoma metastasis. The result of the FNAB that was performed with the suspicion of metastasis from the LN with a 13 mm of long axis whose hilus was not observed was reported as malignant cytological findings consistent with papillary thyroid carcinoma metastasis.

Pathological examination was reported as papillary microcarcinoma; classical variant at the right lobe; multinodular goiter at the right and left lobes; one metastatic and eight reactive LNs in the right central area; two metastatic and ten reactive LNs at the left central area; three metastatic LNs at right level III; and 13 reactive LNs at right level III and level IV. A microcarcinoma focus of 6 mm was identified at the upper medial portion of the right lobe of the thyroid gland; it had intrathyroidal localization. According to the AJCC/UICC TNM system, the patient was staged as T1N1bM0, stage IVA [3].

As there were not any findings of advanced disease or invasion of peripheral tissues during USG evaluation, further investigations such as CT, MRI, or PET were not considered (ATA Recommendation (R) 33 (A) and (B) [1]).

The patient was discussed at the endocrine council. Upon the decision of the endocrine council, the patient underwent bilateral total thyroidectomy and bilateral central and right modified levels III and IV lateral neck dissection with a diagnosis of metastatic papillary thyroid carcinoma. Intraoperative evaluation showed the majority of the right thyroid as extended to the subclavicular area and the anterior mediastinum (Fig. 35.2).

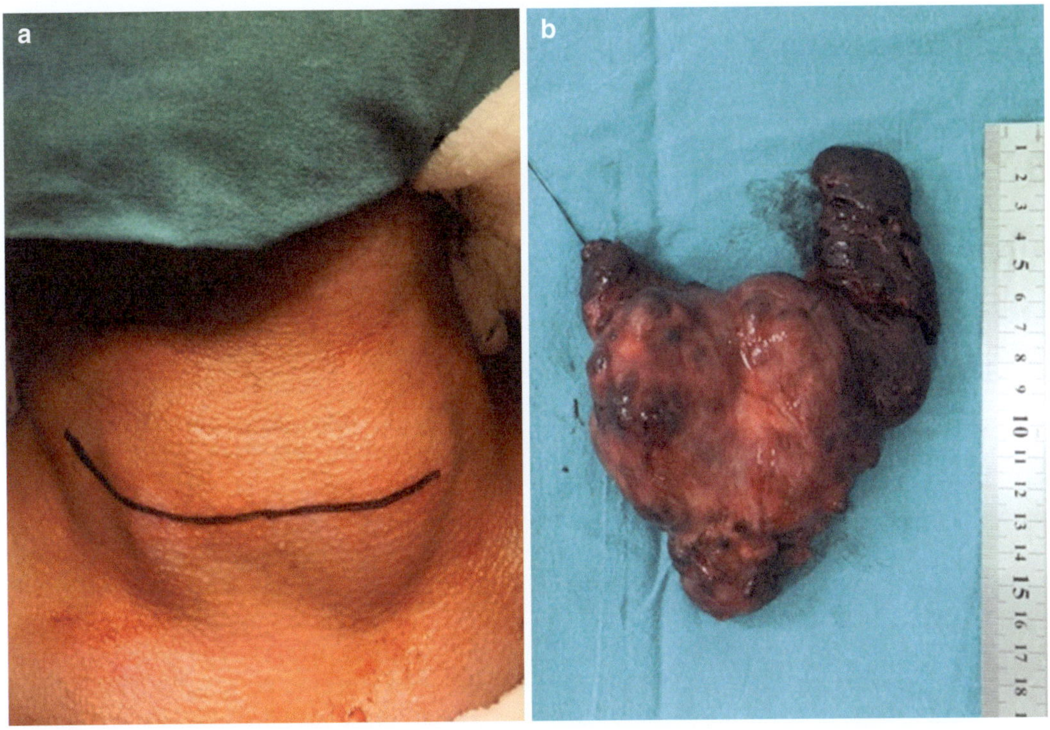

Fig. 35.2 Neck incision (left) and thyroidectomy specimen (right)

35.2 Discussion

Bilateral total thyroidectomy is the standard surgical procedure for metastatic thyroid cancers. In this section, the definition and the extent of neck dissection will be discussed for thyroid cancer patients with lateral neck metastases.

Since the first description of the radical neck dissection by George Crile almost a century ago, many variations and modifications of the procedure have been discovered. These include the functional neck dissection, the modified radical neck dissection, and various selective neck dissections. The surgical management of thyroid cancer patients with metastatic regional lymph nodes continues to be a challenge.

The otorhinolaryngologist Osvaldo Suarez and the anatomist Pedro Ara have described the functional neck dissection for the first time while the whole world was still performing radical neck dissections under the influence of Halsted. Several variations and modifications have been described for radical neck dissection. These are functional and modified radical neck dissections and various selective neck dissections.

After 1991, neck dissections were reclassified in 2002. Today, the classification made in 2002 is still valid. Nowadays, we do not type modified radical neck dissections, we define the structures we protect with the new classification. Moreover, we do not classify selective neck dissections anymore. We only define the region we remove (Table 35.1).

In the year 2002, revised neck dissection classification is published; the level limits also changed. To describe the boundaries between levels II and III, the horizontal level determined by the lower border of the hyoid bone is used instead of the carotid bifurcation. Instead of linking the superior part of the omohyoid muscle to describe the border between levels III and IV, the horizontal level is determined by the inferior border of the cricoid cartilage (Fig. 35.3).

Table 35.1 Changes in neck dissection classification

1991 classification	2002 classification
1. Radical neck dissection	1. Radical neck dissection
2. Modified radical neck dissection (types 1, 2, and 3)	2. Modified radical neck dissection. No typing with numbering; only protected structures are specified
3. Selective neck dissection (a) Supraomohyoid (b) Lateral (c) Posterolateral (d) Anterior	3. Selective neck dissection. No special naming, selective neck dissection, and removed levels, sublevels, or other groups of nodes are written in brackets
4. Extended neck dissection	4. Extended neck dissection

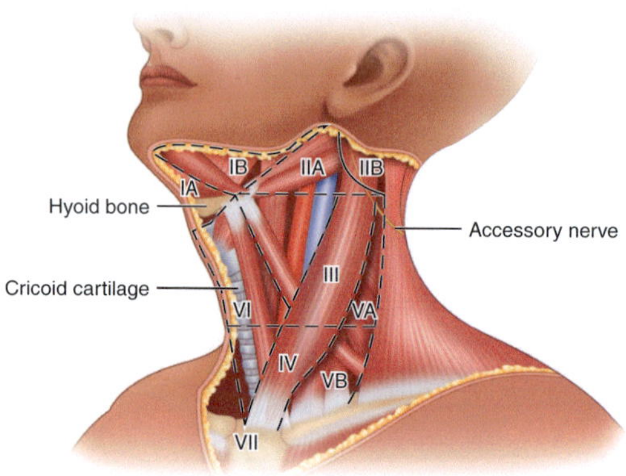

Fig. 35.3 Topographic anatomy of neck dissection

Selective neck dissection defines a cervical lymphadenectomy where one or more of the lymph node groups that are routinely removed in the radical neck dissection are preserved. The removal of lymph node groups is based on metastatic patterns, and these are predictable relative to the primary disease site.

The role of therapeutic lymph node dissection for the treatment of thyroid cancer nodal metastases is well accepted for cN1 disease [4–7].

35.3 Could the Lymphatic Drainage of the Tumor Show a Change Based on Its Location Within the Thyroid Gland? At Which Level Should the Neck Dissection Be Performed?

The lymphatics appearing from the inferior-medial aspect of thyroid lobes go after the course of the inferior thyroid veins and empty into the primary echelon nodes in pretracheal, paratracheal (level IV), and lower jugular regions (level IV) [8]. They secondarily drain into the nodes of the anterior-superior mediastinum (level VII) and rarely into the lower mediastinal nodes. The lymphatics stemming from the lateral aspect of the gland follow the middle thyroid vein and empty into jugular lymph nodes (levels II, III, IV). The lymphatics from the superior aspect of the gland and the isthmus drain into prelaryngeal (Delphian) and jugular lymph nodes, particularly to the midjugular nodes (Level III) [8].

However, lymphatic metastases in the thyroid do not always follow this spreading plan. Skip metastases can be seen in thyroid cancers. Metastases to the lateral lymph nodes without metastasis to the central LNs have been reported in 9.6–45% of the cases in the literature [9, 10]. Skip lateral cervical metastasis can even reach 33% in microcarcinomas [11]. Interestingly, although the tumor was a classical variant of papillary microcarcinoma, in this case, both the bilateral central and right cervical regions harbored metastases.

Metastases in the cervical lymphatic chain are most commonly seen in level IV (52%), to be followed by III (45%), V (33%), and II (30%). In very advanced disease, metastasis in level I is seen only after all other neck compartments have been very intensely involved and particularly if level II is involved [9] ATA R37 [1].

Lateral cervical lymph nodes (compartments II–V), level VII (anterior mediastinum), and rarely level I may be involved in thyroid cancer. Unproven prophylactic lymph node dissections are likely to lead to unwanted morbidity. Dralle developed the technique of compartment-oriented microdissection of the central and lateral

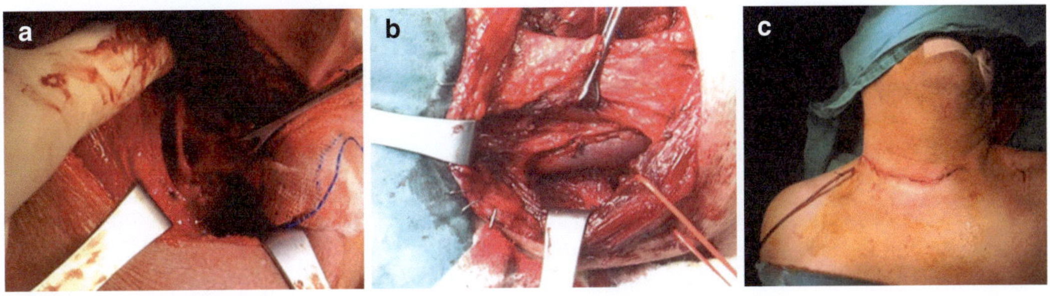

Fig. 35.4 (**a–c**) Therapeutic central neck dissection (**a**), lateral neck dissection (**b**, **c**)

compartments in patients with thyroid carcinoma in the early 1990s; this technique then became a consensus-backed part of the guidelines [12, 13]. Thus, in patients with no signs of lymph node metastasis, it is acceptable not to perform lymph node dissection for two reasons: (1) to minimize the risk of intraoperative injury to the marginal mandibular branch of the facial nerve and (2) to prevent associated functional impairments to the accessory nerve [13]. The ATA 2015 guide also provided a comment supporting this view. In clinically proven cases of nodal disease with preoperative USG and FNAB or thyroglobulin (Tg) measurements, compartment lymph node dissection during surgery may reduce the risk of relapses and possible mortality [1]. Neither clinical examination nor USG evaluation revealed any metastatic findings in other areas of the neck in our patient. Following the current literature, the patient was evaluated intraoperatively, and only levels III and IV selective compartment lymph node dissection were performed (Fig. 35.4a–c).

Medullary thyroid cancer (MTC) is less frequently encountered, and only treatment option is surgery for MTC patients; in involvements of levels II–VII, or even in extensive level II involvement, levels I–VII therapeutic lateral neck dissection should be performed.

35.4 Follow-Up and Outcome

The case was discussed at a multidisciplinary endocrine council. The decision was that the patient would complete the healing period and wait for TSH levels to rise to allow for radioactive iodine treatment (RAT) and to receive 150 mCi I-131 treatment approximately a month later. No residual activity was detected in whole-body iodine scintigraphy performed after administration of 150 mCi RAT. The patient who is currently in the third month after RAT is being followed up with TSH suppression therapy. Replacement therapy was started with 100 μgm levothyroxine. At the end of the third month, the last measured value of TSH was 0.75 for TSH, and then levothyroxine dose was increased to 125 μgm.

According to the ATA 2009 Risk Stratification System with Proposed Modifications, the patient is in the intermediate-risk class (Because of clinical N1 or >5 pathologic N1 with all involved lymph nodes <3 cm in the largest dimension, proposed modifications were not present in the original 2009 initial risk stratification system. See ATA guidelines' sections [B19]–[B23] and recommendation 48B) [1]. If a total thyroidectomy and RAT were performed, an excellent response was usually defined as a TSH-stimulated Tg of <1 ng/mL in the absence of structural or functional evidence of disease (and in the absence of anti-Tg antibodies) [14–16]. An excellent response to initial therapy is achieved in 86–91% of ATA low-risk patients, 57–63% of ATA intermediate-risk patients, and 14–16% of ATA high-risk patients [14–16]. The target TSH value is below 0.1 uIU/mL; Tg value is <0.2 ng/mL [1]. TSH and Tg levels were monitored 1 month after the surgery and every 6 months after that, and a decision was made to perform the follow-up with USG twice a year. The objective of the treatment is to obtain an excellent response. The excellent response is defined as no clinical, biochemical, or structural evidence of disease [1].

The preceding recommendations should be interpreted based on available surgical experience and literature data; for patients with small tumors without capsular or lymphovascular invasion who are clinically cN0, the balance of risk and benefit may favor thyroid lobectomy and close intraoperative inspection of the central compartment, with intraoperative detailed control, and the operative plan adjusted to total thyroidectomy with compartmental dissection only in the presence of involved lymph nodes. However, the fact that the patient cannot receive RAI I-131 therapy should be taken into consideration.

What Can We Learn from This Case?

- The level of regional lymphatic spread in thyroid cancer is independent of tumor size and its location in the thyroid.
- Histological type of the tumor, the age of the patient, the size of the tumor, and the presence of a capsular invasion might increase lymphatic metastasis in thyroid cancers.
- In treatment, cervical lymphatic dissection has a place only in clinically proven metastatic disease.
- In clinically proven cases of metastatic nodal disease with preoperative USG and FNAB or Tg washout, surgical dissection is the appropriate treatment choice.
- In clinically proven cases of metastatic nodal disease, rather than the dissection of all levels, selective dissection can be applied only to the compartments that are involved.
- Surgical resection with compartmental node dissection may decrease the risk of recurrence and possibly mortality for patients with clinically evident nodal disease on the preoperative US and nodal FNA cytology or Tg washout measurement or at the time of surgery [17–19].
- In medullary thyroid cancer, bilateral central dissection and dissection of all neck levels on the side of involvement are the standard treatment option.

References

1. Haugen BR, Alexander EK, Bible KC, Doherty GM, Mandel SJ, Nikiforov YE, et al. American Thyroid Association management guidelines for adult patients with thyroid nodules and differentiated thyroid cancer the American Thyroid Association guidelines task force on thyroid nodules and differentiated thyroid cancer. Thyroid. 2016;26:1–133. https://doi.org/10.1089/thy.2015.0020.
2. Crippa S, Mazzucchelli L, Cibas ES, Ali SZ. The Bethesda System for reporting thyroid fine-needle aspiration specimens. Am J Clin Pathol. 2010;134(2):343–4.
3. Edge SB, Compton CC. The American Joint Committee on Cancer: the 7th edition of the AJCC cancer staging manual and the future of TNM. Ann Surg Oncol. 2010;17:1471–4.
4. Podnos YD, Smith D, Wagman LD, Ellenhorn JD. The implication of lymph node metastasis on survival in patients with well-differentiated thyroid cancer. Am Surg. 2005;71:731–4.
5. Lang BH, Wong KP, Wan KY, Lo CY. Impact of routine unilateral central neck dissection on preablative and postablative stimulated thyroglobulin levels after total thyroidectomy in papillary thyroid carcinoma. Ann Surg Oncol. 2012;19:60–7. 347.
6. Wang TS, Evans DB, Fareau GG, Carroll T, Yen TW. Effect of prophylactic central compartment neck dissection on serum thyroglobulin and recommendations for adjuvant radioactive iodine in patients with differentiated thyroid cancer. Ann Surg Oncol. 2012;19:4217–22.
7. Carty SE, Cooper DS, Doherty GM, Duh QY, Kloos RT, Mandel SJ, et al. Consensus statement on the terminology and classification of central neck dissection for thyroid cancer. Thyroid. 2009;19:1153–8.
8. Medina JE, Hefetz AK. Lateral neck dissection: indications. In: Randolph GW, editor. Surgery of the thyroids and parathyroid glands. Philadelphia: Elsevier; 2013. p. 382–8.
9. Roh JL, Kim JM, Park CI. Lateral cervical lymph node metastases from papillary thyroid carcinoma: pattern of nodal metastases and optimal strategy for neck dissection. Ann Surg Oncol. 2008;15:1177–82. https://doi.org/10.1245/s10434-008-9813-5. Epub 2008 Feb 6.
10. Machens A, Hauptmann S, Dralle H. Lymph node dissection in the lateral neck for completion in central node-positive papillary thyroid cancer. Surgery. 2009;145:176–81. https://doi.org/10.1016/j.surg.2008.09.003. Epub 2008 Nov 29.
11. Ito Y, Miyauchi A. Lateral lymph node dissection guided by preoperative and intraoperative findings in differentiated thyroid carcinoma. World J Surg. 2008;32:729–39.
12. Dralle H, Musholt TJ, Schabram J, Steinmüller T, Frilling A, Simon D, et al. German Association of Endocrine Surgeons practice guideline for the surgical management of malignant thyroid tumors.

Langenbeck's Arch Surg. 2013;398:347–75. https://doi.org/10.1007/s00423-013-1057-6. Epub 2013 Mar 3.

13. Stack BC Jr, Ferris RL, Goldenberg D, Haymart M, Shaha A, Sheth S, et al. American Thyroid Association consensus review and statement regarding the anatomy, terminology, and rationale for lateral neck dissection in differentiated thyroid cancer. Thyroid. 2012;22:501–8. https://doi.org/10.1089/thy.2011.0312. Epub 2012 Mar.
14. Tuttle RM, Tala H, Shah J, Leboeuf R, Ghossein R, Gonen M, et al. Estimating risk of recurrence in differentiated thyroid cancer after total thyroidectomy and radioactive iodine remnant ablation: using response to therapy variables to modify the initial risk estimates predicted by the new American Thyroid Association staging system. Thyroid. 2010;20:1341–9.
15. Vaisman F, Momesso D, Bulzico DA, Pessoa CH, Dias F, Corbo R, et al. Spontaneous remission in thyroid cancer patients after biochemical incomplete response to initial therapy. Clin Endocrinol. 2012;77:132–8.
16. Castagna MG, Maino F, Cipri C, Belardini V, Theodoropoulou A, Cevenini G, et al. Delayed risk stratification, to include the response to initial treatment (surgery and radioiodine ablation), has better outcome predictivity in differentiated thyroid cancer patients. Eur J Endocrinol. 2011;165:441–6.
17. Kupferman ME, Weinstock YE, Santillan AA, Mishra A, Roberts D, Clayman GL, et al. Predictors of level V metastasis in well-differentiated thyroid cancer. Head Neck. 2008;30:1469–74. https://doi.org/10.1002/hed.20904.
18. Lee J, Sung TY, Nam KH, Chung WY, Soh EY, Park CS. Is level IIb lymph node dissection always necessary in N1b papillary thyroid carcinoma patients? World J Surg. 2008;32:716–21.
19. Lee BJ, Wang SG, Lee JC, Son SM, Kim IJ, Kim YK. Level IIb lymph node metastasis in neck dissection for papillary thyroid carcinoma. Arch Otolaryngol Head Neck Surg. 2007;133:1028–30.

36 Prophylactic Unilateral Neck Dissection for Differentiated Thyroid Cancer

Serap Erel

Abstract

The extent of dissection for differentiated thyroid cancer in the neck is a balance between the greater morbidity of more extensive neck dissection and the possibility of leaving residual untreated metastatic lymph nodes. Therapeutic unilateral nodal dissection is performed for cN1b disease. In order to prevent morbidities and to prevent overtreatment, it is suggested that risk factors of ipsilateral and contralateral central lymph node metastases should be considered while planning the extent of central lymph node dissection in patients with cN0 and unilateral papillary thyroid cancer upon preoperative neck ultrasound.

36.1 Case Presentation

A 33-year-old male patient presented with anterior neck swelling which gradually increased in size during the last year. It was not painful, and there were no skin changes overlying the skin and no other swelling. He did not complain of obstructing symptoms like shortness of breath or difficulty in swallowing. He denied any hypo- or hyperthyroid symptoms. He has no history of radiation exposure and family history of thyroid cancer. He initially presented to another hospital early this year where thyroid ultrasound (USG) revealed a nodule in his right lobe of the thyroid with suspicious features for malignancy. Then, he was referred for USG-guided fine needle aspiration cytology (FNAC) to another hospital.

Physical examination revealed a solitary 2-cm swelling to the right of the midline just above the manubrium. The swelling was firm and smooth. There were no associated palpable lymph nodes. General examination revealed no further abnormalities. His serum levels of thyroid-stimulating hormone (TSH) and free thyroxine were normal.

Neck USG showed that the dimensions of the right lobe of the thyroid gland were 16 × 18 × 63 mm and left lobe were 12 × 17 × 46 mm. The right lobe contained hypoechoic nodule with a size of 19 × 13 × 7 mm, located in the lower pole which has central microcalcifications together with central and peripheric vascularization. The lesion had minimal capsular invasion at its inferior border. No pathological lymph node was noted in the neck. USG-guided FNAC of the nodule was found as suspicious for papillary carcinoma (Bethesda category V). He was subsequently offered total thyroidectomy with prophylactic central lymph node dissection (CLND) because of the presence of capsular invasion. The patient was a teacher; he was very anxious about his voice change

S. Erel
General Surgery, Ankara Education and Research Hospital, University of Health Sciences, Ankara, Turkey

T. Özülker et al. (eds.), *Thyroid and Parathyroid Diseases*, https://doi.org/10.1007/978-3-319-78476-2_36

possibility after the surgery. Intraoperative recurrent nerve monitoring was used.

We performed a standard Kocher incision; the skin flaps were prepared, and the sternocleidomastoid muscle was lateralized. At exploration, there was a nodule with cystic components at the right lobe. We identified the Delphian and prelaryngeal lymph nodes anterior to the cricothyroid membrane. We sent the Delphian node for frozen section; the result was benign. We decided to perform unilateral CLND only. We started from the tumor-bearing right lobe, by preserving superior parathyroid gland, cranial dissection was completed. We routinely first elevated the thyroid gland because superior retraction of the thyroid gland allows removal of peri-recurrent nerve nodes and peritracheal lymph nodes from the medial part of the common carotid artery to its origin at the branching point of the innominate trunk (Fig. 36.1). In this region, dissection may be performed from lateral to medial by preserving the recurrent laryngeal nerve.

The total thyroidectomy was completed en bloc with paratracheal and pretracheal lymph nodes and removing the isthmus from the pretracheal fascia. Because perioperative appearance and size of the lymph nodes were not pathologic, we did not send any of the lymph nodes for frozen section from this region. The intraoperative recurrent nerve monitoring system, unfortunately, was unhelpful because of technical problems. Therefore, we especially paid maximum attention to preserve the nerves on both sides. He had no any voice changes and no any hypocalcemia symptoms postoperatively. He was discharged from the hospital with suppressive doses of levothyroxine on the second postoperative day.

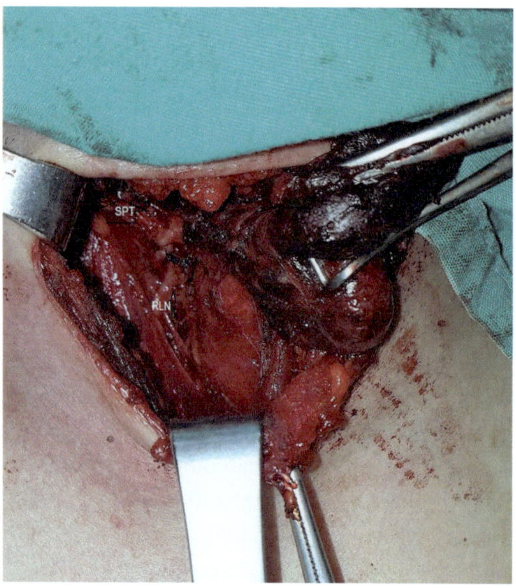

Fig. 36.1 Superior retraction of the thyroid gland allows removal of peri-recurrent nerve nodes and peritracheal lymph nodes. *RLN* recurrent laryngeal nerve, *SPT* superior parathyroid gland

The histopathologic evaluation confirmed the diagnosis of papillary cancer at the right-sided nodule with a largest diameter of 17 mm with minimal capsule invasion. Three out of ten lymph nodes of the central compartment were positive for metastasis. According to pathology report TNM classification of the tumor was pT1b, N1a, M0 and was classified as in low-intermediate risk group which consists of patients with T1-3, N1a, M0, Mx [1, 2, 3].

He proceeded to receive radioactive iodine ablation therapy. The post-therapy whole-body 131-I scan showed no radioiodine uptake in the thyroid bed. The suppressive doses of levothyroxine were administered to maintain a TSH of <0.01 μU/mL. Postoperative thyroglobulin (Tg) was 0.18 ng/mL, and Tg antibody was <15 U/mL at 5 months.

36.2 Discussion

This case illustrates many of the issues and difficulties encountered in the management of patients with papillary thyroid cancers (PTC) who were clinically negative (cN0). Although the patient was cN0 and there were no any suspicious lymph nodes at surgical exploration, three lymph nodes were found to be metastatic in the central region. Because of minimal capsular invasion, we have planned prophylactic CLND. In order to reduce postoperative morbidities, we have performed prophylactic CLND only in the ipsilateral and pretracheal regions, sparing the contralateral central neck. We have used frozen section analysis for the decision of not performing contralateral CLND.

Although therapeutic compartment-oriented CLND is the standard treatment for patients with clinical nodal involvement (cN1), the role, the indications, and the extension for therapeutic or prophylactic CLND in patients with clinically node-negative (cN0) neoplasms remain controversial [1–3]. The most important morbidities associated with CLND consist of recurrent laryngeal nerve damage and hypocalcemia related to parathyroid hypofunction or accidental parathyroidectomy [4–6]. In order to prevent morbidities and to prevent overtreatment, it is suggested that risk factors of ipsilateral and contralateral central lymph node metastases (CLNM) should be considered while planning the extent of CLND in patients with cN0 and unilateral PTC upon preoperative ultrasonography [7]. According to ATA 2015, thyroidectomy without prophylactic CLND is appropriate for small (T1 or T2), noninvasive, cN0 PTC and for most follicular cancers [8].

There are many studies identifying clinical and pathologic factors that may predict CLNM in cN0; unfortunately, the results were inconsistent [9]. The high incidence of CLNM and low sensitivity of USG and computerized tomography (CT) make it challenging to determine which factors are associated with subclinical CLNM. The low sensitivity of USG and CT may be due to the small size of the CLNM and presence of the intact thyroid gland which may increase the difficulty of examining posterior lymph nodes around the recurrent laryngeal nerve by USG [10]. USG-guided FNAC, performed to obtain both cytology and Tg determination, is commonly considered as the best available technique for the early diagnosis of differentiated thyroid CLNM. This technique is hampered by a 6–8% false-negative rate [11]. A short-axis diameter greater than 8 mm in level II and 5 mm for levels III, IV, and VI raises the suspicion of malignancy [12]. It is not able to detect every metastatic lymph node in the central compartment. Because of the small size and overlying thyroid gland itself, FNAC from the central neck has limited value. It can be performed in large lymph nodes which may have been already reported as suspicious at USG.

The efficacy of routine sentinel lymph node biopsy (SLNB) is controversial, and it is not widely used in the management of occult metastases in PTC. Although some authors have reported high sensitivities for SLNB, it is of limited use in the management of clinically node-negative papillary thyroid carcinoma because of low sensitivity and a high false-negative rate [13, 14]. Careful examination of central lymph nodes by palpation and inspection for morphological changes during the operation may be helpful to identify suspicious lymph nodes for frozen section [14]. In some cases, CLNM which are not suspicious in preoperative imaging can be detected during thyroidectomy by palpation or inspection, and this may guide surgeon for therapeutic CLND [15]. Enlarged lymph nodes exceeding 5 mm, and those with dark discoloration or hardness on palpation, were defined as suspicious metastatic lymph nodes. Ji et al. found out that the ability of the surgeon using intraoperative palpation and inspection to detect small metastatic lymph nodes not detected by preoperative imaging and to guide therapeutic CLND has limited value due to low sensitivity and specificity [14]. They reported that only the hardness of lymph nodes has a relatively high positive predictive value for lymph node metastasis. If there is any suspicious lymph node in the pretreacheal region, it should be sent for frozen section analysis because if the Delphian node is positive, ipsilateral and bilateral CLNM risk is found to be higher [16].

The technique of CLND differs on both sides. On the right, lymph nodes are distributed both anterior and posterior to the recurrent laryngeal nerve, whereas on the left, lymph nodes lie anteriorly. Thus, dissection of the right side of compartment VI is technically more demanding than the dissection of the left side. The dissection of the paratracheal nodes is best performed by initially identifying the recurrent laryngeal nerve at the base of the neck and then proceeding cranially. The lower parathyroid glands should be identified and preserved before starting the lymph node dissection. Thymus preservation should be the rule in prophylactic CLND. When there is massive nodal involvement requiring a bilateral therapeutic CLND, thymectomy and parathyroidectomy might be the part of the operation [17].

In many meta-analyses, an elevated risk of CLNM was found significantly associated with male sex, age >45 years, and tumor size >2 cm for PTC and >0.5 cm for papillary microcarcinoma, multifocality, location of primary tumor in the central area and low lobe, lymphovascular invasion, capsular invasion, and extrathyroidal extension, but not with thyroid bilaterality and chronic lymphocytic thyroiditis [1–3]. Several oncogenes (p53, BRAF) are also associated with nodal involvement [1].

A validated nomogram utilizing readily available preoperative variables has been developed to give a predicted probability of CLNM in patients presenting with PTC. This nomogram may help guide surgical decision-making in PTC [18, 19]. All nomograms should be used as a supplement to clinical knowledge and not as a substitute for clinical judgment or common sense.

36.2.1 Future

Favorable outcomes of prophylactic CLND were not clearly defined yet; therefore, in the treatment of PTC patients with cN0, it is not indicated, and more prospective, well-designed randomized controlled studies are required in order to demonstrate its clinical significance and prognostic impact. In order to identify high-risk patients who will benefit from CLND, more precise criteria should be investigated for preoperative assessment and decision for a tailored surgery. Validated nomograms may be more helpful for decision of prophylactic or therapeutic CLND.

What Can We Learn from This Case?

- Optimized and tailored surgery is becoming the mainstay of treatment. It is still difficult to define any precise factors for the decision of prophylactic CLND in cN0 PTC patients. A prospective randomized controlled study does not seem to be feasible because of the low rate of recurrence and morbidity.
- Prophylactic CLND ipsilateral to the tumor associated with total thyroidectomy may represent an effective strategy for reducing the rate of permanent hypoparathyroidism.
- Concomitant completion contralateral paratracheal lymph node neck dissection should be performed if the lymph node metastasis was reported at frozen section pathology analysis. This approach enables the surgeon to perform bilateral CLND to patients with intraoperative pathological findings of lymph node metastases.
- Although Delphian lymph node frozen section analysis was benign, there might be positive lymph nodes at final pathology report of central dissection.

References

1. Gambardella C, Tartaglia E, Nunziata A, Izzo G, Siciliano G, Cavallo F, et al. Clinical significance of prophylactic central compartment neckdissection in the treatment of clinically node-negative papillary thyroid cancer patients. World J Surg Oncol. 2016;14:247. https://doi.org/10.1186/s12957-016-1003-5.
2. Sun W, Lan X, Zhang H, Dong W, Wang Z, He L, et al. Risk factors for central lymph node metastasis in CN0 papillary thyroid carcinoma: a systematic review and meta-analysis. PLoS One. 2015;10(10):e0139021. https://doi.org/10.1371/journal.pone.0139021.

3. Ma B, Wang Y, Yang S, Ji Q. Predictive factors for central lymph node metastasis in patients with cN0 papillary thyroid carcinoma: a systematic review and meta-analysis. Int J Surg. 2016;28:153–61. https://doi.org/10.1016/j.ijsu.2016.02.093.
4. Giugliano G, Proh M, Gibelli B, Grosso E, Tagliabue M, De Fiori E, et al. Central neck dissection in differentiated thyroid cancer: technical notes. Acta Otorhinolaryngol Ital. 2014;34:9–14.
5. De Crea C, Raffaelli M, Sessa L, Lombardi CP, Bellantone R. Surgical approach to level VI in papillary thyroid carcinoma: an overview. Updates Surg. 2017;69:205–9. https://doi.org/10.1007/s13304-017-0468-2.
6. Giordano D, Valcavi R, Thompson GB, Pedroni C, Renna L, Gradoni P, et al. Complications of central neck dissection in patients with papillary thyroid carcinoma: results of a study on 1087 patients and review of the literature. Thyroid. 2012;22:911–7. https://doi.org/10.1089/thy.2012.0011.
7. Lee KE, Chung IY, Kang E, Koo do H, Kim KH, Kim SW, et al. Ipsilateral and contralateral central lymph node metastasis in papillary thyroid cancer: patterns and predictive factors of nodal metastasis. Head Neck. 2013;35:672–6. https://doi.org/10.1002/hed.23016.
8. Haugen BR, Alexander EK, Bible KC, Doherty GM, Mandel SJ, Nikiforov YE, et al. 2015 American Thyroid Association management guidelines for adult patients with thyroid nodules and differentiated thyroid cancer: the American Thyroid Association guidelines task force on thyroid nodules and differentiated thyroid cancer. Thyroid. 2016;26:1–133. https://doi.org/10.1089/thy.2015.0020.
9. Chen Q, Zou XH, Wei T, Huang QS, Sun YH, Zhu JQ. Prediction of ipsilateral andcontralateral central lymph node metastasis in unilateral papillary thyroid carcinoma: a retrospective study. Gland Surg. 2015;4:288–94. https://doi.org/10.3978/j.issn.2227-684X.2015.05.06.
10. Lee DW, Ji YB, Sung ES, Park JS, Lee YJ, Park DW, et al. Roles of ultrasonography and computed tomography in the surgical management of cervical lymph node metastases in papillary thyroid carcinoma. Eur J Surg Oncol. 2013;39:191–6. https://doi.org/10.1016/j.ejso.2012.07.119.
11. Pacini F, Fugazzola L, Lippi F, Ceccarelli C, Centoni R, Miccoli P, et al. Detection of thyroglobulin in fine needle aspirates of nonthyroidal neck masses: a clue to the diagnosis of metastatic differentiated thyroid cancer. J Clin Endocrinol Metab. 1992;74:1401–4.
12. Leenhardt L, Erdogan MF, Hegedus L, Mandel SJ, Paschke R, Rago T, et al. 2013 European thyroid association guidelines for cervical ultrasound scan and ultrasound-guided techniques in the postoperative management of patients with thyroid cancer. Eur Thyroid J. 2013;2:147–59. https://doi.org/10.1159/000354537.
13. Balasubramanian SP, Harrison BJ. Systematic review and meta-analysis of sentinel node biopsy in thyroid cancer. Br J Surg. 2011;98:334–44. https://doi.org/10.1002/bjs.7425.
14. Ji YB, Lee DW, Song CM, Kim KR, Park CW, Tae K. Accuracy of intraoperative determination of central node metastasis by the surgeon in papillary thyroid carcinoma. Otolaryngol Head Neck Surg. 2014;150:542–7. https://doi.org/10.1177/0194599813519405.
15. Shen WT, Ogawa L, Ruan D, Suh I, Duh QY, Clark O. Central neck lymph node dissection for papillary thyroid cancer: the reliability of surgeon judgment in predicting which patients will benefit. Surgery. 2010;148:398–403. https://doi.org/10.1016/j.surg.2010.03.021.
16. Zheng GB, Hao SL, Liu XC, Ning JY, Wu GC, Wang D, et al. The clinical significance of Delphian lymph node metastasis in papillary thyroid cancer. Zhonghua Er Bi Yan Hou Tou Jing Wai Ke Za Zhi. 2016;51:842–5. https://doi.org/10.3760/cma.j.issn.1673-0860.2016.11.008.
17. Sitges-Serra A, Lorente L, Mateu G, Sancho JJ. Therapy of Endocrine Disease: central neck dissection: a step forward in the treatment of papillary thyroid cancer. Eur J Endocrinol. 2015;173:199–206. https://doi.org/10.1530/EJE-15-0481.
18. Thompson AM, Turner RM, Hayen A, Aniss A, Jalaty S, Learoyd DL, et al. A preoperative nomogram for the prediction of ipsilateral central compartment lymph node metastases in papillary thyroid cancer. Thyroid. 2014;24:675–82. https://doi.org/10.1089/thy.2013.0224.
19. Hei H, Song Y, Qin J. A nomogram predicting contralateral central neck lymph node metastasis for papillary thyroid carcinoma. J Surg Oncol. 2016;114:703–7. https://doi.org/10.1002/jso.24403.

37 Surgical Treatment of Locally Advanced Papillary Thyroid Cancer

Fatih Tunca

Abstract

Although the majority of the differentiated thyroid carcinomas belong to low-risk group, 10–15% of these tumors present with locally advanced disease. Aerodigestive tract invasion is one of the challenging problems in these patients. Here we have reported a patient who presented with stage IV tracheal invasion of thyroid cancer and underwent bilateral total thyroidectomy, central neck dissection, bilateral modified radical neck dissection, and tracheal resection and primary anastomosis. The histopathologic examination revealed multicentric papillary thyroid carcinoma of diffuse sclerosing variant. The tumor was 6.5 cm with diffuse lymphovascular invasion and extrathyroidal extension. Ten of the dissected 25 lymph nodes were metastatic. Diffuse angiolymphatic and cartilage invasion was found on partial tracheal resection specimen with negative surgical margins. The patient received postoperative adjuvant radioiodine treatment. On the postoperative 6th month, nodal recurrence was detected at lateral neck region level II, and segmental level II lymphadenectomy was performed.

F. Tunca
Division of Endocrine Surgery, Istanbul University, Istanbul Medical Faculty, Istanbul, Turkey

37.1 Case Presentation

A 38-year-old male patient presented with cervical mass and hemoptysis in February 2016. He had no family history of thyroid cancer or history of head and neck irradiation. Physical examination revealed a firm and fixed mass located on the isthmus and bilateral cervicolateral lymphadenomegaly. The size of the isthmic mass was estimated as 6 cm by physical examination. His thyroid function tests were all within normal ranges. Neck ultrasonography (USG) revealed an isthmic nodule expanding through the left thyroid lobe with USG features highly suspicious for malignancy and bilateral multiple cervicolateral lymph nodes which had characteristics of metastatic nodes. The fine needle aspiration biopsy (FNAB) of both the nodule and the suspicious lymph nodes was reported as papillary thyroid carcinoma (PTC). According to the history of hemoptysis, we preferred to perform a cervical magnetic resonance imaging (MRI). The MRI revealed an isthmic thyroid mass invading both the anterior and the left tracheal wall and protruding into the tracheal lumen (Fig. 37.1) and also bilateral cervical pathologic lymph nodes at levels II, III, IV, and V (Fig. 37.2). Vocal cords were normal in the preoperative laryngoscopic examination, and the intraluminal extension of the tumor was evaluated by tracheoscopic examination. We performed bilateral total thyroidectomy, central lymph node dissection, bilateral modified

T. Özülker et al. (eds.), *Thyroid and Parathyroid Diseases*, https://doi.org/10.1007/978-3-319-78476-2_37

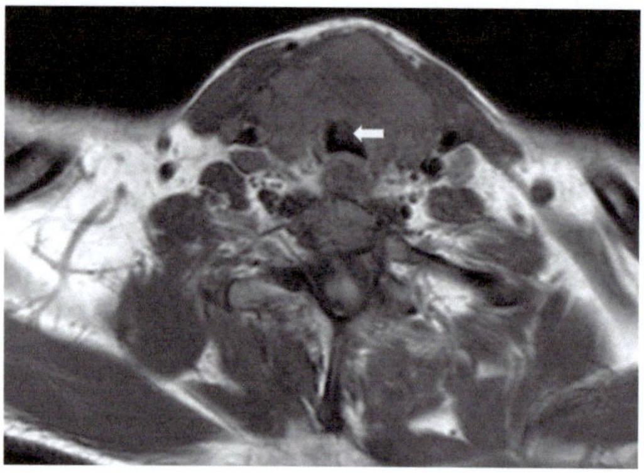

Fig. 37.1 MRI showing the gross transmucosal involvement by thyroid carcinoma

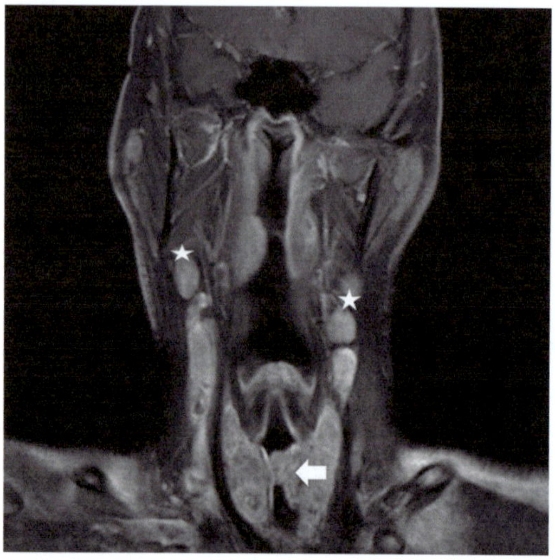

Fig. 37.2 Both transmucosal involvement (arrow) and bilateral metastatic cervical lymph nodes (stars) showed on MRI

radical neck dissection, and tracheal resection with primary anastomosis (Fig. 37.3) followed by an end-to-end anastomosis. Bilateral recurrent laryngeal nerves were identified and monitored by using continuous intraoperative nerve monitoring (CIONM). Postoperative laryngeal examination showed the function of both vocal cords was normal.

Pathological findings: Histopathologic examination revealed multicentric PTC of diffuse sclerosing variant. The maximum diameter of the tumor was 6.5 cm with diffuse lymphovascular invasion and extrathyroidal extension. Ten of the

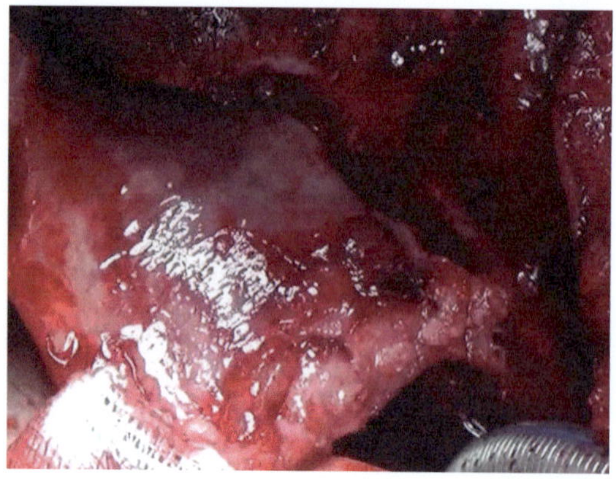

Fig. 37.3 Intraoperative image of tracheal involvement on the resection material

dissected 25 lymph nodes were metastatic. Diffuse angiolymphatic and cartilage invasion was found on partial tracheal resection specimen with negative surgical margins.

The patient was classified as stage I according to the TNM staging system (age < 45, T4a, N1b, M0); nevertheless according to the ATA Risk Stratification System with Proposed Modifications, the patient was classified as ATA high risk because of the gross extrathyroidal extension (ETE) (pT4).

37.2 Discussion

37.2.1 Evaluation and Diagnosis

Most of the patients with PTC have an excellent prognosis. However, 10–15% of these tumors can show aggressive behavior, such as local invasion, resistance to treatment, distant metastasis, and increased mortality [1]. ETE has the greatest negative impact on prognosis, with 10-year overall survival rates dropping to 45% in patients who have ETE compared with 91% for those who do not have ETE [2]. In a review of 262 patients with invasive thyroid cancer, the most commonly involved structures included the strap muscles (53%), recurrent laryngeal nerve (47%), trachea (37%), esophagus (21%), lateral neck structures including the great vessels and vagus nerve (30%), and larynx (12%) [3]. Tracheal invasion is the major ETE in our patient.

Aerodigestive tract invasion may present with prominent symptoms that direct the clinicians to the site of invasion, such as hoarseness, stridor, hemoptysis, and dysphagia [4]. In patients with a fixed neck mass and stiffness, cough, and hoarseness, preoperative laryngoscopic examination is critical. However, most of the patients with a vocal cord paralysis may present without voice changes due to compensatory function of the contralateral cord [5]. In the recent years as a part of nerve monitoring, preoperative laryngoscopic examination has become a routine preoperative examination which should be done in all patients. Hemoptysis, stridor, or dyspnea could be the symptoms of an airway invasion, and dysphagia could be the result of esophageal compression or invasion. In such cases, radiologic imaging including computerized tomography (CT) or MRI may help to evaluate the extent of the disease in the neck, laryngeal or tracheal involvement, and/or intraluminal extension. Due to the history of hemoptysis in our patient, we performed MRI to stage the tracheal invasion to plan the surgical management.

Imaging modalities also provide information about the mediastinal extension of the disease. Occasionally, the patient may require a tracheobronchoscopy or esophagoscopy to evaluate the presence of gross mucosal involvement. As a standard radiological imaging, USG should be combined with FNAB to confirm the diagnosis of a malignant thyroid mass preoperatively.

37.2.2 Management

In patients with locally advanced PTC, the most commonly involved structures include the strap muscles, recurrent laryngeal nerve, trachea, esophagus, lateral neck structures including the great vessels and vagus nerve, and larynx [3].

37.2.2.1 Strap Muscle Invasion

The strap muscle invasion is the common form of ETE according to the close relationship of the structures. Only strap muscle invasion does not worsen the prognosis, and the goal of the surgical treatment is to resect the invaded portion of the strap muscle with negative surgical margins [6, 7].

37.2.2.2 Recurrent Laryngeal Nerve Invasion

The recurrent laryngeal nerve (RLN) invasion occurs in 25–47% of the invasive cases [5, 8]. If the RLN is paralyzed on preoperative laryngoscopic examination and found to be invaded intraoperatively, en bloc resection of the RLN with the thyroid cancer is the treatment of choice. However, we have to keep in mind that RLN paralysis could be related to pressure on the nerve without invasion in some cases, and dissection and preservation of the nerve have some potential for nerve recovery [8, 9]. In case of both, vocal cord functions were normal preoperatively; the decision to sacrifice the nerve is challenging. In such cases, the nerve should be sacrificed, if preservation requires leaving gross tumor behind. However, before sacrificing the RLN, surgeon has to be sure that the opposite RLN is not invaded by the tumor and that it can be preserved. Several studies have demonstrated that intraoperative nerve monitoring reduces the risk of permanent nerve injury and bilateral vocal cord paralysis rate in patients with thyroid cancer and for reoperative settings [10, 11]. Intraoperative nerve monitoring will give prognostic information about the opposite nerve function during the surgery. With a functioning RLN adherent to thyroid cancer but can be pealed clearly or if the nerve could be preserved just leaving microscopic disease, then the nerve should be spared [7, 12]. In these cases, there are no differences in survival between patients in whom the nerve is resected when compared with patients in whom the nerves are preserved as long as patients receive postoperative RAI [9].

37.2.2.3 Laryngotracheal Invasion

The trachea is the third common invasion site following the strap muscle and RLN occurring up to 37% of the locally advanced thyroid carcinomas. Of these patients, laryngeal involvement only occurs in 12% [3].

The surgical options for laryngeal involvement are peeling or shave procedures, partial laryngectomy, and total laryngectomy. Shaving the tumor from the cartilage could be performed in thyroid cancers invading the laryngeal cartilage without intraluminal involvement. Several retrospective studies including patients with laryngeal involvement have shown no difference in survival between radical resection, and shave procedures in case of all gross disease are completely resected [3, 4, 6]. The main purpose of the treatment is to preserve laryngeal function. In some cases, the laryngeal framework may need to be resected. Up to 50% of the external laryngeal framework could be resected with internal laryngeal preservation [13]. In patients with only one side has been invaded, partial laryngectomy is an appropriate surgical option [14]. Total laryngectomy is a rare indication in patients with thyroid cancer involvement; however, total laryngectomy could be performed in patients with the recurrent disease with an invasion through the laryngeal lumen or cricothyroid area. Early cricoid cartilage invasion can be treated by shave excision [15].

The tracheal invasion has been more extensively studied due to its more frequent manner relative to laryngeal involvement. However, a few staging systems have been introduced to describe the extent of invasion for planning the surgical treatment options. Shin et al. [16] generated a pathologic staging system in PTC based on the depth of tracheal invasion. McCaffrey [17] has also constituted a staging system for aerodigestive tract involvement by well-differentiated thyroid carcinoma based on the depth of invasion. In stage I, tumor is placed entirely within the thyroid capsule without any invasion. In stage II, tumor invades the perichondrium or firmly abuts the muscle but does not invade into the cartilage or deeply into the muscular layer. In stage III disease, tumor invades through the perichondrium into the cartilage or deeply into muscle, but submucosa is not involved. In stage IV disease, tumor invades through the perichondrium and cartilage or through the muscle, deforms the submucosa, but does not penetrate the mucosa, and gross transmucosal invasion of the tumor is classified as stage V disease. McCaffrey recommended total thyroidectomy for stage I disease; complete gross removal by total thyroidectomy and shave partial thickness excision for stage II and III diseases; and complete aerodigestive tract resection for stages IV and V [17].

In several retrospective studies, authors have reported similar survival and recurrence rates between radical resection and shave procedures when all gross disease resection is completely achieved in patients with laryngotracheal involvement [3, 4, 6, 18]. Segal et al. [19] reported that they showed similar survival rates comparing conservative procedures followed by radioiodine treatment and aggressive techniques. And they reported less perioperative mortality and lower overall morbidity in the conservative group. In the study of Nishida et al. [20], authors reported higher recurrence rates and shorter overall survival in patients with Shin's stage II or higher stages with subtotal resection without airway resection. Nevertheless, several others have reported higher recurrence rates [13] and worse survival [13, 21] in patients undergoing conservative resection for tracheal invasion. The disease-free and overall survival are worse in patients with tracheal recurrence following shave procedures when compared with patients undergoing tracheal resection at the initial surgical procedure [12].

In cases with destroyed tracheal cartilage or tumoral invasion into the trachea, more aggressive treatment other than shaving procedures should be considered. Shaving procedures are likely to leave macroscopic residual disease in such patients. In patients with limited involvement of an anterior or laterally located tumor, window resection could be a treatment of choice. After the resection closure options could be primary closure or closure with strep muscle and periosteum [6, 7, 13]. Sleeve resection and reanastomosis are needed in patients with more than one tracheal ring to be excised. Window resection is not a suitable technique for tumors with intraluminal involvement and if the tumor invades both anterior and lateral tracheal walls. In such cases circumferential tracheal resection and primary anastomosis are required. A total of 5–6 cm of the trachea can be resected and primarily reanastomosed without tracheal or laryngeal mobilization [6].

37.2.2.4 Esophageal Invasion

Esophageal invasion most commonly occurs in association with tracheal invasion, although it can also occur from extracapsular spread from paratracheal or paraoesophageal lymph nodes [12]. The mucosa of the esophagus is resistant to direct tumoral invasion. Tumor invasion usually confined to the muscular layer of the esophagus, without mucosal or submucosal extension [3]. Resection of the involved tissue with negative surgical margins avoiding esophageal entry is the treatment of choice in such cases. If a full-thickness defect occurred during the resection, a tension-free watertight primary closure could be performed, in patients with healthy and nonirradiated tissue. Segmental resection is needed in patients with full-thickness or circumferential esophageal involvement. In such cases, reconstructive options include myocutaneous pedicled flap, fascial or fasciocutaneous flap, or gastric, colonic, or jejunal tissue transfer [13].

37.2.2.5 Adjuvant Treatment

Patients with locally advanced thyroid cancer have an increased risk for postoperative local recurrences, regional nodal recurrence, and distant metastasis. Thyroid-stimulating hormone suppression (TSH) and radioiodine ablation treatment (RAT) are the mainstay postoperative adjuvant treatments in patients with differentiated thyroid carcinoma. However, patients with locally advanced thyroid carcinoma often have tumors of aggressive histology, and the role of RAI is not well defined in some aggressive subtypes. For patients with only anterior strap muscle invasion and complete tumor resection, no additional therapy may be required. In case of risk for residual microscopic disease or with significant local invasion into the larynx, trachea, recurrent laryngeal nerve or esophagus, external beam radiotherapy (EBRT) is another adjuvant treatment option. EBRT improve locoregional control in these patients with differentiated thyroid cancer [6, 7, 12]. Classic chemotherapy regimens including doxorubicin have partial response rates with poor long-term outcomes. In the recent years, targeted therapies such as RET kinase inhibitors, B-RAF mutation targeting drugs, retinoids, and histone deacetylase treatments have emerged as an attractive treatment strategy in RAI refractory DTC patients with locally advanced disease. However, The American Thyroid Association (ATA) 2015 guideline weakly recommends that kinase inhibitor therapy should be considered in RAI refractory DTC patients with metastatic, rapidly progressive, symptomatic, and/or imminently threatening disease not otherwise amenable to local control using other approaches.

37.3 Follow-Up and Outcome

The patient was classified as high risk because of gross ETE according to the ATA Risk Stratification System with Proposed Modifications. Serum-stimulated thyroglobulin (sTg) and TSH level was 24 ng/mL and 78 mIU/L, respectively, on the postoperative 3rd week. The patient was scheduled for 150 mCi RAI treatment. On the postoperative 6th month, serum Tg level was >1 ng/mL with suppressive TSH levels. The patient was reevaluated with neck USG, and USG revealed two suspicious level II lymph nodes. Then the patient underwent a second operation for segmental lymph node dissection. Two of nine dissected lymph nodes were metastatic. Then the patient scheduled for another 150 mCi RAI treatment with thyrogen (rhTSH). Negative images were obtained on the post-ablation whole-body scan. However, the suppressed Tg level is still >1 ng/mL. According to the dynamic risk stratification scheme, patient was classified as biochemical incomplete response to treatment which has 20% risk to develop structural disease.

37.4 Future

Locally advanced thyroid carcinomas are mostly associated with aggressive subtypes of differentiated thyroid cancers. In such cases, surgical treatment and adjuvant therapies with RAI ablation and EBRT could be insufficient. Future studies on targeted therapies are needed to investigate if these treatments might provide a better long-term outcome.

What Can We Learn from This Case?

- Laryngotracheal invasion should be considered in patients with nodular goiter presenting with hemoptysis.
- In such cases, preoperative CT or MRI and laryngo-bronchoscopic examination could be performed to evaluate tracheal invasion and plan the extent of tracheal resection.
- A total of 5–6 cm of the trachea can be resected and primarily reanastomosed without tracheal or laryngeal mobilization.
- According to the high recurrence risk in these locally advanced thyroid carcinomas, patients should be followed up closely. Patients have to be reevaluated if the stimulated Tg levels >10 ng/mL or Tg levels >1 ng/mL on thyroxin treatment.

References

1. Cody HS 3rd., Shah JP. Locally invasive, well-differentiated thyroid cancer: 22 years; experience at Memorial Sloan-Kettering Cancer Center. Am J Surg. 1981;42:480–3.
2. Andersen PE, Kinsella J, Loree TR, Shaha AR, Shah JP. Differentiated carcinoma of the thyroid with extra-thyroidal extension. Am J Surg. 1995;170:467–70.
3. McCaffrey TV, Bergstralh EJ, Hay ID. Locally invasive papillary thyroid carcinoma: 1940–1990. Head Neck. 1994;16:165–72. https://doi.org/10.1002/hed.288016021.
4. McCaffrey TV, Lipton RJ. Thyroid carcinoma invading the upper aerodigestive system. Laryngoscope. 1990;100:824–30. https://doi.org/10.1288/00005537-199008000-00006.
5. Randolph GW, Kamani D. The importance of preoperative laryngoscopy in patients undergoing thyroidectomy: voice, vocal cord function, and the preoperative detection of invasive thyroid malignancy. Surgery. 2006;139:357–62. https://doi.org/10.1016/j.surg.2005.08.009.
6. Czaja JM, McCaffrey TV. The surgical management of laryngotracheal invasion by well-differentiated papillary thyroid carcinoma. Arch Otolaryngol Head Neck Surg. 1997;123:484–90. https://doi.org/10.1001/archotol.1997.01900050030003.
7. Patel KN, Shaha AR. Locally advanced thyroid cancer. Curr Opin Otolaryngol Head Neck Surg. 2005;13:112–6. Review. https://doi.org/10.1097/01.moo.0000156161.82671.43.
8. Chiang FY, Wang LF, Huang YF, Lee KW, Kuo WR. Recurrent laryngeal nerve palsy after thyroidectomy with routine identification of the recurrent laryngeal nerve. Surgery. 2005;137:342–7. https://doi.org/10.1016/j.surg.2004.09.008.
9. Falk SA, McCaffrey TV. Management of the recurrent laryngeal nerve in suspected and proven thyroid cancer. Otolaryngol Head Neck Surg. 1995;113:42–8. https://doi.org/10.1016/S0194-59989570143-5.
10. Chan WF, Lang BH, Lo CY. The role of intraoperative neuromonitoring of recurrent laryngeal nerve during thyroidectomy: a comparative study on 1000 nerves at risk. Surgery. 2006;140:866–72. https://doi.org/10.1016/j.surg.2006.07.017.
11. Dralle H, Sekulla C, Haerting J, Timmermann W, Neumann HJ, Kruse E, et al. Risk factors of paralysis and functional outcome after recurrent laryngeal nerve monitoring in thyroid surgery. Surgery. 2004;136:1310–22. https://doi.org/10.1016/j.surg.2004.07.018.
12. Price DL, Wong RJ, Randolph GW. Invasive thyroid cancer: management of the trachea and esophagus. Otolaryngol Clin N Am. 2008;41:1155–68. https://doi.org/10.1016/j.otc.2008.08.002.
13. Friedman M, Danielzadeh JA, Caldarelli DD. Treatment of patients with carcinoma of the thyroid invading the airway. Arch Otolaryngol Head Neck Surg. 1994;120:1377–81. https://doi.org/10.1001/archotol.1994.01880360071013.
14. Ballantyne AJ. Resections of the upper aerodigestive tract for locally invasive thyroid cancer. Am J Surg. 1994;168:636–9. https://doi.org/10.1016/S0002-9610(05)80136-9.
15. Donnelly MJ, Timon CI, McShane DP. The role of total laryngectomy in the management of intraluminal upper airway invasion by well-differentiated thyroid carcinoma. Ear Nose Throat J. 1994;73:659–62.
16. Shin DH, Mark EJ, Suen HC, Grillo HC. Pathologic staging of papillary carcinoma of the thyroid with airway invasion based on the anatomic manner of extension to the trachea: a clinicopathologic study based on 22 patients who underwent thyroidectomy and airway resection. Hum Pathol. 1993;24:866–70.
17. McCaffrey JC. Aerodigestive tract invasion by well differentiated thyroid carcinoma: diagnosis, management, prognosis, and biology. Laryngoscope. 2006;116:1–11. https://doi.org/10.1097/01.MLG.0000200428.26975.86.
18. An SY, Kim KH. Surgical management of locally advanced thyroid cancer. Curr Opin Otolaryngol Head Neck Surg. 2010;18:119–23. https://doi.org/10.1097/MOO.0b013e3283374d84.
19. Segal K, Shpitzer T, Hazan A, Bachar G, Marshak G, Popovtzer A. Invasive well-differentiated thyroid carcinoma: effect of treatment modalities on outcome. Otolaryngol Head Neck Surg. 2006;134:819–22. https://doi.org/10.1016/j.otohns.2005.11.040.
20. Nishida T, Nakao K, Hamaji M. Differentiated thyroid carcinoma with airway invasion: indication for tracheal resection based on the extent of cancer invasion. J Thorac Cardiovasc Surg. 1997;114:84–92. https://doi.org/10.1016/S0022-5223(97)70120-X.
21. Kasperbauer JL. Locally advanced thyroid carcinoma. Ann Otol Rhinol Laryngol. 2004;113:749–53. https://doi.org/10.1177/000348940411300914.

Completion Thyroidectomy in a Patient with Differentiated Thyroid Cancer

38

Serdar Özbaş and Seyfettin Ilgan

Abstract

A considerable number of patients, undergoing less than total or near-total thyroidectomy as an initial surgical treatment, will need reoperation for incidentally found thyroid carcinoma on final histopathology to provide complete resection of possible multicentric disease or to allow for efficient radioiodine therapy. In the 2015 American Thyroid Association guidelines for the management of thyroid cancer, completion thyroidectomy was offered to patients for whom a bilateral thyroidectomy would have been recommended had the diagnosis been available before the initial surgery. Older age (>45 years), contralateral suspicious thyroid nodules, a personal history of radiation therapy to the head and neck, and the existence of familial differentiated thyroid cancer should be taken into account to recommend a bilateral procedure to facilitate either radioiodine therapy or follow-up. Since a significant proportion of thyroid surgery is still being performed by low-volume surgeons, the discovery of large remnant tissue even after so-called total thyroidectomy is not a rare issue. To enhance the safety and success of completion thyroidectomies, new technologies and guiding methods are being used more often including intraoperative nerve monitoring, preoperative and intraoperative USG mapping, and gamma surgical probe.

S. Özbaş (✉)
Department of Surgery, Güven Hospital, Ankara, Turkey

S. Ilgan
Department of Nuclear Medicine, Güven Hospital, Ankara, Turkey

38.1 Case Presentation

A 37-year-old woman presented to an endocrinology clinic of a state hospital with palpitation and weight loss for 2 months. Her thyroid function tests (TFT) revealed hyperthyroidism. Thyroid ultrasonography (USG) and scintigraphy confirmed the diagnosis of toxic multinodular goiter with the largest nodule being 2.5 cm in size in the left thyroid lobe. She has been given antithyroid medication and a fine needle aspiration biopsy (FNAB) performed from the left lobe several weeks later. The result of FNAB was reported as atypia of undetermined significance (Bethesda category III). Upon normalization of TFT, she has been referred to general surgery department of the same hospital and underwent so-called total thyroidectomy in November 2012. The final pathology revealed a 2.5 cm unifocal follicular variant of papillary cancer in the left lobe with no extrathyroidal extension and no evidence of venous or lymphatic invasion. No lymph nodes were removed at the time of surgery.

T. Özülker et al. (eds.), *Thyroid and Parathyroid Diseases*, https://doi.org/10.1007/978-3-319-78476-2_38

She has been scheduled for radioactive iodine (RAI) ablation, and L-thyroxin treatment stopped for 4 weeks for endogenous TSH stimulation. After 1 month, her physician realized that her TSH level did not increase. She had a serum TSH of 7.04 μIU/mL, and thyroglobulin (Tg) level was 13.8 ng/mL without Tg antibodies. Afterward, she had a thyroid scintigraphy that showed residual thyroid tissue on the left thyroid bed. Completion thyroidectomy was offered to her for an effective RAI ablation, and she was referred to our clinic for further evaluation and surgery.

A comprehensive USG of the neck during the first visit in our center revealed three different foci of residual thyroid tissue in left thyroid bed, 1.7 cc in total volume (Figs. 38.1, 38.2, and 38.3).

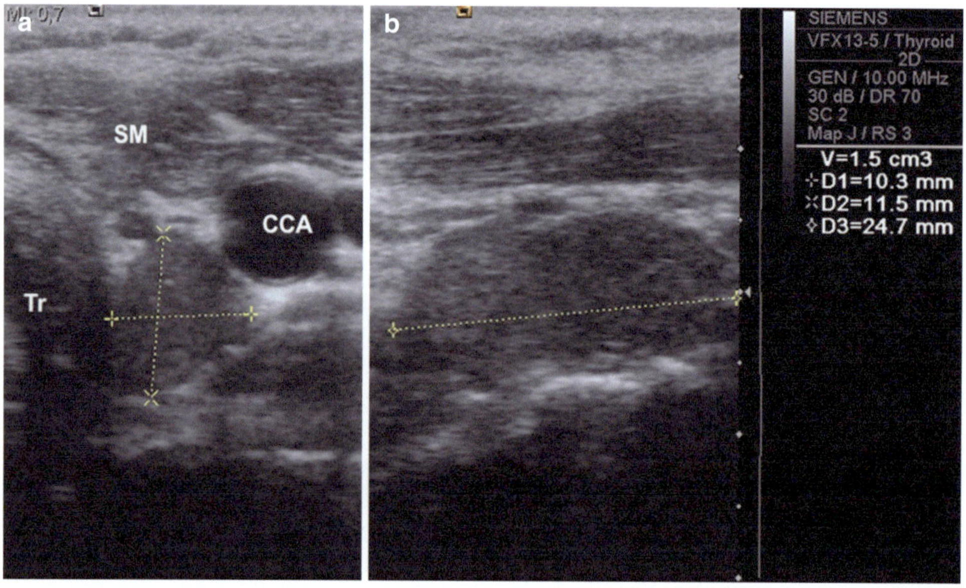

Fig. 38.1 Axial (**a**) and longitudinal (**b**) sonograms of residual thyroid tissues in left thyroid bed as three different foci (hair-cross). *SM* strap muscles, *Tr* trachea, *IJV* internal jugular vein, *CCA* common carotid artery

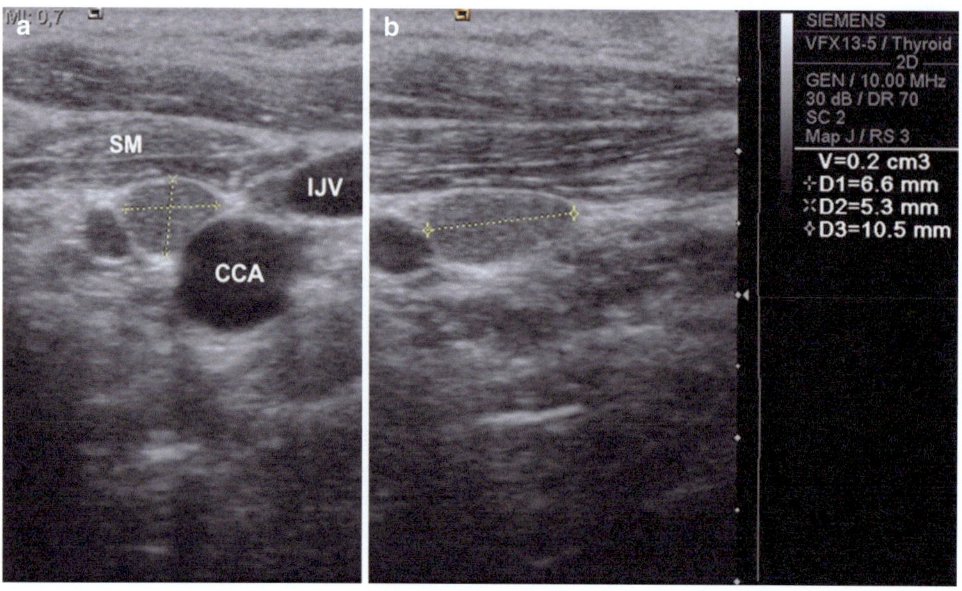

Fig. 38.2 Axial (**a**) and longitudinal (**b**) sonograms of residual thyroid tissues in left thyroid bed as three different foci (hair-cross). *SM* strap muscles, *Tr* trachea, *IJV* internal jugular vein, *CCA* common carotid artery

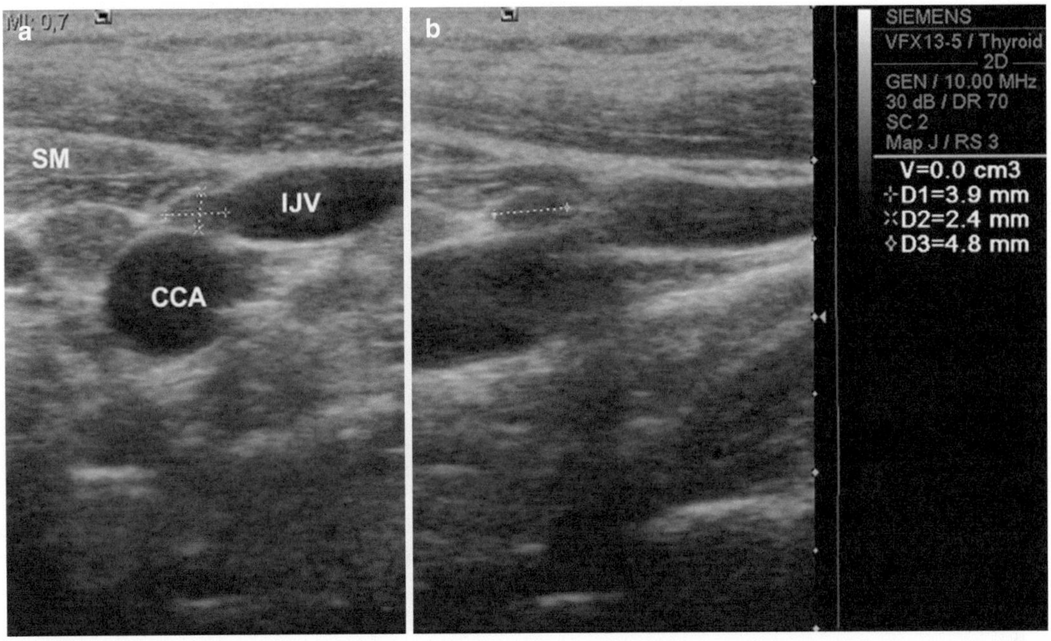

Fig. 38.3 Axial (**a**) and longitudinal (**b**) sonograms of residual thyroid tissues in left thyroid bed as three different foci (hair-cross). *SM* strap muscles, *Tr* trachea, *IJV* internal jugular vein, *CCA* common carotid artery

Residual thyroid tissues were in homogenous echotexture, and no nodules were appreciated within the remnant tissues. In February 2013, completion thyroidectomy with prophylactic central lymph node dissection is performed under intraoperative electrophysiological nerve monitoring and by using radioguided occult lesion localization (ROLL) technique. The final pathology revealed diffuse hyperplasia and six lymph nodes from central compartment without any metastatic involvement.

38.2 Discussion

Although our aim for this chapter is to discuss completion thyroidectomy in differentiated thyroid cancer (DTC), first of all, we want to comment on the diagnostic procedures in this patient. When evaluating the risk of cancer, it has been accepted that a solitary nodule had a higher likelihood of malignancy than did a non-solitary nodule. However, in agreement with the other studies, the risk of malignancy per patient was the same and independent of the number of nodules [1]. In a review and meta-analysis by Brito et al. [2], the risk of malignancy is found to be slightly higher in a solitary nodule compared with an individual nodule as part of a multinodular goiter. They also concluded that, this is mostly true in iodine-deficient populations [2].

Multiple thyroid nodules >1 cm may require FNAB, based on sonographic risk criteria of each nodule. A diagnostic USG in experienced hands is the most critical issue to decide which nodule needs to be biopsied especially in patients with multinodular goiter. The FNAB of the dominant or largest nodule might only be appropriate if all the nodules have similar USG features. Otherwise, applying only size criteria may lead to misdiagnosis in multinodular goiter [3]. Radionuclide scanning may also be considered in patients with hyperthyroidism to identify hyper- and hypofunctioning nodules to avoid sampling of hyperactive nodules since they rarely harbor malignancy. The patients with scintigraphic findings suggesting nodularity need to be correlated with USG to prove both presence of concordant nodule and nonfunctioning nodules which meet USG criteria for FNAB [4]. In our patient, we were not quite sure whether biopsied nodule, in fact, the same one with malignant histopathology.

Decisions regarding the extent of surgery for Bethesda category III nodules are influenced by several factors including size and number of the nodules, family history of thyroid cancer, history of personal radiation exposure, USG pattern, patient preference, the presence of contralateral nodularity, and coexistent hyperthyroidism [5–9]. These risk factors impact the decision of thyroid lobectomy with the possible need for subsequent completion thyroidectomy versus total thyroidectomy up front. In our case, although the initial operation was reported as total thyroidectomy, the subsequent neck USG and scintigraphy revealed that she had right total, left subtotal thyroidectomy leaving a remnant tissue of nearly 2 g on the tumor side. It is possible that the surgical team might plan to do a near-total thyroidectomy; however, the remnant thyroid tissue was too much to call near-total thyroidectomy for this case.

Thyroid lobectomy alone may be sufficient initial treatment for low-risk papillary and follicular carcinomas; however, the treatment team may choose total thyroidectomy to enable RAI therapy or to enhance follow-up based upon disease features and/or patient preferences [10]. The term completion thyroidectomy is usually used for second operations after an initial lobectomy on one side in the current literature. However, all revision surgeries after less than total and near-total thyroidectomy could also be referred as completion thyroidectomy. The subtotal procedures, either bilateral or unilateral, is not recommended for any thyroid pathology in the 2015 American Thyroid Association (ATA) guideline. For patients who have thyroid cancer >1 and <4 cm without extrathyroidal extension, and without clinical evidence of any lymph node metastases, the initial surgical procedure may be either a bilateral procedure (near-total or total thyroidectomy) or a unilateral lobectomy [10].

A considerable number of patients, undergoing less than total or near-total thyroidectomy as an initial surgical treatment, will need reoperation for incidentally found thyroid carcinoma on final histopathology to provide complete resection of possible multicentric disease or to allow for efficient RAI therapy. In the 2015 ATA guidelines for the management of thyroid cancer, completion thyroidectomy was offered to patients for whom a bilateral thyroidectomy would have been recommended had the diagnosis been available before the initial surgery [10]. Older age (>45 years), contralateral suspicious thyroid nodules, a personal history of radiation therapy to the head and neck, and the existence of familial differentiated thyroid cancer should be taken into account to recommend a bilateral procedure to facilitate either RAI therapy or follow-up [11, 12]. Patients with indeterminate nodules who have a bilateral nodular disease, those with significant medical comorbidities, or those who prefer to undergo bilateral thyroidectomy to avoid the possibility of requiring a future surgery on the contralateral lobe, may undergo total or near-total thyroidectomy, assuming completion thyroidectomy would be recommended if the indeterminate nodule proved malignant following the first operation.

Since a large proportion of thyroid surgery is still being performed by low-volume surgeons, the discovery of large remnant tissue even after so-called total thyroidectomy is not a rare issue. Patients who are in need of a completion thyroidectomy frequently prefer or referred to high-volume surgeons or specialized endocrine surgery units to optimize oncologic outcomes. However, it is still likely that amount of remnant thyroid tissue after completion thyroidectomy is greater than total thyroidectomy procedures due to nature of difficulty of revision surgeries even in experienced hands [13]. Therefore the completeness of these types of operations is often doubtful especially in patients with more than one foci of residual tissue in different sizes like in our case. The timing of completion thyroidectomy is another critical issue. It is recommended that reoperations should be either performed within a week of the first operation or at least 2–3 months later.

There is still controversy for routine central lymph node dissection (CLND) in DTC. Central lymph node metastasis has been shown to be associated with an increased risk of locoregional recurrence but not with overall survival [13]. Therapeutic CLND should be included if the lymph nodes are clinically involved. The advantage of prophylactic CLND argues against its application in reoperations. CLND also provides information about the use of adjuvant RAI [14]. It may improve the posttreatment Tg levels and decrease the need for repeated RAI treatments. In our previously published reports, the positivity of CLND was more than 40% in papillary thyroid cancer, and complications of this procedure are not more than the total thyroidectomies [15, 16].

As we mentioned before, the need for radioiodine remnant ablation is one of the major reasons to recommend completion thyroidectomy in some patients in whom the diagnosis of thyroid cancer is not known preoperatively. In this scenario, the decision to recommend completion thyroidectomy would depend on whether postoperative radioiodine therapy was deemed to be appropriate for the patient's risk of recurrence and death. However, RAI ablation after completion thyroidectomy is not recommended on a routine basis and could be reserved for selected cases.

The ablation of the remaining lobe with RAI has been used as an alternative to completion thyroidectomy [17, 18]. There are limited data regarding the long-term outcomes of this approach. The data suggest similar clinical outcomes with a slightly higher proportion of patients with persistent detectable Tg. This approach may be helpful in patients for whom completion thyroidectomy carries some increased risk and for whom a delay in the length of time required to achieve the destruction of the normal thyroid, which follows RAI (as opposed to surgical resection), is acceptable.

To enhance the safety and success of completion thyroidectomies, new technologies and guiding methods are being used more often including intraoperative nerve monitoring, preoperative and intraoperative USG mapping, and gamma surgical probe. Since normal thyroid tissue is avid for several radiopharmaceuticals (Tc-99m pertechnetate, I-123, or I-131), finding residual thyroid tissue with the radioguided surgery after systemic application of one of these agents seems very useful though it is not unanimously agreed [19]. Doubts result from differences in physical properties of applied radiopharmaceutical and methodology including the type of isotope used, timing of surgery, and the type of device used.

We would also like to comment on the ROLL technique. It is a new localization technique that was originally described for nonpalpable breast lesions. The technique depends on direct injection of a small quantity of Tc-99m-labeled particles (macroaggregated albumin, colloid, etc.) into the lesion under radiographic or USG guidance. Recently, the ROLL technique was used for nonpalpable nodal recurrences of thyroid cancer in the lateral and central cervical compartments as well as for a limited number of parathyroid adenomas [20, 21]. As the ROLL technique does not depend on the systemic application of the radiotracer and the concentrating ability of lesions, we found this technique to be extremely helpful in selected clinical problems in the cervical region. We, therefore, use the ROLL technique on a routine basis for patients with primary hyperparathyroidism as well as for recurrent papillary thyroid carcinoma in central and lateral cervical compartments. Radioguided surgery with ROLL seems more advantageous than systemic applications of radiopharmaceuticals since technique requires considerably less amount of radioactivity, does not depend on the concentrating ability of lesions, and does not include background activity.

The large remnant that triggers completion thyroidectomy is referred to as residual tissue >2 g in the literature [22]. The size of the thyroid remnant is an important determinant predicting hypothyroidism and total thyroid ablation with I-131. For the RAI ablation therapy to be effective, the preferred TSH level should be higher than 30 μIU/mL. It has been reported that patients with a higher preoperative TSH level, smaller body surface area adjusted volume, fewer ipsilateral nodules, and thyroiditis had a greater risk of hypothyroidism after hemithyroidectomy [23]. Functionally, any size of remnant could be defined as "large remnant" if TSH level does not increase to expected levels within a reasonable time (4–6 weeks) after stopping of levothyroxine replacement.

38.3 Follow-Up and Outcome

She returned to home after completion thyroidectomy with CLND, and her primary physicians planned RAI ablation with 100 mCi (3700 MBq). During the follow-up in October 2013, she had a body scan that showed no uptake in the neck or anywhere else in the body. Annual monitoring of serum Tg and neck ultrasound was recommended to her with the maintenance of serum TSH in the low normal range. She has now been followed up for 4 years without any evidence of recurrent disease. For the last 2 years, she was taking 112.5 μg of levothyroxine per day, and her serum TSH was below 1 mU/L, and Tg < 0.1 ng/mL without Tg antibodies.

What Can We Learn from This Case?

- USG is very helpful to evaluate the sonographic risk pattern of each nodule. It has to be kept in mind that multiple thyroid nodules >1 cm may require aspiration, based on the sonographic pattern. Both USG and FNAB have great success in experienced hands.
- Similarly, since total thyroidectomy is often recommended for patients with a more advanced disease, with postoperative radioiodine remnant ablation in mind, the typical patient for whom lobectomy would be recommended would not be a candidate for radioiodine, even if thyroid cancer were discovered on final pathology.
- One of the reasons to perform completion thyroidectomy is to enable the patient to receive RAI ablative therapy, and a less compelling reason may be that follow-up with Tg measurements may be less ambiguous in patients who have been thyroidectomized.
- Patients with low-risk thyroid cancer who have undergone thyroid lobectomy can be followed by serum thyroglobulin and neck ultrasound.

References

1. Frates MC, Benson CB, Doubilet PM, Kunreuther E, Contreras M, Cibas ES, et al. Prevalence and distribution of carcinoma in patients with solitary and multiple thyroid nodules on sonography. J Clin Endocrinol Metab. 2006;91:3411–7.
2. Brito JP, Yarur AJ, Prokop LJ, McIver B, Murad MH, Montori VM. Prevalence of thyroid cancer in multinodular goiter versus single nodule: a systematic review and meta-analysis. Thyroid. 2013;23:449–55. https://doi.org/10.1089/thy.2012.0156.
3. Papini E, Guglielmi R, Bianchini A, Crescenzi A, Taccogna S, Nardi F, et al. Risk of malignancy in nonpalpable thyroid nodules: predictive value of ultrasound and color-Doppler features. J Clin Endocrinol Metab. 2002;87:1941–6.
4. Langer JE, Agarwal R, Zhuang H, Huang SS, Mandel SJ. Correlation of findings from iodine 123 scan and ultrasonography in the recommendation for thyroid fine-needle aspiration biopsy. Endocr Pract. 2011;17:699–706. https://doi.org/10.4158/EP10382.OR.
5. Yoo WS, Choi HS, Cho SW, Moon JH, Kim KW, Park HJ, et al. The role of ultrasound findings in the management of thyroid nodules with atypia or follicular lesions of undetermined significance. Clin Endocrinol. 2014;80:735–42. https://doi.org/10.1111/cen.12348.
6. Gweon HM, Son EJ, Youk JH, Kim JA. Thyroid nodules with Bethesda system III cytology: can ultrasonography guide the next step? Ann Surg Oncol. 2013;20:3083–8. https://doi.org/10.1245/s10434-013-2990-x.
7. Stojadinovic A, Peoples GE, Libutti SK, Henry LR, Eberhardt J, Howard RS, et al. Development of a clinical decision model for thyroid nodules. BMC Surg. 2009;9:12. https://doi.org/10.1186/1471-2482-9-12.
8. Goldstein RE, Netterville JL, Burkey B, Johnson JE. Implications of follicular neoplasms, atypia, and lesions suspicious for malignancy diagnosed by fine-needle aspiration of thyroid nodules. Ann Surg. 2002;235:656–62.
9. Mehta RS, Carty SE, Ohori NP, Hodak SP, Coyne C, LeBeau SO, et al. Nodule size is an independent predictor of malignancy in mutation-negative nodules with follicular lesion of undetermined significance cytology. Surgery. 2013;154:730–6. https://doi.org/10.1016/j.surg.2013.05.015.
10. Haugen BR, Alexander EK, Bible KC, Doherty GM, Mandel SJ, Nikiforov YE, et al. 2015 American Thyroid Association management guidelines for adult patients with thyroid nodules and differentiated thyroid cancer: the American Thyroid Association guidelines task force on thyroid nodules and differentiated thyroid cancer. Thyroid. 2016;26:1–133. https://doi.org/10.1089/thy.2015.0020.
11. Matsuzu K, Sugino K, Masudo K, Nagahama M, Kitagawa W, Shibuya H, et al. Thyroid lobectomy for

papillary thyroid cancer: long-term follow-up study of 1,088 cases. World J Surg. 2014;38:68–79. https://doi.org/10.1007/s00268-013-2224-1.

12. Nixon IJ, Ganly I, Patel SG, Palmer FL, Whitcher MM, Tuttle RM, et al. Thyroid lobectomy for treatment of well differentiated intrathyroid malignancy. Surgery. 2012;151:571–9. https://doi.org/10.1016/j.surg.2011.08.016.
13. Oltmann SC, Schneider DF, Leverson G, Sivashanmugam T, Chen H, Sippel RS. Radioactive iodine remnant uptake after completion thyroidectomy: not such a complete cancer operation. Ann Surg Oncol. 2014;21:1379–83. https://doi.org/10.1245/s10434-013-3450-3.
14. Wang TS, Evans DB, Fareau GG, Carroll T, Yen TW. Effect of prophylactic central compartment neck dissection on serum thyroglobulin and recommendations for adjuvant radioactive iodine in patients with differentiated thyroid cancer. Ann Surg Oncol. 2012;19:4217–22. https://doi.org/10.1245/s10434-012-2594-x.
15. Soylu L, Aydin OU, Ozbas S, Bilezikci B, Ilgan S, Gursoy A, et al. The impact of the multifocality and histologic subtype of papillary thyroid carcinoma on central compartment lymph node metastasis. Eur Rev Med Pharmacol Sci. 2016;20:3972–9.
16. Aydin OU, Soylu L, Ozbas S, Ilgan S, Bilezikci B, Gursoy A, et al. The risk of hypoparathyroidism after central compartment lymph node dissection in the surgical treatment of pT1, N0 thyroid papillary carcinoma. Eur Rev Med Pharmacol Sci. 2016;20:1781–7.
17. Barbesino G, Goldfarb M, Parangi S, Yang J, Ross DS, Daniels GH. Thyroid lobe ablation with radioactive iodine as an alternative to completion thyroidectomy after hemithyroidectomy in patients with follicular thyroid carcinoma: long-term follow-up. Thyroid. 2012;22:369–76. https://doi.org/10.1089/thy.2011.0198.
18. Santra A, Bal S, Mahargan S, Bal C. Long-term outcome of lobar ablation versus completion thyroidectomy in differentiated thyroid cancer. Nucl Med Commun. 2011;32:52–8. https://doi.org/10.1097/MNM.0b013e328340e74c.
19. Erbil Y, Barbaros U, Deveci U, Kaya H, Bozbora A, Ozbey N, et al. Gamma probe-guided surgery for revision thyroidectomy: in comparison with conventional technique. J Endocrinol Investig. 2005;28:583–8.
20. Ilgan S, Ozbas S, Bilezikci B, Sengezer T, Aydin OU, Gursoy A, et al. Radioguided occult lesion localization for minimally invasive parathyroidectomy: technical consideration and feasibility. Nucl Med Commun. 2014;35:1167–74. https://doi.org/10.1097/MNM.0000000000000188.
21. Ilgan S, Oztürk E, Yildiz R, Emer O, Ayan A, Görgülü S, et al. Combination of preoperative ultrasonographic mapping and radioguided occult lesion localization in patients with locally recurrent/persistent papillary thyroid carcinoma: a practical method for central compartment reoperations. Clin Nucl Med. 2010;35:847–52. https://doi.org/10.1097/RLU.0b013e3181f48403.
22. Robert JA, Mazzaferri EL. I-131 therapy in a patient with a large thyroid remnant. In: Robert JA, Mazzaferri EL, editors. Essentials of thyroid cancer management. New York: Springer; 2005. p. 257–60.
23. Lang BH, Wong CKH, Wong KP, Chu KK, Shek TWH. Effect of thyroid remnant volume on the risk of hypothyroidism after hemithyroidectomy: a prospective study. Ann Surg Oncol. 2017;24:1525–32. https://doi.org/10.1245/s10434-016-5743-9.

39 FDG PET/CT in the Initial Staging of Differentiated Thyroid Cancer

Gülin Uçmak and B. Büşra Demirel

Abstract

Differentiated thyroid carcinoma (DTC) is the most frequent thyroid neoplasm and has an excellent prognosis with low mortality rate. Despite the good prognosis, distant metastasis at the time of diagnosis is the poorest prognostic factor in patients with DTC. It is important to consider the most efficient combination of treatments in the initial workup of these high-risk patients. If metastasis were found earlier, some patients might subsequently experience a reduction in tumor burden that may ensure therapy success and significant improvement in progression-free survival. F-18 FDG PET/CT has a valuable role in the initial workup of high-risk patients after total thyroidectomy. In the current guidelines, FDG PET/CT is considered as a significant prognostic tool to determine the patients at highest risk for rapid disease progression and a sensitive method to detect surgically resectable disease for the selection of the patients who may benefit from curative surgery and finally a reliable indicator of therapy response. In conclusion, FDG PET/CT may alter the first-choice treatment modality instead prior to radioiodine ablation therapy (RAT) and may provide the decision for surgery or radiation treatment of FDG-positive metastatic foci; it can provide efficiency of adjuvant RAT due to the reduction of tumor burden and also may contribute an improvement of survival.

39.1 Case Presentation

A 51-year-old male patient was referred to our department for further treatment with the diagnosis of metastatic papillary thyroid cancer (PTC) after resection of the frontal bone lesion. His past medical history was negative for known malignancy. No pathologic finding was observed except a nodule with 2 cm diameter in the left thyroid lobe on magnetic resonance imaging (MRI) and ultrasonography (USG) which were performed for exploring the neck. Then the patient underwent total thyroidectomy with central compartment dissection. Histopathological analysis of the tumor in the left thyroid lobe was compatible with PTC with 3.6 × 3 cm in size and with the poor histopathologic feature of extracapsular tumor invasion. Postoperatively serum thyroglobulin (Tg) level under TSH suppression was 671 ng/mL. There was no abnormal finding on neck USG. The patient underwent F-18

G. Uçmak (✉) · B. B. Demirel
Department of Nuclear Medicine, University of Health Sciences (SBÜ) Dr. Abdurrahman Yurtaslan Ankara Oncology Training and Research Hospital, Ankara, Turkey

T. Özülker et al. (eds.), *Thyroid and Parathyroid Diseases*, https://doi.org/10.1007/978-3-319-78476-2_39

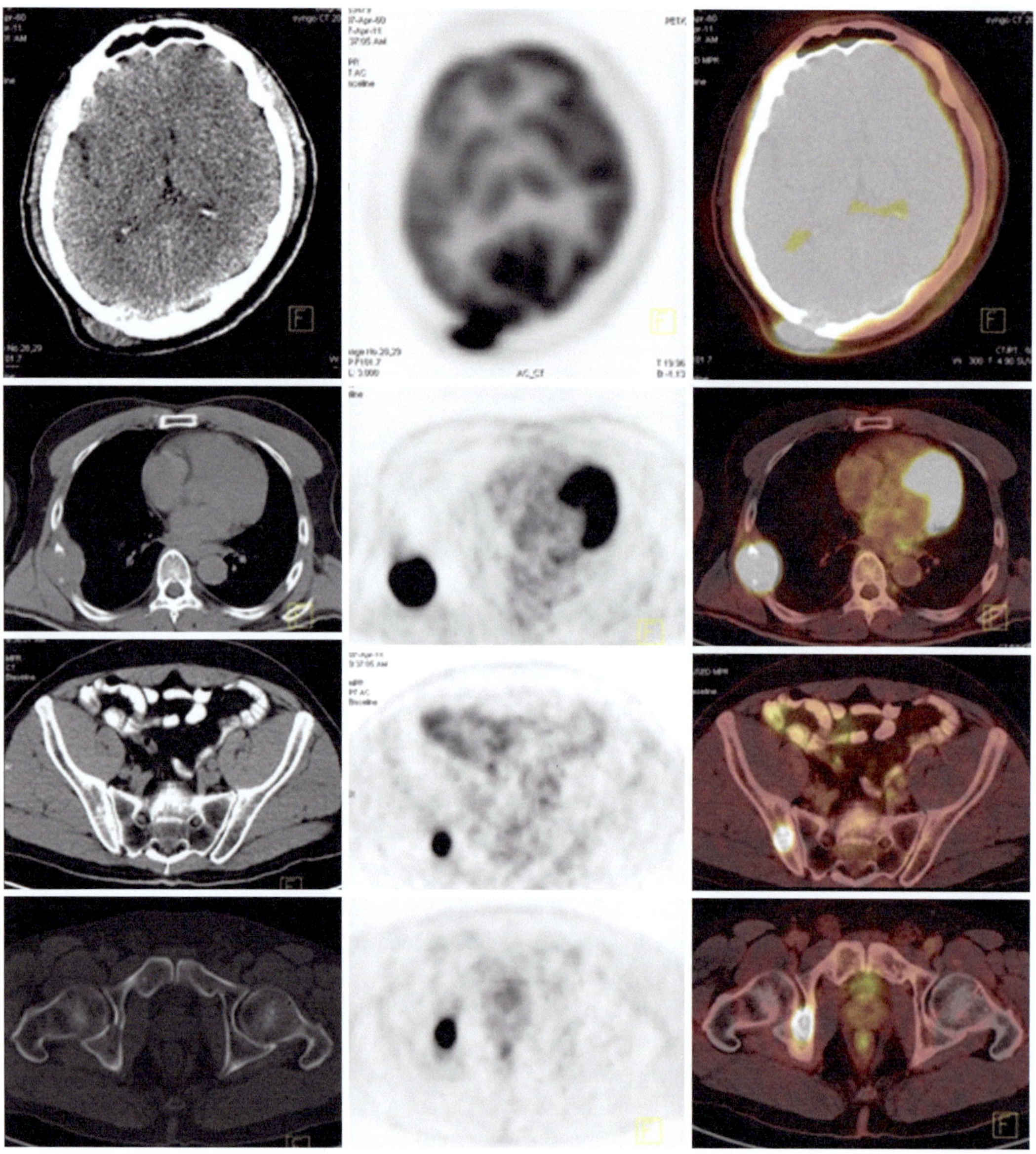

Fig. 39.1 Axial slices of the initial FDG PET/CT scan demonstrated intense FDG uptake in the right occipital region of the calvarium, destructive mass in the right thoracic wall, in the posterior right iliac bone, and in the right acetabulum

fluorodeoxyglucose (FDG) positron emission tomography/computed tomography (PET/CT) for initial staging. On PET/CT, pathological FDG accumulations were seen in left frontoparietal (SUVmax, 17.74) and right occipitotemporal (SUVmax, 37.66) regions of the calvarium. In addition, intense FDG accumulations were observed in the destructive mass lesions located on right thoracic wall (SUVmax, 33.10), right iliac bone (SUVmax, 21.56), and right acetabulum (SUVmax, 18.41) with cortical thinning (Figs. 39.1 and 39.2a).

In the light of PET/CT findings, the patient underwent surgery for bone metastasis in calvarium and the mass located in right thoracic wall for cytoreduction. External beam radiation therapy (EBRT) was administered to the cranium and right acetabulum with palliative intent. Following

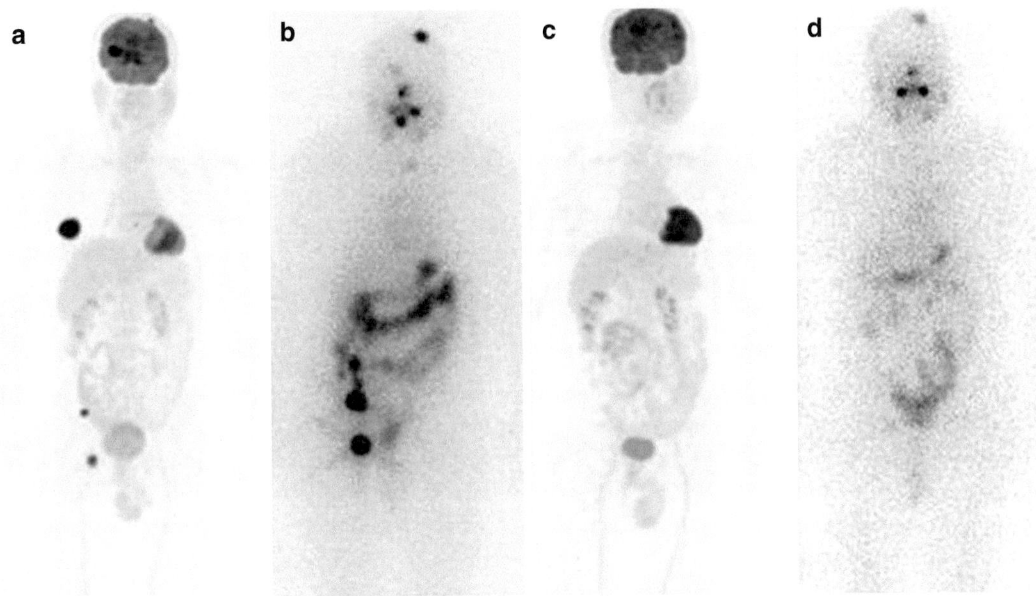

Fig. 39.2 (**a**) demonstrates FDG PET/CT MIP image performed for initial staging. Intense FDG accumulations are clearly observed in left frontoparietal and right occipitotemporal regions in calvarium. In addition, intense FDG accumulations are seen corresponding to the destructive mass lesion on the right thoracic wall and bone metastasis in the right iliac bone and right acetabulum. In (**b**), post-therapy WBS with radioiodine uptake in metastatic deposits is demonstrated. (**c** and **d**) demonstrate follow-up PET/CT and the final post-therapy WBS after 350 mCi of I-131. There is no pathological FDG uptake with regard to metastatic lesions. On the final post-therapy WBS, only slight activity accumulations on the left frontoparietal region and right acetabulum

radiation therapy, a dose of 250 mCi (9.2 GBq) radioiodine ablation therapy (RAT) was administered while serum TSH was >150 μIU/mL and Tg was 668 ng/mL. Recombinant TSH stimulation was not used, and TSH elevation was achieved by thyroid hormone withdrawal prior to adjuvant treatment as recommended by guidelines. Premedication with oral corticosteroids, anti-emetics, and careful hydration was given prior to RAT. Post-therapy whole-body scan (WBS) performed 4 days after therapy demonstrated slight radioiodine uptake in thyroid remnant and intense uptake in left parietal, right frontoparietal, right occipitotemporal, and right hemi-pelvis (Fig. 39.2b).

In a period of 46 months, the patient received a total cumulative dose of 1250 mCi RAI on four consecutive sequences with careful monitoring of bone marrow reserve. Following each consecutive therapy, Tg level both on and off L-thyroxine declined gradually. On the final post-therapy WBS, which was acquired 4 days after the administration of 350 mCi, slight radioiodine uptake was still present only in the left frontal region and right acetabulum, and serum Tg with endogenous TSH stimulation decreased to 24 ng/mL (Fig. 39.2d). In addition, no pathological FDG uptake was seen on post-therapy follow-up PET/CT (Fig. 39.2c).

39.2 Discussion

Differentiated thyroid carcinoma (DTC) is the most frequent thyroid neoplasm and has an excellent prognosis with a mortality rate less than 10% [1]. Despite the good prognosis, distant metastasis at the time of diagnosis is the poorest prognostic factor in patients with DTC. The cancer-specific mortality in patients with distant metastases varies from 36 to 47% at 5 years, rising even further to approximately 70% at 15 years [2, 3]. The prevalence of distant metastasis is 10–15% in patients with DTC, while, in this subgroup of metastatic DTC patients, the distant metastases are present at diagnosis in 50% of the patients. The frequency of individuals diagnosed with DTC presenting initially with distant metastatic disease is 1–9% [4]. The most frequent sites of distant metastases are the lung and bone, with a prevalence of 50–60% and 20–30%, respectively. Liver, brain, and skin metastases, which are much rare, are found in about 3% of patients at the time of diagnosis with a widespread metastatic disease [5, 6]. In our case, multiple bone metastases were present at the time of diagnosis in keeping with the literature.

Although the most common treatment is RAT, the management of metastatic DTC requires an integrated approach including both directed and systemic therapies such as surgery, EBRT, chemotherapy, and targeted treatment agents if the disease becomes iodine refractory. It is important to consider the most efficient combination of treatments in initial workup of high-risk patients. If metastasis were found earlier, some patients might subsequently experience a reduction in tumor burden that may provide treatment success and significant improvement in progression-free survival [4].

Whole-body scan (WBS) after RAT with rising Tg level can demonstrate distant metastasis earlier [7]. However, in a subgroup of metastatic patients, post-therapy I-131 WBS may be false negative and may not demonstrate the overall extent of disease due to tumor heterogeneity. F-18 FDG PET/CT has a valuable role in the initial workup of high-risk patients after total thyroidectomy. FDG PET/CT is widely used in the postsurgical follow-up of DTC, particularly in patients with negative I-131 WBS despite elevated Tg levels.

It is mostly accepted that FDG uptake in DTC related to the loss of differentiated features and associates with aggressive behavior. In patients with FDG-positive recurrences, both progression-free survival and overall survival decrease compared to patients with FDG-negative tumors [8–10]. The current ATA guideline suggests that FDG PET/CT should be used when Tg levels >10 ng/mL with negative I-131 WBS [11]. PET/CT scanning may also be considered as a part of initial staging in poorly differentiated thyroid cancers and invasive Hürthle cell carcinomas, especially those with other evidence of disease on imaging or because of elevated serum Tg levels. In addition, PET/CT is considered a significant prognostic tool to determine patients at highest risk for rapid disease progression, a sensitive method to detect surgically resectable disease for the selection of patients who may benefit from curative surgery select and finally a reliable indicator of posttreatment response following therapy [8–11].

In daily practice, the decision on the timing of FDG PET/CT imaging should be individualized for each patient, considering not only Tg levels and I-131 WBS results but also the individual risk on the basis of histopathological and clinical characteristics [12]. In the presented case, FDG PET/CT performed at initial workup prior to RAT provided accurate staging with the detection of surgically amenable lesions. Aggressive cytoreductive surgeries followed by EBRT provided a significant reduction in tumor burden and enhanced the efficacy of RAT in our patient. Recently few studies have investigated the role of FDG PET/CT in the initial evaluation of patients with DTC [13–16]. It was reported that FDG PET/CT concurrent with RAT could detect unexpected abnormal accumulations in 33% of the patients, who have locoregional recurrence and cervical lymph node metastasis [13]. In another study, FDG PET/CT was performed about 1 week after the first RAT in the high-risk patient group, and they found that 29% of patients had positive PET/CT findings and the treatment strategy for 21% of patients changed [14]. Similarly, FDG-positive additional lesions were found in 14% of intermediate-risk to high-risk patients, in a previous study, and the authors indicate that the treatment was changed in 10% of their patients [15]. FDG PET/CT and Tg levels were found as predictors of progression-free survival, in a recent study, which included newly diagnosed DTC patients [16]. In this study, it was suggested that FDG PET/CT has an independent prognostic role, with a better progression-free survival in patients with negative I-131 WBS. FDG uptake in metastatic patients with DTC is a major negative predictive value for response to RAT and an independent prognostic factor for survival [9, 17]. It can also determine metastatic lesions with high FDG uptake that may be more aggressive and should be targeted for therapy or close monitoring. In consequence, FDG PET/CT may alter the first-choice treatment modality instead prior to radioiodine therapy and may ensure the decision for surgical removal or radiation treatment of metastatic foci with FDG uptake; it can provide efficiency of adjuvant RAT due to reduced tumor load and also may contribute an improvement of survival.

39.3 Follow-Up and Outcome

The patient is on follow-up for 6 years in our clinic with stable serum Tg level about 2.5 ng/mL under TSH suppression with no radiological abnormal finding.

What Can We Learn from This Case?

- FDG PET/CT is widely used in the follow-up of DTC patients with increasing Tg levels and negative WBS.
- FDG PET/CT has a most valuable role in initial workup of high-risk DTC patients.
- Metastatic lesions with high FDG uptake may be more aggressive, and if possible, they should be removed before RAT in consequence of FDG findings.
- Combined treatments such as surgery, EBRT, and targeted therapies also should be performed in this group of patients and may contribute an improvement of progression-free survival and overall survival.
- As a molecular imaging method, FDG PET/CT may predict the initial radioiodine therapy response and improve risk stratification in the initial workup in high-risk DTC patients.

References

1. Durante C, Haddy N, Baudin E, Leboulleux S, Hartl D, Travagli JP, et al. Long-term outcome of 444 patients with distant metastases from papillary and follicular thyroid carcinoma: benefits and limits of radioiodine therapy. J Clin Endocrinol Metab. 2006;91:2892–9. https://doi.org/10.1210/jc.2005-2838.
2. Smith SA, Hay ID, Goellner JR, Ryan JJ, McConahey WM. Mortality from papillary thyroid carcinoma. A case-control study of 56 lethal cases. Cancer. 1988;62:1381–8.
3. Akslen LA, Haldorsen T, Thoresen SO, Glattre E. Survival and causes of death in thyroid cancer: a population-based study of 2479 cases from Norway. Cancer Res. 1991;51:1234–41.
4. Sampson E, Brierley JD, Le LW, Rotstein L, Tsang RW. Clinical management and outcome of papillary and follicular (differentiated) thyroid cancer presenting with distant metastasis at diagnosis. Cancer. 2007;110:1451–6. https://doi.org/10.1002/cncr.22956.
5. Schlumberger M, Challeton C, De Vathaire F, Travagli JP, Gardet P, Lumbroso JD, et al. Radioactive iodine treatment and external radiotherapy for lung and bone metastases from thyroid carcinoma. J Nucl Med. 1996;37:598–605.
6. Ozata M, Suzuki S, Miyamoto T, Liu RT, Fierro-Renoy F, DeGroot LJ. Serum thyroglobulin in the follow-up of patients with treated differentiated thyroid cancer. J Clin Endocrinol Metab. 1994;79:98–105.
7. Lind P, Kohlfürst S. Respective roles of thyroglobulin, radioiodine imaging, and positron emission tomography in the assessment of thyroid cancer. Semin Nucl Med. 2006;36(3):194–205. https://doi.org/10.1053/j.Sem.Nucl.Med.2006.03.002.
8. Vural GU, Akkas BE, Ercakmak N, Basu S, Alavi A. Prognostic significance of FDG PET/CT on the follow-up of patients of differentiated thyroid carcinoma with negative 131I whole-body scan and elevated thyroglobulin levels: correlation with clinical and histopathologic characteristics and long-term follow-up data. Clin Nucl Med. 2012;37:953–9. https://doi.org/10.1097/RLU.0b013e31825b2057.
9. Akkas BE, Demirel BB, Vural GU. Prognostic factors affecting disease-specific survival in patients with recurrent and/or metastatic differentiated thyroid carcinoma detected by positron emission tomography/computed tomography. Thyroid. 2014;24(2):287–95. https://doi.org/10.1089/thy.2013.0195.
10. Robbins RJ, Wan Q, Grewal RK, Reibke R, Gonen M, Strauss HW, et al. Real-time prognosis for metastatic thyroid carcinoma based on 2-[18F]fluoro-2-deoxy-D-glucose-positron emission tomography scanning. J Clin Endocrinol Metab. 2006;91:498–505. https://doi.org/10.1210/jc.2005-1534.
11. Haugen BR, Alexander EK, Bible KC, Doherty GM, Mandel SJ, Nikiforov YE, et al. 2015 American Thyroid Association management guidelines for adult

patients with thyroid nodules and differentiated thyroid cancer: the American Thyroid Association guidelines task force on thyroid nodules and differentiated thyroid cancer. Thyroid. 2016;26(1):1–133. https://doi.org/10.1089/thy.2015.0020.
12. Abraham T, Schöder H. Thyroid cancer—indications and opportunities for positron emission tomography/computed tomography imaging. Semin Nucl Med. 2011;41:121–38. https://doi.org/10.1053/j.semnuclmed.2010.10.006.
13. Iwano S, Kato K, Ito S, Tsuchiya K, Naganawa S. FDG-PET performed concurrently with initial I-131 ablation for differentiated thyroid cancer. Ann Nucl Med. 2012;26:207–13. https://doi.org/10.1007/s12149-011-0559-y.
14. Rosenbaum-Krumme SJ, Gorges R, Bockisch A, Binse I. 18F-FDG PET/CT changes therapy management in high-risk DTC after first radioiodine therapy. Eur J Nucl Med Mol Imaging. 2012;39:1373–80. https://doi.org/10.1007/s00259-012-2065-4.
15. Lee JW, Lee SM, Lee DH, Kim YJ. Clinical utility of 18F-FDG PET/CT concurrent with therapy in intermediate-to-high-risk patients with differentiated thyroid cancer: dual-center experience with 286 patients. J Nucl Med. 2013;54:1230–6. https://doi.org/10.2967/jnumed.112.117119.
16. Pace L, Klain M, Salvatore B, Nicolai E, Zampella E, Assante R, et al. Prognostic role of 18F-FDG PET/CT in the postoperative evaluation of differentiated thyroid cancer patients. Clin Nucl Med. 2015;40(2):111–5. https://doi.org/10.1097/RLU.0000000000000621.
17. Deandreis D, Al Ghuzlan A, Leboulleux S, Lacroix L, Garsi JP, Talbot M, et al. Do histological, immunohistochemical, and metabolic (radioiodine and fluorodeoxyglucose uptakes) patterns of metastatic thyroid cancer correlate with patient outcome? Endocr Relat Cancer. 2011;18:159–69. https://doi.org/10.1677/ERC-10-0233.

A Case of a Papillary Thyroid Cancer with Gross Residual Disease After Surgery

40

Ülkem Yararbaş and Zehra Özcan

Abstract

Locally advanced disease accounts for 5–15% of the differentiated thyroid cancer (DTC) patients. Although surgical excision of the entire primary lesion is aimed for the optimum disease management, incomplete resections may occur especially in patients having invasions to recurrent laryngeal nerve, respiratory tract, esophagus, or major vessels. Radioactive iodine (RAI) treatment is the primary adjuvant therapy modality in high-risk DTC cases. In cases with RAI-resistant disease, external beam radiotherapy (EBRT) may be an alternative. However, its role is debated due to the lack of prospective data and also conflicting results in retrospective studies. Since EBRT may have some severe side effects, the consequences of uncontrolled disease and the potential complications of EBRT should be considered comparatively.

40.1 Case Presentation

Seventy-two years old male patient with a neck mass was operated in 2005. Histopathological analysis revealed 2.5 cm, moderately differentiated papillary thyroid carcinoma. The tumor was infiltrated to the trachea. Resection of the tumor was incomplete, and technically completion of the thyroidectomy was not found to be possible. According to AJCC 7th Edition/TNM classification system differentiated thyroid carcinoma, the patient was classified as stage IVa (T4aN0M0). The patient received 200 mCi (7.4 GBq) of radioiodine therapy three times during the postoperative period. Radioiodine scans showed persistent residual thyroid tissue in each post-therapeutic scan. Unfortunately, the patient was lost to clinical follow-up and disappeared for an almost 10 years.

In 2015, the patient was admitted to our institution with respiratory problems. Serum Tg level was elevated, and neck USG showed lymph nodes in the left side. ^{18}F-FDG PET/CT scan was performed in order to demonstrate the extent of the disease and showed hypermetabolic residual thyroid lesion and hypermetabolic lymph nodes in the left cervical region (levels 2, 3, 4) and in right lung hilum. There were also multiple parenchymal nodules in lungs bilaterally. The patient received two consecutive radioiodine therapies 200 mCi (7.4 GBq) courses with 1-year interval. Post-therapy scans showed findings in accordance with previous PET/CT. Tg level was greater than 300 ng/ml both in TSH suppression or L-thyroxine withdrawal periods.

Ü. Yararbaş (✉) · Z. Özcan
Ege University School of Medicine, Department of Nuclear Medicine, Izmir, Turkey

T. Özülker et al. (eds.), *Thyroid and Parathyroid Diseases*, https://doi.org/10.1007/978-3-319-78476-2_40

40.2 Discussion

With the amelioration of technical aspect and wider use of diagnostic tools and also the increasing incidence of the disease, the number of diagnosed differentiated thyroid carcinoma (DTC) is increasing worldwide. Although the majority of the cases present with small, intrathyroidal lesions, locally advanced disease is not rare and consists 5–15% of the DTC patients [1]. The standard management of DTC includes surgery, radioactive iodine therapy (RAI), and thyroid-stimulating hormone (TSH) suppression. Complete resection of the primary tumor is a major determinant of the outcome. RAI and TSH suppression steps have a complementary role with the aim of minimizing disease recurrence rate and metastatic spread risk [2]. Additionally, in patients who had successful ablative RAI postoperatively, follow-up using thyroglobulin is more reliable. Although meta-analysis shows conflicting results on the necessity of routine postoperative ablative RAI treatment in low-risk patients, there is agreement on the use of RAI treatment in patients with distant metastasis and gross extrathyroidal extension [3, 4].

Regarding surgical approach, there is consensus on performing "shave" procedure in case of minimal visceral invasion and "full-thickness excision" for the transmural invasion of the trachea or esophagus. In case of intermediate invasions to superficial layers without submucosal involvement, recent studies recommend less aggressive surgical approaches accompanied by postoperative adjuvant therapies [1]. Additionally, resection of locally invasive thyroid cancers involving recurrent laryngeal nerve, respiratory tract, esophagus, major vessels, or strap muscles is not always technically possible.

Incomplete resection of gross disease is well known to have an unfavorable effect on prognosis [1, 5]. In the study of Hay et al. in a large study group consisting of 2444 thyroid papillary carcinoma cases with a median follow-up period of 15 years, disease-specific mortality rate was found to be 4% and was observed in patients having the distant metastatic disease and gross residual disease persisting after resection [6]. Locally advanced disease and therefore gross residual disease following surgery occur especially in patients having unfavorable prognostic factors consisting of advanced age and aggressive histological subtypes including columnar, Hurthle cell, tall cell, insular variants, and tumors bearing poorly differentiated components [7, 8]. Although RAI treatment is the primary adjuvant therapy modality in high-risk DTC cases, RAI-resistant disease is usually associated with similar risk factors causing aggressive disease. External beam radiotherapy (EBRT) is an alternative when locoregional disease control has not been achieved using surgery and RAI. Due to lack of prospective data and also conflicting results in retrospective studies, the role of EBRT is debated [9]. However, guidelines recommend the use of EBRT in selective cases [2, 10].

In 2016 the Endocrine Surgery Committee of the American Head and Neck Society reported recommendations that are based on literature review and expert opinions regarding the use of EBRT for locoregional control in DTC. According to this report, in the management of gross residual or unresectable locoregional disease, EBRT is recommended except for patients younger than 45 years old with a limited gross disease that shows RAI avidity [8]. The study of Chow et al. that is one of the works forming the basis of the American Head and Neck Society recommendations showed a 10-year locoregional recurrence-free survival of 63% using EBRT and 24% without EBRT in 217 papillary carcinoma cases ($p < 0.001$) [11].

Besides the conflicting results on the benefit of EBRT, another concern is the adverse effects of EBRT. Both the location of the thyroid gland close to central neck structures and upper mediastinum and the necessity of a wide therapy field with irregular margins complicate EBRT [12]. The acute phase complications include dermal reactions, oral mucositis, pharyngitis, laryngitis, xerostomia, and dysphagia. In the late phase, fibrosis in regional muscles and soft tissues, tracheal and esophageal stenosis, chronic dysphagia, chronic laryngeal edema, and xerostomia may develop. Radiation pneumonitis may also evolve if lung parenchyma is included in the radiotherapy field [13].

In general, the EBRT can be performed with curative, adjuvant, or palliative purposes. In DTC, since even patients with unresectable disease or distant metastases will have relatively long survival when compared with other oncological diseases, the consequences of uncontrolled disease and the potential complications of EBRT should be considered comparatively.

Intensity-modulated radiation therapy (IMRT) which may spare critical organs and enable dose intensification is a relatively new technique. Reduction in radiation exposure to normal tissues reduces complications. Using IMRT, Schwartz et al. reported a severe late morbidity rate of 2%, which is significantly less than conventional techniques with a 12% serious complication rate [12]. In the same study, IMRT was not found to have an impact on survival rates.

40.3 Follow-Up and Clinical Course

Currently, the patient is 87 years old. He is stable with the disease. Regarding RAI therapy, following a cumulative dose of 1 Ci, imaging studies and Tg levels do not show a dramatic response to radioiodine. When slow progression of the disease and potential complications of EBRT are considered together in this particular patient, EBRT is not currently performed. However, EBRT appears to be an option in cases with gross invasive residual tumors.

What Can We Learn from This Case?

- We encounter gross residual disease in a small fraction of cases with differentiated thyroid cancer in our clinical practice. Fortunately, as in the case described in this section, most of the cases have a slow progression. Review of the literature shows that EBRT must be considered as a complementary therapy modality in cases with refractory disease to radioiodine. Side effects of EBRT and progression rate of the residual disease should be considered together.

References

1. Nixon IJ, Simo R, Newbold K, Rinaldo A, Suarez C, Kowalski LP, et al. Management of invasive differentiated thyroid cancer. Thyroid. 2016;26:1156–66. https://doi.org/10.1089/thy.2016.0064.
2. Haugen BR, Alexander EK, Bible KC, Doherty GM, Mandel SJ, Nikiforov YE, et al. 2015 American Thyroid Association management guidelines for adult patients with thyroid nodules and differentiated thyroid cancer: the American Thyroid Association guidelines task force on thyroid nodules and differentiated thyroid cancer. Thyroid. 2016;26:1–133. https://doi.org/10.1089/thy.2015.0020.
3. Sawka AM, Thephamongkhol K, Brouwers M, Thabane L, Browman G, Gerstein HC. A systematic review and meta-analysis of radioactive iodine remnant ablation for well-differentiated thyroid cancer. J Clin Endocrinol Metab. 2002;89:3668–76.
4. Sacks W, Fung CH, Chang JR, Waxman A, Braunstein GD. The effectiveness of radioactive iodine for treatment of low-risk thyroid cancer: a systematic analysis of the peer-reviewed literature from 1966 to April 2008. Thyroid. 2010;20:1235–45. https://doi.org/10.1089/thy.2009.0455.
5. Kowalski LP, Filho JG. Results of the treatment of locally invasive thyroid carcinoma. Head Neck. 2002;24(4):340.
6. Hay ID, Thompson GB, Grant CS, Bergstralh EJ, Dvorak CE, Gorman CA, et al. Papillary thyroid carcinoma managed at the Mayo Clinic during six decades (1940–1999): temporal trends in initial therapy and long-term outcome in 2444 consecutively treated patients. World J Surg. 2002;26:879–85.
7. Fatourechi V, Hay ID, Javedan H, Wiseman GA, Mullan BP, Gorman CA. Lack of impact of radioiodine therapy in tg-positive, diagnostic whole-body scan-negative patients with follicular cell-derived thyroid cancer. J Clin Endocrinol Metab. 2002;87:1521–6.
8. Kiess AP, Agrawal N, Brierley JD, Duvvuri U, Ferris RL, Genden E, et al. External-beam radiotherapy for differentiated thyroid cancer locoregional control: a statement of the American Head and Neck Society. Head Neck. 2016;38:493–8. https://doi.org/10.1002/hed.24357.
9. Fussey JM, Crunkhorn R, Tedla M, Weickert MO, Mehanna H. External beam radiotherapy in differentiated thyroid carcinoma: a systematic review. Head Neck. 2016;38:2297–305.
10. Perros P, Colley S, Boelaert K, Evans C, Evans RM, Gerrard GE, et al. British Thyroid Association guidelines for the management of thyroid cancer. Clin Endocrinol. 2014;81(Suppl):1.
11. Chow SM, Yau S, Kwan CK, Poon PC, Law SC. Local and regional control in patients with papillary thyroid carcinoma: specific indications of external radiotherapy and radioactive iodine according to T and N categories in AJCC 6th edition. Endocr Relat Cancer. 2006;13:1159–72.11.

12. Schwartz DL, Lobo MJ, Ang KK, Morrison WH, Rosenthal DI, Ahamad A, et al. Postoperative external beam radiotherapy for differentiated thyroid cancer: outcomes and morbidity with conformal treatment. Int J Radiat Oncol Biol Phys. 2009;74:1083–91. https://doi.org/10.1016/j.ijrobp.2008.09.023.
13. Tuttle RM, Rondeau G, Lee NY. A risk-adapted approach to the use of radioactive iodine and external beam radiation in the treatment of well-differentiated thyroid cancer. Cancer Control. 2011;18:89–95.

41 The Effect of Positive Surgical Margins After Thyroidectomy on Patient Prognosis in Cases with Differentiated Thyroid Carcinoma

Gülin Uçmak and Burcu Esen Akkaş

Abstract

The presence of gross/macroscopic positive margins and incomplete resection has long been recognized as significant risk factors for disease recurrence in patients with differentiated thyroid carcinoma (DTC). However, this is less clear for patients with microscopic positive margin when other significant risk factors are not present. In this chapter, two cases are presented in order to discuss the impact of microscopically involved surgical margins on disease recurrence.

41.1 Case Presentations

41.1.1 Case 1

A 55-year-old female patient was referred to our Nuclear Medicine Department after total thyroidectomy with a diagnosis of multifocal papillary thyroid cancer for clinical management and the evaluation of radioiodine treatment. Tumors were present in both lobes, and tumor sizes were 15 mm and 2 mm. On pathology report, surgical margins were reported as involved by tumor cells.

G. Uçmak (✉) · B. E. Akkaş
Department of Nuclear Medicine, University of Health Sciences (SBÜ) Dr. Abdurrahman Yurtaslan Ankara Oncology Training and Research Hospital, Ankara, Turkey

On thyroid scan performed after the i.v. administration of 5 mCi Tc99m-pertechnetate, activity accumulations compatible with small thyroid residues were seen in thyroid bed. Neck ultrasound (USG) revealed small residues on thyroid lobes and no enlarged lymph nodes were seen in the central and lateral compartments. The patient was not receiving any thyroid replacement. Her thyroid function test results were as follows: free triiodothyronine (FT3) level of 0.7 pg/mL (reference range, 2.50–4.30 pg/mL), free thyroxine (FT4) level of 0.4 ng/dL (reference range, 0.90–1.70 ng/dL), and thyroid-stimulating hormone (TSH) level of 54.2 μIU/mL (reference range, 0.35–5.00 μIU/mL). Serum thyroglobulin (Tg) level was 78.3 ng/mL. Anti-thyroglobulin antibodies were within normal ranges.

An ablative I-131 dose of 150 mCi was chosen for serum Tg level which was relatively high and out of proportion to the residual thyroid tissue on neck ultrasound. On post-therapy whole-body scan (WBS), intense I-131 uptake was detected reflecting the residual tissues on thyroid bed, and no abnormal uptake related to metastatic disease was seen throughout the body. After therapy, the patient was discharged from hospital with L-thyroxin replacement treatment. A follow-up visit was conducted 3 months after the ablation therapy. Clinical examination and neck ultrasound (USG) were performed; serum TSH, non-stimulated Tg, anti-Tg antibody levels, and complete blood counts were checked during follow-up visits.

T. Özülker et al. (eds.), *Thyroid and Parathyroid Diseases*, https://doi.org/10.1007/978-3-319-78476-2_41

Response to therapy was assessed based on Tg values following after ablation therapy. Serum Tg was 12.2 ng/mL on the first follow-up visit on L-thyroxine therapy. Neck USG was negative for the local disease. A ^{18}F-FDG positron emission tomography/computed tomography (PET/CT) was also negative for residual and/or metastatic disease (Fig. 41.1a).

A therapy dose of 200 mCi I-131 was given 9 months after the initial dose while serum TSH and Tg were 93.4 μIU/mL and 31.9 ng/mL, respectively. No pathological radioiodine uptake was seen on post-therapy images (Fig. 41.1b).

41.1.1.1 Follow-Up and Outcome

On follow-up visits, serum Tg declined to 2.5 ng/mL on L-thyroxine and remained stable in the range of 2–3 ng/mL during the follow-up period of 3 years. The patient is alive with a stable but not localized disease (incomplete biochemical response) with a serum Tg of 2.5 ng/mL under L-thyroxine suppression.

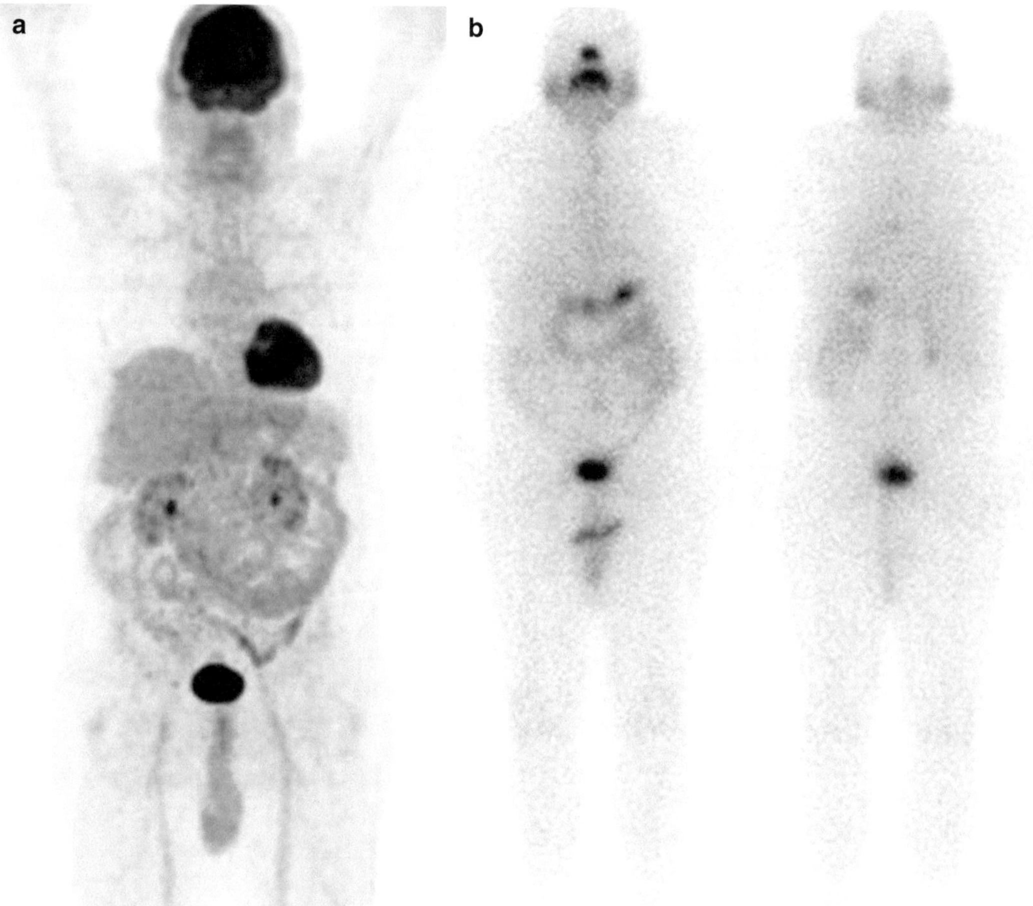

Fig. 41.1 ^{18}F-FDG PET/CT maximum intensity projection (MIP) image in (**a**) and the whole-body scan after administration of 200 mCi I-131. (**b**) Physiological uptakes are observed on both images with no pathological uptake reflecting residual or metastatic disease

41.1.2 Case 2

A 60-year-old female patient was referred to our Nuclear Medicine Department after total thyroidectomy for clinical management and the evaluation of radioiodine treatment. Two tumor types were defined in the pathology report. A follicular variant of papillary thyroid cancer, 10 mm in size, was present in the left lobe and poorly differentiated insular carcinoma with 3 mm in size in right lobe was seen. In addition, surgical margins were involved by tumor cells.

On thyroid scan performed after the i.v. administration of 5 mCi Tc99m-pertechnetate, small thyroid gland residues were seen on both sides of thyroid bed. Neck USG revealed small residues on thyroid lobes and no enlarged lymph nodes were seen in the central and lateral compartments. Serum TSH level was 75.2 μIU/mL (reference range, 0.35–5.00 μIU/mL), and Tg level was 1.02 ng/mL; Anti-TG antibodies were within normal ranges.

An ablative I-131 dose of 120 mCi was given orally in an isolated room in our department. The post-therapy whole-body scan (WBS) was acquired 4 days later. Intense I-131 uptake was detected reflecting the residual tissues on thyroid bed, and no abnormal uptake related to metastatic disease was seen throughout the body. After therapy, the patient was discharged from the hospital with L-thyroxin replacement treatment.

41.1.2.1 Follow-Up and Outcome

A follow-up visit was conducted 3 months after the ablation therapy. Clinical examination and neck USG were performed; serum TSH, non-stimulated Tg, anti-Tg antibody levels, and complete blood counts were checked during follow-up visits. Response to therapy was assessed based on Tg values following after ablation therapy. Serum Tg was undetectable on the first follow-up visit on L-thyroxine therapy. Neck USG was negative for the local disease. On the annual control, iodine WBS performed 48 h after the administration of 5 mCi I-131 revealed physiological biodistribution of radioiodine. The patient is considered cured and is still under follow-up with L-thyroxine suppression therapy for 6 years.

41.2 Discussion

Differentiated thyroid cancer (DTC) is the most common endocrine malignancy. In many centers throughout the world, clinical management of patients with DTC has based on a risk-stratified approach, supported by the major consensus guidelines of the American Thyroid Association (ATA) and European Thyroid Association (ETA) [1, 2]. Total thyroidectomy and radioiodine remnant ablation are the mainstays of treatment in patients with DTC. It is well recognized that radioiodine remnant ablation facilitates the follow-up of DTC and reduces the risk of local recurrences.

The prognosis of DTC is generally excellent when appropriate treatment is given. The 10-year overall cause-specific survival for DTC patients is known as 85% even for patients with distant metastasis [3]. However, the lifetime recurrence rate is relatively high, reaching to 30% [4]. Incomplete resection and residual tumor burden after thyroidectomy are among the most important risk factors for local recurrences and increased morbidity. According to American Thyroid Association, minimal extrathyroidal extension of the tumor indicates an intermediate risk for local recurrence (5–20% risk) [1]. However, it is not clear whether a microscopic positive margin found only on final pathology has similar implications on patient outcomes like the gross positive margins.

The "margin" is defined as the outer aspect of the tissue and/or inked edge of the specimen. The determination of margin status is represented by the evaluation of the relationship of the tumor to the inked edge of the specimen. However, the thyroid capsule is not a real anatomical structure. Based on the autopsy series; it is shown that the thyroid capsule may be missing or focally incomplete in many thyroid glands [5].

It may be considered that patients with positive microscopic margins may have more advanced tumors and may have increased risk for disease recurrence than those with negative microscopic margins. Lang et al. evaluated the impact of involved margins and locations (anterior vs. posterior) on disease recurrence [6]. They reported that posterior margins involved with tumor cells did appear to increase disease recurrence, whereas an anterior involved margin did not [6]. Kluijfhout et al. reported in their series of patients with T1–T2 tumors, 11% of patients had a microscopic positive margin found on pathology examination, and this finding alone did not increase the chance of recurrence compared with those with a negative margin [7].

Although it is recommended that a positive margin must be mentioned in the final pathology report, studies on the effect of positive margins and outcome in large series of patients with long-term follow-up are lacking. Indeed, there is not enough data to date on the prognostic value of close margins as an independent or co-variable.

There is still controversy about the term "microscopic residual tumor." Patients with microscopic incomplete tumor resection after surgery are classified as a high-risk group according to the ATA guidelines, and several retrospective reports have shown that external beam radiotherapy is of benefit in high-risk patients [1]. However, the term microscopic residual tumor must be well clarified according to whether the tumor remained limited to the thyroid gland with only positive surgical margins or the microscopic tumor is left in the margins of the specimen of extrathyroidal areas. The two situations may have a significant influence on the patient outcome and must be taken into account when determining the risk stratification on initial management individually.

The pathologists report that the existence of tumor at the margin (i.e., capsule and/or ink) does not correlate to incomplete excision as is in other organs where there is continuity of the entire viscera such that a real surgical and pathologic margin exists (www.cap.org) [8]. After corrected for other significant factors, involved margins may not be accounted for an independent factor for DFS.

However, the extrathyroidal extension may reflect a worse prognosis. The diagnosis of extensive extrathyroidal extension is straightforward and is usually established clinically; however, the histological diagnosis of minimal extrathyroidal extension may be problematic and subjective since the thyroid gland does not have a well-defined capsule.

There are many well recognized poor prognostic factors for patients with DTC. With appropriate risk stratification both before and closely after thyroidectomy, patients with increased risk of local recurrences and patients who are confronted with tumors with aggressive clinical behavior may be identified successfully. Of these, as a reliable marker for tumor burden, serum Tg levels, in the absence of circulating Anti-Tg antibodies, may account for one of the most significant factors to tailor treatment for selected patients who may need aggressive therapies and close monitoring. There is a significant association between residual tumor and serum Tg levels. Vural et al. reported that among patients with recurrent DTC, serum Tg was significantly higher in patients who had extrathyroidal spread at the time of diagnosis [9].

Measurement of serum Tg has emerged as the most accurate means of detecting persistent or recurrent tumor on follow-up [9]. Tg levels either on L-thyroxine therapy or not indicate the residual tumor burden after thyroidectomy and may be used to tailor therapy. There is a close relation between the serum Tg level after withdrawal of thyroid hormone treatment and tumor mass, as appreciated by the total surface and the total volume of metastatic foci. Furthermore, patients with higher serum Tg levels more frequently had an extracapsular extension and persistent foci of uptake on postoperative 131I-WBS, indicating a more extended disease [10].

The clinician must be alert for residual or recurrent tumor if serum Tg level remains relatively high and out of proportion to the residual thyroid tissue. Despite the numerous studies performed to correlate the values of postoperative Tg, the optimal cutoff value for postoperative serum Tg to guide radioiodine ablation decision-making has been unclear. Since there is inseparable integrity between Tg production and tumor differentiation, the real existence of "an optimal Tg level" may be questionable. Serum Tg level indicative of recurrence may vary within a wide range due to tumor heterogeneity or underlying genetic factors that may play a role in prognosis.

From this point of view, the term "out of proportion to the residual tissue or identified residual disease" used to define serum Tg levels seems as a more reasonable and rationale term to indicate recurrent or persistent disease for Tg levels. However, it is important to realize that not all patients have Tg-producing tumors. It is a well-known phenomenon that dedifferentiation process may lead to loss of Tg production. In addition, although very rare, a little percent of patients with differentiated thyroid cancer may have undetectable or reduced serum Tg levels at the time of diagnosis [11]. In such situations, Tg retesting with different immunoassays may be advisory in ruling out these pitfalls in a large majority of patients.

The cases presented in this chapter demonstrate the significant difference with regard to clinical behavior of the tumors and response to radioiodine ablation even they have almost similar tumor characteristics. Both were age-matched female patients with papillary carcinomas that have similar tumor sizes with differentiated features. Herein, it is important to note that case 2 had insular-type thyroid cancer which is associated with aggressive clinical behavior and poor prognosis. Despite the higher initial dose selected for radioiodine ablation and the second dose was given on follow-up and the lack of poor prognostic variant of thyroid cancer, a complete biochemical response could not be achieved in case 1. On the contrary, a successful therapy response could be achieved in case 2 by ablation therapy despite the presence of insular thyroid cancer. In fact, two patients differed significantly with respect to postoperative serum Tg levels. Case 1 presented with high serum Tg level (78.3 ng/mL) under TSH stimulation which was indicative of residual tumor burden, whereas case 2 had significantly low serum TG level (1.02 ng/mL).

In this chapter, we presented two cases with papillary thyroid carcinoma that have almost similar histopathological features with regard to tumor histology, tumor size, and microscopic margin involvement but have completely different outcomes. Despite the postoperative radiological findings that define almost similar residues on thyroid bed, serum Tg levels were strikingly different between our patients. Although there is still controversy about the impact of residual microscopic disease on disease-free survival (DFS) in patients with DTC, we considered that poorer DFS reported in patients with positive surgical margins may be more related to more advanced local and nodal disease rather than the presence of involved microscopic margins solely.

What Can We Learn from This Case?

- Thyroid gland does not have a well-defined structural capsule.
- The microscopically involved surgical margin is completely different from extrathyroidal invasion and seems to have a negligible effect on patient prognosis.
- Postoperative Tg level under TSH stimulation is an important factor in risk stratification of patients with differentiated thyroid carcinoma.

References

1. Haugen BR, Alexander EK, Bible KC, Doherty GM, Mandel SJ, Nikiforov YE, et al. 2015 American Thyroid Association management guidelines for adult patients with thyroid nodules and differentiated thyroid cancer: the American Thyroid Association guidelines task force on thyroid nodules and differentiated thyroid cancer. Thyroid. 2016;26:1–133.
2. Pacini F, Schlumberger M, Dralle H, Elisei R, Smit JW, Wiersinga W. European consensus for the management of patients with differentiated thyroid carcinoma of the follicular epithelium. Eur J Endocrinol. 2006;154:787–803.
3. Mazzaferri EL, Kloos RT. Clinical review 128: current approaches to primary therapy for papillary and follicular thyroid cancer. J Clin Endocrinol Metab. 2001;86:1447–63.
4. Mazzaferri EL, Jhiang SM. Long-term impact of initial surgical and medical therapy on papillary and follicular thyroid cancer. Am J Med. 1994;97:418–28.
5. Komorowski RA, Hanson GA. Occult thyroid pathology in the young adult: an autopsy study of 138 patients without clinical thyroid disease. Hum Pathol. 1988;19:689–96.
6. Lang BH, Shek TW, Wan KY. Does microscopically involved margin increase disease recurrence after

curative surgery in papillary thyroid carcinoma? J Surg Oncol. 2016;113:635–9. https://doi.org/10.1002/jso.2419.

7. Kluijfhout WP, Pasternak JD, Kwon JS, Lim J, Shen WT, Gosnell JE, et al. Microscopic positive tumor margin does not increase the risk of recurrence in patients with T1-T2 well-differentiated thyroid cancer. Ann Surg Oncol. 2016;23:1446–51. https://doi.org/10.1245/s10434-015-4998-x.
8. Seethala RR, Asa SL, Carty SE, Hodak SP, McHugh JB, Richardson MS, et al. College of American Pathologist. Protocol for the examination of specimens from patients with carcinomas of the thyroid gland. 2017. http://www.cap.org/ShowProperty?nodePath=/UCMCon/Contribution%20Folders/WebContent/pdf/cp-thyroid-17protocol-4000.pdf. Accessed 28 June 2017.
9. Vural GU, Akkas BE, Ercakmak N, Basu S, Alavi A. Prognostic significance of FDG PET/CT on the follow-up of patients of differentiated thyroid carcinoma with negative 131I whole-body scan and elevated thyroglobulin levels: correlation with clinical and histopathologic characteristics and long-term follow-up data. Clin Nucl Med. 2012;37:953–9. https://doi.org/10.1097/RLU.0b013e31825b2057.
10. Bachelot A, Cailleux AF, Klain M, Baudin E, Ricard M, Bellon N, et al. Relationship between tumor burden and serum thyroglobulin level in patients with papillary and follicular thyroid carcinoma. Thyroid. 2002;12:707–11.
11. Giovanella L, Ceriani L, Ghelfo A, Maffioli M, Keller F. Preoperative undetectable serum thyroglobulin in differentiated thyroid carcinoma: incidence, causes and management strategy. Clin Endocrinol. 2007;67:547.

42 Low-Dose Radioiodine Therapy in Well-Differentiated Thyroid Carcinoma

Zehra Özcan and Ülkem Yararbaş

Abstract

Thyroid carcinomas are usually diagnosed in small sizes and accepted as low-risk disease without disease-related mortality. However, there has been still controversy regarding the optimal management of differentiated thyroid carcinoma both in surgical technique and the use of radioactive iodine ablation. Moreover, there is also uncertainty about what activity should be administered for ablative purposes. In the current case, after completing almost 7 years of clinical follow-up without evidence of disease recurrence, low-dose radioactive ablation in thyroid cancer patients is discussed under the relevant literature.

42.1 Case Presentation

A 53-year-old female with a history of nodular thyroid disease on both lobes was referred for diagnostic evaluation. An ultrasound-guided needle biopsy revealed suspicious findings suggesting malignancy. She underwent bilateral thyroidectomy. Surgical specimen revealed three foci of follicular variant of papillary carcinoma with diameters of 1.2, 0.6 and 0.3 cm distributed over left and right lobes. There was no evidence of cervical lymph node involvement and extra-thyroidal extension. According to the AJCC/UICC TNM system noted in ATA guideline 2015, she was defined as T2N0M0 and stage I [1]. Postoperative TSH was 57.05 μIU/mL (normal range: 0.35–5.50) and Tg was 3.82 ng/mL (normal range: 1.6–60). Anti-thyroglobulin antibody levels were not elevated. Two months after thyroidectomy, she received 29.7 mCi (1100 MBq) radioactive ablation therapy.

42.2 Discussion

Postsurgical radioactive iodine treatment has been playing an important role in differentiated thyroid carcinoma. It aims to destroy residual thyroid tissue therefore eliminating thyroglobulin secretion and iodine accumulation which are used as biomarkers in the follow-up setting [2–4]. However, there is no consensus regarding the amount of activity for ablation therapy [5, 6]. Mostly given in fixed doses, the low activity of

Z. Özcan (✉) · Ü. Yararbaş
Ege University School of Medicine, Department of Nuclear Medicine, Izmir, Turkey

T. Özülker et al. (eds.), *Thyroid and Parathyroid Diseases*, https://doi.org/10.1007/978-3-319-78476-2_42

I-131 ranged from 800 to 1100 MBq. Due to the potential side effects in the acute period after I-131 therapy such as salivary gland dysfunction or long-term carcinogenetic effects, there has been a trend to manage with low iodine doses in patients with low-risk DTC. Moreover, this approach has practical advantages as there is no need for hospitalization and decreased costs as well. In the revised guidelines by ATA in 2015, this approach has appeared as a strong recommendation with high quality evidence, and it has been stated that low-dose I-131 remnant ablation has been generally favoured in patients with low-risk or intermediate-risk profile who had total thyroidectomy [1]. It has also been well-established that ablation therapy may not be indicated in patients with micropapillary carcinoma without high-risk features. In their meta-analysis reviewing nine randomized trials, Cheng et al. documented that low-dose strategy with 1100 MBq I-131 was sufficient to achieve remnant ablation with similar efficacy to 3700 MBq radioiodine activity [7]. While focusing on the success rate of ablation dose, they have found that 3700 MBq activity provided 7% higher rate than 1100 MBq activity if the negative I-131 scan was used alone (RR, 0.93, [0.87, 0.98]; *p*: 0.16). However, the authors have concluded that this high rate of ablation might not be remarkable when side effects of high dose or hospital stay are taken into account [7]. On the other hand, in the study of Fallahi et al., the difference between the success rates of 1100 and 3700 MBq was significant (39 vs 68%, respectively) [8]. It seems that the extent of thyroid surgery, patient selection and criteria used in defining successful ablation may be responsible for these different rates. It has also been found that a single 800 MBq I-131 provided 58% success rate in low-risk DTC when negative ultrasound, undetectable Tg and negative iodine uptake or scan is defined as successful ablative treatment [9]. However, most of the studies did not provide data for long-term effects, as the assessment of ablation success was limited for 6–12 months. Regarding the therapeutic outcome in the long term in a prospective comparison of 1100, 2200 and 3700 MBq I-131, respectively, Kukulska et al. have demonstrated no significant differences in the 5 years efficacy [10]. However, the number of patients requiring a second course of radioiodine was higher in patients who received initially low activity. While focusing on success rate and long-term clinical outcome, Han et al. showed that low-dose RAI therapy equally well-performed in patients with small DTC having an extra-thyroidal extension [11]. No significant difference was found between the low- and high-dose groups. More importantly, clinical recurrence was not observed in both groups in the follow-up after a median of 7.2 years. Overall, the published data so far implied that successful ablation rate provided with 1100 MBq was not inferior to 3700 MBq I-131. The results were also similar in trials using recombinant TSH (rhTSH) during preparation prior to I-131 ablation [12, 13]. Mallick et al. conducted a randomized study comparing low- and high-dose radioiodine treatment combined with thyroid hormone withdrawal or thyrotropin alfa [12]. The authors showed that remnant ablation was similarly successful in groups receiving low-dose and high-dose treatment (85.0% and 88.9%, respectively). The success rate was also almost similar to those with thyrotropin alfa and thyroid hormone withdrawal groups (87.1% and 86.7%, respectively). However, higher rate of adverse effects including neck pain and nausea was noted in patients undergoing high-dose treatment. In agreement with these results, the randomized prospective study of Schlumberger et al. also indicated that low-dose RAI ablative therapy in combination with rhTSH represents an effective and attractive option providing good quality of life [13]. The use of rhTSH instead of T4 withdrawal has the advantage of eliminating hypothyroidism before ablation therefore improves the quality of daily life. In ATA guideline 2015, rhTSH is recommended strongly with the moderate quality of evidence in ATA low-risk and intermediate-risk patients without extensive lymph node involvement in whom ablation therapy is planned [1]. It is stated that rhTSH provides superior shorter-term quality of life, non-inferiority of remnant ablation and potentially no remarkable difference in the long-term outcomes. Moreover, recently Wang et al. published a retrospective data covering patients also with extra-thyroidal extension and positive lymph nodes [14]. They have found that 1100 MBq activity was not inferior to high-dose ablation even in patients with microscopic ETE and pre-ablative stimulated serum Tg <5 ng/mL irrespective of the lymph node metastases. This observation was parallel with the published data of Rosaria et al. showing that low-dose ablation was efficient in a group of patients with stage T3 and/or N1 papillary thyroid carcinoma [15]. On the other hand, some authors underline the lack of long-term prospective studies and, therefore, propose not to change standard 3700 MBq ablation dose particularly given the trend towards less aggressive surgery which results in more remnant thyroid tissue [6]. It is suggested that individualized dose assessment fitting to the patient needs considering long-term surveillance and quality of life with a lower cost should be integrated in clinical practice.

42.3 Follow-Up and Clinical Course

In the current case, low-dose ablative therapy provided success rate after a single course of RAI. Whole-body scan obtained at 12 months after remnant ablation was negative in agreement with undetectable serum Tg level (Figs. 42.1 and 42.2). She continued with L-thyroxine treatment and currently completed 7 years of therapy without evidence of recurrent disease. At the final clinical visit, serum Tg was <0.1 ng/mL when she is on T4 and neck ultrasound obtained yearly was negative supporting long-term efficacy of low-dose ablation therapy.

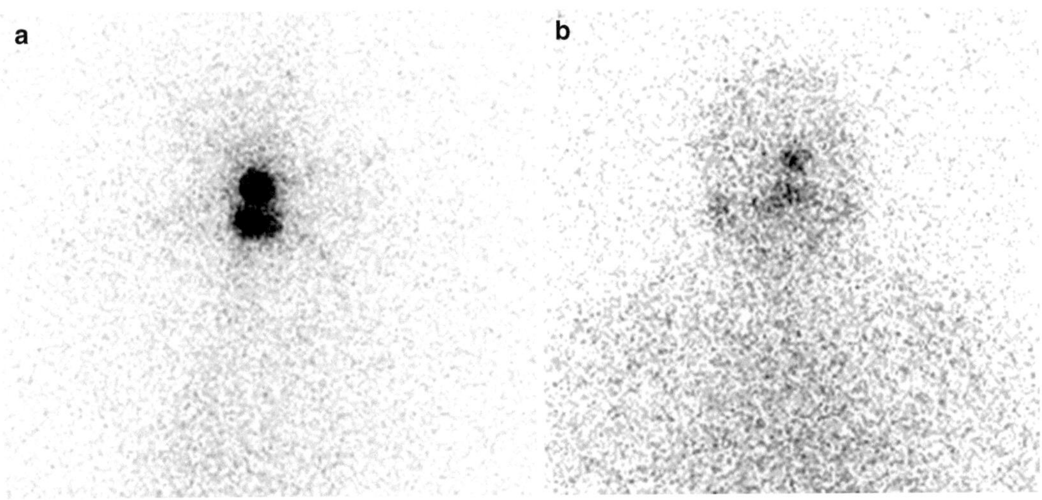

Fig. 42.1 Post-ablative I-131 scan (**a**) showing iodine accumulation in thyroid bed and follow-up diagnostic I-131 at 12 months is presented. Follow-up scan (**b**) obtained while T4 off, shows no evidence of remnant tissue in agreement with undetectable serum Tg

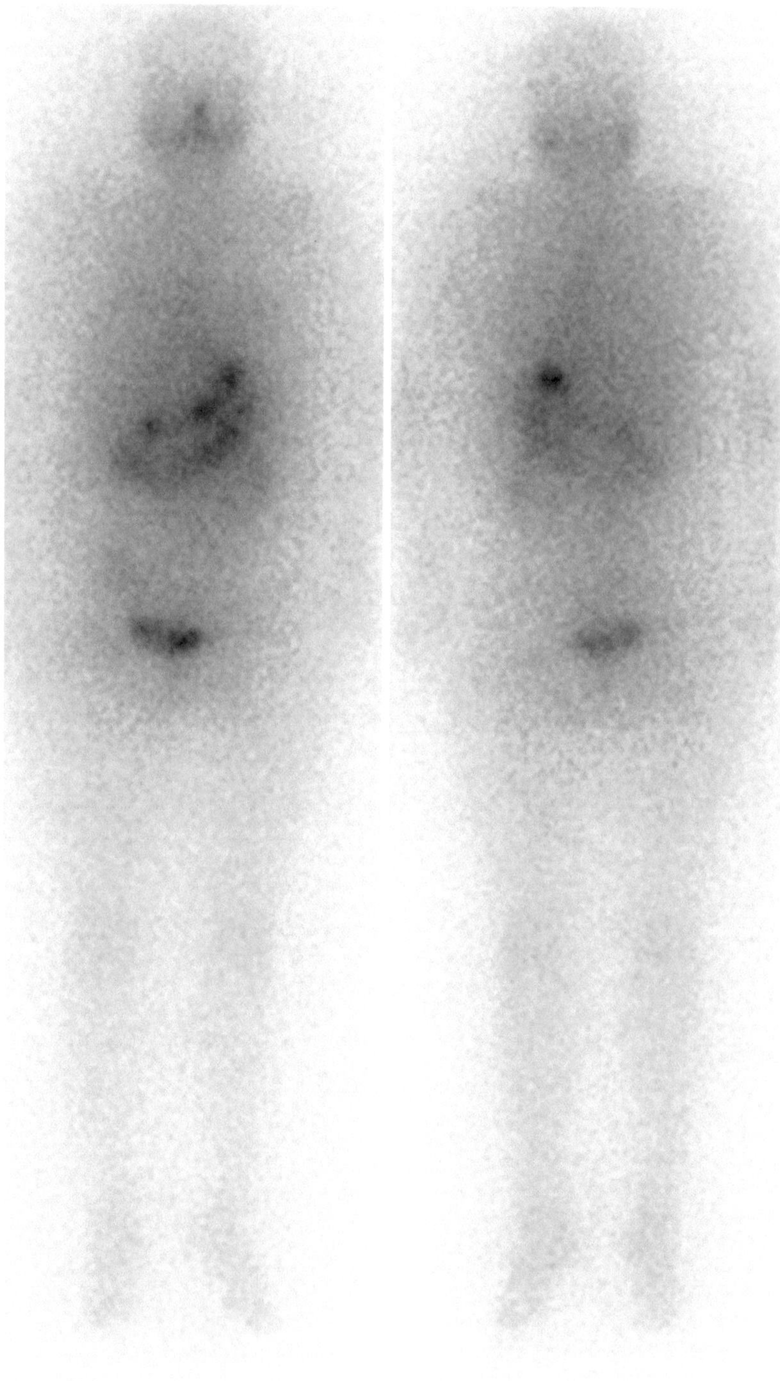

Fig. 42.2 Diagnostic whole-body scan obtained at 12 months after remnant ablation with radioiodine

What Can We Learn from This Case?

- Ablation therapy with low-dose RAI provides similar success rate in comparison with high dose in patients with low-risk DTC.
- This approach has the advantages of fewer side effects in the early post-treatment, short hospital stay and reduced medical costs. While long-term prospective studies are limited, late occurrence of secondary neoplasms theoretically will also be of less concern when low-dose RAI is given.
- The current literature shows also promising results for low-dose ablation therapy combined with rhTSH instead of T4 withdrawal. This approach, when available, may be a reasonable option as symptoms of hypothyroid state before RAI is eliminated.

References

1. Haugen BR, Sawka AM, Alexander EK, Bible KC, Caturegli P, Doherty GM, et al. American Thyroid Association guidelines on the management of thyroid nodules and differentiated thyroid cancer task force review and recommendation on the proposed renaming of encapsulated follicular variant papillary thyroid carcinoma without invasion to noninvasive follicular thyroid neoplasm with papillary-like nuclear features. Thyroid. 2017;27:481–3. https://doi.org/10.1089/thy.2016.0628.
2. Mazzaferri EL. Thyroid remnant 131I ablation for papillary and follicular thyroid carcinoma. Thyroidology. 1997;7:265–71.
3. Goldsmith SJ. To ablate or not to ablate: issues and evidence involved in 131I ablation of residual thyroid tissue in patients with differentiated thyroid carcinoma. Semin Nucl Med. 2011;41:96–104.
4. Gulec S, Kuker R. Radioactive iodine remnant ablation: the beta-knife completion thyroidectomy. Mol Imaging Radionucl Ther. 2017;26(Suppl 1):16–23. https://doi.org/10.4274/2017.26.suppl.03.
5. Haymart MR, Esfandiari NH, Stang MT, Sosa JA. Controversies in the management of low-risk differentiated thyroid cancer. Endocr Rev. 2017;38:351–78. https://doi.org/10.1210/er.2017-00067.
6. Blumhardt R, Wolin EA, Phillips WT, Salman UA, Walker RC, Stack BC Jr, et al. Current controversies in the initial post-surgical radioactive iodine therapy for thyroid cancer: a narrative review. Endocr Relat Cancer. 2014;21:R473–84. https://doi.org/10.1530/ERC-14-0286.
7. Cheng W, Ma C, Fu H, Li J, Chen S, Wu S, Wang H. Low- or high-dose radioiodine remnant ablation for differentiated thyroid carcinoma: a meta-analysis. J Clin Endocrinol Metab. 2013;98:1353–60. https://doi.org/10.1210/jc.2012-3682.
8. Fallahi B, Beiki D, Takavar A, Fard-Esfahani A, Gilani KA, Saghari M, et al. Low versus high radioiodine dose in postoperative ablation of residual thyroid tissue in patients with differentiated thyroid carcinoma: a large randomized clinical trial. Nucl Med Commun. 2012;33:275–82. https://doi.org/10.1097/MNM.0b013e32834e306a.
9. Caglar M, Bozkurt FM, Akca CK, Vargol SE, Bayraktar M, Ugur O, et al. Comparison of 800 and 3700 MBq iodine-131 for the postoperative ablation of thyroid remnant in patients with low-risk differentiated thyroid cancer. Nucl Med Commun. 2012;33:268–74. https://doi.org/10.1097/MNM.0b013e32834ec5d6.
10. Kukulska A, Krajewska J, Gawkowska-Suwińska M, Puch Z, Paliczka-Cieslik E, Roskosz J, et al. Radioiodine thyroid remnant ablation in patients with differentiated thyroid carcinoma (DTC): prospective comparison of long-term outcomes of treatment with 30, 60 and 100 mCi. Thyroid Res. 2010;31:9. https://doi.org/10.1186/1756-6614-3-9.
11. Han JM, Kim WG, Kim TY, Jeon MJ, Ryu JS, Song DE, et al. Effects of low-dose and high-dose postoperative radioiodine therapy on the clinical outcome in patients with small differentiated thyroid cancer having microscopic extrathyroidal extension. Thyroid. 2014;24:820–5. https://doi.org/10.1089/thy.2013.0362.
12. Mallick U, Harmer C, Yap B, Wadsley J, Clarke S, Moss L, et al. Ablation with low-dose radioiodine and thyrotropin alfa in thyroid cancer. N Engl J Med. 2012;366:1674–85. https://doi.org/10.1056/NEJMoa1109589.
13. Schlumberger M, Catargi B, Borget I, Deandreis D, Zerdoud S, Bridji B, et al. Strategies of radioiodine ablation in patients with low-risk thyroid cancer. N Engl J Med. 2012;366:1663–73. https://doi.org/10.1056/NEJMoa1108586.
14. Wang C, Zhao T, Li H, Gao W, Lin Y. Low activity versus high activity: noninferior response to radioiodine therapy in differentiated patients with extrathyroid extension. Nucl Med Commun. 2017;38:366–71. https://doi.org/10.1097/MNM.0000000000000666.
15. Rosário PW, Calsolari MR. Thyroid ablation with 1.1 GBq (30 mCi) iodine-131 in patients with papillary thyroid carcinoma at intermediate risk for recurrence. Thyroid. 2014;24:826–31. https://doi.org/10.1089/thy.2013.0479.

43 Dosimetric Approach in Metastatic Differentiated Thyroid Cancer and Hyperthyroidism

Haluk B. Sayman, Nami Yeyin, and Mohammad Abuqbeitah

Abstract

Radioiodine (^{131}I) therapy has been widely used for well-differentiated thyroid cancer and its metastases for many years. Two approaches, namely, *empirical dosage* and *dosimetry-based* methods, are currently utilized to manage the therapeutic iodine activity.

Empirical dosage is based on the physician's rating to suggest appropriate activity within a certain range of without individualized dose planning. On the other hand, dosimetry-based approach implicates effective activity administration leaning on specific activity regulated by the organs at risk.

In this report, we propose and define dosimetry-based treatment with examples of differentiated thyroid cancer and hyperthyroidism cases.

Our results indicated that the implementation of dosimetry protocol might help to administer larger amounts of activity controlled by critical organ dose limits, thereby delivering lethal dose to tumors with no toxicity. It is also well demonstrated that dosimetric approach is favorable for hyperthyroid patients in order to deliver right amount of radioiodine activity for efficient therapeutical response.

43.1 Introduction

Radioiodine (^{131}I) therapy has been widely used for well-differentiated thyroid cancer and its metastases for many years. Its main purpose is to destroy thyroid gland residues and possible distant metastases after near-total thyroidectomy. Two approaches are currently utilized to manage the therapeutic iodine activity for differentiated thyroid cancer treatment; these are *empirical dosage* and *dosimetry-based* methods.

Empirical dosage is the most widespread strategy and based on the physician's rating to suggest appropriate activity within a certain range of GBqs (normally 1.11–9.25 GBq) without individualized dose planning.

Unlikely, dosimetry approach implicates effective activity administration leaning on specific activity regulated by the organs at risk. Personalized dosimetric studies have been introduced early since 1962 by Benua et al. In their study, red marrow was reported as critical organ, and the radiation dose was limited to 2 Gy after radioiodine therapy of thyroid cancer. Most often,

H. B. Sayman (✉) · N. Yeyin · M. Abuqbeitah
Department of Nuclear Medicine,
Cerrahpaşa Medical Faculty, Istanbul University,
Istanbul, Turkey

T. Özülker et al. (eds.), *Thyroid and Parathyroid Diseases*, https://doi.org/10.1007/978-3-319-78476-2_43

the critical amount of radioiodine activity is required in cases of differentiated thyroid cancer (DTC) with metastases.

Maxon et al. [1] reported a comprehensive study for tumor dose and related response. In this study, the relationship between the delivered radiation dose to the target tissue and the clinical outcome was evaluated in 76 patients after radioiodine therapy. Briefly, the desired clinical outcomes were successfully achieved in patients receiving approximately 300 Gy for residual thyroid tissue and a minimum of 80 Gy for metastatic thyroid cancer.

43.2 Dosimetry Methods

43.2.1 Thyroid Ablation Dosimetry

MIRD (Medical Internal Radiation Dose) method is the most common technique to calculate the absorbed dose of thyroid residues. Accordingly, the amount of activity required to deliver 300 Gy for ablation can be calculated using these equations:

$$D_t = \sum_s \widetilde{A}_t \cdot S_{t \leftarrow S}$$

$$S_{t \leftarrow S} = \frac{k \sum_i n_i E_i \phi_i}{m_t}$$

$\widetilde{A}$ is the cumulative activity, $S_{t \leftarrow S}$ dose factor Gy/MBq-s [dose from source (s) to target (t)], n energy abundance per nuclear decay, E radiation energy (MeV), ϕ fraction of energy absorption by the target, m mass of the target organ (kg), and k dose constant (Gy-kg/MBq-s-MeV)

The cumulative activity $\widetilde{A}$ accounts for the total number of I-131 disintegrations in the remaining tissue. Thyroid uptake probe device might be easily operated to pursue the uptake and elimination of the radioactivity. Dosimetry commences with oral administration of ~100 μCi ^{131}I. Subsequent measures are then recorded from the neck and thigh at several time marks following administration (2, 24, 72, 144, 168 h). The obtained counts are used to derive the amount of corresponding activity to the measurement time. Finally, fitting curves are generated over time activity plots (Fig. 43.1). Finally,

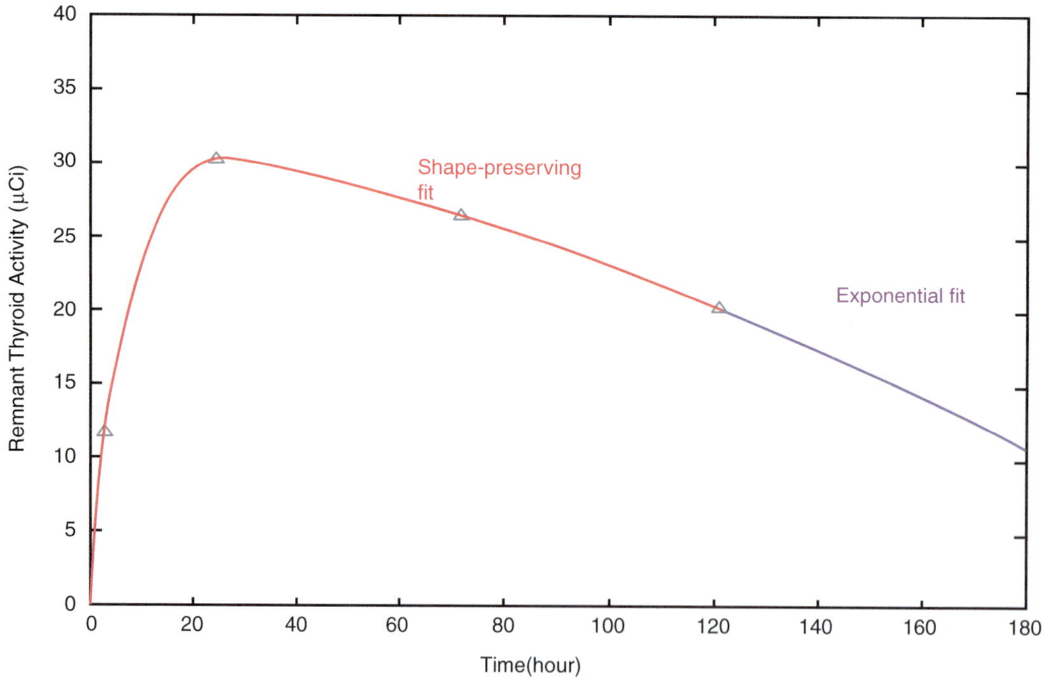

Fig. 43.1 Thyroid uptake over time (shape-preserving fit). After the last measurement point, the activity release was evaluated with physical decay (exponential fitting)

fitting curves are generated over time activity plots , to find the cumulative activity (area under the curve) (Fig. 43.1). It should be kept in mind that the activity after the last measurement time is assumed to have sole physical decay.

The *S* factors of variable residual tissue volumes can be reproduced by fitting the known volume with a corresponding specific dose values generated by Monte Carlo simulations. The volume of thyroid tissue can be estimated by radiological modalities such as CT, MR, etc. or planar scintigraphy. Finally, unit density sphere model is the readily available method for sphere-like dose calculations with a density of 1 g/cm^3.

43.2.2 Metastatic Thyroid Cancer Dosimetry

Treatment of metastatic differentiated thyroid cancer implies administration of larger amount of iodine activities. Thus, application of this regime ought to be performed without exceeding the maximum tolerated dose of the organ at risk, which is red marrow. In general, MIRD method is widely applied for calculating the absorbed dose of red marrow and consequently the maximum safe activity that delivers 2 Gy to red marrow. The following equation below reported by Wessels et al. [2] can also be used to estimate red marrow dose:

$$D_{\text{Rm}} = D_{\text{Rm}}(\text{self}) + D_{\text{Rm}}(\text{Cross})$$

$$D_{\text{Rm}} = \breve{A}_{\text{bl}} \times \frac{\text{RMECFF}}{1-\text{HCT}} \times \left(\frac{1.5}{5.2}\right) \times S_{\text{RM}\leftarrow\text{RM}} \times \frac{70}{M_{\text{wb patient}}}$$

$$D_{\text{Rmcross}} = \left\{ \breve{A}\text{wb} - \left[\breve{A}_{\text{bl}}\right] \times \frac{\text{RMECFF}}{1-\text{HCT}} \left(\frac{1.5}{70}\right) \times M_{\text{wb}} \right\} \times S_{(\text{Rm}\leftarrow\text{RB})}$$

$$S_{(\text{Rm}\leftarrow\text{RB})} = \begin{cases} S(\text{RM}\leftarrow\text{WB}) \times \left(\dfrac{1}{1-\left(\dfrac{1.5}{70}\right)} \right) \\ -S(\text{RM}\leftarrow\text{RM}) \times \left(\dfrac{\left(\dfrac{1.5}{70}\right)}{1-\left(\dfrac{1.5}{70}\right)} \right) \end{cases}$$

D_{Rm} is the red marrow dose, $\breve{A}_{\text{bl}}$ blood cumulative activity in the blood, HCT hematocrit value, $S_{(\text{RM} \leftarrow \text{RM})}$ bone marrow self-dose factor for man phantom (0.00001725 mGy/MBq-s), M_{wb} patient weight, $\breve{A}_{\text{wb}}$ total body cumulative activity, $[\breve{A}_{\text{bl}}]$ blood cumulative activity concentration [kg^{-1}], and $S_{(\text{Rm}\leftarrow\text{WB})}$ *S* dose factor of whole body to bone marrow. Such a correction should be made to express *S* value for the remainder of body as mass dependent when using Wessels et al. model. So $S_{(\text{Rm} \leftarrow \text{RB})}$ can be expressed as $(3.26 \times 10^{-5}/\text{M}_{\text{wb patient}})$.

Ultimately, the predicted absorbed dose is depending on the accumulated activity and the range of energy release in the target. To note that some references exclusively recommend incorporating whole blood cumulated activity for accurate red marrow self-dose estimation in radioiodine therapy.

43.3 Case Study of Metastatic Thyroid Cancer Dosimetry

A 19-year-old female patient previously had been treated for follicular thyroid cancer and later visited the department for the periodical follow-up. The blood tests showed an elevated Tg level (74 ng/ml) in addition to large bone lesions detected in the pelvis and sternum on the ^{131}I whole-body scintigraphy.

The patient was subjected to pre-therapeutic dosimetry protocol to optimize an effective, safe activity. Approximately 74 MBq of radioiodine was measured using a dose calibrator (Capintec

CRzC25, Florham Park, NJ, USA). After a few hours of fasting, the radiotracer was administered orally, and the patient was isolated in a lead shielded room. Patients abstained from consuming food or drink and micturition during the first 2 h after radiotracer administration in order to perform the first whole-body scintigraphy. Blood samples were withdrawn in conjunction with scintigraphy and kept in heparinized tubes. Whole-body scintigraphy was acquired with 10 cm/min scan speed using dual-detector gamma camera equipped with high-energy parallel hole collimator (Siemens Symbia T16, Erlangen, Germany). Settings of single 364 KeV energy photopeak, 15% window width, and matrix size of 256 × 1024 were selected for imaging parameters. Series of whole-body scintigraphy were carried out at 6, 24, 48, 72, and 96 h following radioiodine administration (Fig. 43.2). SPECT/CT acquisition was performed on the region with enhanced uptake to estimate the lesion volume via fused SPECT/CT slices. Volume determination was made by 3D iso-contour technique and the threshold adjusted to 40% for all lesions. Blood samples (2 ml) were collected further after scintigraphy and kept for measurement under uniform background. An aliquot of 0.5 ml was withdrawn from each blood sample and counted. Then decay-corrected counts were multiplied by a calibration factor which was found experimentally using an ^{131}I phantom. OLINDA/EXM code was used for absorbed dose calculation of red marrow and lesions. No scatter or spilled out correction was applied.

Red marrow dose was calculated 0.087 mGy/MBq, and thereby the maximum safe activity was 310 mCi with respect to the dose limit of red marrow (2 Gy). The absorbed doses of both sternal and pelvic lesions were 9 and 11 Gy, respectively. The decided activity for therapy was 150 mCi in which the expected dose to red marrow would be 0.97 Gy and the delivered dose to both lesions would be 675 and 825 Gy, respectively. The Tg value after therapy was 1.02 ng/ml, and the lesions showed complete regression.

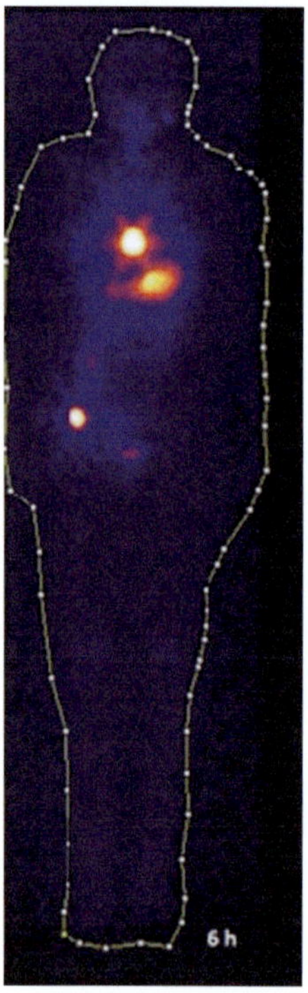

Fig. 43.2 Whole-body scintigraphy after 48 h

43.4 Case Study of Hyperthyroidism Dosimetry

The 34-year-old female patient was diagnosed with Graves' disease and referred to radioiodine therapy. The blood tests showed TSH level 0.01 μIU/ml, FT3 level 30 pg/ml, and FT4 level was 3.45 ng/dl. Dosimetry-based therapy plan was organized involving radiotracer administration of 0.3 MBq and quantitated by thyroid uptake probe. Five uptake measurements were acquired over 1 week, and the volume of the thyroid gland was measured by ultrasound. The activity turnover in thyroid gland was very slow, where the effective half-life was calculated as 180 h. Dose calculation was made relying on the whole gland volume and the activity residence time. Accordingly, the administered activity was calculated as 7 mCi to deliver 200 Gy for an efficient therapeutical response.

43.5 Discussion and Conclusion

The implementation of dosimetry protocol might help to administer larger amounts of activity controlled by red marrow dose limit, thereby delivering a lethal dose to tumors with no toxicity. On the other hand, empirical dosage regime is deemed simple and practical but blind to consider the individuality of patients. Moreover, subsequent therapies with low doses induce lesion uptake reduction and suboptimal response. This might support the rationale of maximum activity administration equal/or somewhat less than the estimated maximum safe activity for patients with distal metastases. In condition of thyroid ablation, dosimetry-oriented therapy interestingly demonstrated optimum response with low activity level that would replace the traditionally followed criteria of excessive needless doses.

A set of relevant limitations should be addressed under the dosimetry concept, such as lesion's structure and heterogeneity or nonuniform dose distribution in the targeted tumors. However, pretreatment dosimetry provides useful information about the radioiodine biokinetics in blood, whole body, and cancerous lesions. Furthermore, the joining red marrow and lesion dosimetry approaches seem worthwhile to optimize the prescribed activity and to avoid unnecessary exposure to the internal organs.

Ultimately, patient-specific therapy is more advantageous to the empirical regime as higher activities can be safely administered in one strike instead of multiple therapies with low activities and deteriorated outcomes.

References

1. Maxon HR, Thomas SR, Hertzberg VS, Kereiakes JG, Chen IW, Sperling MI, Saenger EL. Relation between effective radiation dose and outcome of radioiodine therapy for thyroid cancer. N Engl J Med. 1983;309:937–41. https://doi.org/10.1056/NEJM198310203091601.
2. Wessels BW, Bolch WE, Bouchet LG, Breitz HB, DeNardo GL, Meredith RF. Bone marrow dosimetry using blood-based models for radiolabeled antibody therapy: a multiinstitutional comparison. J Nucl Med. 2004;45:1725–33.

44

Anti-thyroglobulin Antibody Positivity During Follow-Up of a Patient with Differentiated Thyroid Cancer

Gülin Uçmak and B. Büşra Demirel

Abstract

Serum thyroglobulin (Tg) measurement is the most important and sensitive marker of persistent and/or recurrent disease in the follow-up of differentiated thyroid cancer (DTC) after total thyroidectomy and radioiodine ablation of remnant tissue. However, in the presence of increased level of serum anti-thyroglobulin antibody (TgAb), serum Tg cannot be used reliably as a tumor marker of DTC. On the follow-up of patients with DTC, the standard and useful practice is measuring the levels of both Tg and TgAb. The main source of TgAb positivity is lymphocytic infiltration of thyroid tissue. The increased level of TgAb is also associated with continuing lymphocytic memory cell reply or a low load of thyroid remnant. In patients with a preexisting autoimmune thyroid disease, most of them lose their TgAb positivity during the period up to 2–3 years on follow-up in association with the disappearance of thyroid tissue and its antigenic components after total thyroidectomy and RAI ablation. Therefore, prolonged positive TgAb levels or being positive in follow-up may indicate the recurrent and/or metastatic disease and may be a prognostic indicator of worse outcome. In case of persistent and/or rising TgAb positivity with undetectable Tg levels, especially without preexisting autoimmune thyroiditis, patients must be monitored closely and examined by imaging modalities such as neck ultrasound, and/or CT, MR, and F-18 FDG PET/CT for recurrence.

G. Uçmak (✉) · B. B. Demirel
Department of Nuclear Medicine, University of Health Sciences (SBÜ) Dr. Abdurrahman Yurtaslan Ankara Oncology Training and Research Hospital, Ankara, Turkey

44.1 Case Presentation

A 69-year-old female patient, diagnosed with papillary thyroid cancer with areas of poorly differentiated features and vascular invasion, without lymph node metastasis and lymphocytic infiltration of thyroid tissue, was referred to our clinic for radioiodine ablation therapy (RAT) following total thyroidectomy. At the time of diagnosis, stimulated serum thyroglobulin (Tg) level was 464 ng/ml, and anti-thyroglobulin antibody (TgAb) level was <20 IU/ml. Because of the poor histopathological parameters and high postoperative serum Tg level, the patient was considered in high-risk group and received 200 mCi (7.4 GBq) RAT.

T. Özülker et al. (eds.), *Thyroid and Parathyroid Diseases*, https://doi.org/10.1007/978-3-319-78476-2_44

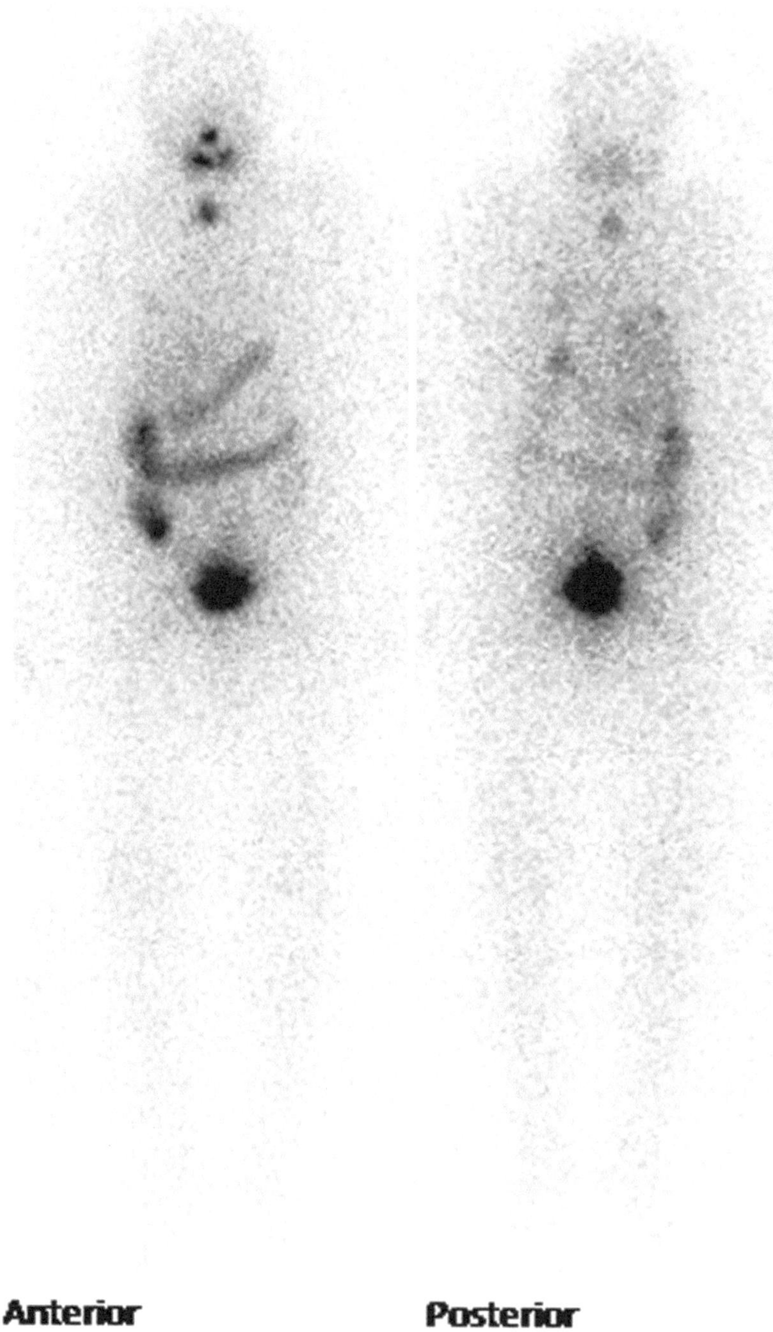

Fig. 44.1 Focal radioiodine uptake in thyroid bed and heterogeneous thoracic uptake suspicious for lung metastasis were seen on anterior and posterior images of WBS acquired after 200 mCi radioiodine ablation treatment

On the post-therapy whole body scan (WBS), focal iodine uptake in right thyroid lobe site and heterogeneous thoracic uptake suspicious of lung metastasis were seen (Fig. 44.1). On follow-up, serum Tg and TgAb levels were 16 ng/ml and 31 IU/ml on L-thyroxine therapy, respectively. One year after the first radioiodine (RAI) treatment, a 250 mCi (9.2 GBq) dose of I-131 was administered for the persistence of high Tg level. On posttreatment scan, iodine uptake was seen only in the thyroid bed.

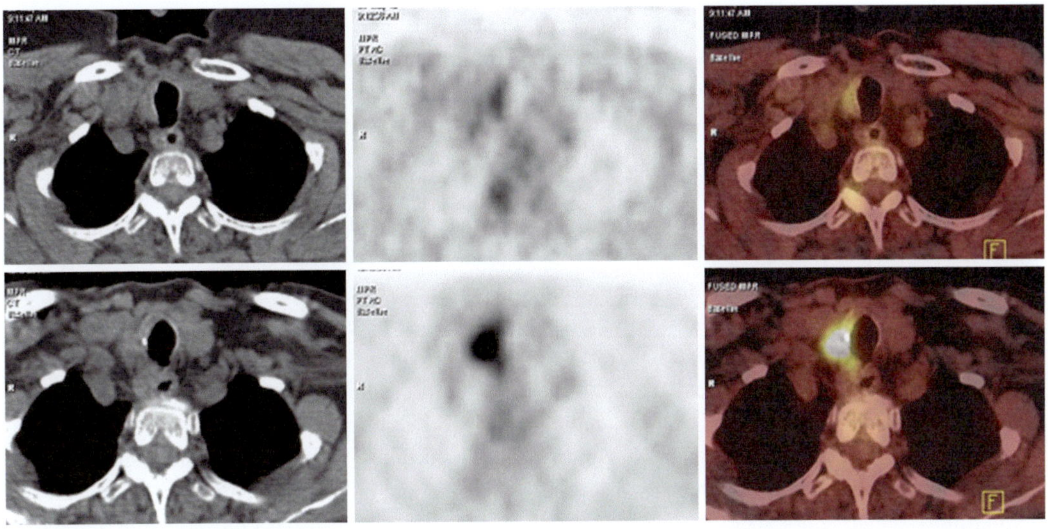

Fig. 44.2 Upper row demonstrates axial slices of initial FDG PET/CT study which was performed to evaluate the cause of TgAb manifestation seen on follow-up with undetectable Tg levels. A hypermetabolic soft tissue lesion with ill-defined margins was observed in the right paratracheal region (SUVmax: 4.09) matching local recurrence. On follow-up PET/CT (lower row), significant increase in size and metabolic activity was observed on the right paratracheal lesion (SUVmax: 7.91). The patient was referred to surgery following the final progress

On follow-up, 15 months after diagnosis, suppressed Tg levels decreased to <0.2 ng/ml and TgAb increased to 192 IU/ml. No abnormal finding was seen on neck ultrasound (USG). The patient underwent F-18 FDG (fluorodeoxyglucose) positron emission tomography/computed tomography (PET/CT) imaging in order to evaluate the etiology of progressively rising TgAb level on follow-up. On PET/CT, a hypermetabolic soft tissue lesion with ill-defined margins was observed in the right paratracheal area (SUVmax: 4.09) (Fig. 44.2). Surgery was not planned due to the millimetric size of the lesion and surgical morbidity. A 250 mCi RAI dose was given in consensus with surgeons and nuclear medicine physicians. At that time, stimulated serum Tg was 136 ng/dl, and TgAb level was 2418 IU/ml. The iodine uptake on thyroid bed was similar to previous post-therapy scans. No abnormal finding was observed in concurrent neck USG. A follow-up PET/CT was acquired to monitor treatment response. On PET/CT, a significant increase in size and metabolic activity was observed in the right paratracheal lesion (SUVmax: 7.91) (Fig. 44.2).

44.2 Discussion

Serum thyroglobulin (Tg) measurement is the most important and sensitive marker of persistent and/or recurrent disease in the follow-up of differentiated thyroid cancer (DTC) after total thyroidectomy and RAI ablation of remnant tissue [1]. However, the presence of increased levels of serum TgAb is more frequently observed in patients with DTC than in general population, and TgAb positivity is known to influence the accurate measurement of serum Tg [2, 3]. Serum Tg cannot be used reliably as a tumor marker of DTC in the presence of TgAb [4]. It is a standard and useful practice to measure the levels of both Tg and TgAb in the follow-up of DTC.

Lymphocytic infiltration of thyroid tissue is the main source of TgAb presence, and the production of TgAb is related to the immune system. The increased level of TgAb is also associated with continuing lymphocytic memory cell reply or low load of thyroid remnant [5]. It was reported that detectable TgAb level is observed in 10–25% of the patients with DTC [2]. Recurrent disease is also determined approximately in 20–30% in these patients [6]. Most of the patients with a pre-existing autoimmune thyroid disease lose their TgAb positivity during the follow-up in association with the disappearance of thyroid tissue and its antigenic components after total thyroidectomy and RAI ablation. The median disappearance time is about 3 years for TgAb [7]. Therefore, sustained positive or increasing TgAb levels may indicate recurrent and/or metastatic disease and may be a prognostic indicator of poor outcome as observed in our patient [8]. Although it is reported that increased TgAb can be used as an alternative of the tumor marker of DTC, TgAb cannot replace Tg, because TgAb indicates the activity of the immune system [1]. Moreover, TgAb is neither more sensitive nor specific than increased Tg level in estimating persistent disease.

There is no accepted consensus on the management and follow-up in patients with negative Tg but increased TgAb after thyroidectomy and RAT in DTC. Therefore, both Tg and TgAb measurements might be useful during follow-up in patients with DTC. It is a clinically challenging problem to manage patients, who persistently have increased TgAb, and these patients may require individualized management. Thus, it might be emphasized that if TgAb levels proceed persistently high or have a tendency to rise in follow-up, detailed research should be carried out to detect possible recurrent disease. It is especially important in patients with negative Tg and negative I-131 whole body scan (WBS) who don't have preexisting autoimmune thyroid disease and underwent thyroidectomy followed by RAI ablation at least 3 years ago. In our case, TgAb was negative at the time of diagnosis, but it turned out to be positive 15 months after diagnosis and persistently increased on follow-up.

Iodine-131 WBS is the most commonly used imaging study in the evaluation of remnant tissue and metastatic disease in patients with DTC. The specificity of I-131 WBS is 96–100%, and sensitivity range is between 45% and 75% [9]. However, many patients with increased Tg or TgAb have negative WBS in the presence of residual-recurrent and/or metastatic disease. The reasons for negative WBS may be small lesion volume and insufficient TSH stimulation. Because of limited spatial resolution of I-131 scan, small lesions can be missed. I-131 WBS also may be negative or unable to determine metastasis in low or dedifferentiated tumors. Neck USG is still the primary imaging modality to detect tumor recurrence and/or regional lymph nodes in DTC. But its accuracy is dependent on the physician and is not able to detect distant disease. The method of choice to image iodine negative or dedifferentiated tumors and to determine the extent of disease is F-18 FDG PET/CT [10, 11].

According to the American Thyroid Association (ATA) guidelines, F-18 FDG PET/CT is clinically useful for the detection of regional lymph node metastasis or distant metastasis in patients with TSH stimulated serum Tg levels higher than 10 ng/ml after RAT [10]. It is reported that the sensitivity of FDG PET for detection of metastasis in case of elevated Tg for all patients was 77%, and in case of elevated Tg but negative WBS it increased to 88% [9]. However, there are few publications about the usefulness of F-18 FDG PET/CT in patients with increased TgAb. According to the ATA guidelines, in patients with undetectable Tg levels but with persistent TgAb, the level of serum Tg cannot be reliably assessed, and F-18 FDG-PET may localize disease in some of them [10]. Recently in a study, the sensitivity, specificity, and accuracy of F-18 FDG PET/CT were 71%, 100%, and 78%, respectively, for detection of recurrence in patients with increased TgAb and negative radioiodine scan [12]. In few studies, no relation was seen between serum TgAb level and FDG PET/CT findings, and it was observed that Tg level was increased while TgAb level was stable under TSH stimulation as seen in our case [13, 14]. Also, timing measurement of TgAb may have an effect on the prevalence of positive TgAb levels in patients with DTC after treatment. Previous studies demonstrated that elevated TgAb levels were decreased to undetectable levels on 2–3 years after thyroidectomy followed by radioiodine therapy in most of the patients [7, 15]. The rapid decrease of TgAb levels along with therapy might be a favorable indicator whereas persistently high TgAb levels might account for the evidence of recurrent disease and a poor prognosis. However, the cutoff value for positive TgAb has not been determined in previously published studies, and various TgAb levels ranging between 6 IU/ml and 140 IU/ml have been reported [3, 15, 16]. It must be kept in mind that TgAb positivity may not be directly correlated with the tumor load and it indicates the activity of the immune system. Nevertheless, the patient who has elevated TgAb levels, especially without preexisting autoimmune thyroiditis, must be monitored closely for the recurrent disease on follow-up.

44.3 Follow-Up and Outcome

Due to radiological progression and biochemical progression with pathologically increased TgAb levels, the patient was referred to surgery for recurrent disease.

What Can We Learn from This Case?

- Serum TgAb levels must be monitored combined with serum Tg levels in the postsurgical staging and on follow-up of patients with differentiated thyroid cancers.
- Serum Tg levels cannot be reliable in the presence of TgAb positivity, and persistently increased TgAb levels may indicate recurrent and/or metastatic disease. However, TgAb cannot replace Tg as a marker for tumor recurrence since TgAb may arise from the activity of the immune system particularly in the early follow-up period up to 2–3 years.
- In case of persistent and/or rising TgAb positivity with undetectable Tg levels, patients must be carefully examined by imaging modalities such as neck USG, and/or CT, MR, and F-18 FDG PET/CT for recurrence.

References

1. Verburg FA, Luster M, Cupini C, Chiovato L, Duntas L, Elisei R, et al. Implications of thyroglobulin antibody positivity in patients with differentiated thyroid cancer: a clinical position statement. Thyroid. 2013;23:1211–25. https://doi.org/10.1089/thy.2012.0606.
2. Spencer CA. Clinical review: clinical utility of thyroglobulin antibody (TgAb) measurements for patients with differentiated thyroid cancers (DTC). J Clin Endocrinol Metab. 2011;96:3615–27. https://doi.org/10.1210/jc.2011-1740.
3. Seo JH, Lee SW, Ahn BC, Lee J. Recurrence detection in differentiated thyroid cancer patients with elevated serum level of antithyroglobulin antibody: special emphasis on using 18F-FDG PET/CT. Clin Endocrinol. 2010;72:558–63. https://doi.org/10.1111/j.1365-2265.2009.03693.x.
4. Spencer CA. Challenges of serum thyroglobulin (Tg) measurement in the presence of Tg autoantibodies. J Clin Endocrinol Metab. 2004;89:3702–4. https://doi.org/10.1210/jc.2004-0986.
5. Spencer CA, Takeuchi M, Kazarosyan M, Wang CC, Guttler RB, Singer PA, et al. Serum thyroglobulin autoantibodies: prevalence, influence on serum thyroglobulin measurement, and prognostic significance in patients with differentiated thyroid carcinoma. J Clin Endocrinol Metab. 1998;83:1121–7.
6. Rubello D, Casara D. Clinical meaning of circulating ATG in differentiated thyroid cancer: a prospective study. J Nucl Med. 1992;33:1478–80.
7. Chiovato L, Latrofa F, Braverman L, Pacini F, Capezzone M, Masserini L, et al. Disappearance of humoral thyroid autoimmunity after complete removal of thyroid antigens. Ann Intern Med. 2003;139:346–51.
8. Durante C, Montesano T, Orlandi F, Torlontano M, Puxeddu E, Attard M, et al. Clinical aggressiveness and long-term outcome in patients with papillary thyroid cancer and circulating anti-thyroglobulin autoantibodies. Thyroid. 2014;24:1139–45. https://doi.org/10.1089/thy.2013.0698.
9. Lind P, Kohlfürst S. Respective roles of thyroglobulin, radioiodine imaging, and positron emission tomography in the assessment of thyroid cancer. Semin Nucl Med. 2006;36:194–205. https://doi.org/10.1053/j.semnuclmed.2006.03.002.
10. Haugen BR, Alexander EK, Bible KC, Doherty GM, Mandel SJ, Nikiforov YE, et al. 2015 American Thyroid Association management guidelines for adult patients with thyroid nodules and differentiated thyroid cancer: the American Thyroid Association guidelines task force on thyroid nodules and differentiated thyroid cancer. Thyroid. 2016;26:1–133. https://doi.org/10.1089/thy.2015.0020.
11. Vural GU, Akkas BE, Ercakmak N, Basu S, Alavi A. Prognostic significance of FDG PET/CT on

the follow-up of patients of differentiated thyroid carcinoma with negative 131I whole-body scan and elevated thyroglobulin levels: correlation with clinical and histopathologic characteristics and long-term follow-up data. Clin Nucl Med. 2012;37:953–9. https://doi.org/10.1097/RLU.0b013e31825b2057.

12. Choi SJ, Jung KP, Lee SS, Park S, Lee SM, Bae SK. Clinical usefulness of F-18 FDG PET/CT in papillary thyroid cancer with negative radioiodine scan and elevated thyroglobulin level or positive anti-thyroglobulin antibody. Nucl Med Mol Imaging. 2016;50:130–6. https://doi.org/10.1007/s13139-015-0378-5.
13. Leboulleux S, Schroeder PR, Busaidy NL, Auperin A, Corone C, Jacene HA, et al. Assessment of the incremental value of recombinant thyrotropin stimulation before FDG PET/CT imaging to localize residual differentiated thyroid cancer. J Clin Endocrinol Metab. 2009;94:1310–6. https://doi.org/10.1210/jc.2008-1747.
14. Moreno Ortega E, Vallejo Casas JA, Mena Bares LM, del Real Núñez R, Maza Muret FR, Hidalgo Ramos FJ, et al. Response of thyroglobulin, antithyroglobulin antibodies, TSH, FT4 and total T3 after rhTSH stimulation in differentiated thyroid carcinoma. Rev Esp Med Nucl. 2008;27:253–8.
15. Görges R, Maniecki M, Jentzen W, Sheu SN, Mann K, Bockisch A, et al. Development and clinical impact of thyroglobulin antibodies in patients with differentiated thyroid carcinoma during the first 3 years after thyroidectomy. Eur J Endocrinol. 2005;153:49–55. https://doi.org/10.1530/eje.1.01940.
16. Aras G, Gültekin SS, Küçük NO. The additive clinical value of combined thyroglobulin and antithyroglobulin antibody measurements to define persistent and recurrent disease in patients with differentiated thyroid cancer. Nucl Med Commun. 2008;29:880–4. https://doi.org/10.1097/MNM.0b013e328308e079.

A Patient with Differentiated Thyroid Cancer with Tg Values Constantly Above Normal but Not Increasing Gradually

45

Çiğdem Soydal and Elgin Özkan

Abstract

A 46-year-old female patient with an euthyroid multinodular goiter underwent fine needle aspiration biopsy because ultrasound examination indicated a thyroid malignancy. In the postoperative evaluation of thyroidectomy material, a papillary thyroid carcinoma was detected in the right thyroid lobe with a maximum 2.2 cm diameter (T2N0Mx). The patient received radioiodine ablation treatment with 3700 MBq (100 mCi) iodine-131. Six months after RAT, diagnostic whole-body scintigraphy was performed with 185 MBq (5 mCi) I-131. Serum-stimulated Tg levels were 3.47 ng/mL, and I-131 scintigraphy results were normal. Neck ultrasound and computed tomography of the thorax were performed to search possible recurrent disease. There was no cervical lymph node or lung metastases.

Ç. Soydal (✉)
Department of Nuclear Medicine, Ankara University School of Medicine, Ankara, Turkey

E. Özkan
Department of Nuclear Medicine, Medical Faculty of Ankara University, Ankara, Turkey

45.1 Case Presentation

A 46-year-old female patient with an euthyroid multinodular goiter underwent fine needle aspiration biopsy (FNAB) because ultrasound (USG) examination indicated a thyroid malignancy. After confirmation of thyroid carcinoma, the patient underwent total thyroidectomy. A papillary thyroid carcinoma was detected in the right thyroid lobe with a maximum 2.2 cm diameter (T2N0Mx). The patient received radioiodine ablation treatment (RAT) with 3700 MBq (100 mCi) iodine-131 (I-131). Six months after RAT, diagnostic whole-body scintigraphy was performed with 185 MBq (5 mCi) I-131. Serum-stimulated Tg levels were 3.47 ng/mL, and I-131 scintigraphy results were normal (Fig. 45.1). Neck USG and computed tomography (CT) of the thorax were performed to search possible recurrent disease. Cervical lymph node or lung metastases could not be revealed.

45.1.1 Assessment in the Light of the Literature

Although ATA 2015 guideline and initial risk stratification systems indicated that the patient had stage II disease and belonged to low-risk group, her serum Tg levels were detected higher than expected after initial treatment [1]. After total thyroidectomy followed by RAT, serum-

T. Özülker et al. (eds.), *Thyroid and Parathyroid Diseases*, https://doi.org/10.1007/978-3-319-78476-2_45

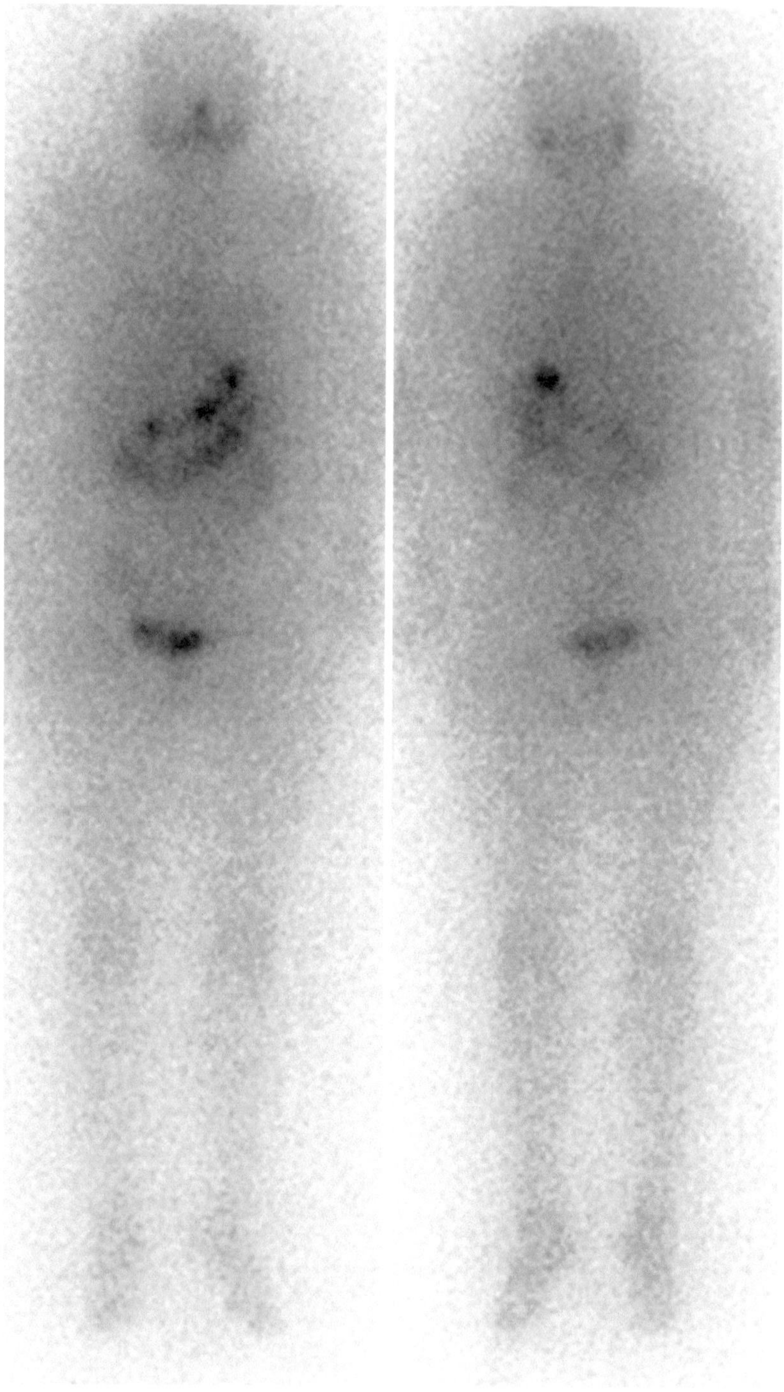

Fig. 45.1 The planar image of diagnostic I-131 scintigraphy

stimulated Tg levels were expected to decrease to <1 ng/mL [2]. It is known that serum Tg measurements are highly sensitive markers for follow-up of differentiated thyroid cancer patients [3]. In the last decade, a dynamic risk estimation system has been developed [4–7]. This system has attempted to reduce the discordance between the initial risk stratification system and later biochemical or structural findings related to residual/recurrent disease during follow-up. Dynamic risk stratification system has been widely accepted and is established within the ATA 2015 guideline. Elevated stimulated Tg levels between 1 and 10 ng/mL and suppressed Tg levels <1 ng/mL without accompanying structural recurrent or residual disease have been described as acceptable response. Additionally, suppressed Tg levels >1 ng/mL, stimulated Tg levels >10 ng/mL, rising Tg levels, or persistent or newly identified disease on cross-sectional and/or nuclear medicine imaging has been described as incomplete response [4]. During the 6-year follow-up period with our patient, serum Tg levels under TSH suppression therapy were at undetectable levels and stimulated Tg levels were ranged between 3 and 5 ng/mL. However, any recurrent or residual disease could not be shown. In patients with an acceptable response, 15–20% of them will have a structural disease identified during follow-up. Thus, patients with acceptable responses are recommended to have follow-up serial imaging and Tg monitoring. Similar to our patient, nonspecific Tg elevation will likely be stable or resolve [8, 9]. Because most recurrences are located in the neck, USG and serum Tg measurements are the recommended monitoring methods in indeterminate response cases. After initial evaluation CT of the thorax, ^{18}F-FDG PET/CT should be considered in patients with an increase in serum Tg levels. In our patient, we could not show the reason for serum Tg elevation. However, because indeterminate biochemical response indicates a high risk for recurrent disease, we have followed up closely. Despite close follow-up, the reason for serum Tg elevation could not be revealed in that case. Serum TSH level of the patient was suppressed under 0.1 ng/mL because of the high risk of recurrence based on the ATA 2015 guidelines.

45.1.2 The Future

Today with our present imaging tools and radiotracers, we cannot show the cause of Tg elevation in patients with indeterminate responses. A couple of possible causes may be microscopic residual or recurrent disease. More sensitive imaging technologies or alternative tracers (e.g., the PET tracer I-124) could further determine if microscopic diseases are the cause of Tg elevation. Because of its high sensitivity in comparison to I-123 and I-131, I-124 could potentially be used to detect small metastatic tissue [10–12]. Another development that could be beneficial in the same patient group is combined PET/MRI systems [13, 14]. Due to the high sensitivity of MRI in soft tissue, small recurrences in the thyroid bed could be detected.

What Can We Learn from This Case?

- Observed elevated Tg levels between 1 and 10 without accompanying structural recurrent or residual disease are described as an indeterminate response.
- 15–20% of patients with an indeterminate response will have structural disease identified during follow-up.
- Patients with indeterminate responses are recommended to undergo serial imaging and Tg monitoring.
- Because most disease recurrences will be located in the neck, USG and serum Tg measurements are the recommended monitoring methods for indeterminate response cases.

References

1. Haugen BR, Alexander EK, Bible KC, Doherty GM, Mandel SJ, Nikiforov YE, et al. American Thyroid Association management guidelines for adult patients with thyroid nodules and differentiated thyroid cancer the American Thyroid Association guidelines task force on thyroid nodules and differentiated thyroid cancer. Thyroid. 2015;2016(26):1–159. https://doi.org/10.1089/thy.2015.0020.
2. Matthews TJ, Chua E, Gargya A, Clark J, Gao K, Elliott M. Elevated serum thyroglobulin levels at the time of ablative radioactive iodine therapy indicate a worse prognosis in thyroid cancer: an Australian retrospective cohort study. J Laryngol Otol. 2016;130(Suppl 4):50–3. https://doi.org/10.1017/S0022215116008331.
3. Miyauchi A, Kudo T, Miya A, Kobayashi K, Ito Y, Takamura Y, et al. Prognostic impact of serum

thyroglobulin doubling-time under thyrotropin suppression in patients with papillary thyroid carcinoma who underwent total thyroidectomy. Thyroid. 2011;21:707–16. https://doi.org/10.1089/thy.2010.0355.

4. Tuttle RM, Tala H, Shah J, Leboeuf R, Ghossein R, Gonen M, et al. Estimating the risk of recurrence in differentiated thyroid cancer after total thyroidectomy and radioactive iodine remnant ablation: using response to therapy variables to modify the initial risk estimates predicted by the new American Thyroid Association staging system. Thyroid. 2010;20:1341–9. https://doi.org/10.1089/thy.2010.0178.
5. Park S, Kim WG, Song E, Oh HS, Kim M, Kwon H, et al. Dynamic risk stratification for predicting recurrence in patients with differentiated thyroid cancer treated without radioactive iodine remnant ablation therapy. Thyroid. 2017;27:524–30. https://doi.org/10.1089/thy.2016.0477.
6. Morosán YJ, Parisi C, Urrutia MA, Rosmarin M, Schnitman M, Serrano L, et al. Dynamic prediction of the risk of recurrence in patients over 60 years of age with differentiated thyroid carcinoma. Arch Endocrinol Metab. 2016;60:348–54. https://doi.org/10.1590/2359-3997000000146.
7. Omry-Orbach G. Risk stratification in differentiated thyroid cancer: an ongoing process. Rambam Maimonides Med J. 2016;28:7. https://doi.org/10.5041/RMMJ.
8. Vaisman F, Momesso D, Bulzico DA, Pessoa CH, Dias F, et al. Spontaneous remission in thyroid cancer patients after biochemical incomplete response to initial therapy. Clin Endocrinol. 2012;77:132–8. https://doi.org/10.1111/j.1365-2265.2012.04342.x.
9. Durante C, Montesano T, Attard M, Torlontano M, Monzani F, Costante G, PTC Study Group, et al. Long-term surveillance of papillary thyroid cancer patients who do not undergo postoperative radioiodine remnant ablation: is there a role for serum thyroglobulin measurement? J Clin Endocrinol Metab. 2012;97:2748–53. https://doi.org/10.1210/jc.2012-1123.
10. Dercle L, Deandreis D, Terroir M, Leboulleux S, Lumbroso J, Schlumberger M. Evaluation of (124)I PET/CT and (124)I PET/MRI in the management of patients with differentiated thyroid cancer. Eur J Nucl Med Mol Imaging. 2016;43:1006–10. https://doi.org/10.1007/s00259-016-3334-4.
11. Santhanam P, Taieb D, Solnes L, Marashdeh W, Ladenson PW. Utility of I 124 PET/CT in identifying radioiodine avid lesions in differentiated thyroid cancer; a systematic review and meta-analysis. Clin Endocrinol. 2017;86:645–51. https://doi.org/10.1111/cen.13306.
12. Kuker R, Sztejnberg M, Gulec S. I-124 imaging, and dosimetry. Mol Imaging Radionucl Ther. 2016;5:66–73. https://doi.org/10.4274/2017.26.
13. Binse I, Poeppel TD, Ruhlmann M, Gomez B, Umutlu L, Bockisch A, et al. Imaging with (124) I in differentiated thyroid carcinoma: is PET/MRI superior to PET/CT? Eur J Nucl Med Mol Imaging. 2016;43:1011–7. https://doi.org/10.1007/s00259-015-3288-y.
14. Vrachimis A, Burg MC, Wenning C, Allkemper T, Weckesser M, Schäfers M, et al. [(18)F]FDG PET/CT outperforms [(18)F]FDG PET/MRI in differentiated thyroid cancer. Eur J Nucl Med Mol Imaging. 2016;43:212–20. https://doi.org/10.1007/s00259-015-3195-2.

46 A Patient with Papillary Thyroid Carcinoma and Biochemical Incomplete Response with Gradually Increasing Tg Values and Negative Imaging Studies

Çiğdem Soydal and Elgin Özkan

Abstract

A 61-year-old asymptomatic female patient having no risk factors for thyroid carcinoma underwent neck ultrasound. Following a diagnosis of papillary thyroid cancer (PTC) by fine needle aspiration biopsy, the patient underwent total thyroidectomy and right lateral neck lymph node dissection. Histopathological examination of the surgical specimen revealed two PTC foci in the right thyroidal lobe that were 4 cm and 0.1 cm in diameter. The patient received radioiodine ablation treatment (RAT) with 5550 MBq (150 mCi) iodine-131 (I-131) 3 months after the operation. Six months after RAT, diagnostic whole-body scintigraphy was performed with endogenous TSH stimulation with 185 MBq I-131. Serum TSH-stimulated Tg levels were 66.55 ng/mL, and I-131 scintigraphy revealed the absence of any pathological uptake. Neck ultrasound (US) and computed tomography (CT) of the thorax were normal. A ^{18}F-FDG PET/BT was planned to search for possible recurrent disease, but it was determined normal. Serum thyroglobulin levels gradually increased to 89.79 ng/mL during the 8-year follow-up period. Several neck USGs, thorax CTs, and one additional ^{18}F-FDG PET/CT were performed. Finally, cranial CT and Tc-99^{m} MDP bone scintigraphy were performed. No residual or metastatic tissue detected so far.

Ç. Soydal (✉)
Department of Nuclear Medicine, Ankara University School of Medicine, Ankara, Turkey

E. Özkan
Department of Nuclear Medicine, Medical Faculty of Ankara University, Ankara, Turkey

46.1 Case Presentation

A 61-year-old asymptomatic female patient having no risk factors for thyroid carcinoma underwent neck ultrasound (USG). A hypoechoic thyroid nodule 4 cm in diameter and accompanying multiple enlarged right lateral compartment lymph nodes were detected. Following a diagnosis of papillary thyroid cancer (PTC) by fine needle aspiration biopsy (FNAB), the patient underwent total thyroidectomy and right lateral neck lymph node dissection. Histopathological examination of the surgical specimen revealed two PTC foci in the right thyroidal lobe that were 4 cm and 0.1 cm in diameter. Additionally, three metastatic lymph nodes were detected in the right lateral compartment, with the largest

T. Özülker et al. (eds.), *Thyroid and Parathyroid Diseases*, https://doi.org/10.1007/978-3-319-78476-2_46

being 2 cm in diameter (T2N1bMx, ATA intermediate risk group). The patient received radioiodine ablation treatment (RAT) with 5550 MBq (150 mCi) iodine-131 (I-131) 3 months after the operation. During RAT, serum thyroglobulin (Tg) levels were measured as 81.95 ng/mL. Posttreatment scintigraphy revealed several foci of radioiodine uptake in the thyroid bed. Six months after RAT, diagnostic whole-body scintigraphy was performed with endogenous TSH

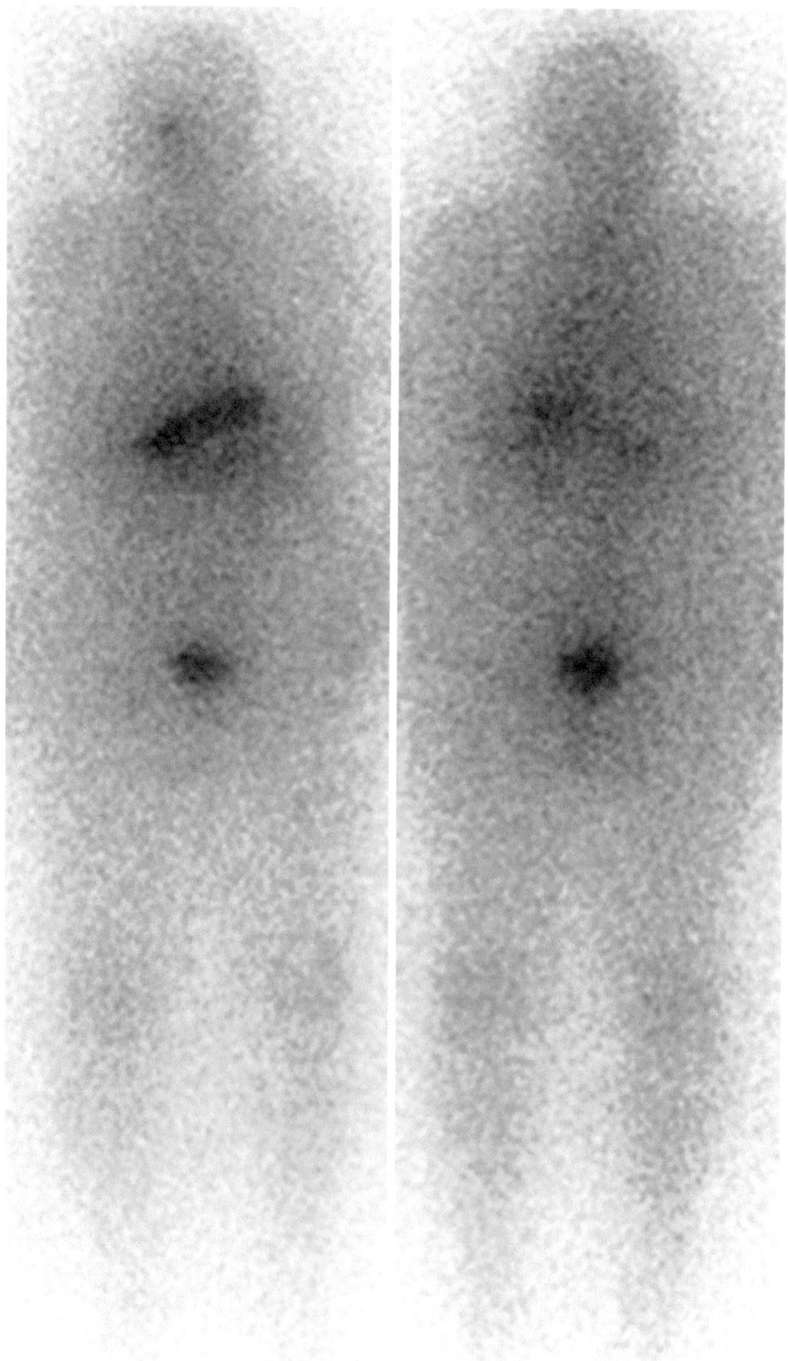

Fig. 46.1 Planar whole-body image of diagnostic I-131 scintigraphy

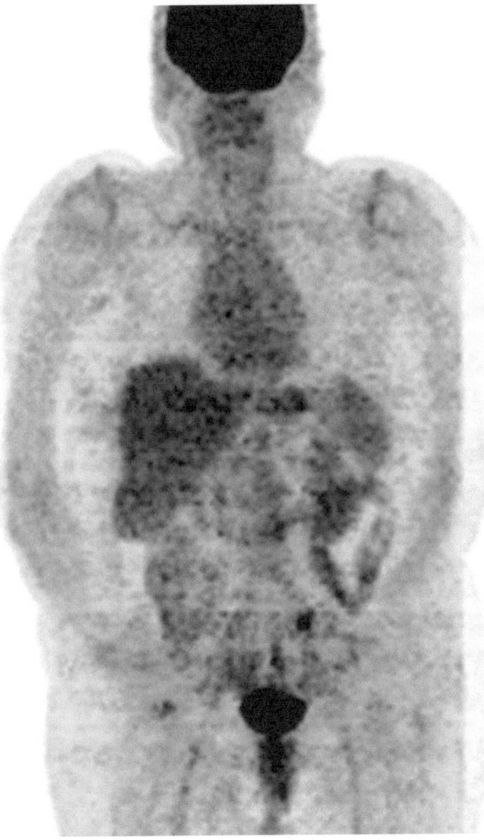

Fig. 46.2 Maximum intensity projection ^{18}F-FDG PET/CT image

stimulation with 185 MBq (5 mCi) I-131. Serum TSH-stimulated Tg levels were 66.55 ng/mL, and I-131 scintigraphy revealed the absence of any pathological uptake (Fig. 46.1). There was no pathology in the neck USG and computed tomography (CT) of the thorax. An ^{18}F-FDG PET/BT was planned to search for possible recurrent disease, but it was determined normal (Fig. 46.2). A second dose of radioiodine treatment (7400 MBq (200 mCi)) was administered to treat possible millimetric metastatic tissue. However, no pathological uptake was seen on whole-body scintigraphy 1 week after radioiodine treatment. Serum Tg levels gradually increased to 89.79 ng/mL during the 8-year follow-up period. Several neck USGs, thorax CTs, and one additional ^{18}F-FDG PET/CT were performed. Finally, cranial CT and Tc-99^{m} MDP bone scintigraphy were performed. No residual or metastatic tissue detected so far.

46.2 Discussion

Elevated serum Tg levels during the first radioiodine treatment were reported as a poor prognostic factor [1, 2]. However, early transient elevation in serum Tg levels after RAT also has been described [3]. A short period of decreased Tg serum levels is expected in patients after a successful ablation. For this reason, Tg measurement is a highly sensitive marker for monitoring treatment response and detecting residuals from metastatic disease in well-differentiated thyroid cancer patients. In patients with persistently elevated Tg serum levels, neck USG, thorax CT, and ^{18}F-FDG PET/CT are the imaging tools to detect possible metastatic disease [4]. Recently, combined ^{18}F-FDG PET/CT and magnetic resonance imaging (MRI) of the neck were recommended to patients who have negative results from initial imaging methods [5, 6]. According to the ATA 2015 guidelines, suppressed Tg serum levels >1 ng/mL or stimulated Tg levels >10 nm/mL or rising anti-Tg antibody levels and absence of localized disease can be categorized as a biochemical incomplete response [7]. Despite the development of imaging tools, the cause of the elevation of Tg serum levels could not be elucidated in some of the patients. In addition to Tg levels, Tg doubling time is another controversial prognostic factor. Some have claimed that Tg doubling time is an independent prognostic factor [7]. Contrarily, Rössing et al. recently reported that Tg doubling time was not a prognostic factor and is only important in patients with high tumor burden [8]. Close follow-up of patients under serum TSH suppression is recommended because they are at high risk for disease recurrence [9]. Persistently elevated serum Tg levels after total thyroidectomy and RAT might be related to residual diseased tissue from insufficient surgical resection or unsuccessful ablation treatment. Neck USG should be the first choice for imaging and evaluating thyroidal bed and neck lymph nodes. Following evaluation of the neck, it is also important to check the patient for possible distant organ metastases. As such, CT of the patient's thorax was performed to evaluate the lungs for possible metastases. After those initial imaging methods,

^{18}F-FDG PET/CT could be performed in I-131-negative and Tg-positive patients. However, the cause of Tg elevation was not detected in our patient after initial imaging. Thus, a second high dose of radioiodine was administered to treat possible microscopic metastatic disease and to decrease Tg levels. A limited number of patients became to have undetectable Tg levels after repeated empiric radioiodine treatments have been reported. Leboulleux et al. administered a second dose of radioiodine treatment in only 1 out of 23 patients. This patient became I-131 negative with undetectable stimulated Tg levels [10]. We did not observe any decrease in Tg serum levels after the second dose of radioiodine. After searching for possible brain and bone metastases, cranial CT and bone scintigraphy tests were found normal. In that patient, we could not determine the cause of Tg elevation. However, because incomplete biochemical response indicates a high risk for recurrent disease, we followed up closely and still could not figure out the cause of elevated Tg. The serum TSH levels of the patient were suppressed under 0.1 ng/mL because of the high risk of recurrence.

46.2.1 The Future

Recently, a few studies were reported on the effects of the Ga-68 DOTA-peptide PET/CT in radioiodine-negative thyroid cancer patients. Previous work has also evaluated the appropriateness of peptide receptor radionuclide treatment with Lu-177 DOTA-peptides [11, 12]. Another novel PET tracer for the same patient group is iodine-124. Because of its high sensitivity in comparison to I-123 and I-131 due to improved resolution during PET imaging, I-124 can detect small metastatic tissue [13]. A recent meta-analysis reported that I-124 PET/CT identifies more lesions than posttreatment scans [14]. Kuker et al. recommended I-124 PET due to its higher sensitivity and spatial resolution compared to standard gamma scintigraphy, which can aid in the detection of recurrent or metastatic disease and provide more accurate measurements of metabolic tumor volumes [15]. In the future, the role of new PET tracers should be examined in patients with elevated serum Tg levels that are under follow-up. Additionally, a combination of PET and MRI imaging will be able to increase the sensitivity of detection of recurrent disease in neck and bone tissue [16, 17].

References

1. Matthews TJ, Chua E, Gargya A, Clark J, Gao K, Elliott M. Elevated serum thyroglobulin levels at the time of ablative radioactive iodine therapy indicate a worse prognosis in thyroid cancer: an Australian retrospective cohort study. J Laryngol Otol. 2016;130:50–3. https://doi.org/10.1017/S0022215116008331.
2. Park HJ, Jeong GC, Kwon SY, Min JJ, Bom HS, Park KS, et al. Stimulated serum thyroglobulin level at the time of first dose of radioactive iodine therapy is the most predictive factor for therapeutic failure in patients with papillary thyroid carcinoma. Nucl Med Mol Imaging. 2014;48:255–61. https://doi.org/10.1007/s13139-014-0282-4.
3. Stevic I, Dembinski TC, Pathak KA, Leslie WD. Transient early increase in thyroglobulin levels post-radioiodine ablation in patients with differentiated thyroid cancer. Clin Biochem. 2015;48:658–61. https://doi.org/10.1007/s13139-014-0282-4.
4. Wiebel JL, Esfandiari NH, Papaleontiou M, Worden FP, Haymart MR. Evaluating positron emission tomography use in differentiated thyroid cancer. Thyroid. 2015;25:1026–32. https://doi.org/10.1089/thy.2015.0062.
5. Hempel JM, Kloeckner R, Krick S, Pinto Dos Santos D, Schadmand-Fischer S, Boeßert P, et al. Impact of combined FDG-PET/CT and MRI on the detection of local recurrence and nodal metastases in thyroid cancer. Cancer Imaging. 2016;3:37. https://doi.org/10.1186/s40644-016-0096-y.
6. Riola-Parada C, García-Cañamaque L, Pérez-Dueñas V, Garcerant-Tafur M, Carreras-Delgado JL. Simultaneous PET/MRI vs PET/CT in oncology. A systematic review. Rev Esp Med Nucl Imagen Mol. 2016;35:306–12. https://doi.org/10.1016/j.remn.2016.06.001.
7. Miyauchi A, Kudo T, Miya A, Kobayashi K, Ito Y, Takamura Y, et al. Prognostic impact of serum thyroglobulin doubling-time under thyrotropin suppression in patients with papillary thyroid carcinoma who underwent total thyroidectomy. Thyroid. 2011;21:707–16. https://doi.org/10.1089/thy.2010.0355.
8. Rössing RM, Jentzen W, Nagarajah J, Bockisch A, Görges R. Serum thyroglobulin doubling time in progressive thyroid cancer. Thyroid. 2016;26:1712–8. https://doi.org/10.1089/thy.2016.0031.

9. Haugen BR, Alexander EK, Bible KC, Doherty GM, Mandel SJ, Nikiforov YE, et al. 2015 American Thyroid Association management guidelines for adult patients with thyroid nodules and differentiated thyroid cancer the American Thyroid Association guidelines task force on thyroid nodules and differentiated thyroid cancer. Thyroid. 2016;26:1–159. https://doi.org/10.1089/thy.2015.0020.
10. Leboulleux S, El Bez I, Borget I, Elleuch M, Déandreis D, Al Ghuzlan A, et al. Postradioiodine treatment whole-body scan in the era of 18-fluorodeoxyglucose positron emission tomography for differentiated thyroid carcinoma with elevated serum thyroglobulin levels. Thyroid. 2012;22:832–8. https://doi.org/10.1089/thy.2012.0081.
11. Vrachimis A, Stegger L, Wenning C, Noto B, Burg MC, Konnert JR, Allkemper T, et al. (68)Ga DOTATATE PET/MRI and [(18)F]FDG PET/CT are complementary and superior to diffusion-weighted MR imaging for radioactive-iodine-refractory differentiated thyroid cancer. Eur J Nucl Med Mol Imaging. 2016;43:1765–72. https://doi.org/10.1007/s00259-016-3378-5.
12. Elboğa U, Ozkaya M, Sayiner ZA, Çelen YZ. Lu-177 labelled peptide treatment for radioiodine refractory differentiated thyroid carcinoma. BMJ Case Rep. 2016. https://doi.org/10.1136/bcr-2015-213627.
13. Dercle L, Deandreis D, Terroir M, Leboulleux S, Lumbroso J, Schlumberger M. Evaluation of (124)I PET/CT and (124)I PET/MRI in the management of patients with differentiated thyroid cancer. Eur J Nucl Med Mol Imaging. 2016;43:1006–10. https://doi.org/10.1007/s00259-016-3334-4.
14. Santhanam P, Taieb D, Solnes L, Marashdeh W, Ladenson PW. Utility of I 124 PET/CT in identifying radioiodine avid lesions in differentiated thyroid cancer; a systematic review and meta-analysis. Clin Endocrinol. 2017;86(5):645–51. https://doi.org/10.1111/cen.13306.
15. Kuker R, Sztejnberg M, Gulec S. I-124 imaging and dosimetry. Mol Imaging Radionucl Ther. 2016;5:66–73. https://doi.org/10.4274/2017.26.suppl.07.
16. Binse I, Poeppel TD, Ruhlmann M, Gomez B, Umutlu L, Bockisch A, et al. Imaging with (124)I in differentiated thyroid carcinoma: is PET/MRI superior to PET/CT? Eur J Nucl Med Mol Imaging. 2016;43:1011–7. https://doi.org/10.1007/s00259-015-3288-y.
17. Vrachimis A, Burg MC, Wenning C, Allkemper T, Weckesser M, Schäfers M, et al. [(18)F]FDG PET/CT outperforms [(18)F]FDG PET/MRI in differentiated thyroid cancer. Eur J Nucl Med Mol Imaging. 2016;43:212–20. https://doi.org/10.1007/s00259-015-3195-2.

47 Rosiglitazone Effect on Radioiodine Uptake in a Case of Dedifferentiated Thyroid Carcinoma

Gülin Uçmak and Burcu Esen Akkaş

Abstract

Differentiated thyroid cancer may lose its differential characteristics and transform to a less-differentiated form that does not concentrate radioiodine. These tumors represent an aggressive tumor type and may necessitate alternative therapies. Various attempts have been made to augment iodine uptake and to redifferentiate tumors in order to regain benefit from radioiodine therapy. Thiazolidinediones, such as rosiglitazone, act by binding to peroxisome proliferator-activated receptors (PPARs) and have also shown promise in the redifferentiation treatment of dedifferentiated thyroid carcinomas as antiproliferative and apoptosis-inducing agents. In this section, the effect of rosiglitazone is discussed in a case with dedifferentiated thyroid cancer.

47.1 Case Presentation

A 59-year-old female with follicular variant of papillary thyroid carcinoma (FVPTC) with tumor size of 2 cm referred to our Nuclear Medicine Department for evaluation of radioiodine (I-131) treatment following bilateral total thyroidectomy. The tumor had some poor histopathological parameters such as vascular invasion, perineural invasion, and extension to perithyroidal soft tissues. Postoperatively, on thyroid scintigraphy, small residual tissues were observed on the thyroid bed. There was no abnormal finding on neck ultrasound (USG). Serum thyroglobulin (Tg) level was 171 ng/ml, and anti-thyroglobulin antibody (Tg-Ab) level was <20 μIU/ml IU/ml under TSH stimulation (>100 μIU/ml). The TNM stage was considered as T3N0M0 in the year 2006. The patient was regarded as in high-risk group because of the existence of poor histopathological parameters and high postoperative serum Tg level. Therefore, a 200 mCi dose of I-131 treatment was planned.

I-131 treatment was administered orally while serum TSH was >100 μIU/ml and Tg and Tg-Ab were 198 ng/ml and <20 μIU/ml, respectively. Premedication with low-dose oral corticosteroids, H2-receptor antagonists, antiemetics, and anti-inflammatory medication was given, and careful hydration was performed during hospitalization. On post-therapy whole-body scan (WBS) conducted 4 days after therapy, intense I-131 uptakes on the thyroid bed and right upper mediastinum were observed. L-Thyroxine replacement therapy was started 72 h after radioiodine therapy.

G. Uçmak (✉) · B. E. Akkaş
Department of Nuclear Medicine, University of Health Sciences (SBÜ) Dr. Abdurrahman Yurtaslan Ankara Oncology Training and Research Hospital, Ankara, Turkey

T. Özülker et al. (eds.), *Thyroid and Parathyroid Diseases*, https://doi.org/10.1007/978-3-319-78476-2_47

On follow-up, the patient was examined while on L-thyroxine replacement therapy 3 months after I-131 treatment. Serum TSH level was 0.02 µIU/ml, and Tg level was 9.66 ng/ml. Computed tomography (CT) of the thorax was acquired to evaluate the origin of elevated Tg level under TSH suppression. On thorax CT, a right paratracheal lymph node with 10 mm in size and several pulmonary nodules suspected of metastases in the right lung were detected.

A second dose of 250 mCi was administered 11 months after the initial I-131 treatment dose. Laboratory findings were as follows: serum TSH >100 µIU/ml, Tg 176 ng/ml, and Tg-Ab <20 µIU/ml. Recombinant TSH stimulation was not used, and TSH elevation was achieved by thyroid hormone withdrawal prior to adjuvant treatment as recommended by ATA guidelines. On post-therapy WBS, performed on 4 days after I-131 treatment, no uptake was seen on the thyroid bed and neck, but slight uptake was observed on both the hemithorax and right site of the upper mediastinum.

On routine follow-up visits, serum Tg level remained persistently elevated (10.2 ng/ml on L-thyroxine therapy). The patient underwent F-18 FDG (fluorodeoxyglucose) positron-emission tomography/computed tomography (PET/CT) imaging in order to evaluate the origin of persistently elevated Tg level while prominent I-131 uptake was not seen on follow-up. On PET/CT, mild FDG uptake was seen in some of the multiple pulmonary nodules which are 2–5 mm in size and right paratracheal lymph node 10 mm in size on the mediastinum correlated to metastases of thyroid cancer.

Surgery and local treatment were not considered as suitable therapeutic options due to multiplicity of pulmonary nodules. Therefore, the third radioiodine treatment with a dose of 250 mCi was planned with careful monitoring of bone marrow reserve 10 months after the final I-131 treatment. At the time of treatment, serum TSH and Tg were 51.2 µIU/ml and 46.3 ng/ml, respectively. On post-therapy scan, faint uptake was seen on the left hemithorax in the middle zone (Fig. 47.1a).

The patient received a total cumulative dose of 700 mCi I-131 treatment on three consecutive sequences in 3 years. The patient was closely monitored for bone marrow reserve and side effects. Careful clinical support was given during treatments and on follow-up. However, despite consecutive radioiodine therapies, serum Tg level, both on and off L-thyroxine replacement, remained persistently elevated. In addition, radioiodine uptake was negligible on unresectable tumoral deposits on the final post-therapy WBS.

Rosiglitazone (RZ) treatment as a peroxisome proliferator-activated receptor (PPAR) gamma agonist was planned on consensus with the oncologist and nuclear medicine physicians and approved by the Ethic Committee of our hospital. Written informed consent was obtained from the patient before the onset of treatment.

RZ treatment was performed with 4 mg per day for 2 weeks and then 8 mg per day for 6 weeks. The patient was evaluated at baseline and monitored biweekly by laboratory tests including fasting blood glucose, cholesterol, liver, and cardiac function tests and physical examination for toxicity and side effects of the drug. Serum Tg levels on and off L-thyroxine therapy were recorded before and after RZ treatment. The patient has well-tolerated RZ treatment, with no symptoms of hypoglycemia or change in liver function tests and cardiac functions. We did not observe any side effects other than a mild headache and nausea.

On L-thyroxine therapy, serum Tg level decreased to 4.05 ng/ml (TSH 0.67 µIU/ml) and 5.08 ng/ml (TSH 0.74 µIU/ml) from 10.2 ng/ml on the first and second month, respectively, following RZ treatment in the absence of anti-Tg antibodies (Tg-Ab).

L-Thyroxine therapy was discontinued after RZ treatment, and 300 mCi I-131 treatment as the last dose was planned. The dose of 300 mCi I-131 treatment was given 1 month after discontinuing RZ and 1 year after the final I-131 treatment.

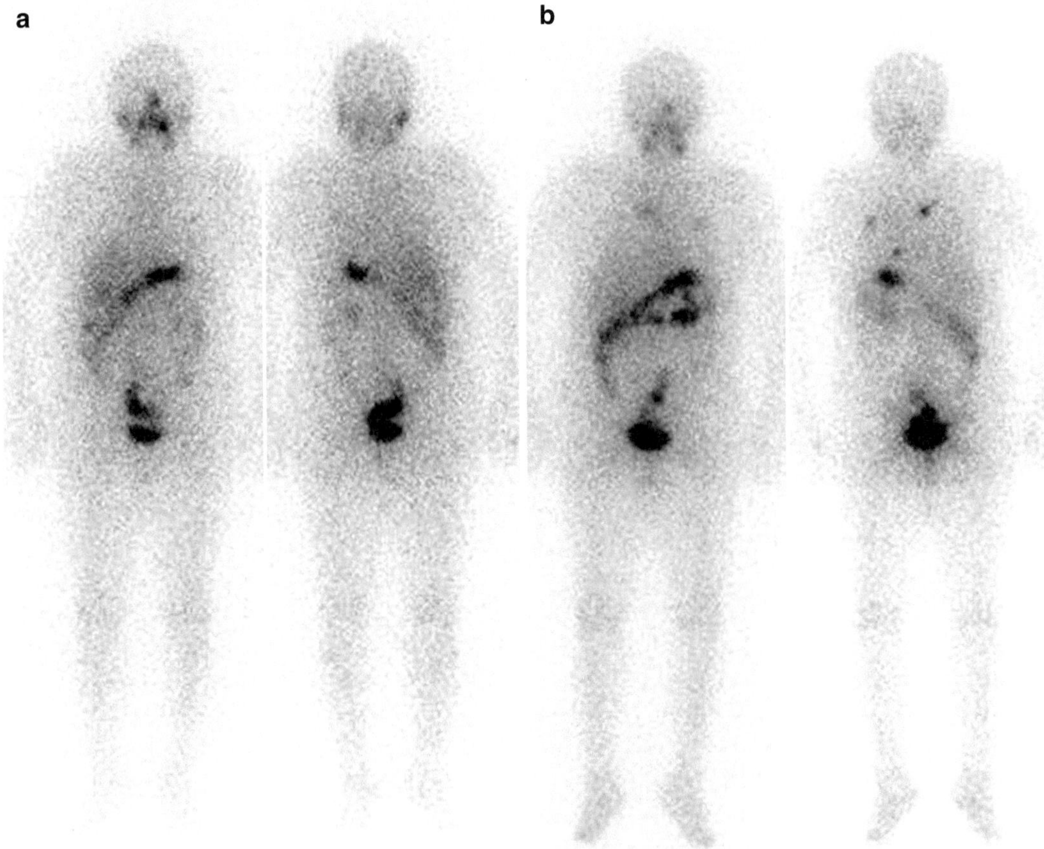

Fig. 47.1 The figure demonstrates the comparison of anterior and posterior post-therapy radioiodine WBS before (in column A) and after (in column B) RZ treatment. (**a**) On post-therapy WBS before RZ, faint uptake is seen on the left hemithorax in the middle zone. (**b**) On post-therapy WBS after RZ, multiple focal uptakes are seen in bilateral lung zones related to lung metastasis of thyroid cancer. Note the marked increase in radioiodine uptake after RZ demonstrated on post-therapy WBS

At the time of treatment, serum TSH was 146 μIU/ml, and Tg was 93.1 ng/ml. Although serum Tg level was elevated compared to the previous therapy, it was considered as a biochemical response as TSH stimulation was significantly stronger during the last therapy (51 μIU/ml vs. 146 μIU/ml). On post-therapy WBS performed 4 days after therapy, markedly intense multiple focal uptakes were seen in bilateral lung zones that may be prominently related to lung metastasis of thyroid cancer (Fig. 47.1b). Uptake in pulmonary nodules was significantly more prominent both in size and in intensity compared to the post-therapy scan before RZ treatment.

47.2 Follow-Up and Outcome

Serum Tg level on L-thyroxine therapy was stable (3–4 ng/ml) in the absence of serum Tg-Ab. According to RECIST 1.1 criteria, the patient had stable disease during 4 years after RZ and the last I-131 treatment [1]. However, in the fifth year after RZ treatment, serum Tg-Ab was elevated (from <20 to 872 μIU/ml) while serum Tg was 0.5 ng/ml. The patient was evaluated by comparative thorax CT and then by F-18 FDG PET/CT. Lung nodules were stable on thorax CT and PET/CT. However, a hypermetabolic (SUVmax: 14.58) hypodense mass lesion, 4 cm in size, was observed in the liver which may be prominently related to the malignant metastatic process in addition to a hypermetabolic mediastinal lymph node in which FDG uptake was significantly increased compared to the previous PET/CT (SUVmax: 28.38). Surgery was planned; however, the patient refused all invasive procedures such as biopsy and surgery and did not come to any other follow-up visit.

47.3 Discussion

Thyroid cancer is the most common endocrine malignancy. Differentiated thyroid cancers (DTC), which include papillary, follicular, and Hurthle cell carcinoma subtypes, constitute the vast majority of thyroid cancers. The prognosis of DTC is generally good, with a 10-year survival rate of 85% [2].

Radioiodine (RAI) is widely used for diagnosis and therapy of DTC for more than 70 years as the first theranostic agent. The accumulation of radioiodine in cancer cells was not fully understood until 1996 when the sodium iodide symporter (NIS) was first identified by Dai et al. [3]. Iodide uptake occurs across the membrane of the cancer cells as well as thyroid follicular cells through an active transporter process mediated by the NIS gene [3]. NIS activity provides the molecular basis for RAI therapy in DTC. While most cases of DTC are curable with the use of surgery and radioactive iodine ablation of the remaining thyroid remnant, prognosis worsens, and treatment options become limited when DTC becomes RAI-refractory. On average, about 25–50% of locally advanced/metastatic patients become refractory to RAI (RAI-R) [4].When RAI becomes ineffective against DTC, 5-year survival decreases to 50% and 10-year survival to <10% [5, 6].

The RAI-R status is related to decreased expression of the NIS and diminished targeting of NIS to the membrane of cancer cells or both [7, 8]. Genetic changes in DTC, such as mutations of BRAF and RAS genes and RET rearrangements, decrease NIS mRNA [9]. The finding of an elevated Tg or Tg-Ab with negative radioiodine scan is highly indicative of non-radioiodine avid residual or recurrent disease. If Tg is out of proportion to the amount of disease or symptoms, other imaging modalities include MR of the brain, CT, bone scan and F-18 FDG PET/CT is indicated to evaluate disease extent [10].

In the past, an empiric treatment was used in such patients, but recent studies have shown that F-18 FDG PET/CT imaging is more sensitive and should be performed as the first-line approach, with empiric RAI treatment being considered only for those patients with no detectable FDG uptake [11, 12].

In our case, F-18 FDG PET/CT imaging was performed in order to evaluate the origin of persistently elevated Tg level despite the absence of I-131 uptake on follow-up. On PET/CT, mild FDG uptake was seen in some pulmonary nodules and mediastinal lymph node corresponding to metastases of thyroid cancer.

The expressions of NIS and glucose transporter-1 (Glut-1) are inversely related, and they reflect the biological characteristics of cancer differentiation. In particular, it appears that with the dedifferentiation process; the NIS expression decreases, Glut-1 expression increases, and this situation associates with poor prognosis [12, 13]. Since radioiodine is no longer a therapy option for non-iodine avid thyroid cancer, alternative therapy strategies are needed.

Localized radioiodine-refractory thyroid cancer can be treated with surgery, stereotactic external beam radiotherapy, chemoembolization, or radioembolization. However, systemic or targeted therapies with tyrosine kinase inhibitors (TKIs) become crucial in systemic disease. Re-induction of thyroid-specific enzymes in order to restore NIS function using compounds such as retinoic acids, peroxisome proliferator-activated receptor gamma (PPARγ) agonists, HDAC inhibitors (valproic acid and carbamazepine), PI3K/AKT inhibitors, and MEK/ERK inhibitors has been evaluated in clinical trials [14]. To enhance radioiodine accumulation in RAI-R, retinoic acid has been used for more than 20 years to increase NIS expression [15]. Although retinoic acid has the potential to increase iodine uptake in cell lines, researchers have reported that the clinical response to radioiodine treatment after retinoic acid administration was only marginal or negligible for the augmentation of iodine accumulation and concentration in the tumor tissue was limited [16].

PPARγ is a nuclear hormone receptor transcription factor that regulates cellular growth and differentiation. PPARγ ligands inhibit growth in PTC cell lines [17]. Thiazolidinediones (TZDs), including rosiglitazone, pioglitazone, and ciglitazone which are used in type II diabetes as they reduce insulin resistance, are high-affinity ligands for the PPARγ [18].

First evidence for augmented RAI uptake upon treatment with rosiglitazone was reported by Philips et al. in five patients with dedifferentiated thyroid cancer [19]. They stated that RZ treatment increased the production of Tg in some patients with thyroid cancer; however, RZ could rarely restore significant iodine trapping. Frohlich et al. reported that another glitazone, troglitazone, increased NIS expression and radioiodine uptake [20]. Park et al. also observed upregulation of NIS mRNA after troglitazone treatment in both DTC and anaplastic thyroid cancer cells [21].

In our case, as a response to RZ treatment, serum Tg level decreased to 4.05 ng/ml and 5.08 ng/ml from 10.2 ng/ml on L-thyroxine therapy on the first and second months following RZ treatment and was stayed stable (3–4 ng/ml) during the first 4 years. In addition, on the post-radioiodine therapy scan performed after RZ treatment, we observed increased I-131 uptake and significant iodine trapping. Tg level is a reliable marker for recurrent or persistent disease and response to therapy in patients with DTC. However, it is unclear whether redifferentiation agents could increase Tg level as a result of a differentiation process in follicular cell origin or elevation of Tg results from tumor progression [22]. In another pilot study, 5 of 9 patients with progressive DTC improved lesion-absorbed dose per administered activity on I-124 PET/CT, and three had decreased lesion size after therapeutic I-131 application following RZ treatment for 6 months [23]. They observed that the elevation in serum Tg was more notable on the third month after therapy compared to the measure on the sixth month. Today, it is questionable whether serum Tg can be used as a response marker after RZ treatment and the most accurate measurement duration after RZ treatment is still unclear.

Another unclear issue is the correlation of PPARγ status and RZ effect on improvement of iodine uptake. Tepmongkol et al. investigated that there was a correspondence between the effect of RZ and the degree of staining for PPARγ within thyroid expression [24]. However, Kebebew et al. found no difference in PPARγ expression between patients who restored iodine uptake and those who did not. They reported that 25% of patients showed positive radioiodine uptake after RZ treatment; however, this result did not provide a clinically significant response to iodine-refractory DTC on long-term follow-up [22]. Rearrangements of PPARγ/PAX8 occur in 36–45.5% of follicular thyroid cancer and in 37.5% of papillary thyroid cancer with follicular variant [25, 26].

In our case, the histopathological status of PPARγ expression in tumor samples before RZ treatment was not determined. However, our patient with papillary thyroid cancer with follicular variant demonstrated markedly intense iodine uptake throughout the metastases corresponding to restored iodine uptake. In addition, the disease progression was stopped with time to progression of 4 years after RZ treatment. However, on the fifth year after RZ treatment, increase in serum Tg-Ab and progressive disease were observed. Up to date, the current literature lacks controlled case series with a longer time of follow-up period after RZ treatment. In general, the observation time remained limited to less than 1 year.

Rosiglitazone has been taken off the market in Europe and restricted in the USA due to cardiovascular side effects in long-term diabetes mellitus therapy in September 2010 [27]. Another glitazone, pioglitazone, was evaluated by Rosenbaum-Krumme SJ et al. in five patients but showed no increase in lesion-absorbed dose of I-131 [28]. They concluded that pioglitazone revealed some positive effects in radioiodine-negative and progressive DTC patients, but it did not fulfill the expectations given by the results of rosiglitazone therapy. On the contrary, Dobson et al. showed promising results that pioglitazone was highly therapeutic and prevented metastasis in mice by the thyroid-specific expression of PAX8-PPARγ fusion protein and homozygous deletion of phosphatase and tensin homolog [29]. Based on these data, a phase II clinical trial of pioglitazone in follicular variant of PTC is being reassessed (NCT01655719). As pioglitazone was already approved by FDA and has a better toxicity profile than other targeted agents, such as TKIs, positive results of the trial would indicate that pioglitazone may be a good therapeutic option for patients with RR-DTC [30].

As a summary, up to date, PPAR gamma agonists have shown disappointing results in recent clinical trials. However, it can be said that in these studies, selection of redifferentiation agents was not performed according to tumor characterization. Today, we know that all thyroid tumors differ widely from each other in terms of histology and genetic profile with the absence or presence of various mutations and different signaling pathways throughout the tumor. We believe that by using advanced knowledge on tumor genetic profile and histopathological data on a patient-based approach, appropriate selection of redifferentiation agents or combining redifferentiation agents with certain targeted therapies may increase the effectiveness of redifferentiation treatment and provide better progression-free survival. We consider that further clinical trials are needed on an individual-based approach to understand the mechanisms of dedifferentiation with regard to genetic profile and biological behavior of the tumor in order to better target and treat the tumor.

What Can We Learn from This Case?

- Differentiated thyroid cancer may lose its differential characteristics and transform to a less-differentiated form that do not concentrate radioiodine. These tumors represent an aggressive tumor type and may necessitate alternative therapies. When RAI becomes ineffective against DTC, 5-year survival decreases to 50% and 10-year survival to <10%.
- Thiazolidinediones, such as rosiglitazone, act by binding to peroxisome proliferator-activated receptors (PPARs) and show promise in the redifferentiation treatment of dedifferentiated thyroid carcinomas as anti-proliferative and apoptosis inducing agents.
- Thyroid tumors differ widely from each other in terms of histology, genetic profile with absence or presence of various mutations and different signaling pathways throughout the tumor.
- Dedifferentiating agents must be planned on a patient based approach with regard to genetic profile and biological behavior of the tumor in order to better target and treat the tumor.

References

1. Eisenhauer EA, Therasse P, Bogaerts J, Schwartz LH, Sargent D, Ford R, et al. New response evaluation criteria in solid tumours: revised RECIST guideline (version 1.1). Eur J Cancer. 2009;45:228–47.
2. Eustatia-Rutten CF, Corssmit EP, Biermasz NR, Pereira AM, Romijn JA, Smit JW. Survival and death causes in differentiated thyroid carcinoma. J Clin Endocrinol Metab. 2006;91:313–9.
3. Dai G, Levy O, Carrasco N. Cloning and characterization of the thyroid iodide transporter. Nature. 1996;379:458–60.
4. Schlumberger M, Tubiana M, De Vathaire F, Hill C, Gardet P, Travagli J, et al. Long-term results of treatment of 283 patients with lung and bone metastases from differentiated thyroid carcinoma. J Clin Endocrinol Metab. 1986;63:960–7.
5. Capdevila J, Argiles G, Rodriguez-Frexinos V, Nunez I, Tabernero J. New approaches in the management of radioiodine-refractory thyroid cancer: the molecular targeted therapy era. Discov Med. 2010;9:153–62.
6. Durante C, Haddy N, Baudin E, Leboulleux S, Hartl D, Travagli JP, et al. Long-term outcome of 444 patients with distant metastases from papillary and follicular thyroid carcinoma: benefits and limits of radioiodine therapy. J Clin Endocrinol Metab. 2006;91:2892–9.
7. Spitzweg C, Bible KC, Hofbauer LC, Morris JC. Advanced radioiodine-refractory differentiated thyroid cancer: the sodium iodide symporter and other emerging therapeutic targets. Lancet Diabetes Endocrinol. 2014;2:830–42. https://doi.org/10.1016/S2213-8587(14)70051-8.

8. Oh SW, Paeng JC, Chung J. New strategies for combined radioiodine therapy in refractory thyroid cancer. J Korean Thyroid Assoc. 2015;8:26–35.
9. Riesco-Eizaguirre G, Gutierrez-Martinez P, Garcia-Cabezas MA, Nistal M, Santisteban P. The oncogene BRAF V600E is associated with a high risk of recurrence and less differentiated papillary thyroid carcinoma due to the impairment of Na+/I– targeting to the membrane. Endocr Relat Cancer. 2006;13:257–69.
10. Haugen BR, Alexander EK, Bible KC, Doherty GM, Mandel SJ, Nikiforov YE, et al. 2015 American Thyroid Association management guidelines for adult patients with thyroid nodules and differentiated thyroid cancer: the American Thyroid Association guidelines task force on thyroid nodules and differentiated thyroid cancer. Thyroid. 2016;26:1–133. https://doi.org/10.1089/thy.2015.0020.
11. Rosario PW, Mourão GF, dos Santos JB, Calsolari MR. Is empirical radioactive iodine therapy still a valid approach to patients with thyroid cancer and elevated thyroglobulin? Thyroid. 2014;24:533–6. https://doi.org/10.1089/thy.2013.0427.
12. Vural GU, Akkas BE, Ercakmak N, Basu S, Alavi A. Prognostic significance of FDG PET/CT on the follow-up of patients of differentiated thyroid carcinoma with negative 131I whole-body scan and elevated thyroglobulin levels: correlation with clinical and histopathologic characteristics and long-term follow-up data. Clin Nucl Med. 2012;37:953–9. https://doi.org/10.1097/RLU.0b013e31825b2057.
13. Chung JK, Youn HW, Kang JH, Lee HY, Kang KW. Sodium iodide symporter and the radioiodine treatment of thyroid carcinoma. Nucl Med Mol Imaging. 2010;44:4–14. https://doi.org/10.1007/s13139-009-0016-1.
14. Rothenberg SM, McFadden DG, Palmer EL, Daniels GH, Wirth LJ. Redifferentiation of iodine-refractory BRAF V600E-mutant metastatic papillary thyroid cancer with dabrafenib. Clin Cancer Res. 2015;21:1028–35. https://doi.org/10.1158/1078-0432.CCR-14-2915.
15. Schreck R, Schnieders F, Schmutzler C, Köhrle J. Retinoids stimulate type I 50-deiodinase activity in human follicular thyroid carcinoma cell lines. J Clin Endocrinol Metab. 1994;79:791–8.
16. Oh SW, Moon SH, Park DJ, Cho BY, Jung KC, Lee DS, et al. Combined therapy with 131I and retinoic acid in Korean patients with radioiodine-refractory papillary thyroid cancer. Eur J Nucl Med Mol Imaging. 2011;38:1798–805. https://doi.org/10.1007/s00259-011-1849-2.
17. Ohta K, Endo T, Haraguchi K, Hershman JM, Onaya T. Ligands for peroxisome proliferator-activated receptor gamma inhibit growth and induce apoptosis of human papillary thyroid carcinoma cells. J Clin Endocrinol Metab. 2001;86:2170–7.
18. Day C. Thiazolidinediones a new class of antidiabetic drugs. Diabet Med. 1999;16:179–92.
19. Philips JC, Petite C, Willi JP, Buchegger F, Meier CA. Effect of peroxisome proliferator-activated receptor gamma agonist, rosiglitazone, on dedifferentiated thyroid cancers. Nucl Med Commun. 2004;25:1183–6.
20. Frohlich E, Machicao F, Wahl R. Action of thiazolidinediones on differentiation, proliferation and apoptosis of normal and transformed thyrocytes in culture. Endocr Relat Cancer. 2005;12:291–303.
21. Park JW, Zarnegar R, Kanauchi H, Wong MG, Hyun WC, Ginzinger DG, et al. Troglitazone, the peroxisome proliferator-activated receptor-gamma agonist, induces antiproliferation and redifferentiation in human thyroid cancer cell lines. Thyroid. 2005;15:222–31. https://doi.org/10.1089/thy.2005.15.222.
22. Kebebew E, Lindsay S, Clark OH, Woeber KA, Hawkins R, Greenspan FS. Results of rosiglitazone therapy in patients with thyroglobulin-positive and radioiodine-negative advanced differentiated thyroid cancer. Thyroid. 2009;19:953–6. https://doi.org/10.1089/thy.2008.0371.
23. Rosenbaum-Krumme SJ, Freudenberg LS, Jentzen W, Bockisch A, Nagarajah J. Effects of rosiglitazone on radioiodine negative and progressive differentiated thyroid carcinoma as assessed by ^{124}I PET/CT imaging. Clin Nucl Med. 2012;37:e47–52. https://doi.org/10.1097/RLU.0b013e3182443ca6.
24. Tepmongkol S, Keelawat S, Honsawek S, Ruangvejvorachai P. Rosiglitazone effect on radioiodine uptake in thyroid carcinoma patients with high thyroglobulin but negative total body scan: a correlation with the expression of peroxisome proliferator-activated receptor-gamma. Thyroid. 2008;18:697–704. https://doi.org/10.1089/thy.2008.0056.
25. Castro P, Rebocho AP, Soares RJ, Magalhaes J, Roque L, Trovisco V, et al. PAX8-PPARgamma rearrangement is frequently detected in the follicular variant of papillary thyroid carcinoma. J Clin Endocrinol Metab. 2006;91:213–20.
26. Nikiforova MN, Lynch RA, Biddinger PW, Alexander EK, Dorn GW 2nd, Tallini G, et al. RAS point mutations and PAX8-PPAR gamma rearrangement in thyroid tumors: evidence for distinct molecular pathways in thyroid follicular carcinoma. J Clin Endocrinol Metab. 2003;88:2318–26.
27. Graham DJ, Ouellet-Hellstrom R, MaCurdy TE, Ali F, Sholley C, Worrall C, et al. Risk of acute myocardial infarction, stroke, heart failure, and death in elderly Medicare patients treated with rosiglitazone or pioglitazone. JAMA. 2010;304:411–8. https://doi.org/10.1001/jama.2010.920.
28. Rosenbaum-Krumme SJ, Bockisch A, Nagarajah J. Pioglitazone therapy in progressive differentiated thyroid carcinoma. Nuklearmedizin. 2012;51:111–5. https://doi.org/10.3413/Nukmed-0474-12-01.
29. Dobson ME, Diallo-Krou E, Grachtchouk V, Yu J, Colby LA, Wilkinson JE, et al. Pioglitazone induces a proadipogenic antitumor response in mice with PAX8-PPARgamma fusion protein thyroid carcinoma. Endocrinology. 2011;152(11):4455–65. https://doi.org/10.1210/en.2011-1178.
30. Raman P, Koenig RJ. Pax-8-PPAR-gamma fusion protein in thyroid carcinoma. Nat Rev Endocrinol. 2014;10:616–23. https://doi.org/10.1038/nrendo.2014.115.

48 Management of Recurrent Lymph Nodes in Central and Lateral Neck in the Follow-Up of Differentiated Thyroid Carcinoma

Seyfettin Ilgan

Abstract

Despite excellent overall prognosis, up to 40% of patients with papillary thyroid cancer (PTC) will have persistent or recurrent disease, mostly in lateral (53%) or central (28%) cervical lymph nodes. Local and regional recurrences continue to be treated by surgical excision with or without adjuvant radioiodine treatment, especially in potentially curable patients. Discovery of nonpalpable nodal recurrences in the central and lateral neck have been increased considerably with the evolving role of ultrasonography in the follow-up of patients with PTC. However, the management of impalpable or indolent locoregional recurrences of PTC continues to be more controversial. Despite arguments over survival benefit of reoperations, 19–73% remission rates have been reported based on Tg levels with compartment-oriented reoperations. The correct delineation of the disease preoperatively and the use of new techniques facilitating identification of recurrent laryngeal nerve and metastatic foci during surgery are essential parts of therapeutic success.

S. Ilgan
Department of Nuclear Medicine, Güven Hospital, Ankara, Turkey

48.1 Case Presentation

A 33-year-old woman with papillary thyroid carcinoma (PTC) presented to our hospital for evaluation of gradually increasing Tg levels under suppression therapy. Two years previously, she had been diagnosed with multinodular goiter at an outside institution and fine needle aspiration biopsy (FNAB) of dominant nodule reported as benign. After discussion, she had been selected for lobectomy for giant nodule on the left thyroid lobe. Lobectomy material had been submitted to examination of frozen sections, and surgery had switched to total thyroidectomy upon detection of a 1.2 cm PTC in the left lobe. The final pathology had revealed unifocal, intrathyroidal classical variant of PTC with lymphovascular invasion. No lymph node had been removed at the time of surgery. She had been given 100 mCi (3700 MBq) of radioactive iodine (I-131) 4 weeks after surgery under endogenous TSH stimulation. The patient had a serum TSH of 71.68 mIU/L and thyroglobulin (Tg) of 282.1 ng/mL without Tg antibodies during treatment. The post-therapy scan had shown uptake only in the left thyroid bed with no extracervical uptake.

Three months after the I-131 treatment, serum Tg level was found high (23.29 ng/mL) under T4 suppression, and neck ultrasonography (USG) discovered metastatic lymph nodes in the left

T. Özülker et al. (eds.), *Thyroid and Parathyroid Diseases*, https://doi.org/10.1007/978-3-319-78476-2_48

lateral cervical chain. The patient had undergone left lateral neck dissection, and final pathology revealed 6 metastatic lymph nodes out of 26 resected, largest being in level IV and 2.7 cm in size. Six weeks after neck dissection, Tg level was found 2.22 ng/mL under suppression and second high dose (150 mCi, 5500 Mbq) I-131 has been offered to her. The patient had a serum TSH of 104 mIU/L, and Tg of 143.6 ng/mL at the time of I-131 treatment. The post-therapy scan has shown no pathologic uptake in the cervical and extracervical regions. The patient's non-stimulated Tg levels gradually increased from 3.04 to 8.0 ng/mL within several months.

A comprehensive USG of the neck during the first visit in our center revealed multiple pathologic lymph nodes in both thyroid bed; largest one measured 1.0 cm in size. Central lymph nodes were seen predominantly in the left paratracheal region (Fig. 48.1), ipsilateral to primary tumor. There was no suspicious lymph node in previously dissected left neck and right cervical chain. FNAB and Tg washout of dominant suspicious lymph node in left paratracheal region confirmed papillary carcinoma metastasis. She was scheduled for bilateral therapeutic central lymph node dissection. To guide the surgeon during the operation, a neck map showing anatomical relations was drawn, and biopsy-proven and suspicious lymph nodes were plotted on that sketch (Fig. 48.2). In the morning of surgery, most superior (biopsied one) and most inferior metastatic lymph nodes in both central neck were injected with Tc-99m-labeled macroaggregated albumin under USG guidance as described previously [1]. Bilateral central neck dissection was carried out as a comprehensive compartment dissection. With the guidance of intraoperative gamma probe, it was confirmed that pathological lymph nodes which were marked with radioguided occult lesion localization (ROLL) technique remained in dissection material and not left inside. Intraoperative electrophysiological nerve monitoring was also employed.

The final pathology revealed eight metastatic nodes (three in the right paratracheal and five in left paratracheal) out of 13 resected, largest being biopsied one and having a size of 1.1 cm. Histopathological type of metastasis reported as classical variant of PTC and two of the metastatic lymph nodes showed extranodal extension. The clinicopathologic stage of disease in our case was interpreted as follows:

- T1aN1bMx (Stage I) per the AJCC/TNM VIII system [2]
- American Thyroid Association (ATA 2015) intermediate risk of recurrence [3]

48.2 Discussion

Despite excellent overall prognosis, up to 40% of patients with PTC will have persistent or recurrent disease, mostly in lateral (53%) or central (28%) cervical lymph nodes [4, 5]. Local and regional recurrences continue to be treated by surgical excision with or without adjuvant radioiodine treatment, especially in potentially curable patients [6, 7]. Discovery of nonpalpable nodal recurrences in the central and lateral neck has been increased considerably with the evolving role of USG in the follow-up of patients with PTC. However, the management of impalpable or indolent locoregional recurrences of PTC continues to be more controversial. Despite arguments over survival benefit of reoperations, 19–73% remission rates have been reported based on Tg levels with compartment-oriented reoperations [8–10].

Despite ongoing debate on the prognostic significance and the optimal management of regional lymph node metastases in patients with well-differentiated thyroid carcinoma, reported data suggest that survival of patients is adversely affected by lymph node metastases and local recurrences [5, 7]. Radioiodine avid metastatic tumor foci could be treated effectively with I-131 providing radiation dose high enough (8000 cGy) to kill the tumor, whereas response rate is very limited for low radiation doses (3500 cGy) [11]. Although surgery represents the main treatment modality especially for iodine-negative recurrences, reoperation for persistent or recurrent PTC is complicated and requires more experience. Extensive scarring, because

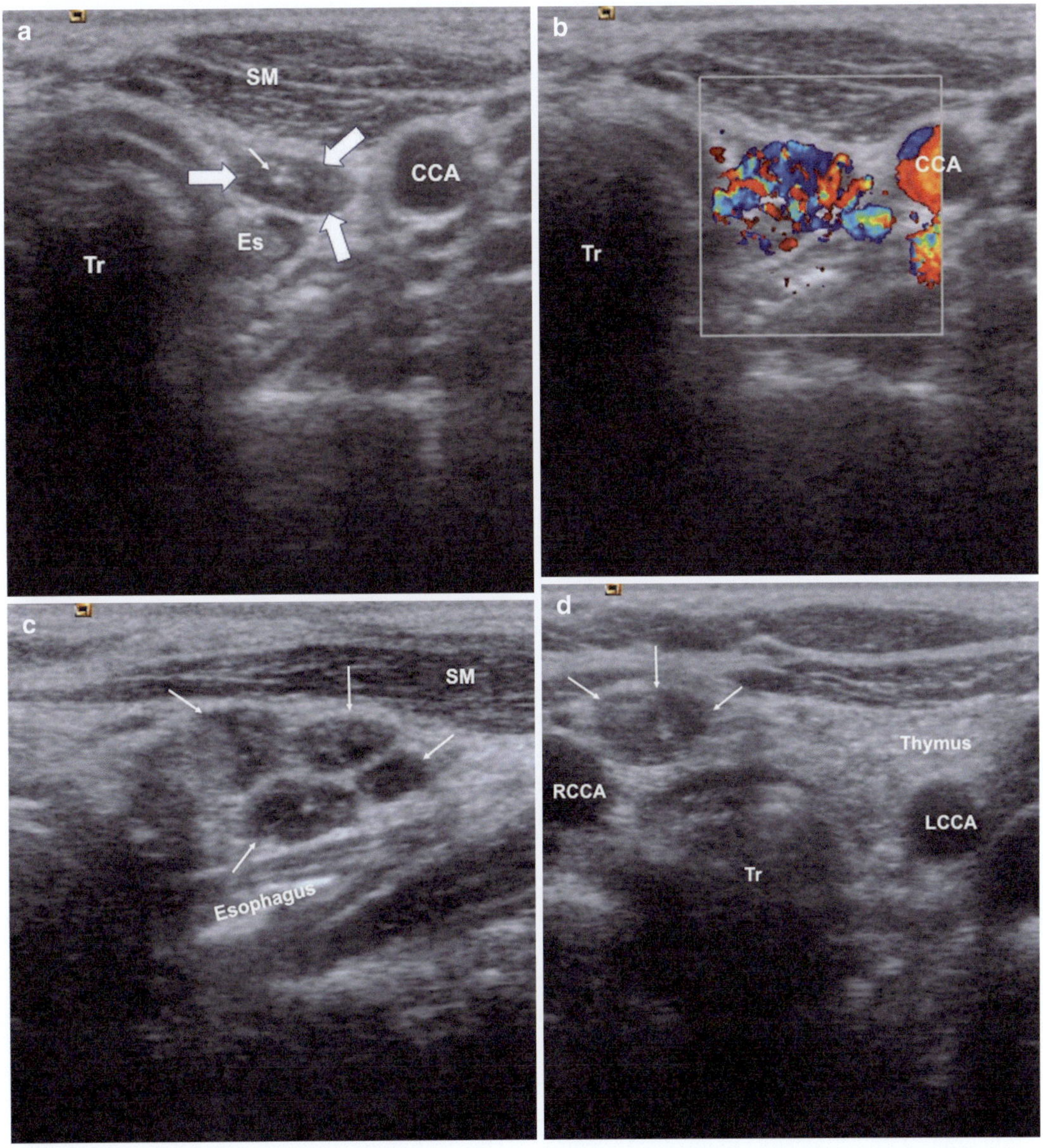

Fig. 48.1 Axial gray scale (**a**) and Doppler (**b**) sonograms of left paratracheal lymph node (thick arrows) showing microcalcifications (thin arrow) and markedly increased vascularity, consistent with nodal metastases. (**c**) Longitudinal sonogram of left paratracheal region shows multiple lymph nodes (arrows) presenting similar features. (**d**) Axial sonogram of deep central compartment shows another metastatic lymph node right to the midline at the level of thyrothymic ligament (arrows) and thymus. *SM* strap muscles, *Tr* trachea, *Es* esophagus, *CCA* common carotid artery, *RCCA* right CCA, *LCCA* left CCA

of previous surgical interventions, considerably increases the incidence of operative complications. Being aware of potential morbidities including hypoparathyroidism (1–13%), recurrent laryngeal nerve (RLN) paralysis (1–12%), Horner syndrome (0.8–1.0%), spinal accessory nerve paralysis (0.7–1.0%), chyle leak (0.2–1.0%), and superior laryngeal nerve deficit and scar [12], sufficient data exist to believe that surgery still represents the key treatment for known recurrent/persistent disease even they are able to concentrate radioactive iodine [9, 10, 13]. Furthermore, progression of recurrent/persistent disease in central compartment might eventually

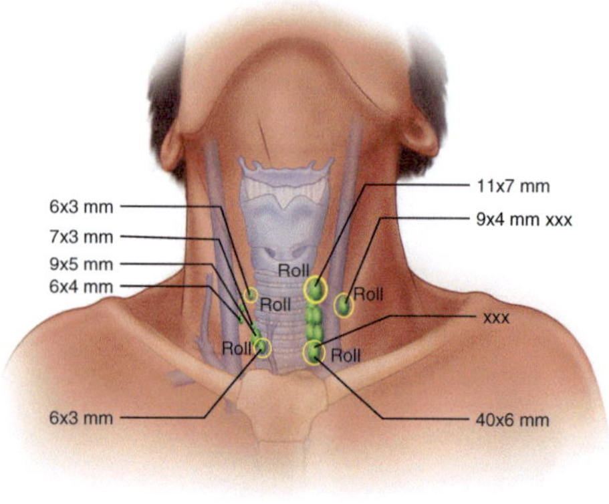

Fig. 48.2 Preoperative US mapping of neck showing metastatic lymph nodes in both central compartments. Reference points such as previous surgical scar, clavicle, sternum, trachea, thyroid cartilage, common carotid artery, etc. shown on the hand drawing as well as injected lymph nodes

result in RLN paralysis and tracheal, laryngeal, or esophageal invasion making timely surgical intervention more critical. Therefore, it has been advocated that efforts should be made to avoid central compartment reoperation by performing a definitive and more radical initial surgical treatment [14].

The ATA 2015 guideline states that therapeutic central compartment (level VI) neck dissection for patients with clinically involved central nodes should accompany total thyroidectomy to provide clearance of disease from the central neck. On the other hand, prophylactic central compartment neck dissection (ipsilateral or bilateral) was recommended in patients with papillary thyroid carcinoma with clinically uninvolved central neck lymph nodes (cN0) who have advanced primary tumors (T3 or T4) or clinically involved lateral neck nodes (cN1b) or if the information will be used to plan further steps in therapy.

The ATA 2015 guideline also do advise therapeutic compartmental central and/or lateral neck dissection in a previously operated compartment for patients with biopsy-proven persistent or recurrent disease for central neck nodes ≥8 mm and lateral neck nodes ≥10 mm in the smallest dimension that can be localized on anatomic imaging [3]. Decision making on timing of surgery mainly based on size criteria in ATA guideline, assuming all the recurrences below this size threshold as low-volume disease. Although indolent nodal disease, even larger than 1 cm, can be managed through active surveillance, multiple factors in addition to size should be taken into account when considering surgical intervention, including existence of high-grade histology, radioiodine avidity, Tg doubling time, and the number of lymph nodes involved (metastatic burden).

It appears that surgical success of reoperations with acceptable complication rates mainly depends on the availability of surgical expertise on revision thyroid cancer surgery. Moreover, correct delineation of the disease preoperatively and the use of new techniques facilitating identification of RLN and metastatic foci during surgery are essential parts of therapeutic success.

With the increasing number of patients discovered with subcentimeter nodal recurrences, the failure to find and remove the recognized recurrences is becoming another risk of reoperations. To improve the surgical success and reduce the complication rates, several methods have been described including preoperative USG mapping [9], intraoperative USG [15], same day USG guidance [16], USG-guided needle localization [17, 18], hook needle-guided excision [19], USG-guided dye injection [20], and radioguided surgery (RGS) [8, 21–24].

ROLL technique which is originally described for breast lesions [25] was also used for nodal recurrences of thyroid cancer in lateral [26] and central compartments [1]. The technique depends on direct inoculation of a small quantity of Tc-99m-labeled particles (macroaggregated albumin, colloid, etc.) into the lesion under radiographic or USG guidance. Since ROLL technique does not depend on the systemic application of the radiotracer and existence of concentrating ability of metastatic lesions, we found this technique noteworthy. Furthermore, it provides best possible lesion to background count ratio during RGS with negligible radiation doses to the operator. We, therefore, use combined preoperative USG mapping with ROLL in patients with PTC recurrences in central compartment.

48.2.1 Management

Despite previous two surgeries, due to increasing Tg levels and apparently, iodine-negative multiple lymph node metastases in central compartment, she was subjected to surgical treatment again. Both central and lateral lymph node metastases were not respected before first surgery and during intraoperative assessment. Most frequently, locoregional nodal disease is the result of incomplete initial surgical treatment, and efforts should be concentrated on timely identification of the presence of cervical lymph node metastasis prior and during first surgery.

Since the patient had undergone thyroid surgery with the intention of lobectomy due to giant benign nodule, central and lateral nodal metastases have been missed during presurgical workup. However, USG examination of known or suspected thyroid nodule should always include the survey of the cervical lymph nodes for detection of possible nodal disease.

Inappropriately high Tg levels after first I-131 treatment have led to the discovery of lateral cervical metastases in our patient. Unfortunately, central nodal metastases have been missed before and during the lateral neck dissection. In general, central compartment is the first nodal basin for metastasis, and skip nodal metastasis is rare and limited to mostly upper pole tumors [27]. Therefore, existence of lateral neck metastasis could have been led to prophylactic central compartment neck dissection (ipsilateral or bilateral) with lateral neck dissection as advised in guidelines.

48.2.2 Follow-Up and Outcome

Since she has been given two high dose RAI treatment and no significant uptake has been appreciated on posttreatment I-131 whole body scans previously, follow-up without additional I-131 treatment recommended to her by our multidisciplinary endocrine tumor board. At 6-week follow-up after last surgery, TSH was 0.04 μIU/mL, and Tg level was 0.158 ng/mL without Tg antibodies.

She was 35 years old and nulliparous by the time of third surgery. She and her husband have been attempting pregnancy before the diagnosis of thyroid cancer. They have been advised to postpone pregnancy for 6 months after each radioiodine treatment. Based on excellent response to surgical treatment, she and her husband encouraged to conceive. She got pregnant two months after final surgery and gave birth to a healthy boy 2 years before. Her Tg levels stayed under <0.2 ng/mL during the pregnancy, and she has been under active surveillance for a few millimetric lymph node in the right central compartment for 4 years now. Last follow-up visit, performed a month before the preparation of this manuscript, revealed serum TSH of 0.107 mIU/L, Tg of 0.132 ng/mL without Tg antibodies and confirmed the stability of millimetric right paratracheal lymph nodes.

What Can We Learn from This Case?

- USG examination of known or suspected thyroid nodule should always include the survey of the cervical lymph nodes for detection of possible nodal disease.
- Surgery still represents the main treatment for known recurrent/persistent disease even they are iodine avid.
- The surgical success of reoperations with acceptable complication rates depends on the availability of surgical expertise on revision thyroid cancer surgery. Correct delineation of the disease preoperatively and the use of new techniques facilitating identification of RLN and metastatic foci during surgery are essential parts of therapeutic success.
- Reoperations of recurrent lateral neck metastasis should include prophylactic central compartment neck dissection (ipsilateral or bilateral) if it is not performed during first surgery.
- Adjuvant radioiodine treatment is not standard in recurrent thyroid carcinoma and could be safely omitted in patients with excellent biochemical and structural response to surgical treatment.

References

1. Ilgan S, Oztürk E, Yildiz R, Emer O, Ayan A, Görgülü S, et al. Combination of preoperative ultrasonographic mapping and radioguided occult lesion localization in patients with locally recurrent/persistent papillary thyroid carcinoma: a practical method for central compartment reoperations. Clin Nucl Med. 2010;35:847–52. https://doi.org/10.1097/RLU.0b013e3181f48403.
2. Amin MB, Edge SB, Greene FL, Compton CC, Gershenwald JE, Brookland RK, et al., editors. AJCC cancer staging manual. 8th ed. New York: Springer; 2017.
3. Haugen BR, Alexander EK, Bible KC, Doherty GM, Mandel SJ, Nikiforov YE, et al. 2015 American Thyroid Association management guidelines for adult patients with thyroid nodules and differentiated thyroid cancer: the American Thyroid Association guidelines task force on thyroid nodules and differentiated thyroid cancer. Thyroid. 2016;26:1–133. https://doi.org/10.1089/thy.2015.0020.
4. Mazzaferri EL. Papillary thyroid carcinoma: factors influencing prognosis and current therapy. Sem Oncol. 1987;14:315–32.
5. Coburn M, Teates D, Wanebo HJ. Recurrent thyroid cancer: role of surgery versus radioactive iodine (I-131). Ann Surg. 1994;6:587–95.
6. Noguchi M, Kumaki T, Taniya T, Segawa M, Nakano T, Ohta N, et al. Impact of neck dissection on survival in well-differentiated thyroid cancer: a multivariate analysis of 218 cases. Int Surg. 1990;75:220–4.
7. Hughes CJ, Shaha AR, Shah JP, Loree TR. Impact of lymph node metastasis in differentiated carcinoma of the thyroid: a matched-pair analysis. Head Neck. 1996;18:127–32.
8. Travagli JP, Cailleux AF, Ricard M. Combination of radioiodine (131I) and probe-guided surgery for persistent or recurrent thyroid carcinoma. J Clin Endocrinol Metab. 1998;83:2675–80. https://doi.org/10.1210/jcem.83.8.5014.
9. Bin Yousef HM, Alzahrani AS, Al Sobhi SS, Al SH, Chaudhari MA, Raef HM. Preoperative neck ultrasonographic mapping for recurrent/persistent papillary thyroid cancer. World J Surg. 2004;28:1110–4. https://doi.org/10.1007/s00268-004-7636-5.
10. Alzahrani AS, Raef H, Sultan A, Al Sobhi S, Ingemansson S, Ahmed M, et al. Impact of cervical lymph node dissection on serum TG and the course of disease in TG-positive, radioactive iodine whole body scan-negative recurrent/persistent papillary thyroid cancer. J Endocrinol Investig. 2002;25:526–31.
11. Maxon HR, Thomas SR, Hertzberg VS, Kereiakes JG, Chen IW, Sperling MI, et al. Relation between effective radiation dose and outcome of radioiodine therapy for thyroid cancer. N Engl J Med. 1983;309:937–41.
12. Kim MK, Mandel SH, Baloch Z, Livolsi VA, Langer JE, Didonato L, et al. Morbidity following central compartment reoperation for recurrent or persistent thyroid cancer. Arch Otolaryngol Head Neck Surg. 2004;130:1214–6. https://doi.org/10.1001/archotol.130.10.1214.
13. Tubiana M, Schlumberger M, Rougier P, Laplanche A, Benhamou E, Gardet P, et al. Long-term results and prognostic factors in patients with differentiated thyroid carcinoma. Cancer. 1985;55:794–804.
14. Wilson DB, Staren ED, Prinz RA. Thyroid reoperations: indications and risks. Am Surg. 1998;64:674–8.
15. Karwowski JK, Jeffrey RB, McDougall IR, Weigel RJ. Intraoperative ultrasonography improves identification of recurrent thyroid cancer. Surgery. 2002;132:924–9. https://doi.org/10.1067/msy.2002.128478.
16. McCoy KL, Yim JH, Tublin ME, Burmeister LA, Ogilvie JB, Carty SE. Same-day ultrasound guidance in reoperation for locally recurrent papillary thyroid cancer. Surgery. 2007;142:965–72. https://doi.org/10.1016/j.surg.2007.09.021.
17. Priven I, Schwartz A, Yeh H. Ultrasonographic localization and marking of a small recurrent thyroid papillary carcinoma. Thyroid. 2003;13:663. https://doi.org/10.1089/105072503322240022.
18. Zimmerman P, DaSilva M, Izquierdo R, Cico L, Kort K, Numan P. Intraoperative needle localization during neck reexploration. Am J Surg. 2004;188:92–3. https://doi.org/10.1016/j.amjsurg.2002.11.037.
19. Triponez F, Poder L, Zarnegar R, Goldstein R, Roayaie K, Feldstein V, et al. Hook needle-guided excision of recurrent differentiated thyroid cancer in previously operated neck compartments: a safe technique for small, nonpalpable recurrent disease. J Clin Endocrinol Metab. 2006;91:4943–7. https://doi.org/10.1210/jc.2006-0386.
20. Sippel RS, Elaraj DM, Poder L, Duh QY, Kebebew E, Clark OH. Localization of recurrent thyroid cancer using intraoperative ultrasound-guided dye injection. World J Surg. 2009;33:434–9.
21. Salvatore M, Ruffini V, Reale F. Radio-guided surgery for lymph node recurrences of differentiated thyroid cancer. World J Surg. 2003;27:770–5.
22. Gulec SA, Eckert M, Woltering EA. Gamma probe-guided lymph node dissection (gamma picking) in differentiated thyroid carcinoma. Clin Nucl Med. 2002;27:859–61.
23. Agrawal A, Hall NC, Ringel MD, Povoski SP, Martin EW Jr. Combined use of perioperative TSH-stimulated (18) F-FDG PET/CT imaging and gamma probe radioguided surgery to localize and verify resection of iodine scan-negative recurrent thyroid carcinoma. Laryngoscope. 2008;118:2190–4. https://doi.org/10.1097/MLG.0b013e3181845738.
24. Rubello D, Salvatori M, Casara D, Piotto A, Toniato A, Gross MD, et al. 99mTc-sestamibi radio-guided surgery of loco-regional 131Iodine-negative recurrent thyroid cancer. Eur J Surg Oncol. 2007;33:902–6. https://doi.org/10.1016/j.ejso.2006.12.016.
25. Nadeem R, Chagla LS, Harris O, Desmond S, Thind R, Titterrell C, et al. Occult breast lesions: a comparison between radioguided occult lesion localization

(ROLL) vs. wire-guided lumpectomy (WGL). Breast. 2005;14:283–9. https://doi.org/10.1016/j.breast.2005.04.002.

26. Tukenmez M, Erbil Y, Barbaros U, Dural C, Salmaslioglu A, Aksoy D, et al. Radio-guided nonpalpable metastatic lymph node localization in patients with recurrent thyroid cancer. J Surg Oncol. 2007;96:534–8. https://doi.org/10.1002/jso.20873.
27. Park JH, Lee YS, Kim BW, Chang HS, Park CS. Skip lateral neck node metastases in papillary thyroid carcinoma. World J Surg. 2012;36:743–7. https://doi.org/10.1007/s00268-012-1476-5.

49 Minimally Invasive Follicular Carcinoma

Elgin Özkan and Çiğdem Soydal

Abstract

A 56-year-old male patient with multiple nodules in both thyroid lobes underwent a left lobectomy due to a nodule with a 3.5 cm diameter in the left thyroid lobe. Histopathological examination of the surgical specimen revealed a minimally invasive follicular thyroid carcinoma (MI-FTC) without vascular invasion. After completion thyroidectomy, additional tumor foci were not detected in the right lobe. The patient received radioiodine ablation treatment (RAT) with 3700 MBq (100 mCi) iodine-131 (^{131}I) 2 months after the operation. During the RAT, the serum thyroid-stimulating hormone (TSH) and thyroglobulin (Tg) levels were measured as 30 IU/ml and 19.5 ng/mL, respectively. Six months after the RAT, a diagnostic whole-body scintigraphy with 185 MBq ^{131}I was performed to evaluate the ablation success. The serum-stimulated Tg level was <0.1 ng/mL, and a ^{131}I whole-body scintigraphy was normal. The patient was followed up with neck USGs, serum suppressed and/or stimulated Tg levels, and/or ^{131}I diagnostic whole-body scintigraphies for 10 years. The patient exhibited no clinical evidence of disease at the final follow-up.

E. Özkan (✉)
Department of Nuclear Medicine, Medical Faculty of Ankara University, Ankara, Turkey

Ç. Soydal
Department of Nuclear Medicine, Ankara University School of Medicine, Ankara, Turkey

49.1 Case Presentation

A 56-year-old male patient with multiple nodules in both thyroid lobes underwent a left lobectomy due to a nodule with a 3.5-cm diameter in the left thyroid lobe. Serum thyroid function tests were compatible with euthyroidism. Histopathological examination of the surgical specimen revealed a minimally invasive follicular thyroid carcinoma (MI-FTC) without vascular invasion. The tumor's maximum diameter was 4.5 cm. A completion thyroidectomy was performed based on considerations of the patient's age and the size of the tumor. After the operation, no tumor was detected in the right thyroid lobe. The patient received radioiodine ablation treatment (RAT) with 3700 MBq (100 mCi) iodine-131 (^{131}I) 2 months after the operation. During the RAT, the serum TSH and Tg levels were measured as 30 IU/mL and 19.5 ng/mL, respectively. Radioiodine uptake limited to the thyroid bed was observed on a postablative whole-body scintigraphy. Six months after the RAT, a diagnostic whole-body scintigraphy with 185 MBq (5 mCi) ^{131}I was performed to evaluate the ablation success.

T. Özülker et al. (eds.), *Thyroid and Parathyroid Diseases*, https://doi.org/10.1007/978-3-319-78476-2_49

The serum-stimulated Tg level was <0.1 ng/mL, and an ^{131}I whole-body scintigraphy was normal. The patient has been followed up with at least one neck USG, one additional diagnostic ^{131}I whole-body scintigraphy and assessments of the serum suppressed and/or stimulated Tg levels every 6 months during the first 2 years of follow-up. Later, the patient was followed up with neck USG and assessments of the serum suppressed and/or stimulated Tg levels at 12-month intervals for 10 years. The patient exhibited no clinical evidence of disease at the final follow-up.

49.2 Evaluation and Diagnosis

Follicular thyroid carcinoma (FTC) is the second most common cancer of the thyroid and accounts for approximately 10% of all thyroid cancers [1]. FTC is more common in women, especially during a short period after menopause, and in iodine-insufficient populations [2]. FTC is divided into two categories based on the degree of invasiveness, i.e., minimally invasive (MI) or encapsulated and widely invasive (WI) [3]. According to the risk of recurrence associated with follicular histological features, three risk groups have been defined as very low-risk FTC, low-risk FTC, and high-risk FTC [3–5]. A very low-risk FTC exhibits capsular invasion without vascular invasion, a low-risk FTC exhibits minimal vascular invasion involving <3–4 microscopic vessels, and a high-risk FTC exhibits extensive vascular invasion that often involves extracapsular vessels. Many clinical studies have demonstrated that the ranges of the risk of recurrence for the very low-, low-, and high-risk groups are 1–7%, 1–5%, and 30–55%, respectively [4–8]. D'Avanzo et al. reported different disease-free survival values at 10 years for the three FTC groups, i.e., 98% for an MI-FTC group without vascular invasion, 80% for an MI-FTC group with vascular invasion and with or without capsular invasion, and 38% for a WI-FTC group [9]. MI-FTCs with a very low or low risk have excellent clinical outcomes, and recurrence and distant metastasis are very rare [4, 5, 7–10]. The correct identification of patients who have a risk for recurrence is important for the clinical outcome. In a recent study, Stenson et al. investigated the outcomes of MI-FTCs and identified prognostic parameters for adequate treatment and follow-up [11]. According to this study, combined vascular and capsular invasion, age at surgery of ≥50 years, and male gender are related to the risk of death from MI-FTC. These authors reported that the age at diagnosis and the existence of combined capsular and vascular invasions are important prognostic factors. Our case had two poor risk factors (i.e., male gender and age ≥50 years) at the time of diagnosis. However, there was no vascular invasion. According to the risk groups, the patient was accepted as having a very low-risk FTC. The patient has been followed up for 10 years without clinical recurrence or disease-related mortality. Despite this finding, in the literature, there are some metastatic MI-FTC cases without vascular invasion [5, 12, 13]. For this reason, some authors believe that the currently accepted histological classification might not precisely predict an aggressive clinical course [12]. These authors recommend total thyroidectomy and RAT for all FTCs [12, 14]. A consensus report of the European Society of Endocrine Surgeons indicated that candidates for total thyroidectomy are MI-FTC patients who are ≥45 years of the age at diagnosis, have tumors ≥4 cm, have vascular invasion, are positive for lymph node metastasis, and are positive for distant metastasis. Radioiodine ablation is also recommended for elderly patients (>45 years) and those with large tumors (>4 cm), extensive vascular invasion, and the presence of metastasis or positive lymph nodes [15]. In our case, we applied total thyroidectomy and RAT.

49.3 Management

Histopathological examination is critical for the discrimination of the FTC categories and patient management. First, a lobectomy was performed because of the large nodule on the left lobe. Second, a completion thyroidectomy was performed because of >4 cm tumor and to enable RAT. Thyroid lobectomy alone may be sufficient for low-risk papillary and follicular carcinoma cancers; however, for patients with thyroid cancers >4 cm, a near-total or total thyroidectomy is recommended by the 2015 ATA guidelines [16]. In our case, an MI-FTC without vascular invasion and a 4.5-cm diameter in the left thyroid lobe was reported in the histopathological examination. Completion thyroidectomy was performed to enable RAT based on consideration of the patient's age, the size of the tumor, and the FTC histology. After the operation, no tumor was detected in the right thyroid lobe. Approximately 2 months after the second surgery, a treatment dose of ^{131}I (3700 MBq) was administered, and a total body scan was obtained 6 days later. Radioiodine uptake limited to the thyroid bed was observed on the postablative whole-body scintigraphy. Postoperative diagnostic ^{131}I or ^{123}I scanning can also be performed 4–6 weeks after surgery. In our department, we do not use routine postoperative iodine scintigraphy because of the stunning effect of ^{131}I. Low-dose (37–111 MBq) ^{131}I or alternative isotopes, such as ^{123}I, can be used to avoid or prevent this effect.

49.4 Follow-Up and Outcome

On the first follow-up 6 months after RAT, a diagnostic whole-body scintigraphy was performed with 185 MBq ^{131}I to evaluate the ablation success. The serum-stimulated Tg level was <0.1 ng/mL, and the ^{131}I whole-body scintigraphy was normal. According to the 2015 ATA guidelines, in patients with an excellent response to therapy (i.e., no clinical evidence of a tumor) and especially in those who are at low-risk for recurrence, the serum TSH may be kept within the low reference range (0.5–2 mU/L). In our case, the serum TSH level remained within the low reference range at 0.5 mU/L. The long-term follow-up of differentiated thyroid cancer has two main goals. The first goal is accurate surveillance for possible recurrence. The second goal is the monitoring of thyroxine suppression or replacement therapy. Our patient was followed up with at least one neck USG, one additional diagnostic ^{131}I whole-body scintigraphy, and assessments of the serum suppressed and/or stimulated Tg levels every 6 months during the first 2 years of follow-up. Later, the patient has been followed up with neck USGs and assessments of the serum suppressed and/or stimulated Tg levels at 12-month intervals for 10 years. The patient exhibited no clinical evidence of disease at the final follow-up.

49.5 Future

The correct identification of an MI-FTC is important for disease management. In the future, the role of new molecular panels should be clarified in patients with MI-FTCs.

What Can We Learn from This Case?

- Although MI-FTCs are usually characterized by an excellent prognosis, distant metastasis has been reported in certain cases.
- The correct identification of patients who have a risk for recurrence is important for the clinical outcome.

References

1. Davies L, Welch HG. Current thyroid cancer trends in the United States. JAMA Otolaryngol Head Neck Surg. 2014;140:317–22.
2. Chow SM, Law SC, Mendenhall SK, Au SK, Yau S, Yuen KT, et al. Follicular thyroid carcinoma: prognostic factors and the role of radioiodine. Cancer. 2002;95:488–98.
3. Schlumberger M, Pacini F, Tuttle RM. Thyroid tumors. Pathology of thyroid tumors. Chapter 2. 4th ed. 2015. p. 41–55.
4. Goldstein NS, Czako P, Neill JS. Metastatic minimally invasive (encapsulated) follicular and Hurthle cell thyroid carcinoma: a study of 34 patients. Mol Pathol. 2000;13:123–30.
5. O'Neill CJ, Vaughan L, Learoyd DL, Sidhu SB, Delbridge LW, Sywak MS. Management of follicular thyroid carcinoma should be individualized based on degree of capsular and vascular invasion. Eur J Surg Oncol. 2011;37:181–5.
6. van Heerden JA, Hay ID, Goellner JR, Salomao D, Ebersold JR, Bergstralh EJ, et al. Follicular thyroid carcinoma with capsular invasion alone: a nonthreatening malignancy. Surgery. 1992;112:1130–6.

7. Sugino K, Ito K, Nagahama M, Kitagawa W, Shibuya H, Ohkuwa K, et al. Prognosis and prognostic factors for distant metastases and tumor mortality in follicular thyroid carcinoma. Thyroid. 2011;21(7):751.
8. Huang CC, Hsueh C, Liu FH, Chao TC, Lin JD. Diagnostic and therapeutic strategies for minimally and widely invasive follicular thyroid carcinomas. Surg Oncol. 2011;20:1–6.
9. Lang W, Choritz H, Hundeshagen H. Risk factors in follicular thyroid carcinomas. A retrospective follow-up study covering a 14-year period with emphasis on morphological findings. Am J Surg Pathol. 1986;10:246–55.
10. D'Avanzo A, Treseler P, Ituarte PH, Wong M, Streja L, Greenspan FS, et al. Follicular thyroid carcinoma: histology and prognosis. Cancer. 2004;100:1123–9.
11. Stenson G, Nilsson IL, Mu N, Larsson C, Lundgren CI, Juhlin CC, et al. Minimally invasive follicular thyroid carcinomas: prognostic factors. Endocrine. 2016;53:505–11.
12. Ban EJ, Andrabi A, Grodski S, Yeung M, Mclean C, Serpell J. Follicular thyroid cancer: minimally invasive tumors can give rise to metastases. ANZ J Surg. 2012;82:136–9.
13. Sugino K, Kameyama K, Ito K, Nagahama M, Kitagawa W, Shibuya H, et al. Outcomes and prognostic factors of 251 patients with minimally invasive follicular thyroid carcinoma. Thyroid. 2012;22(8):22798–804.
14. De Crea C, Raffaell M, Sessa L, Ronti S, Fadda G, Bellantone C, et al. Actual incidence and clinical behaviour of follicular thyroid carcinoma: an institutional experience. Sci World J. 2014. https://doi.org/10.1155/2014/952095.
15. Dionigi G, Kraimps JL, Schmid KW, Hermann M, Sheu-Grabellus SY, De Wailly P, et al. Minimally invasive follicular thyroid cancer (MIFTC)-a consensus report of the European Society of Endocrine Surgeons (ESES). Langenbeck's Arch Surg. 2014;399:165–84.
16. Haugen BR, Alexander EK, Bible KC, Doherty GM, Mandel SJ, et al. American Thyroid Association management guidelines for adult patients with thyroid nodules and differentiated thyroid cancer. The American Thyroid Association Guidelines Task Force on thyroid nodules and differentiated thyroid cancer. Thyroid. 2015;26:1–133.

50 Follicular Thyroid Cancer and Bone Metastasis

Elgin Özkan and Çiğdem Soydal

Abstract

A 78-year-old male patient with follicular carcinoma in the left thyroidal lobe with 10 cm diameter received radioiodine ablation treatment (RAT) with 5550 MBq (150 mCi) iodine-131 (^{131}I) 2 months after the operation. During the RAT, the serum thyroglobulin (Tg) level was measured as 252.59 ng/ml. Radioiodine uptake in the thyroid bed and thoracal and pelvic regions was observed on a postablative whole-body scintigraphy. Simultaneous bone scintigraphy was performed. A moderately increased uptake was observed in the right iliac bone. Thoracal and pelvic computed tomographies (CTs) were also performed for further evaluation of the radioiodine uptake in thoracal and pelvic regions. A pathologic soft tissue lesion of 2.5 × 1.5 cm that may have been compatible with a lymphadenopathy on the anterior mediastinum was observed, and a sclerotic bone lesion of 2 cm in diameter that was concordant with metastasis on the right iliac bone was reported on CT. The patient was followed up for 5 years under suppressive dose of LT4 treatment. Serum Tg measurements and pelvic CT and/or MRI were performed periodically. Biochemical and radiological stabilization were detected during the 5-year follow-up period. Additional surgery or local therapy for the bone metastasis was not applied because of the asymptomatic and stable local metastatic disease.

E. Özkan (✉)
Department of Nuclear Medicine, Medical Faculty of Ankara University, Ankara, Turkey

Ç. Soydal
Department of Nuclear Medicine, Ankara University School of Medicine, Ankara, Turkey

50.1 Case Presentation

A 78-year-old male patient with neck mass underwent total thyroidectomy due to a histopathologically demonstrated follicular lesion that was diagnosed by fine needle aspiration biopsy (FNAB). Histopathological examination of the surgical specimen revealed a follicular carcinoma in the left thyroidal lobe with a diameter of 10 cm. Additionally, capsular and extracapsular invasions were detected on the histopathological examination (T4N0Mx). The patient received radioiodine ablation treatment (RAT) with 5550 MBq (150 mCi) iodine-131 (^{131}I) 2 months after the operation. During the RAT, the serum thyroglobulin (Tg) level was measured as 252.59 ng/ml. Radioiodine uptake in the thyroid bed and thoracal and pelvic regions were observed on anterior and posterior postablative whole-body scintigraphy (Fig. 50.1a, b).

T. Özülker et al. (eds.), *Thyroid and Parathyroid Diseases*, https://doi.org/10.1007/978-3-319-78476-2_50

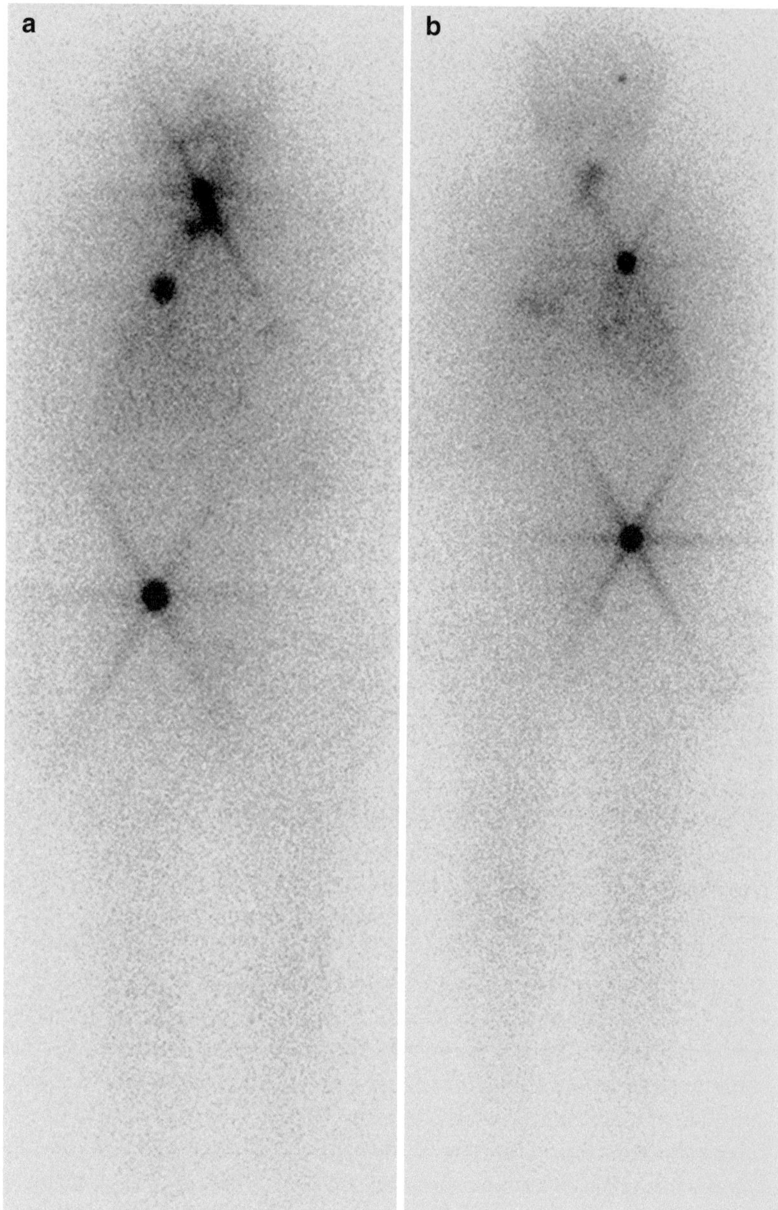

Fig. 50.1 (**a**, **b**) Anterior and posterior images of postablative whole-body scintigraphy following radioiodine ablation treatment (RAT) with high dose iodine-131

Simultaneous bone scintigraphy was performed, and a moderately increased uptake was observed in the right iliac bone. Thoracal and pelvic computed tomographies (CTs) (Figs. 50.2 and 50.3) were also performed for further evaluation of the radioiodine uptake in thoracal and pelvic regions. A pathologic soft tissue lesion of 2.5 × 1.5 cm that may have been compatible with a lymphadenopathy at the anterior mediastinum was observed, and a sclerotic bone lesion of 2 cm in diameter that was concordant with metastasis at the right iliac bone was reported. The patient was followed up for 6 months while under a suppressive-dose LT4 treatment. In the third month, while the TSH level was 0.05 ng/ml, the serum Tg level was 10.03 ng/ml. In the sixth month, while the TSH level was 0.03 ng/ml, the Tg level was 4.68 ng/ml, and simultaneous ^{99m}Tc-MIBI whole-body scintigraphy was performed to evaluate the disease activity. There were no path-

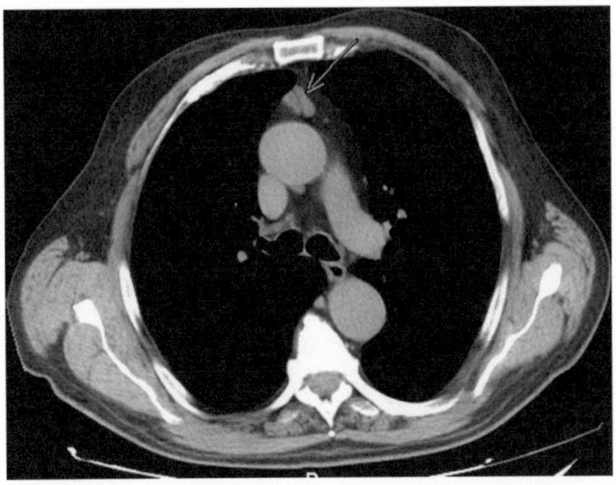

Fig. 50.2 Axial slice of thoracal CT showing pathologic soft tissue lesion at the anterior mediastinum (arrow)

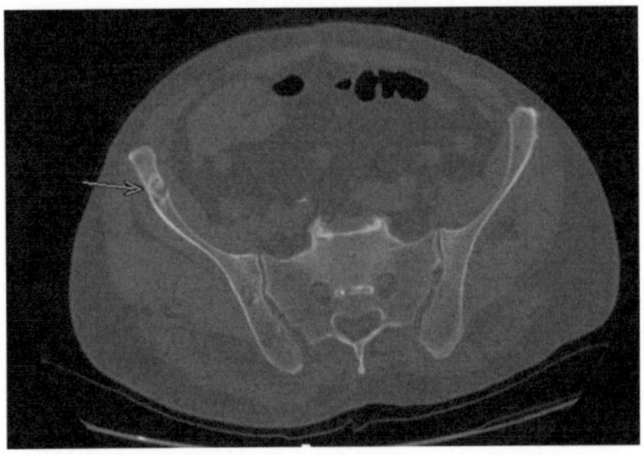

Fig. 50.3 Axial slice of pelvic CT showing sclerotic bone lesion at the right iliac bone

ological findings on the ^{99m}Tc-MIBI whole-body scintigraphy. An ^{18}F-FDG PET/CT was also performed to evaluate the glycolytic activity of the metastases. However, no pathologic FDG uptake was observed on the whole-body PET scan.

50.2 Evaluation and Diagnosis

Follicular thyroid carcinoma (FTC) originates from the thyroid follicular cells, and it is the second most common cancer of the thyroid [1]. FTC usually presents as a solitary thyroid tumor and occurs most commonly in older patients as in our case. Distant metastases, such as those to bones and the lungs, are more likely to develop in patients with FTC than in patients with papillary thyroid cancer due to hematogenous spread [2]. Older patients are at an increased risk of developing distant metastases. High serum Tg levels and initially worse histologic features, such as extensive vascular invasion and extrathyroidal extension, are important indicators of suspected metastasis [3]. The serum Tg levels are higher in patients with bone metastases than in patients with isolated lung involvement [3, 4]. Half of the metastases are initially present and generally identified on postablative whole-body scans as in our case. The remaining patients are discovered after a median follow-up of 3–4 years. Local symptoms, such as pain and swelling and orthopedic complications, are common in up to 85% of patients with bone metastases [2, 5, 6]. Bone metastases are generally purely osteolytic, and radiographic visualizations are often difficult. Bone scintigraphy may reveal decreased or moderately increased uptake. CT and magnetic resonance imaging (MRI) are more successful regarding visualizing bone involvement.

50.3 Management

In cases with radioiodine avidity of the bone metastases, radioiodine treatment is the first-choice treatment. For this reason, our patient received two additional radioiodine treatments. There was radioiodine uptake in the right iliac bone on whole-body scintigraphies after the therapy doses. The patient has been followed up while under suppressive dose of LT4 treatment. Serum Tg measurements and pelvic CT and/or MRI scans have been performed periodically. Biochemical and radiological stabilization were detected during the 5-year follow-up period. Additional surgery or local therapy for the bone metastasis was not applied because of the asymptomatic and stable local metastatic disease. TSH-suppressive thyroid hormone therapy is a preferred therapeutic option for patients with stable or slowly progressing asymptomatic disease [7]. At the end of the 5-year follow-up period, the serum Tg levels began to increase. While the TSH level was 0.05 ng/ml, the serum Tg level was 21.54 ng/ml. No further radioiodine treatment was planned based on considerations of the age of the patient and the total previously received radioiodine therapy dose (cumulative 25,900 MBq). At the time of the preparation of this article, we have planned a new thoracoabdominopelvic CT. If we detect symptomatic, significantly progressive multiple macroscopic diseases, we will evaluate systemic therapy with kinase inhibitors. Tyrosine kinase inhibitors (TKIs) should be considered for radioiodine refractory DTC patients with metastatic, rapidly progressive, symptomatic, and/or imminently threatening disease who are not otherwise amenable to local control using other approaches. However, candidates should be thoroughly counseled on the risks and benefits of this therapy [7]. Additionally, the NCCN guidelines state that lenvatinib or sorafenib should be considered for progressive and/or symptomatic disease with iodine-refractory metastases except for central nervous system metastases [8]. However, TKIs are very expensive and are associated with several adverse events. For this reason, optimal patient selection and management are crucial [9, 10]. ^{18}F-FDG PET/CT imaging can also be performed to identify the disease extent and to predict survival as a prognostic factor. Surgical excision of locoregional disease in curable patients, external beam radiotherapy, or other local treatment options, such as thermal ablation, may also be considered to prevent complications.

50.4 Future

Gene expression profiling can detect evidence regarding aggressive tumor characteristics and the propensity for metastasis. Such profiling and several staining techniques can also apply to FNAB specimens [11, 12]. These approaches could be more frequently used to predict distant metastasis in high-risk patients. The early detection of metastasis can improve the therapeutic results. Recently, a few studies have reported the role of Ga-68 DOTA-peptide PET/CT in the treatment of metastatic thyroid cancer patients. This technique also enables the evaluation of the appropriateness of peptide receptor radionuclide treatment with Lu-177 DOTA-peptides [13]. Another novel PET tracer for the same patient group is iodine-124 (^{124}I). Due to the high sensitivity of this tracer to ^{123}I and ^{131}I and the high resolution of PET imaging, this approach can detect small amounts of metastatic tissue [14]. In the future, the roles of new PET tracers should be clarified for patients under follow-up and with elevated serum Tg levels. The additional benefit of combined PET and MRI imaging will enable an increase in the sensitivity of the detection of recurrent disease in the neck and bones [15].

What Can We Learn from This Case?

- Distant metastases are more common in follicular thyroid carcinoma.
- Especially, older age and poor histopathological factors are important to suspect from metastasis.
- Radioiodine treatment is the first choice of treatment in the case of radioiodine avidity of bone metastases.
- TSH-suppressive thyroid hormone therapy is also a preferred therapy option for patients with stable or slowly progressive asymptomatic disease.
- Surgical excision of locoregional disease in curable patients, external beam radiotherapy, or other local treatment options such as thermal ablation may also be considered to prevent complications.
- Tyrosine kinase inhibitors (TKIs) should be considered in radioiodine refractory DTC patients with metastatic, rapidly progressive, symptomatic, and/or imminently threatening disease not otherwise amenable to local control using other approaches.

References

1. Pacini F, Schlumberger M, Dralle H, Elisei R, Smit JW, Wiersinga W, European Thyroid Cancer Taskforce. European consensus for the management of patients

with differentiated thyroid carcinoma of the follicular epithelium. Eur J Endocrinol. 2006;154:787–803.
2. Durante C, Haddy N, Baudin E, Leboulleux S, Hartl D, Travagli JP, et al. Long-term outcome of 444 patients with distant metastases from papillary and follicular thyroid carcinoma: benefits and limits of radioiodine therapy. J Clin Endocrinol Metab. 2006;91:2892–9.
3. Schlumberger M, Baudin E. Serum thyroglobulin determination in the follow-up of patients with differentiated thyroid carcinoma. Eur J Endocrinol. 1998;138:249–52.
4. Robbins RJ, Srivastava S, Shaha A, Ghossein R, Larson SM, Fleisher M, et al. Factors influencing the basal and recombinant human thyrotropin-stimulated serum thyroglobulin in patients with metastatic thyroid carcinoma. J Clin Endocrinol Metab. 2004;89:6010–6.
5. Bernier MO, Leenhardt L, Hoang C, Aurengo A, Mary JY, Menegaux F, et al. Survival and therapeutic modalities in patients with bone metastasis of differentiated thyroid carcinoma. J Clin Endocrinol Metab. 2001;86:1568–73.
6. Farooki A, Leung V, Tala H, Tuttle RM. Skeletal-related events due to bone metastases from differentiated thyroid cancer. J Clin Endocrinol Metab. 2012;97:2433–9.
7. Haugen BR, Alexander EK, Bible KC, Doherty GM, Mandel SJ, Nikiforov YE, et al. American Thyroid Association Management Guidelines for adult patients with thyroid nodules and differentiated thyroid cancer: The American Thyroid Association Guidelines Task Force on thyroid nodules and differentiated thyroid cancer. Thyroid. 2015;26:1–133. https://doi.org/10.1089/thy.2015.0020.
8. NCCN Clinical Practice Guidelines in Oncology, Thyroid Carcinoma, 2015 Version 2. 2015. NCCN.org.
9. Schlumberger M, Brose M, Elisei R, Leboulleux S, Luster M, Pitoia F, Pacini F. Definition and management of radioactive iodine-refractory differentiated thyroid cancer. Lancet Diabetes Endocrinol. 2014;2:356–8. https://doi.org/10.1016/S2213-8587(13)70215-8.
10. Ito Y, Suzuki S, Ito K, Imai T, Okamoto T, Kitano H, et al. Tyrosine-kinase inhibitors to treat radioiodine-refracted, metastatic, or recurred and progressive differentiated thyroid carcinoma. Endocr J. 2016;63:597–602. https://doi.org/10.1507/endocrj.EJ16-0064.
11. Kebebew E, Weng J, Bauer J, Ranvier G, Clark OH, Duh QY, et al. The prevalence and prognostic value of BRAF mutation in thyroid cancer. Ann Surg. 2007;246:466–70.
12. Vasko V, Espinosa AV, Scouten W, He H, Auer H, Liyanarachchi S, et al. Gene expression and functional evidence of epithelial-to-mesenchymal transition in papillary thyroid carcinoma invasion. Proc Natl Acad Sci. 2007;104(8):2803.
13. Elboğa U, Özkaya M, Sayiner ZA, Çelen YZ. Lu-177 labelled peptide treatment for radioiodine-refractory differentiated thyroid carcinoma. BMJ Case Rep. 2016. https://doi.org/10.1136/bcr-2015-213627.
14. Santhanam P, Taieb D, Solnes L, Marashdeh W, Ladenson PW. Utility of I-124 PET/CT in identifying radioiodine avid lesions in differentiated thyroid cancer: a systematic review and meta-analysis. Clin Endocrinol. 2017;86:645–51. https://doi.org/10.1111/cen.13306.
15. Dercle L, Deandreis D, Terroir M, Leboulleux S, Lumbroso J, Schlumberger M. Evaluation of (124)I PET/CT and (124)I PET/MRI in the management of patients with differentiated thyroid cancer. Eur J Nucl Med Mol Imaging. 2016;43:1006–10.

Differentiated Thyroid Cancer with Brain Metastasis

51

Gülin Uçmak and Burcu Esen Akkaş

Abstract

Differentiated thyroid cancer is associated with favorable prognosis. The presence of distant metastases is generally rare. The most common sites of distant metastases are the lungs and bones followed by the brain and liver. Even with distant metastases, the 10-year survival can reach up to 50% in a majority of patients. However, the prognosis of patients with brain metastases generally differs and associates with cancer-associated mortality. In this chapter, the clinical progression and the diagnosis of brain metastases on follow-up are presented in a patient with papillary thyroid carcinoma.

51.1 Case Presentation

A 46-year-old male patient was referred to our Nuclear Medicine Department after total thyroidectomy with a diagnosis of papillary thyroid cancer for clinical management and the evaluation of radioiodine treatment. The tumor had macroscopical invasion to fat tissues and muscles surrounding the thyroid gland. In addition, there were lymphatic metastases on central and bilateral cervical compartments.

Thyroid scan performed after i.v. administration of 5 mCi Tc-99m pertechnetate was negative for residual thyroid tissue. Neck ultrasound (USG) revealed slightly enlarged superior jugular lymph nodes. The patient was not receiving any thyroid hormone replacement. His thyroid function test results were as follows: Free triiodothyronine (FT3) level was 0.8 pg/ml (reference range, 2.50–4.30 pg/ml), free thyroxine (FT4) level was 0.5 ng/dl (reference range, 0.90–1.70 ng/dl), and thyroid-stimulating hormone (TSH) level was 96.9 µIU/ml (reference range, 0.35–5.00 µIU/ml). Serum thyroglobulin (TG) level was 844 ng/ml. Anti-TG antibodies were within normal ranges.

As serum TG level was significantly elevated, 18-FFDG positron emission tomography/computed tomography (PET/CT) was performed to evaluate disease extent and to stratify patient's risks. Hypermetabolic cervical and mediastinal lymph nodes were detected on PET/CT (SUVmax, 18.4) (Fig. 51.1). In addition, multiple pulmonary nodules which were smaller than 1 cm were seen in both lungs. The patient was discussed in the multidisciplinary tumor board of our hospital for treatment strategies. Cervical and

G. Uçmak (✉) · B. E. Akkaş
Department of Nuclear Medicine, University of Health Sciences (SBÜ) Dr. Abdurrahman Yurtaslan Ankara Oncology Training and Research Hospital, Ankara, Turkey

T. Özülker et al. (eds.), *Thyroid and Parathyroid Diseases*, https://doi.org/10.1007/978-3-319-78476-2_51

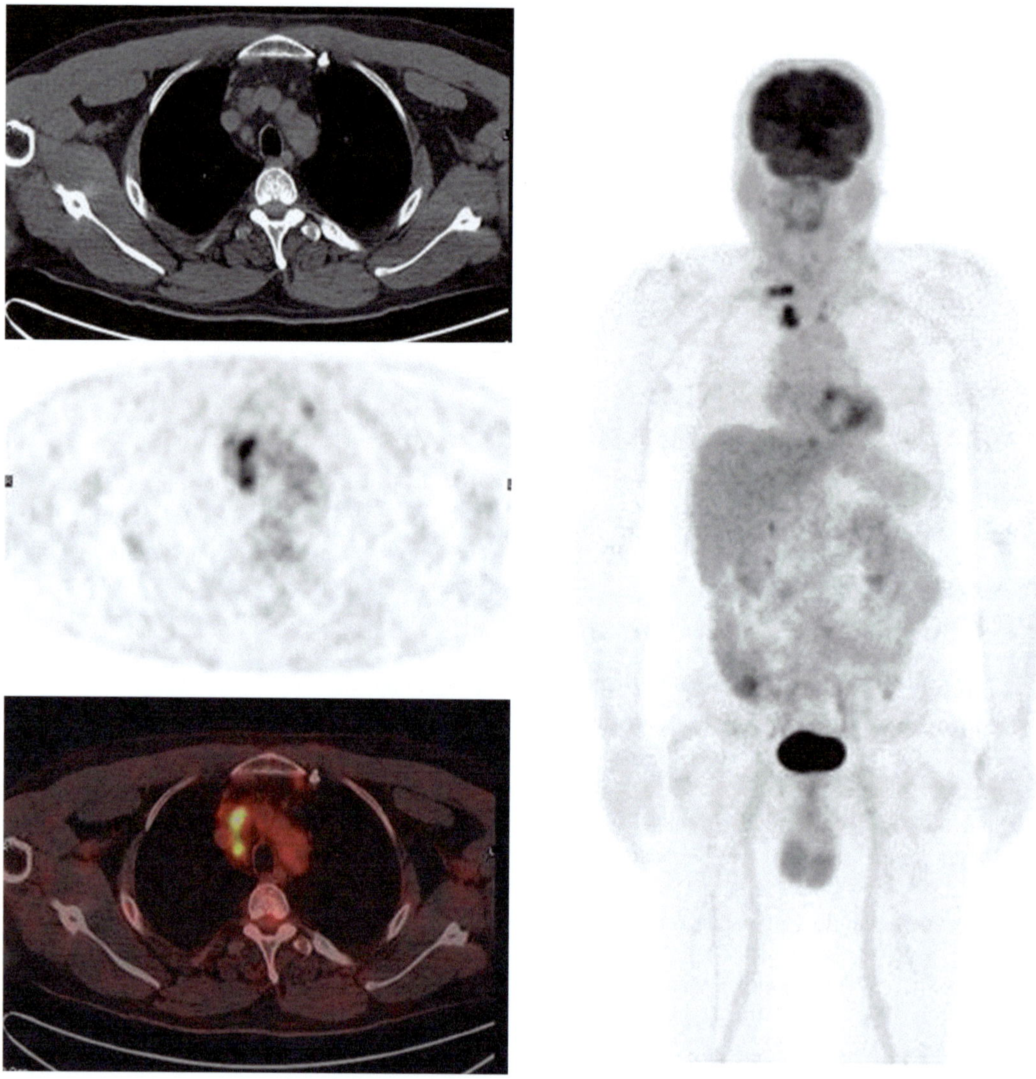

Fig. 51.1 Figure demonstrates staging FDG PET/CT performed after total thyroidectomy. On the left column, axial slices of CT, PET, and fused PET/CT images are given. On the right column, maximum intensity projection image is shown. On PET/CT images, multiple hypermetabolic lymph nodes on right level IV and in mediastinum are seen. The largest mediastinal nodes are 2 cm in size and are located on right paratracheal region with SUVmax of 18.4. Note the intense FDG uptake in the parasternal lymph node which is 3 mm in size

mediastinal hypermetabolic lymph nodes were considered as suitable for surgical resection. In addition, high-dose radioiodine therapy and external beam radiation therapy (EBRT) were planned following surgery. However, the patient refused to have a surgical operation.

A therapy dose of 200 mCi I-131 was chosen for initial therapy. On post-therapy whole-body scan (WBS), intense I-131 uptake was detected reflecting the residual tissues on thyroid bed, and a mild solitary focal uptake was detected on upper mediastinum (Fig. 51.2). After therapy, the patient was discharged from the hospital with L-thyroxin replacement treatment.

A follow-up visit was conducted 3 months after the ablation therapy. Clinical examination and neck USG were performed; serum TSH, non-stimulated TG, anti-TG antibody levels, and complete blood counts were checked during follow-up visits. Response to therapy was assessed

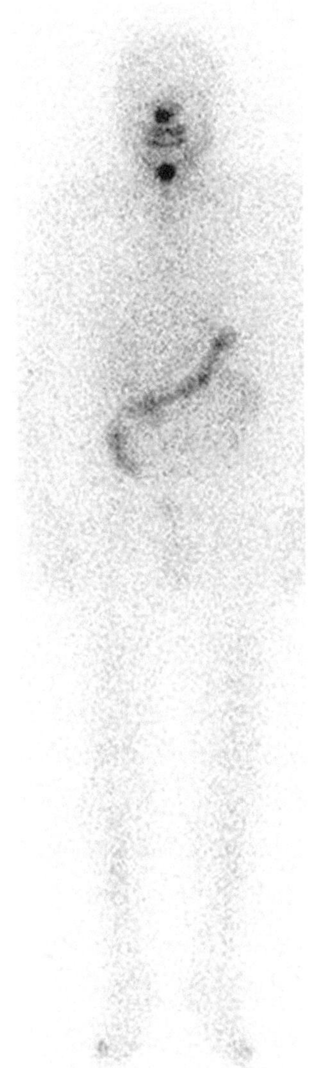

Fig. 51.2 Figure demonstrates the post-therapy WBS following the administration of 200 mCi I-131. Intense iodine uptake is seen on thyroid

based on TG values following after ablation therapy. Serum TG was 65 ng/ml with TSH: 0.1 μIU/ml. Sixty-five Gy EBRT was applied to cervical and mediastinal metastatic lymph nodes. On the control visit 3 months after EBRT, serum TG declined to 20 ng/ml while TSH was 0.1 μIU/ml. Anti-TG antibodies were negative.

The second radioiodine therapy with 250 mCi I131 was given 9 months after the initial therapy dose. Serum TSH was 95 μIU/ml, and TG was 597 ng/ml with no anti-TG antibodies. Post-therapy iodine WBS was negative for pathological iodine uptake. A follow-up PET/CT study performed 6 months after the final iodine therapy and demonstrated a significant reduction in size and metabolic activity in mediastinal lymph nodes. SUVmax declined to 3.12 in hypermetabolic lymph nodes, whereas SUVmax was 18.4 on the previous PET/CT scan.

On the following 4 years after the final iodine treatment, serum TG levels stayed stable within the range 18–25 ng/ml on TSH suppression. However, in the fifth year of follow-up, a sudden progressive TG increase was seen on suppression (25–55 ng/ml, within 6 months). Restaging PET/CT was negative for radiological and metabolic progression. For there were no findings of disease progression on body screening, magnetic resonance imaging (MRI) was acquired for possible brain metastases. On MRI, a 6-mm-sized metastatic mass lesion was seen on left frontal lobe that was isointense on T1-weighted images and hyperintense on T2-weighted images and showed intense contrast enhancement on post-contrast T1-weighted series (Fig. 51.3).

The patient was consulted for neurosurgery for resection of the mass lesion; however stereotactic body radiation therapy (SBRT) was planned on consensus with the tumor board and the patient. Twenty-one Gy SBRT was given in a single fraction to the metastatic lesion. Control MRI was acquired 3 months after SBRT. On MRI, findings compatible with efficient local control were observed.

However, the progressive increase of serum TG was continued, and TG level reached to 91.5 ng/ml 6 months after SBRT on suppression. A restaging PET/CT was acquired. On PET/CT we observed multiple new metastatic lung nodules, some of which have pathological FDG uptake (SUVmax, 2.40) in addition to increase in size of pre-existing nodules and mediastinal lymph nodes. With these findings, the patient was considered as a suitable candidate for targeted therapies as he had iodine-refractory progressive disease. Tyrosine kinase inhibitor therapy was started with oral sorafenib 2 × 400 mg daily. The patient had tolerable side effects such as diarrhea and skin peeling due to sorafenib, but dose adjustment was not needed.

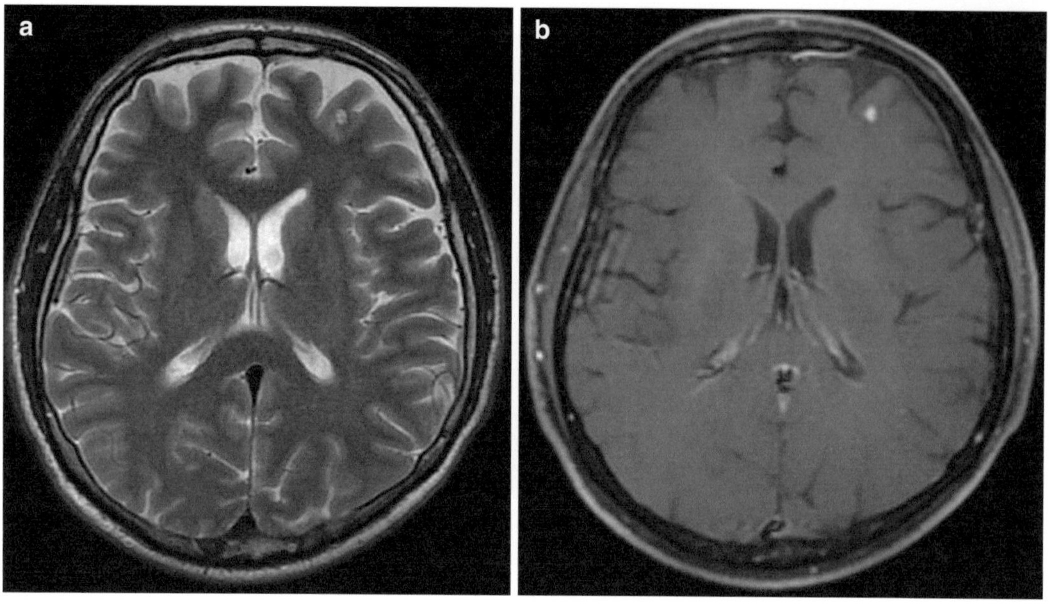

Fig. 51.3 Figure demonstrates the axial slices of MRI imaging. On T2-weighted MRI images (**a**), a hyperintense mass lesion is seen on left frontal lobe which showed increased contrast enhancement on post-contrast T1-weighted series (**b**)

51.2 Follow-Up and Outcome

During 2 years following the onset of sorafenib treatment, control MRI showed findings of local control. However, despite systemic sorafenib treatment, the progression of pulmonary nodules on thorax CT is seen on follow-up. Serum TG levels ranged within 90–161 ng/ml.

As a summary, the patient was diagnosed with local advanced papillary thyroid cancer and had lung metastases and lymph node metastasis in cervical and mediastinum. Following thyroidectomy, the patient received two sequential doses of radioiodine therapy (total dose of 450 mCi) and EBRT to the neck and upper mediastinum. On follow-up, disease stayed stable for 4 years. On the 5th year of follow-up, biochemical progression was seen with stable previous metastatic sites. Cranial MRI imaging detected brain metastases. SBRT was given to the brain, and systemic sorafenib treatment was given due to the progression of lung metastases. In conclusion, 7 years have passed after the initial diagnosis of locally advanced and metastatic papillary cancer, and 2 years have passed after the diagnosis of brain metastases. The patient is still alive with progressive disease and is asymptomatic, and ECOG performance score is 1.

51.3 Discussion

Brain metastases from differentiated thyroid carcinoma (DTC) are rare. The reported frequency is approximately 1% [1–3]. In undifferentiated carcinoma and anaplastic thyroid cancer, the incidence may reach up to 10%. The most common site of brain metastases is hemispheres. Cerebellum, brain stem, and pituitary gland involvement may rarely be seen [4]. Brain metastases may be asymptomatic, or headache, visual disturbances, or symptoms resulting from cerebral edema may be seen.

Since the occurrence of brain metastases from DTC is very rare, there is no specific consensus on how to manage patients with brain metastases from DTC. The choice of therapy must depend on a variety of factors, including performance status of the patient; lifetime expectancy; number, location, and size of brain metastases; the presence or absence of neurological symptoms; suitability for surgical resection; and the chance to control the primary extracranial disease. For solitary brain metastases (SBM) from DTC, in general, surgery remains the preferred treatment modality if applicable [2]. The American Thyroid Association guideline recommends surgery and SBRT as the mainstays of therapy for brain metastases, in addition to radioiodine therapy if the tumors concentrate iodine [5].

Initial treatment for patients with brain metastases includes surgery and radiotherapy, either whole-brain radiotherapy (WBRT) or SBRT. Stereotactic RT is preferred to WBRT because life expectancy in patients with brain metastases may be prolonged, and CyberKnife is generally well tolerated and has fewer side effects compared to WBRT.

In the clinical management of metastatic brain lesions, neurosurgery is severely indicated for patients with >3 cm tumors and patients with smaller tumors but have neurological symptoms due to cerebral edema or compression of vital brain parenchyma. Neurosurgery is generally reserved for patients with limited extracranial metastases and for SBM. However, with the technical improvement in radiation treatment technology, in the new era, CyberKnife may offer considerable outcomes compared to neurosurgery for SBM. For SBM of non-small cell lung cancer, researchers reported that there was no statistical difference between CyberKnife and surgery in terms of overall survival and local disease control [6]. For patients with few brain metastases from DTC, ATA reported that CyberKnife is as effective as surgery and can be repeated in case of diagnosis of new brain lesions [5]. Furthermore, CyberKnife is less invasive, is usually well tolerated, does not significantly increase morbidity, and is more acceptable for patients with SBM particularly for elder patients with comorbid diseases. However, the use of CyberKnife in the treatment of pediatric brain metastases is not well established.

For radioiodine concentrating tumors, radioiodine therapy can be considered as a part of the treatment strategy for brain metastases in a multidisciplinary approach with neurosurgery or RT [7]. When high-dose radioiodine is given, concomitant use of glucocorticoids and anti-edema medications play a pivotal role to prevent the potential TSH-induced increase in tumor size or inflammatory response caused by radioiodine. The use of recombinant TSH stimulation rather than thyroid hormone withdrawal and concomitant corticosteroid therapy may be helpful to avoid prolonged TSH stimulation and significant neurologic symptoms [7].

Particularly in the pediatric population, high-dose radioiodine therapy can provide safe and effective treatment for brain metastasis since pediatric DTC is associated with higher NIS expression in tumor cells than in adults and can accumulate iodine in higher concentrations. In their paper, Vrachimis et al. reported that they succeeded to provide complete remission of all metastases in the brain, bones, lungs, and soft tissues in a 15-year-old girl with oxyphilic variant of papillary thyroid cancer after high-dose radioiodine therapy and maintained over a follow-up period of 7.5 years [8]. For pediatric population, high-dose radioiodine therapy can be considered for the treatment of small brain metastases, if surgery is contraindicated and radiotherapy is to be avoided to minimize adverse effects on the developing brains of children and adolescents. In that context, it is important to premedicate patient with glucocorticoids to minimize the inflammatory effects of radioiodine.

In consensus with our patient, SBRT was applied. Radioiodine therapy was not a therapeutic option for our patient presented here as the tumor was refractory to iodine. Our patient was 46 years old, and even though he did not have any comorbid systemic diseases other than metastatic thyroid cancer, he refused to have neurosurgery and preferred to have SBRT.

Even though the prognosis of DTC with distant metastases is more favorable than the majority of other stage four malignancies, central nervous system involvement associates with poor prognosis. In general, survival decreases to less than 1 year after the diagnosis of involvement in patients with brain metastases [3, 9]. Very rarely, long survival periods up to 10 years are reported in the literature with brain metastases from DTC [10]. Multiple prognostic factors such as the histopathological characteristics of the primary tumor, the avidity of radioiodine, patient age, and comorbid diseases play important role in survival rates. It is suggested that the prognosis of SBM would be better than multiple brain metastases and benefit from more aggressive therapies [11].

The role of systemic therapy, either chemotherapy or targeted therapy, in the management of patients with brain metastases is not well-defined. However, brain metastases on follow-up indicate progressive disease for DTC and may necessitate the administration of systemic targeted therapies to control the extracranial disease. The reason for sorafenib administration for our patient was the need to control the systemic progression other than treatment of BM. Moreover, even data are lacking on the efficacy of systemic targeted therapies such as tyrosine kinase inhibitors for the treatment of BM from DTC; there are published reports suggesting a beneficial role of these agents in the treatment of brain metastases in other malignancies [12, 13].

It is known that patient outcome depends mostly on the progression rate of extracerebral lesions other than the brain metastases [9, 14]. In a recent review, Choi et al. investigated the clinical features and prognostic factors of 37 patients with brain metastases from DTC [14]. They reported that the patients treated for brain metastases had better survival compared to those who were not, but the main reason for disease-caused mortality was lung progression, not the brain metastases [14].

Systemic screening for metastatic disease is important to accurately restage patients with biochemical progression. PET/CT is an effective diagnostic tool to accurately screen distant metastases in patients with iodine-refractory thyroid cancer and to determine patient who would benefit from curative surgery and/or RT [15, 16]. Surgery is crucial to improving progression-free survival. Our group previously analyzed the prognostic factors of patients with distant metastases from DTC and found that surgically amenable disease was the only independent factor in patient prognosis [15]. However, brain metastases, particularly small-volume disease, may be underdiagnosed due to the high physiological glucose uptake in brain parenchyma. Magnetic resonance imaging plays an important role in detecting central nervous system involvement in patients with neurological symptoms. Also, MRI should be included in the clinical workup of patients with locally advanced tumors with poor prognostic histopathological factors, patients with the biochemical progression that cannot be explained by body screening even in the absence of neurological symptoms.

Serum TG is a specific and an extremely useful tumor marker for recurrent disease both with TSH stimulation and suppression. Residual or distant metastatic diseases have been associated with high serum TG levels in DTC. Casco-Diaz et al. evaluated seven patients with brain metastases from DTC [17]. They found that patients with brain metastases had significantly higher levels of TG than those with local or extracranial systemic disease (8.087 vs. 210 ng/ml, respectively). Our patient had significantly high serum TG levels beginning from the initial diagnosis. Although high TG level was a problematic indicator to suspect brain metastases given that our patient had already metastatic disease in lymph nodes and lungs, monitoring the progressive increase in TG with stable previous metastatic sites, we needed to screen for possible brain metastases.

Since the ability to detect small-volume disease and to monitor disease progression has improved significantly, earlier detection of distant metastases and administration of more efficient treatment modalities can provide better outcomes and longer survival periods. Clinicians should consider this risk and investigate the possibility of intracranial involvement as early as possible in patients with metastatic or iodine-refractory DTC in order to minimize clinical deterioration. Surgical resection of all operable metastatic lesions is critical to improving patient survival. As an alternative option, ATA guidelines reports that SBRT is as effective as surgery and can be repeated in case of appearance of new brain lesions [5]. However, the role of multidisciplinary adjuvant treatment following neurosurgery remains unclear [7].

In conclusion, systemic screening for metastatic disease is important to accurately restage patients with biochemical progression. PET/CT is an effective diagnostic tool to screen distant metastases in patients with iodine-refractory thyroid cancer accurately. However, brain metastases, particularly small-volume disease, may be underdiagnosed due to the high physiological glucose uptake in brain parenchyma. In patients with a biochemical progression that cannot be explained by FDG PET/CT imaging, the possibility of brain metastases must be kept in mind. Magnetic resonance imaging plays a pivotal role in detecting central nervous system involvement and should be included in the clinical workup of patients with biochemical progression.

The case presented here had dedifferentiated papillary cancer with cervical and mediastinal lymphatic metastasis and progressed with brain involvement on follow-up. With our meticulous care for distant metastasis screening, the brain lesion was detected while it was a small-volume disease, and with aggressive definitive multidisciplinary treatment, he is still alive and asymptomatic 2 years after the diagnosis of brain metastases. However, we are aware of the worsening clinical outcome of our patient resulting mainly from lung metastases. Further clinical care and alternative therapies such as new targeted modalities, theranostic agents, and/or radiation therapies will be discussed for our patient to prolong event-free survival on follow-up.

What Can We Learn from This Case?

- Serum TG is a specific and an extremely useful tumor marker for the recurrent disease. PET/CT is an effective diagnostic tool to accurately restage patients on follow-up. In patients with the biochemical progression that cannot be explained by FDG PET/CT imaging, the possibility of brain metastases must be kept in mind.
- MRI is crucial in detecting brain metastases from DTC. MRI should be included in the clinical workup of patients with locally advanced tumors with poor prognostic histopathological factors, patients with the biochemical progression that cannot be explained by body screening even in the absence of neurological symptoms, and patients with neurological symptoms on follow-up.
- Treatment options for brain metastases include surgery, RT, and high-dose radioiodine treatment with concomitant glucocorticoids for iodine-avid tumors. The choice of therapy should be tailored to each patient individually.
- Although brain metastases are associated with poor prognosis, the patient outcome depends mostly on the progression rate of extracerebral lesions.
- Local control for brain metastases should be provided. Careful clinical care and individualized alternative therapies should be planned for systemic disease control.

References

1. Clark JR, Lai P, Hall F, Borglund A, Eski S, Freeman JL. Variables predicting distant metastases in thyroid cancer. Laryngoscope. 2005;115:661–7.
2. Henriques de Figueiredo B, Godbert Y, Soubeyran I, Carrat X, Lagarde P, Cazeau A, et al. Brain metastases from thyroid carcinoma. A retrospective study of 21 patients. Thyroid. 2014;24:270–7.

3. Slutzky-Shraga I, Gorshtein A, Popovitzer A, Robenshtok E, Tsvetov G, Akirov A, et al. Clinical characteristics and disease outcome of patients with non-medullary thyroid cancer and brain metastases. Oncol Lett. 2018;15:672–6. https://doi.org/10.3892/ol.2017.7325.
4. Al-Dhahri SF, Al-Amro AS, Al-Shakwer W, Terkawi AS. Cerebellar mass as a primary presentation of papillary thyroid carcinoma: case report and literature review. Head Neck Oncol. 2009;1:23. https://doi.org/10.1186/1758-3284-1-23.
5. Haugen BR, Alexander EK, Bible KC, Doherty GM, Mandel SJ, Nikiforov YE, et al. American Thyroid Association management guidelines for adult patients with thyroid nodules and differentiated thyroid cancer: The American Thyroid Association guidelines task force on thyroid nodules and differentiated thyroid cancer. Thyroid. 2015;26:1–133.
6. Tian LJ, Zhuang HQ, Yuan ZY. A comparison between CyberKnife and neurosurgery in solitary brain metastases from non-small cell lung cancer. Clin Neurol Neurosurg. 2013;115:2009–14. https://doi.org/10.1016/j.clineuro.2013.06.006.
7. McWilliams RR, Giannini C, Hay ID, Atkinson JL, Stafford SL, Buckner JC. Management of brain metastases from thyroid carcinoma: a study of 16 pathologically confirmed cases over 25 years. Cancer. 2003;98:356–62.
8. Vrachimis A, Schmid KW, Jürgens H, Schober O, Weckesser M, Riemann B. Cerebral metastases from thyroid carcinoma: complete remission following radioiodine treatment. Dtsch Arztebl Int. 2013;110:861–6. https://doi.org/10.3238/arztebl.2013.0861.
9. Chiu AC, Delpassand ES, Sherman SI. Prognosis and treatment of brain metastases in thyroid carcinoma. J Clin Endocrinol Metab. 1997;82:3637–42.
10. Miranda ER, Padrão EL, Silva BC, De Marco L, Sarquis MS. Papillary thyroid carcinoma with brain metastases: an unusual 10-year-survival case. Thyroid. 2010;20:657–61. https://doi.org/10.1089/thy.2009.0442.
11. Nieder C, Nestle U, Motaref B, Walter K, Niewald M, Schnabel K. Prognostic factors in brain metastases: should patients be selected for aggressive treatment according to recursive partitioning analysis (RPA) classes? Int J Radiat Oncol Biol Phys. 2000;46:297–302.
12. Soffietti R, Trevisan E, Ruda R. Targeted therapy in brain metastasis. Curr Opin Oncol. 2012;24:679–86.
13. Lin NU. Targeted therapies in brain metastases. Curr Treat Options Neurol. 2014;16:276. https://doi.org/10.1007/s11940-013-0276-z.
14. Choi J, Kim JW, Keum YS, Lee IJ. The largest known survival analysis of patients with brain metastasis from thyroid Cancer based on prognostic groups. PLoS One. 2016;11:e0154739. https://doi.org/10.1371/journal.pone.0154739.
15. Akkas BE, Demirel BB, Vural GU. Prognostic factors affecting disease-specific survival in patients with recurrent and/or metastatic differentiated thyroid carcinoma detected by positron emission tomography/computed tomography. Thyroid. 2014;24:287–95. https://doi.org/10.1089/thy.2013.019.
16. Vural GU, Akkas BE, Ercakmak N, Basu S, Alavi A. Prognostic significance of FDG PET/CT on the follow-up of patients of differentiated thyroid carcinoma with negative 131I whole-body scan and elevated thyroglobulin levels: correlation with clinical and histopathologic characteristics and long-term follow-up data. Clin Nucl Med. 2012;37:953–9. https://doi.org/10.1097/RLU.0b013e31825b2057.
17. Cacho-Diaza B, Cuevas-Ramos D, Spinola-Marono H, Reyes-Soto G, Olvera-Manzanilla E, Monroy-Sosa A, et al. Thyroid cancer brain metastases and thyroglobulin. J Endocrinol Metab. 2016;6:90–4.

Differentiated Thyroid Cancer and Pulmonary Metastasis

52

Çiğdem Soydal and Elgin Özkan

Abstract

A 50-year-old female patient exhibiting hyperthyroidism, with no known risk factors for thyroid cancer, underwent thyroid ultrasound. Multiple thyroid nodules with different echo patterns were detected. A fine needle aspiration biopsy (FNAB) detected a papillary thyroid carcinoma in the cold nodule in the left lobe. The intraoperative evaluation determined that the central compartment lymph nodes were enlarged, so the patient underwent a total thyroidectomy and a bilateral central compartment lymph node dissection. Histopathological examination of the surgical specimen revealed two foci of papillary thyroid carcinomas, 3 and 0.7 cm in size, in both thyroid lobes with extra-thyroidal soft tissue invasion and lymph node metastases (T2N1aMx, ATA intermediate risk group). A 5550 MBq (150 mCi) I-131 dose was administered under endogenous TSH elevation. After 6 months of radioiodine treatment (RAT), diagnostic whole-body scintigraphy was performed with 185 MBq (5 mCi) I-131. Although, there was no pathological uptake at the thyroid bed or any site during whole-body scintigraphy, stimulated Tg serum levels were 140 ng/ml. No pathologic lesion was detected in the neck ultrasound. For this reason, the patient underwent ^{18}F-FDG PET/CT. Multiple ^{18}F-FDG avid lung nodules were identified with a SUVmax of 2.7. Diagnostic computed tomography of the thorax revealed multiple millimetric metastatic nodules in both lungs.

Ç. Soydal (✉)
Department of Nuclear Medicine, Ankara University School of Medicine, Ankara, Turkey

E. Özkan
Department of Nuclear Medicine, Medical Faculty of Ankara University, Ankara, Turkey

52.1 Case Presentation

A 50-year-old female patient exhibiting hyperthyroidism, with no known risk factors for thyroid cancer, underwent thyroid ultrasound (USG). Multiple thyroid nodules with different echo patterns were detected. Additionally, technetium-99m pertechnetate thyroid scintigraphy was performed to evaluate nodule activity. A fine needle aspiration biopsy (FNAB) detected a papillary thyroid carcinoma in the cold nodule in the left lobe. The intraoperative evaluation determined that the central compartment lymph nodes were enlarged, so the patient underwent a total thyroidectomy and a bilateral central compartment lymph node dissection. Histopathological examination of the surgical specimen revealed two foci of papillary thyroid carcinomas, 3 and

T. Özülker et al. (eds.), *Thyroid and Parathyroid Diseases*, https://doi.org/10.1007/978-3-319-78476-2_52

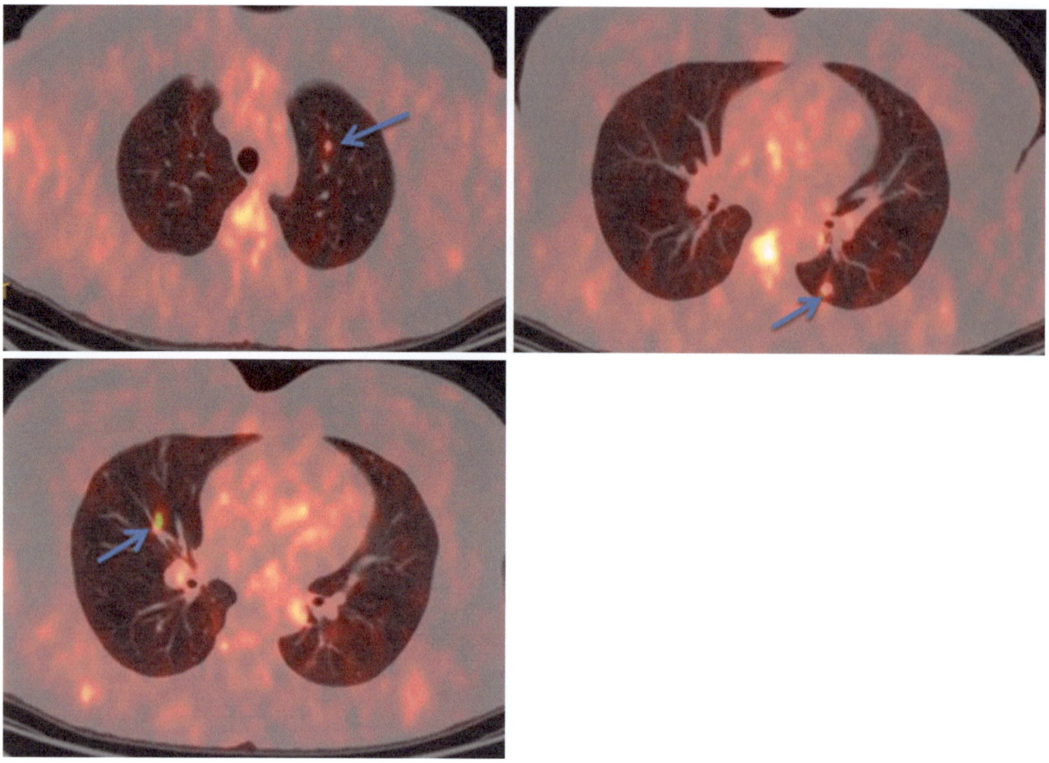

Fig. 52.1 Transaxial fused ^{18}F-FDG PET/CT images of the thorax

0.7 cm in size, in both thyroid lobes with extrathyroidal soft tissue invasion and lymph node metastases (T2N1aMx, ATA intermediate risk group). A 5550 MBq (150 mCi) I-131 dose was administered under endogenous TSH elevation. During treatment, serum Tg levels were measured at 117.3 ng/ml while TSH levels were >30 mIU/l. Post-therapeutic whole-body scintigraphy demonstrated multiple foci of activity in the thyroid bed. After 6 months of radioiodine treatment (RAT), diagnostic whole-body scintigraphy was performed with 185 MBq (5 mCi) I-131. Although there was no pathological uptake in the thyroid bed or any site during whole-body scintigraphy, stimulated Tg serum levels were detected as 140 ng/ml. No pathological conditions were detected in the neck USG. For this reason, the patient underwent ^{18}F-FDG PET/CT. Multiple ^{18}F-FDG avid lung nodules were detected with a SUVmax of 2.7 (Fig. 52.1). Diagnostic computed tomography (CT) of the thorax revealed multiple millimetric metastatic nodules in both lungs (Fig. 52.2).

52.1.1 Evaluation and the Diagnosis

The most common site of metastasis of differentiated thyroid cancer (DTC) is cervical lymph nodes [1]. The lung is the most common site of distant metastases [2, 3]. As such, approximately 10% of patients develop pulmonary metastases. Although the life expectancy of these patients is shortened, most studies report an average survival rate approaching 50% at both 5 and 10 years [4, 5]. The prognostic factors in pulmonary metastasis are tumor histology, radioiodine avidity, and patient age. Additionally, the presence of malignant pleural effusion has been described as a negative prognostic factor [1]. Radiologically, pulmonary metastases may be seen in micronodular or macronodular patterns [6]. Micronodular metastases are usually observed in children, have a miliary and diffuse reticular pattern predominating in the lower lung fields, and are more likely to concentrate radioiodine diffusely. In contrast, macronodular pattern has lesions larger than 0.5 cm with nodules of unequal size, is more frequent in older

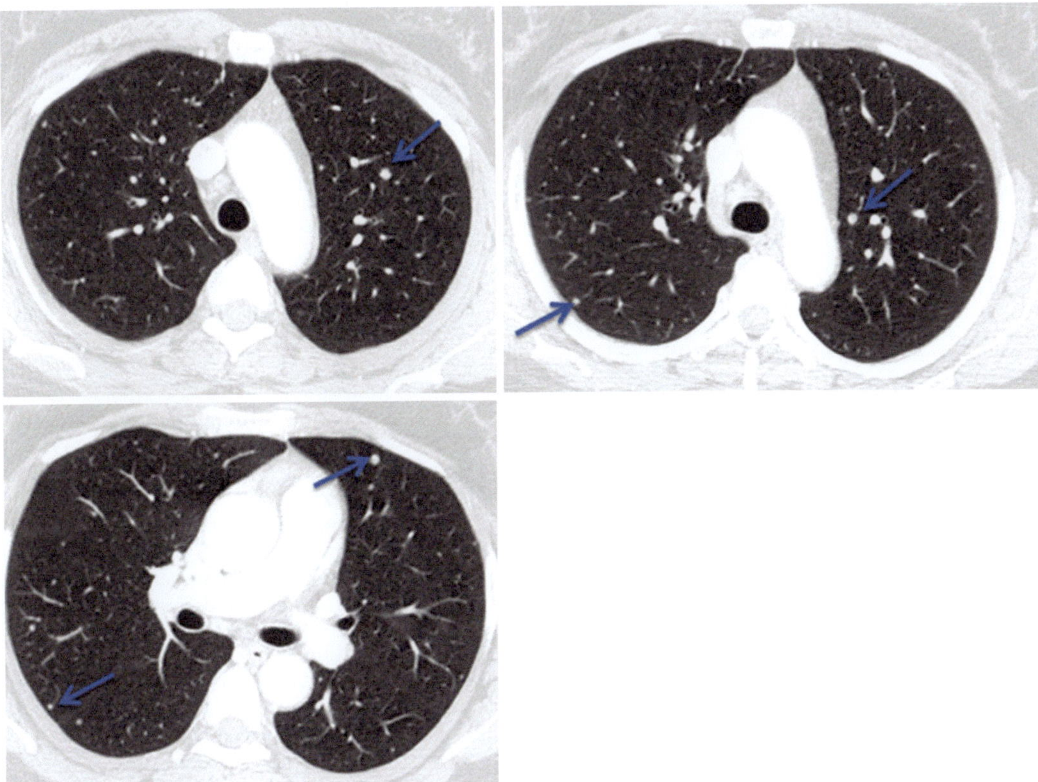

Fig. 52.2 Transaxial diagnostic CT images of the thorax

patients, and exhibits heterogeneous and/or absent radioiodine incorporation [1]. Although they rarely occur, it is important to assess patients for lung metastases because they can elicit an aggressive disease state and lethal complications.

52.1.2 Management

Since lung metastases are highly avid for radioiodine, radioiodine treatment is the choice of treatment. As such, our patient received a second dose of 7400 MBq (200 mCi) radioiodine. However, there was no radioiodine uptake in the lungs as determined by whole-body scintigraphy after the second dose. Following radioiodine treatment, the patient received a suppressive dose of LT4. Serum Tg measurements and thorax CT were performed periodically. Both biochemical and radiological progressions were detected in the second-year control. Because the lung metastases of the patient became non-avid to radioiodine, tyrosine kinase inhibitor treatment was initiated for progressive disease. Tyrosine kinase inhibitors (TKI), a molecular-targeted agent, recently have become available for treatment against radioiodine non-avid or radioiodine-refractory metastatic DTCs [7, 8]. As per the ATA guideline, it is recommended that tyrosine kinase inhibitor therapies should be considered in radioiodine-refractory DTC patients with metastatic, rapidly progressive, symptomatic, and/or imminently threatening disease not otherwise amenable to local control using other approaches. However, candidates should be thoroughly counseled on the risks and benefits of this therapy [9]. Additionally, the NCCN Guidelines state that lenvatinib or sorafenib should be considered for progressive and/or symptomatic disease of iodine-refractory metastases except for central nervous system metastasis [10]. However, TKIs are very expensive and have several adverse side effects. For this reason, optimal patient selection and management are crucial [11].

52.2 Follow-Up and Outcome

The patient has been followed up, and it was determined that biochemical and radiological disease was stable after TKI treatment for 1 year.

52.2.1 The Future

Non-radioiodine avid metastatic thyroid carcinomas are a challenging patient group. Surgical resection can be performed in the case of a limited number of metastases. In addition to tyrosine kinase inhibitors, more targeted treatments should be developed. For example, radionuclide therapy using the Lu-177 DOTA-peptide has been reported as an alternative option. However, large prospective studies with a large number of patients should be designed to reveal the effectiveness of Lu-177 DOTA-peptide treatment.

What Can We Learn from This Case?

- Lung metastasis is detected in approximately 10% of DTC patients.
- Tyrosine kinase inhibitors could be an alternative in the management of radioiodine non-avid or radioiodine-refractory patients.
- Lu-177 DOTA-peptide receptor treatment would be an alternative in Ga-68 DOTA-peptide positive metastases.

References

1. Vassilopoulou-Sellin R. Management of papillary thyroid cancer. Oncology (Williston Park). 1995;9:145–51.
2. Samaan NA, Schultz PN, Hickey RC, Goepfert H, Haynie TP, Johnston DA, et al. The results of various modalities of treatment of well differentiated thyroid cancer: a retrospective review of 1599 patients. J Clin Endocrinol Metab. 1992;75:714–20. https://doi.org/10.1210/jcem.75.3.1517360.
3. Mazzaferri EL. Papillary thyroid carcinoma: factors influencing prognosis and current therapy. Semin Oncol. 1987;14:315–32.
4. Ruegemer JJ, Hay ID, Bergstralh EJ, Ryan JJ, Offord KP, Gorman CA. Distant metastases in differentiated thyroid carcinoma: a multivariate analysis of prognostic variables. J Clin Endocrinol Metab. 1988;67:501–8.
5. Robbins J, Merino MJ, Boice JD Jr, Ron E, Ain KB, Alexander HR, et al. Thyroid cancer: a lethal endocrine neoplasm. Ann Intern Med. 1991;115:133–47.
6. Massin JP, Savoie JC. Pulmonary metastases in differentiated thyroid carcinoma. Cancer. 1984;53:982–92.
7. Brose MS, Nutting CM, Jarzab B, Elisei R, Siena S, Bastholt L, et al. Sorafenib in radioactive iodine-refractory, locally advanced or metastatic differentiated thyroid cancer: a randomized, double-blind, phase 3 trial. Lancet. 2013;384:319–28. https://doi.org/10.1016/S0140-6736(14)60421-9.
8. Schlumberger M, Tahara M, Wirth LJ, Robinson B, Brose MS, Elisei R, et al. Lenvatinib versus placebo in radioiodine-refractory thyroid cancer. N Engl J Med. 2015;372:621–30. https://doi.org/10.1056/NEJMoa1406470.
9. Haugen BR, Alexander EK, Bible KC, Doherty G, Mandel SJ, Nikiforov YE, et al. American Thyroid Association management guidelines for adult patients with thyroid nodules and differentiated thyroid cancer: the American Thyroid Association guidelines task force on thyroid nodules and differentiated thyroid cancer. Thyroid. 2016;26:1–133. https://doi.org/10.1002/cncr.30360.
10. Schlumberger M, Brose M, Elisei R, Leboulleux S, Luster M, Pitoia F, et al. NCCN clinical practice guidelines in oncology, thyroid carcinoma, 2015 version 2, (2015). NCCN.org definition and management of radioactive iodine-refractory differentiated thyroid cancer. Lancet Diabetes Endocrinol. 2014;2:356–8. https://doi.org/10.1016/S2213-8587(13)70215-8.
11. Ito Y, Suzuki S, Ito K, Imai T, Okamoto T, Kitano H, et al. Tyrosine-kinase inhibitors to treat radioiodine-refracted, metastatic, or recurred and progressive differentiated thyroid carcinoma. Endocr J. 2016;30(63):597–602. https://doi.org/10.1507/endocrj.EJ16-0064.

53 Targeted Systemic Therapy May Be Promising in Radioiodine-Refractory Differentiated Thyroid Cancer

Zehra Özcan and Ülkem Yararbaş

Abstract

During the follow-up of a patient with differentiated thyroid carcinoma, Tg elevation without iodine uptake on WB scan was noted. She received an empiric dose of radioiodine to evaluate the possible Tg production site; however, no evidence of uptake was found. PET/CT scan showed pulmonary nodules, some of which were FDG avid. Finally, sorafenib treatment was initiated which is currently at the 22nd month of the follow-up.

53.1 Case Presentation

A 45-year-old female with a history of nodular thyroid disease suspicious for malignancy on the left lobe was referred for surgery. Initially, she underwent left lobectomy, isthmusectomy, and subtotal thyroidectomy on the right side. Surgical specimen revealed papillary carcinoma of 2 cm on the largest dimension, with multicentric involvement including features of both classic and follicular variant tumor cells. Postoperative Doppler ultrasound illustrated remnant tissue on the right lobe and level IV lymph node measuring 20 × 10 mm with tiny calcifications and mixed vascular pattern suspicious for metastatic features. She underwent completion thyroidectomy and lateral lymph node dissection which showed several metastatic lymph nodes (3/32). She was defined as T1bN1bM0 and stage IVa according to the AJCC/UICC TNM system as noted in ATA guideline 2015 [1]. She received high-dose I-131 treatment 150 mCi (5550 MBq), while TSH was 72 μIU/mL and thyroglobulin (Tg) 79 ng/mL. Six months later, she still had an elevated Tg of 66.3 ng/mL without elevation of anti-Tg antibodies. A second dose of 150 mCi (5550 MBq) I-131 was given. Posttreatment whole-body scan revealed a small focus of uptake in the left neck region; no additional focus outside neck was detected. Six months later, diagnostic I-131 scan was obtained while she was T4 off, Tg was 122 ng/mL, and anti-Tg antibodies were normal. Whole-body iodine scan performed under the restriction of iodine intake showed no evidence of functioning thyroid or metastatic tissue. Urine excretion of iodine was also checked to rule out artefactual iodine suppression. Her records were discussed in the thyroid tumor board, and a neck ultrasound and a thorax computerized tomography (CT) or ^{18}F-FDG PET/CT was requested to evaluate the presence of abnormal foci without

Z. Özcan (✉) · Ü. Yararbaş
Department of Nuclear Medicine, Ege University School of Medicine, Izmir, Turkey

T. Özülker et al. (eds.), *Thyroid and Parathyroid Diseases*, https://doi.org/10.1007/978-3-319-78476-2_53

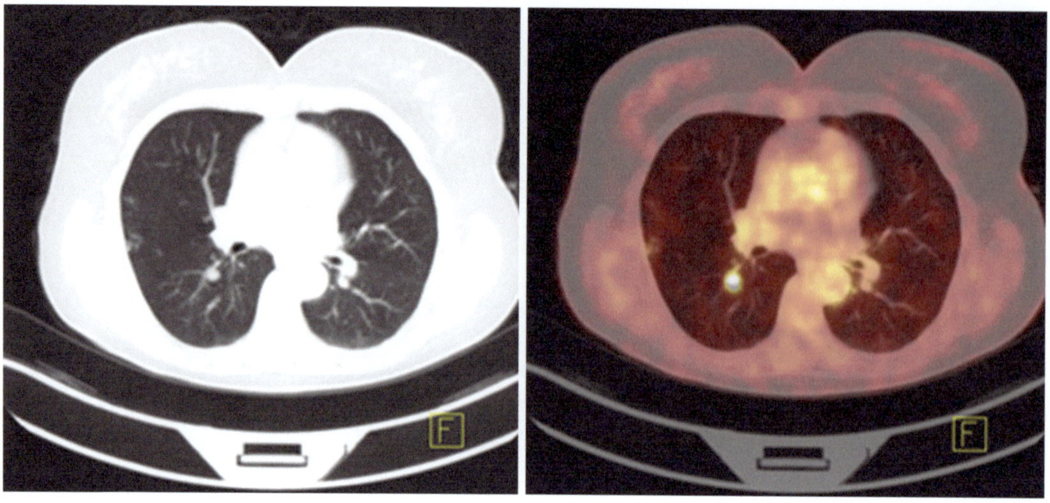

Fig. 53.1 Transaxial CT and fusion ^{18}F-FDG PET/CT scan show tiny nodules with the largest one (9 mm) in the right lung with high FDG uptake (SUV max 21.9)

iodine avidity. Neck ultrasound was normal, but thorax CT (without iv contrast) showed several lung nodules with the largest size of 3 mm that is too small to be characterized. Follow-up CT was suggested to evaluate the stability over time. She received 200 mCi (7400 MBq) iodine-131 treatment. Post-therapeutic scan was found to be negative again. Eight months later, non-stimulated Tg level was 17 ng/mL. ^{18}F-FDG PET/CT scan was obtained to evaluate possible metastatic involvement. ^{18}F-FDG PET/CT scan with low-dose non-contrast CT demonstrated progression of lung nodules in both lungs, some of which were FDG avid (Fig. 53.1). As there is gradual decline but still elevated Tg production, despite the lack of iodine avidity, a final empiric high-dose I-131 [200 mCi (7400 MBq)] was given. However, radioiodine was not taken up by the small lung nodules. Six months later, Tg levels were 164 and 12 ng/mL, respectively, while T4 off and on. So, the total cumulative RAI dose was >600 mCi (>22.2 GBq), obtained during a 5-year period with interval of at least 6 months. Despite slight decline in Tg levels indicating biochemical response, progression of lung nodules on FDG PET/CT without iodine avidity was representing that targeted therapy might be more appropriate to control the disease. She is referred to the oncology department, and sorafenib treatment with a dose of 400 mg twice daily was initiated. She is currently under treatment for 22 months with regular follow-up for every 3 months.

53.2 Discussion

Serum Tg level monitoring and I-131 whole-body scanning are the mainstay of long-term surveillance in patients with differentiated thyroid carcinoma. The absence of iodine accumulation and undetectable Tg levels indicate complete remission of the disease. However, discordance of these two biomarkers may be encountered in some patients due to a variety of reasons [2]. Therefore, it is required to rule out false-positive or false-negative Tg levels related to improper patient preparation prior to the scan, lack of TSH stimulation, and interference with elevated Tg antibodies. The false-negative I-131 scan is assumed to be due to microscopic metastatic disease smaller than scan detectability limits, loss of iodine trapping mechanism, and dedifferentiation. While there is no established consensus in this particular clinical setting, some authors have recommended the use of empiric therapy with high-dose radioiodine [3–8]. It is noted that post-therapy scan might be of value to detect tiny metastatic deposits that are not visible with a diagnostic I-131 WBS [5, 7]. Moreover, a therapeutic goal which can be assessed with a decline in serum Tg levels can be possible in a considerable number of patients [7]. It has also been demonstrated that blind use of high-dose radioiodine has much more beneficial effect in patients with lung metastasis [5] than those with lymphatic involvement particularly when the disease is micrometastatic [7]. On the other hand, due to the lack of scientific evidence obtained from randomized prospective controlled trials, further diagnostic investigations might be indicated for deciding for these patients [9]. FDG PET/CT imaging is the method of choice for a high-risk patient with rising Tg level (>10 ng/mL) and negative iodine scan [1]. PET imaging may also have a role for prognostication of patients with rising Tg or anti-Tg levels without corresponding iodine uptake [10, 11]. As represented in the current case, FDG PET scan has been a powerful tool to locate the disease, directing the patient to therapy according to the extent of metastatic disease. Lack of iodine accumulation in lung nodules on post-therapy scan under TSH stimulation indicated that this patient could be classified as RAI-refractory DTC [1], and there is no further indication of iodine treatment. As the high FDG avidity was indicating less favorable outcome in this scenario, a novel systemic approach with kinase inhibitors can be recommended [1, 12–14]. Phase III trial by Brose et al. showed that sorafenib treatment provides an improvement in progression-free survival and therefore might be a new treatment choice in RAI-refractory patients [15]. For assessing the therapeutic effect, median thyroglobulin level was found to be decreased or stable in this trial. In contrast to this, although derived from a limited number of patients, Benekli et al. have found no correlation between biomarkers and sorafenib efficacy in advanced differentiated and medullary thyroid cancer [16]. So, the current scientific evidence is limited to assess the relationship between therapeutic efficacy of sorafenib and biochemical response. Finally, sorafenib seems to be a promising agent in patients with advanced or iodine-refractory differentiated thyroid carcinoma. However, due to the high probability of side effects that may seriously affect the quality of life, it is imperative to review all benefits and risks of this therapy.

53.3 Follow-Up and Clinical Course

Short term after sorafenib, she described arthralgia symptoms, hypertension, and hand/foot skin reactions. Antihypertensive medication was started after cardiologic counseling. Skin reactions were suppressed well with supportive care. Additional analgesics were effective in arthralgia symptoms. However, she also defined several attacks of diarrhea and fatigue. The dose was decreased to 200 mg/day. When the clinical symptoms were progressing, sorafenib treatment was interrupted for several days and started again. At the end of the 6th month, FDG PET/CT scan showed, when compared to the prior scan, decrease in size of the nodules and decreased FDG uptake indicating therapeutic response (Fig. 53.2). Now the patient completed 22 months of treatment. Despite the adverse effects described above, with short intervals of dose reduction when needed, she is well-tolerating the treatment. For the clinical practice, informing the patient about the side effects and close communication between the doctor and the patient seem to be a key for successful management in patients undergoing sorafenib treatment.

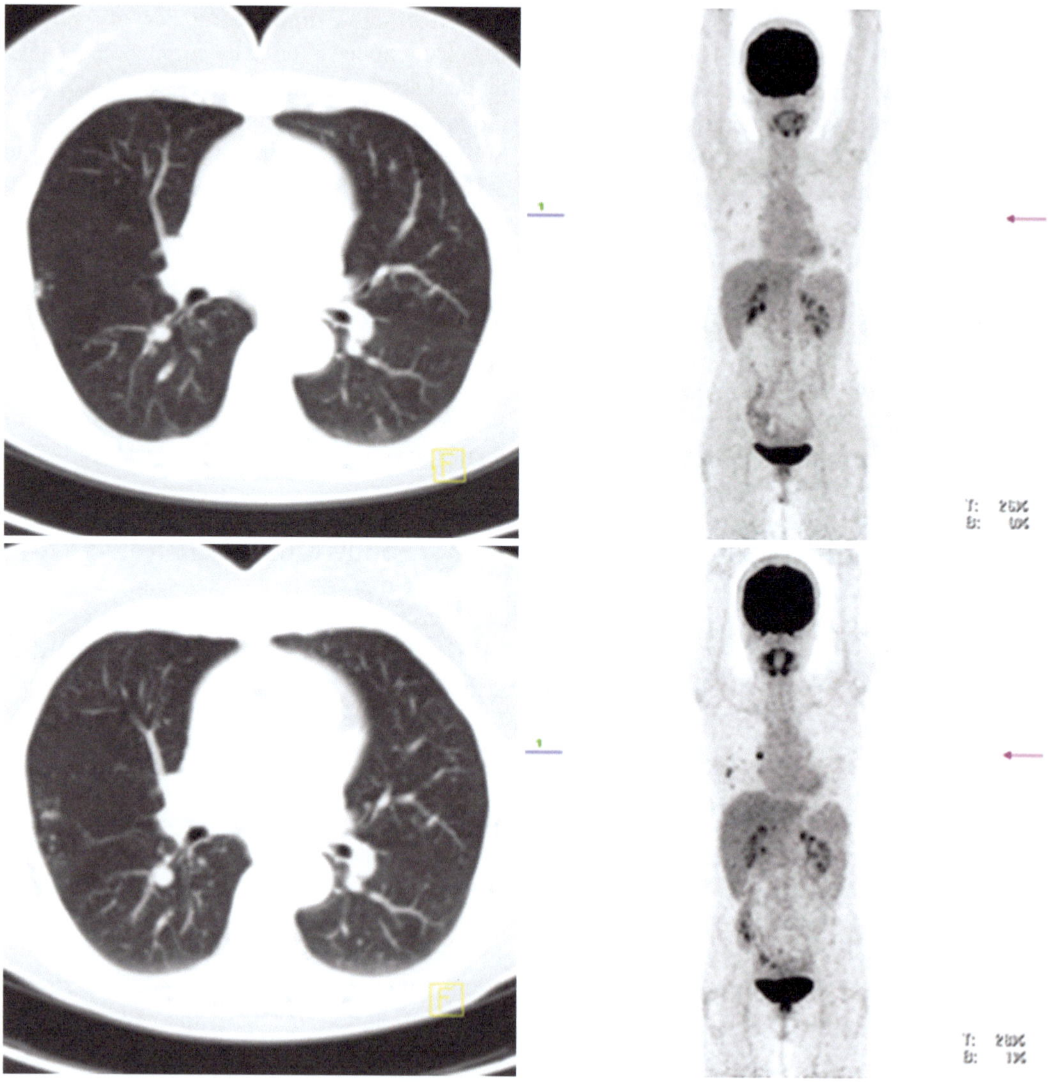

Fig. 53.2 Comparison of MIP image and transaxial CT image of the thorax before (below the line) and 6 months after sorafenib treatment (upper line) shows partial improvement in metastatic lung disease

What Can We Learn from This Case?

- In cases with abnormally elevated Tg levels without abnormal whole-body iodine scan, it is crucial to exclude potential reasons for this discordance such as interaction with anti-thyroglobulin antibodies or false-negative iodine scans due to iodine contamination or improper patient preparation. Neck ultrasound, thorax CT, and PET/CT have been recommended in patients with rising serum Tg levels.
- FDG PET/CT has been mainly indicated for those high-risk patients with elevated Tg levels without corresponding positive iodine uptake. It has the advantage of examining the whole body on a single session

and may also have a prognostic importance as high FDG uptake may be associated with more aggressive behavior and reduced survival rate.

- Targeted therapy with tyrosine kinase inhibitors seems to have a potential in iodine-refractory thyroid carcinomas. However, adverse effects are common. Therefore, proper patient selection, informing the patient about these effects, and offering supportive care with close communication are essential for effective therapy.

References

1. Haugen BR, Sawka AM, Alexander EK, Bible KC, Caturegli P, Doherty GM, et al. American Thyroid Association guidelines on the management of thyroid nodules and differentiated thyroid cancer task force review and recommendation on the proposed renaming of encapsulated follicular variant papillary thyroid carcinoma without invasion to noninvasive follicular thyroid neoplasm with papillary-like nuclear features. Thyroid. 2017;27:481–3. https://doi.org/10.1089/thy.2016.0628.
2. Ma C, Kuang A, Xie J, Ma T. Possible explanations for patients with discordant findings of serum thyroglobulin and 131I whole-body scanning. J Nucl Med. 2005;46:1473–80.
3. Pineda JD, Lee T, Ain K, Robbins J. Iodine-131 therapy for thyroid cancer patients with elevated thyroglobulin and negative diagnostic scan. J Clin Endocrinol Metab. 1995;80:1488–92.
4. de Keizer B, Koppeschaar HP, Zelissen PM, et al. Efficacy of high therapeutic doses of iodine-131 in patients with differentiated thyroid cancer and detectable serum thyroglobulin. Eur J Nucl Med. 2001;28:198–202.
5. Pacini L, Agate R, Elisei M. Outcome of differentiated thyroid cancer with detectable serum Tg and negative ^{131}I whole body scan: comparison of patients treated with high ^{131}I activities versus untreated patients. J Clin Endocrinol Metab. 2001;86:4092–7.
6. Koh JM, Kim ES, Ryu JS, et al. Effects of therapeutic doses of ^{131}I in thyroid papillary carcinoma patients with elevated thyroglobulin level and negative ^{131}I whole-body scan: comparative study. Clin Endocrinol. 2003;58:421–7.
7. Kabasakal L, Selçuk NA, Shafipour H, Ozmen O, Onsel C, Uslu I. Treatment of iodine-negative thyroglobulin-positive thyroid cancer: differences in outcome in patients with macrometastases and patients with micrometastases. Eur J Nucl Med Mol Imaging. 2004;31:1500–4.
8. Ma C, Xie J, Kuang A. Is empiric 131I therapy justified for patients with positive thyroglobulin and negative 131I whole-body scanning results? J Nucl Med. 2005;46:1164–70.
9. Chao M. Management of differentiated thyroid cancer with rising thyroglobulin and negative diagnostic radioiodine whole body scan. Clin Oncol (R Coll Radiol). 2010;22:438–47. https://doi.org/10.1016/j.clon.2010.05.005.
10. Vural GU, Akkas BE, Ercakmak N, Basu S, Alavi A. Prognostic significance of FDG PET/CT on the follow-up of patients of differentiated thyroid carcinoma with negative 131I whole-body scan and elevated thyroglobulin levels: correlation with clinical and histopathologic characteristics and long-term follow-up data. Clin Nucl Med. 2012;37:953–9. https://doi.org/10.1097/RLU.0b013e31825b205.
11. Ozkan E, Aras G, Kucuk NO. Correlation of 18F-FDG PET/CT findings with histopathological results in differentiated thyroid cancer patients who have increased thyroglobulin or antithyroglobulin antibody levels and negative 131I whole-body scan results. Clin Nucl Med. 2013;38:326–31. https://doi.org/10.1097/RLU.0b013e318286827b.
12. Pacini F. Which patient with thyroid cancer deserves systemic therapy and when? Best Pract Res Clin Endocrinol Metab. 2017;31:291–4. https://doi.org/10.1016/j.beem.2017.08.001.
13. Thomas L, Lai SY, Dong W, Feng L, Dadu R, Regone RM, Cabanillas ME. Sorafenib in metastatic thyroid cancer: a systematic review. Oncologist. 2014;19:251–8. https://doi.org/10.1634/theoncologist.2013-0362.
14. Viola D, Valeria L, Molinaro E Agate L, Bottici V, Biagini A, et al. Treatment of advanced thyroid cancer with targeted therapies: ten years of experience. Endocr Relat Cancer. 2016;23:R185–205.
15. Brose MS, Nutting CM, Jarzab B, Elisei R, Siena S, Bastholt L, et al. Sorafenib in radioactive iodine-refractory, locally advanced or metastatic differentiated thyroid cancer: a randomised, double-blind, phase 3 trial. Lancet. 2014;384:319–28. https://doi.org/10.1016/S0140-6736(14)60421-9.
16. Benekli M, Yalcin S, Ozkan M, Elkiran ET, Sevinc A, Cabuk D, et al. Efficacy of sorafenib in advanced differentiated and medullary thyroid cancer: experience in a Turkish population. Onco Targets Ther. 2014;15:1–5. https://doi.org/10.2147/OTT.S70670.

54 Targeted Systemic Therapy in Patients with Radioiodine-Refractory Differentiated Thyroid Cancer

Levent Kabasakal and Onur Erdem Şahin

Abstract

With the common use of imaging modalities such as ultrasonography (USG), the incidence of thyroid cancer has increased in recent years. Most of the thyroid cancers are differentiated thyroid cancers (DTC). In the case of DTC, the ability of cancer cells to concentrate iodine makes radioactive iodine (RAI) therapy possible, which is an effective treatment for DTCs. Surgical operation and RAI treatment give a chance to be cured for many thyroid cancer patients. Nonetheless, resistance to RAI treatment develops in a group of patients, and the prognosis worsens. In RAI-refractory (RAI-R) DTC patients, chemotherapeutic drugs such as doxorubicin and cisplatin have been tried, but no successful results have been obtained. In contrast, multiple kinase inhibitors (MKIs) have provided for RAI-R patients a new treatment option. Sorafenib and lenvatinib have been approved by the FDA for RAI-R DTC patients, and phase studies of other MKIs are ongoing.

In addition to offering a new opportunity for RAI-R patients with reduced treatment options, side effect profile creates difficulties in clinical practice. These side effects can affect the patients' quality of life. For these reasons, treatment of MKIs should be considered in significantly symptomatic patients with rapid progression rather than those with minimal progression or stable, symptom-free patients. Treatment decision should be made by considering patient-based profit-loss rates.

L. Kabasakal (✉) · O. E. Şahin
Department of Nuclear Medicine, Cerrahpaşa Faculty of Medicine, İstanbul University, Istanbul, Turkey
e-mail: lkabasakal@tsnm.org

Case 1 Sixty five-year-old male patient, due to the result of a biopsy taken from thyroid nodule showing suspicious for papillary thyroid cancer and suspicious lymph nodes being observed in his neck, underwent a total thyroidectomy and bilateral neck dissection operation. The pathology results showed multifocal classic type papillary thyroid cancer in the thyroid gland, 2 cm in a diameter, showing thyroid capsule invasion, and 12/24 + metastatic lymph nodes in right-left and upper mediastinal lymphatic stations. The patient's blood panel results upon first application were TSH, 78 uIU/ml; Tg, 286 pg/ml; and anti-Tg, 1.6 ng/dl; ultrasonography (USG) and 18-fluorodeoxyglucose positron emission tomography-computed tomography (18-FDG PET/CT) imaging were requested for the patient. In USG and FDG PET/CT imaging, mass lesions in both retropharyngeal areas that suggested invasion to thyroid cartilage and metastatic lymph nodes in the right posterior cervical lymphatic chain were observed. Upon consultation with surgery, the patient was deemed inoperable. Four cycles of radioiodine (RAI) therapy (cumulated

T. Özülker et al. (eds.), *Thyroid and Parathyroid Diseases*, https://doi.org/10.1007/978-3-319-78476-2_54

activity of 27.75 GBq) were administered between October 2010 and November 2012, and in his 131I-whole-body scintigraphy (WBS) after last treatment, no activity retention was observed in metastatic lesions. Patient's Tg progression was also tracked, and in the new FDG-PET/CT scan, response was observed in some of the existing lesions and progression in others. He was referred to oncology to be evaluated for sorafenib treatment. Having been found suitable for treatment, sorafenib was applied to the patient for 3 months. In the follow-up FDG PET scan after 3 months of sorafenib treatment, lesions in the retropharyngeal region seemed stable, and partial response was observed in the lymph node present in the right cervical lymphatic chain (Fig. 54.1). But because the patient did not want to go on with the treatment due to side effects, treatment was terminated.

Case 2 Sixty two-year-old female patient underwent total thyroidectomy and central neck dissection operation. Pathology results showed classic type papillary cancer in the thyroid gland, 2.2 cm in size, displaying multifocal widespread thyroid capsule invasion. Postoperative blood panel showed TSH, 100 uIU/ml; Tg, 566 pg/ml; and anti-Tg, 2.22 ng/dl; the patient was given two cycles of radioiodine (RAI) therapy (cumulated activity of 14.8 GBq) between February 2011 and August 2011. In the 131I-WBS after the last treatment, high uptake was observed in the thyroid area. In 6-month check-up, upon Tg progression being observed, FDG-PET/CT scan was requested, which showed mass lesion in the right thyroid lobe with the invasion of the trachea and paratracheal metastatic lymph nodes. Upon consulting with endocrine surgeons, the decision was made to operate including partial tracheal resection. In postsurgery check-up, while TSH was 100 uIU/ml, Tg fell to a level of 4.8 pg/ml. After the operation, the patient was given two cycles of radioiodine (RAI) therapy (cumulated activity of 18.5 GBq) between July 2012 and February 2013, and in the 131I-WBS scan after the last treatment, no retention was observed. The patient

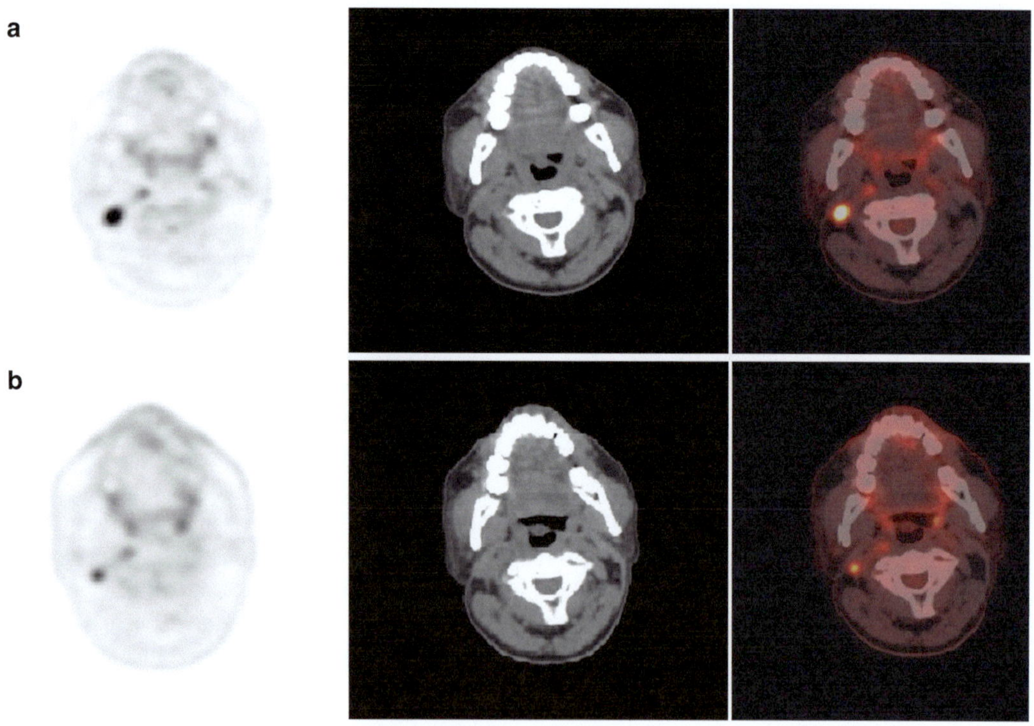

Fig. 54.1 Pretreatment (row **a**) and posttreatment (row **b**) FDG PET/CT images of case 1 (PET, CT, and fusion). FDG PET/CT performed 3 months after sorafenib treatment (**b**) showed partial response of metastatic lymph

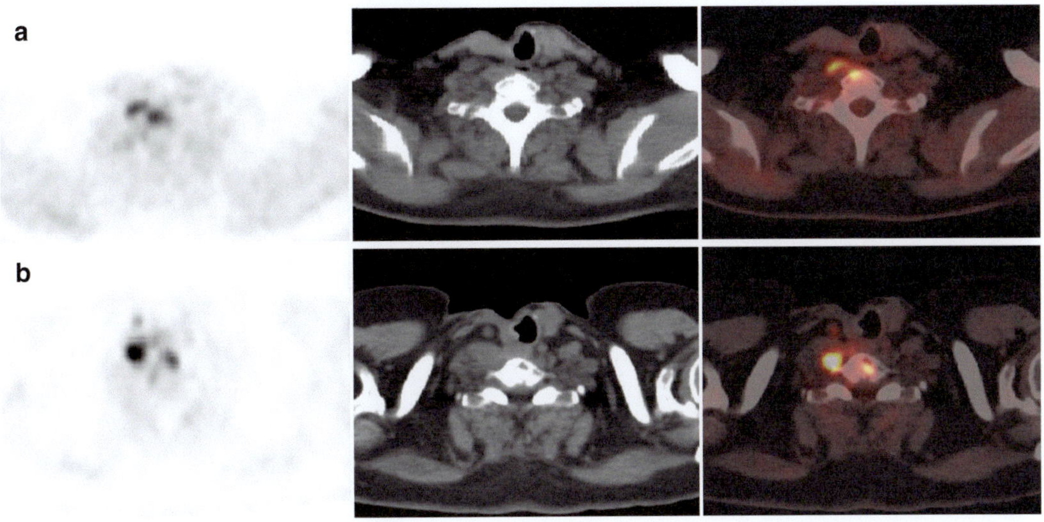

Fig. 54.2 Pretreatment (row **a**) and posttreatment (row **b**) FDG PET/CT images of case 2 (PET, CT, and fusion). FDG PET/CT performed 3 months after sorafenib treatment (**b**) showed progression of metastatic lesions

was put under monitoring, and when Tg level started showing progression, check-up FDG-PET/CT was requested. Imaging results showed multiple lesions consistent with the relapse-metastasis of the primary disease in the neck, upper mediastinum, and C7 vertebrae. In response, the patient was referred to the oncology department to be evaluated for sorafenib treatment. Having been found suitable for treatment, sorafenib was applied to the patient for 3 months. In the follow-up, FDG-PET/CT scan after 3 months of sorafenib treatment, progression in existing lesions, and newly developed bone metastases were observed (Figs. 54.2 and 54.3). Taking into consideration the patient's request, treatment was discontinued, and she was followed up with palliative treatments.

54.1 Discussion

According to data from National Cancer Institute, thyroid cancer makes up 3.4% of all cancer cases observed in the USA in 2017 [1]. Neck USG imaging became more common, and with increasing prevalence of the incidentalomas detected via other radiological imaging, the thyroid cancer frequency has also increased. As it is commonly known, differentiated thyroid cancers (DTC) make up the majority of thyroid cancers. DTCs, which include papillary and follicular thyroid cancers, are rooted in thyrocytes and keep their ability to express sodium iodine symporters. Keeping the ability to concentrate iodine in DTCs has led to the discovery of 131I radioactive iodine (RAI) treatment and become a milestone in DTC treatment. DTCs are known to have fairly good prognoses. The primary approach to DTC treatment is surgical operation along with RAI treatment and TSH suppression, as suggested by guidelines such as American Thyroid Association (ATA) and European Association of Nuclear Medicine (EANM) guidelines. Because of its efficacy and success, RAI treatment, along with surgery, is the most valuable tool in our toolbox in managing DTC patients. Though the revised 2015 version of the ATA guideline puts forward changes in RAI suggestions, RAI is suggested in both postoperation period and cases of relapse, in accordance with the risk classification [2]. On the other hand, for patients whose surgical options are limited and who become refractory to RAI treatment, treatment options are severely narrowed.

According to the ATA guideline classification, not having retention in the 131I-WBS in the malign-metastatic tissue after the first treatment following the appropriate TSH stimulation and

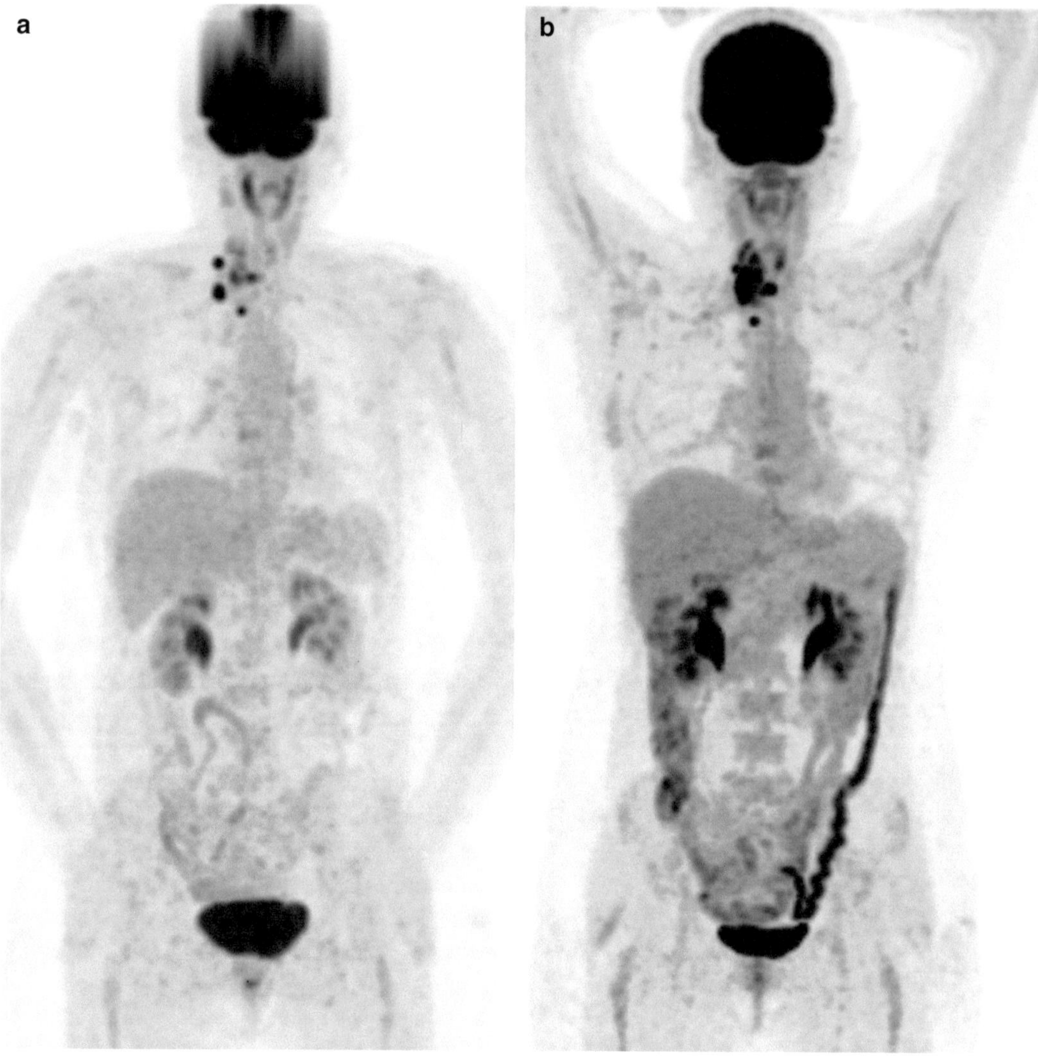

Fig. 54.3 Pretreatment (column **a**) and posttreatment (column **b**) FDG PET MIP images of case 2. The posttreatment FDG PET MIP image showed progression of metastatic lesions

iodine diet, thyroid tissue losing its ability to concentrate RAI over time, observing retention in some lesions and not in others and progressive disease despite there being retention are described as RAI-refractory (RAI-R) DTC [2]. Whereas with DTCs, the disease-specific survival rate is around 85% [3], approximately 10–15% of DTC patients develop distant metastases, and the 10-year disease-specific survival rate falls to about 40% [4]. This rate drops to around 10% for metastatic RAI-refractory DTC [3]. Systemic treatment is considered for metastatic RAI-R DTC patients who have no chance of surgery. Conventional chemotherapeutics like doxorubicin or cisplatin do not produce satisfactory results in these patients, and there is not enough data available [2]. In recent years, the disease's relationship with gene mutations like BRAF and RAS and genetic rearrangements like RET/PTC and PAX8-PPAR having been determined and overexpression of receptors like endothelial growth factor receptor (VEGF-R), fibroblast growth factor receptor (FGF-R), and platelet-derived growth factor receptor (PDGF-R) having come to light have revealed multiple kinase inhibitors (MKI) as a treatment option [5, 6]. MKIs, despite their mechanisms of action not being completely explained yet, affect common targets like VEGFRs, PDGFRs, FGFRs, and RET [6]. Today sorafenib and lenvatinib have been approved by the US Food and Drug Administration (FDA) and European Medicine Agency in the systemic treatment of RAI-R DTC. Apart from that, there are studies available on various other tyrosine kinase inhibitors.

Sorafenib was approved for use on RAI-R DTC with a Phase III trial (DECISION study) involving 417 people [7]. Patients who have been accepted as progressive disease and did not previously receive MKI treatment have been accepted into the study. The median progression-free survival (PFS) in the sorafenib group was found to be significantly higher than that of the placebo group (10.8 vs. 5.8 months; *p:* <0.0001). Hand and foot skin reaction (HFSR) (76.3%), diarrhea (68.6%), alopecia (67.1%), rash or desquamation (50.2%), fatigue (49.8%), weight loss (46.9%), and hypertension (40.6%) made up the most common adverse effects (AEs) related to the disease. Despite most of these are at the level of grade 1 or 2, the most common grade 3 or 4 AEs were HFSR (20.3%), followed by hypertension (9.7%), hypocalcemia (9.2%), weight loss (5.8%), diarrhea (5.8%), and fatigue (5.8%) [7].

Following sorafenib, lenvatinib also received permission for use on RAI-R DTC with a Phase III trial (SELECT study) [8]. Patients who showed progression in the past 13 months and who did not receive MKI or those who only received one regime MKI were accepted into the study, which included a total of 392 patients. The PFS was found to be significantly higher compared to the placebo branch (18.3 vs. 3.6 months; *p:*<0.001). The rate of all AEs (of all grades) related to the treatment was 97.3%, and the rate of AEs of grade 3 or 4 was 75.9%. The most common AE was hypertension (67.8%), followed by diarrhea (59.4%), decreased appetite (50.2%), decreased weight (46.4%), and nausea (41.0%). The AEs that required the highest rate of dose adjustment were diarrhea (22.6%), hypertension (19.9%), proteinuria (18.8%), and decreased appetite (18.0%) [8].

AEs of MKIs and their effect on quality of life constitute the primary problem in their use in RAI-R DTC. In our presented cases, we had to stop the MKIs treatment because of its side effects. Besides, despite their contribution to PFS, their effect on overall survival (OS) is not clear [9]. For these reasons, ATA guidelines suggest that they should be used only in metastatic, rapidly progressive, symptomatic RAI-R DTC cases and/or life-threatening cases with no possibility of local intervention. It states that they can be brought to the forefront in cases that are life-threatening in the short term and require intervention, in cases of symptomatic patients to whom direct treatment cannot be applied or in cases of diffuse disease progression and are avoided in cases of active or recent intestinal disease, poorly controlled hypertension, liver disease, recent cardiovascular event, comorbidities, etc. [2]. It also states that asymptomatic, stable, or minimally progressive patients, those whose possibility of rapid progression is low, who do not have clinically important complications and direct treatment indications can be followed under TSH suppression with radiological imaging, in 3- to 12-month intervals [2].

MKI treatment has created a new treatment option for RAI-R DTC where treatment options are severely limited. Taking into consideration the suggestions and discoveries about these treatments, it's understood that the decision to use MKI treatment must be made carefully. Careful patient choice plays a key role in successful treatment. The patient must especially be thoroughly informed of the side effect that may occur during treatment; this can prevent motivation loss during treatment and will significantly improve patient compliance. Also, having specialists closely follow patients on this matter, quickly identifying adverse effects and early intervention will also contribute positively to patient compliance. Preferring fast-moving, symptomatic RAI-R DTC patients over symptom-free, stable, or minimally progressing patients will not only be useful for patient benefit but also for cost-effectivity.

54.2 The Future

Phase studies or other MKIs like vandetanib, sunitinib, pazopanib, axitinib, or dovitinib in RAI-R DTC treatment are ongoing [10]. More effective MKIs with fewer adverse effects will be promising in RAI-R DTC treatment.

What Can We Learn from This Case?

- RAI treatment and surgery are the most valuable tools for managing disease in DTC patients.
- The survival rate in DTC patients who became refractory to RAI treatment diminishes significantly and causes severe problems in disease management in patients who lose the chance of operation.
- MKI treatment has created a treatment option for RAI-R DTC patients.
- Adverse effect profile constitutes the most important difficulty in using MKI treatment. Therefore, the decision to use this treatment must be made carefully, taking into consideration the profit and loss relation.
- Taking the adverse effect profile into consideration, using MKI treatment on symptomatic and rapidly progressing patients instead of symptom-free, stable, or minimally progressing ones would be more appropriate.
- Before treatment, thoroughly clarifying possible adverse effects for the patient and following them up with physicians experienced in this matter are essential elements that will improve patient compliance.
- MKI treatment in RAI-R DTC patients is a treatment option that can be efficient with the right choice of patient and right timing.

References

1. National Cancer Institute. Surveillance, Epidemiology, and End Results (SEER). SEER stat fact sheets: thyroid cancer. http://seer.cancer.gov/statfacts/html/thyro.html. Accessed 01 July 2017.
2. Haugen BR, Alexander EK, Bible KC, Doherty GM, Mandel SJ, Nikiforov YE, et al. 2015 American Thyroid Association management guidelines for adult patients with thyroid nodules and differentiated thyroid Cancer: the American Thyroid Association guidelines task force on thyroid nodules and differentiated thyroid cancer. Thyroid. 2016;26:1–133. https://doi.org/10.1089/thy.2015.0020.
3. Eustatia-Rutten CF, Corssmit EP, Biermasz NR, Pereira AM, Romijn JA, Smit JW. Survival and death causes in differentiated thyroid carcinoma. J Clin Endocrinol Metab. 2006;91:313–9. https://doi.org/10.1210/jc.2005-1322.
4. O'Neill CJ, Oucharek J, Learoyd D, Sidhu SB. Standard and emerging therapies for metastatic differentiated thyroid cancer. Oncologist. 2010;15:146–56. https://doi.org/10.1634/theoncologist.2009-0190.
5. Nikiforova MN, Nikiforov YE. Molecular genetics of thyroid cancer: implications for diagnosis, treatment and prognosis. Expert Rev Mol Diagn. 2008;8:83–95. https://doi.org/10.1586/14737159.8.1.83.
6. Chow LQ, Santana-Davila R, Pantel A, Roth M, Anderson LN, Failor A, et al. A phase I study of pazopanib in combination with escalating doses of 131I in patients with well-differentiated thyroid carcinoma borderline refractory to radioiodine. PLoS One. 2017;12:e0178325. https://doi.org/10.1371/journal.pone.0178325.
7. Brose MS, Nutting CM, Jarzab B, Elisei R, Siena S, Bastholt L, et al. Sorafenib in locally advanced or metastatic, radioactive iodine-refractory, differentiated thyroid cancer: a randomized, double-blind, phase 3 trial. Lancet. 2014;384:319–28. https://doi.org/10.1016/S0140-6736(14)60421-9.
8. Schlumberger M, Tahara M, Wirth LJ, Robinson B, Brose MS, Elisei R, et al. Lenvatinib versus placebo in radioiodine-refractory thyroid Cancer. N Engl J Med. 2015;372:621–30. https://doi.org/10.1056/NEJMoa1406470.
9. Schmidt A, Iglesias L, Klain M, Pitoia F, Schlumberger MJ. Radioactive iodine-refractory differentiated thyroid cancer: an uncommon but challenging situation. Arch Endocrinol Metab. 2017;61:81–9. https://doi.org/10.1590/2359-3997000000245.
10. Lorusso L, Pieruzzi L, Biagini A, Sabini E, Valerio L, Giani C, et al. Lenvatinib and other tyrosine kinase inhibitors for the treatment of radioiodine refractory, advanced, and progressive thyroid cancer. Onco Targets Ther. 2016;9:6467–77. https://doi.org/10.2147/ott.s84625.

Thyroid Follicular Carcinoma with Iodine-Avid Bone Metastases Showing Mild Uptake on Both ^{18}F-FDG and ^{68}Ga-DOTATOC PET/CT

55

Tevfik Fikret Çermik and Nurhan Ergül

Abstract

Differentiated thyroid carcinoma (DTC) is usually characterized by good prognosis. Radioiodine scan is the first-line diagnostic tool to detect the metastatic disease. In patients with high Tg levels suggesting metastatic disease when radioiodine scan is negative, ^{18}F-fluorodeoxyglucose positron emission tomography/computerized tomography (FDG PET/CT) is reported to be effective in defining the metastatic foci. Another imaging modality is somatostatin receptor imaging with PET/CT which can be used especially when ^{18}F-FDG PET/CT is nondiagnostic. Peptide receptor radionuclide therapy with β-emitting radionuclides may be considered when somatostatin positivity is defined in metastatic lesions. In this case report, a patient with DTC having radioiodine-positive bone metastases showing mild uptake in ^{18}F-FDG PET/CT and ^{68}Ga-DOTATOC PET/CT is presented.

55.1 Case Presentation

A 45-year-old man presenting with low back pain had undergone a lumbar magnetic resonance imaging (MRI) revealing a destructive lesion in the L2 vertebral body. A ^{18}F-fluorodeoxyglucose positron emission tomography/computerized tomography (FDG PET/CT) examination showed high uptake in the vertebral lesion (SUVmax = 8.1) and also a nodular lesion in the left lobe of the thyroid gland with intense uptake (SUVmax = 23.2) (Fig. 55.1). The histopathological examination of the vertebral lesion was consistent with metastasis of thyroid carcinoma. Bilateral total thyroidectomy was performed, and the tumoral lesion in the left lobe measuring approximately 3.8 × 3.5 cm was excised with the diagnosis of follicular carcinoma stage IVc according to the AJCC/TNM VIII system with tumoral capsule invasion and vascular invasion. No metastatic lymph node was excised. The thyroglobulin (Tg) level was 10,527 ng/ml. The patient was treated with 200 mCi I-131 radioiodine therapy. The whole-body scan after therapy revealed some residual thyroid tissue in the thyroidectomy region and also high uptake areas in right upper ribs, lumbar vertebral region, some thoracic vertebrae, and proximal right femur consistent with bone metastases (Fig. 55.2). A control FDG PET/CT scan after 1 month of therapy showed a moderate uptake in the right first rib (SUVmax = 3.5) and low residual uptake in the L2 vertebra (Fig. 55.3). A ^{68}Ga-DOTATOC PET/CT scan was performed to see the option of Lu-177 DOTATOC therapy. There was a low level of somatostatin receptor activity in the right first rib and L2 vertebra (Fig. 55.4). Tg level was

T. F. Çermik · N. Ergül (✉)
University of Health Sciences, İstanbul Training and Research Hospital, Clinic of Nuclear Medicine, Istanbul, Turkey

T. Özülker et al. (eds.), *Thyroid and Parathyroid Diseases*, https://doi.org/10.1007/978-3-319-78476-2_55

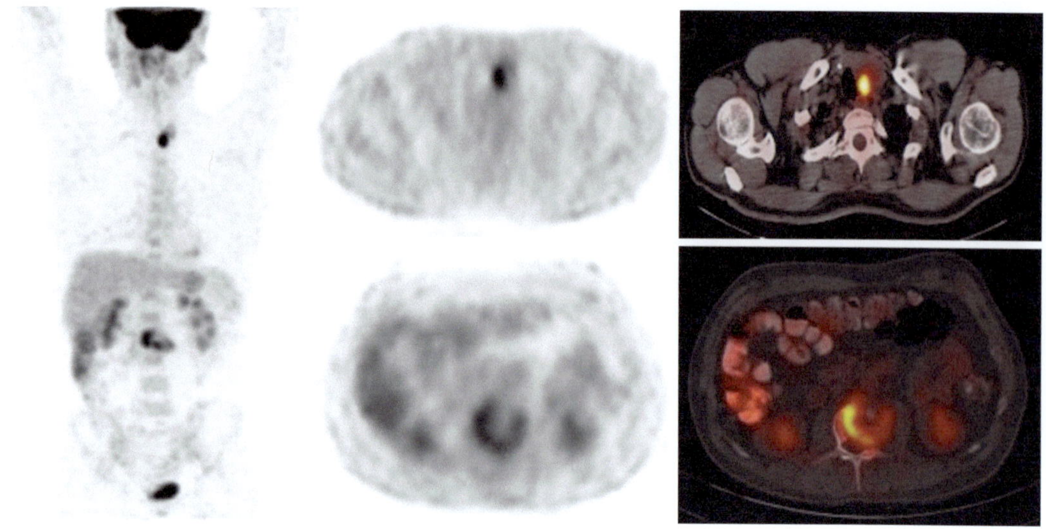

Fig. 55.1 ^{18}F-FDG PET/CT scan before thyroidectomy. Intense uptake in left lobe of thyroid gland. Lytic hypermetabolic lesion in L2 vertebral body

2764 ng/ml after 6 months of therapy, and the second cure of radioiodine therapy with 200 mCi I-131 was administered. The whole-body scan after therapy showed reduced uptake in the right first rib and lumbar vertebra (Fig. 55.5).

55.2 Discussion

Differentiated thyroid carcinoma (DTC), often referred for papillary and follicular types, is usually characterized by good prognosis with a 10-year survival rate of 80% [1]. The standard therapy for DTC and medullary thyroid carcinoma is total or near-total thyroidectomy often followed by ablation of remnant thyroid tissue with I-131 in DTC. The common distant metastasis sites of DTC are lungs, bones, and brain. In the management of initial therapy and follow-up period, measurement of serum Tg levels, ultrasonography (USG) of the neck, and I-131 or I-123 whole-body scintigraphy are used in order to detect the lymphoid or distant metastases. In patients with elevated serum Tg levels and negative radioiodine scan, ^{18}F-FDG PET or PET/CT has been reported to be sensitive for detecting the metastatic sites. In a study comparing the efficacy of I-131 whole-body scan with ^{18}F-FDG PET/CT, it was reported that for organ-basis analysis, radioiodine scan was the best detector for lymph node metastasis (72.4%), while PET/CT was superior to I-131 scintigraphy for detecting metastasis of the bone (85.7% vs. 71.4%) and lung (94.1% vs. 62.7%) [2].

Since the bones are the second common site of metastases from DTC, 99mTc-MDP bone scintigraphy has also been used widely in both staging and follow-up. In a study comparing the ^{18}F-FDG PET and bone scan, the specificity and the overall accuracy of ^{18}F-FDG PET for the diagnosis of bone metastases in patients with DTC were found to be higher than those of 99mTc-bone scintigraphy with a lower incidence of false-positive results [1]. In another study, both I-131 SPECT/CT and ^{18}F-FDG PET/CT were found to be superior to 99mTc-MDP bone scintigraphy for the detection of bone metastases from DTC, and ^{18}F-FDG positivity was the factor predicting a poor prognosis. It was concluded that (99m)Tc-MDP bone scan might be completely replaced by I-131 SPECT/CT in combination with ^{18}F-FDG PET/CT in the management of DTC patients with bone metastases [3].

In metastatic patients at initial staging or in follow-up, repeated therapy with high doses of radioiodine is recommended as long as the metastases are iodine-avid in whole-body scan. In ATA 2015 guideline, it was reported that radioiodine

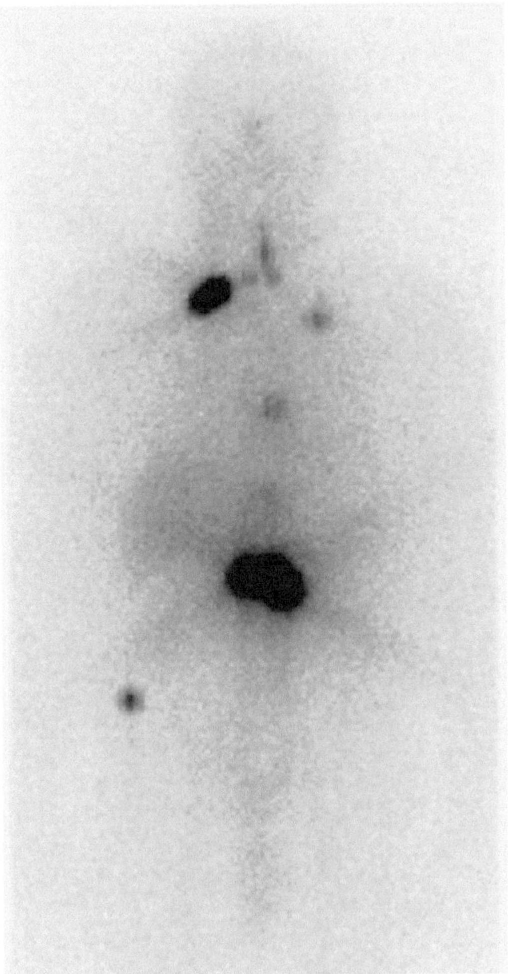

Fig. 55.2 Whole-body scan after 200 mCi radioiodine therapy; intense uptake in right upper ribs, lower dorsal and lumbar vertebral region, and proximal right thigh consistent with bone metastases. There is also some residual activity in thyroidectomy region

therapy for patients with bone metastases is rarely curative, but some patients with iodine-avid bone metastases may benefit from this therapy. For these patients, directed therapies like surgery and external beam radiation therapy and systemic therapy with bone-directed agents should also be considered [4]. However, the dedifferentiation process of the tumor in 20–30% of patients causes the unsuccessful results of radioiodine therapy [5]. In this group of patients that carries a poor prognosis, different targeted therapeutic options are needed. In iodine-negative, ^{18}F-FDG-positive metastatic disease, treatment with chemotherapeutic agents or tyrosine kinase inhibitors that was reported to be associated with poor responses and life-threatening toxicity may be considered.

The somatostatin receptor (SSTR) status of DTC has been investigated in several studies up to date. In a retrospective study with 237 patients with incidental thyroid uptake on ^{68}Ga-DOTATATE PET/CT, 26 (11%) patients had atypical thyroid uptake. Fourteen (54%) of them had focal uptake, and 12 (46%) had diffuse uptake. Of the 14 patients, 3 (21%) were found to have papillary thyroid cancer. The 12 patients with diffusely increased uptake were diagnosed with hypothyroidism, chronic lymphocytic thyroiditis, and nontoxic multinodular goiter [6]. ^{68}Ga-DOTATATE was reported to have a higher lesion uptake in DTC patients and may have a potential advantage over ^{68}Ga-DOTANOC [7].

Non-iodine-avid metastatic lesions of DTC may have SSTR binding potential. The evaluation of SSTR expression of DTC cells with either SPECT or PET using different somatostatin analogs labeled with radionuclides may raise the possibility of therapy with β-emitting radionuclides. It was reported that in metastatic radioiodine-avid DTC, both ^{18}F-FDG and ^{68}Ga-DOTATOC PET show a low rate of lesion visualization and comparable results, whereas in non-iodine-avid patients, FDG PET has much higher lesion detection rates than ^{68}Ga-DOTATOC PET [8]. In another study comparing different somatostatin analogs labeled with ^{68}Ga and ^{18}F-FDG PET in metastases of DTC, FDG PET was positive in 88% of patients, while ^{68}Ga-DOTA-LAN PET was positive in only 35% and ^{68}Ga-DOTATOC in 29%, reflecting the process of dedifferentiation from loss of iodine trapping to loss of SSTR with a concomitant increase in glucose metabolism and more aggressive behavior of the disease [5]. In our patient, we observed high uptake of radioiodine in metastatic bone lesions while there was a mild uptake in both ^{18}F-FDG and ^{68}Ga-DOTATOC PET/CT in metastases, revealing a good differentiation of thyroid cells and a chance of therapy with radioiodine.

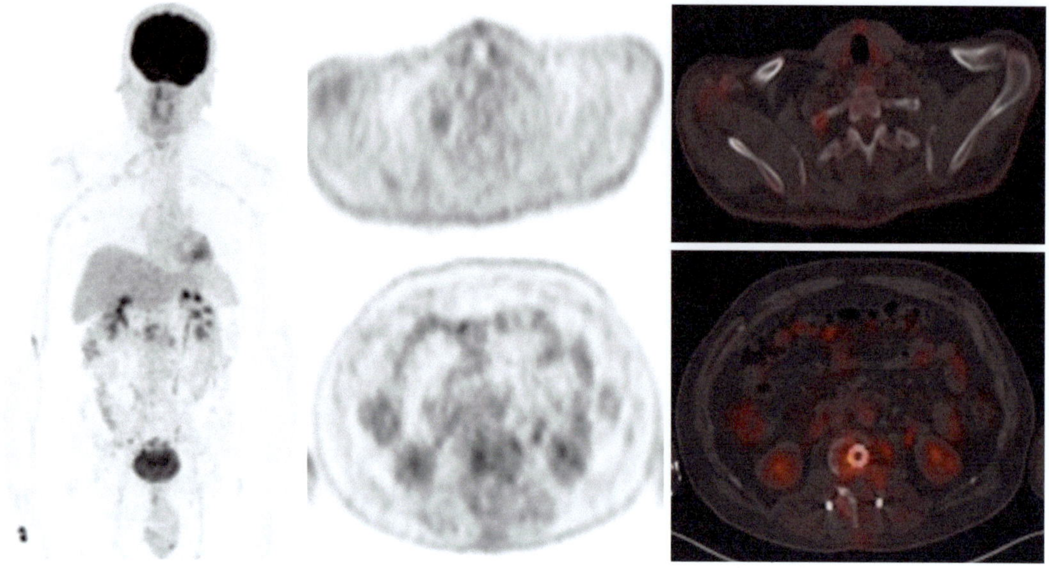

Fig. 55.3 ^{18}F-FDG PET/CT scan after 1 month of therapy. Mild uptake in right first rib and L2 vertebral body

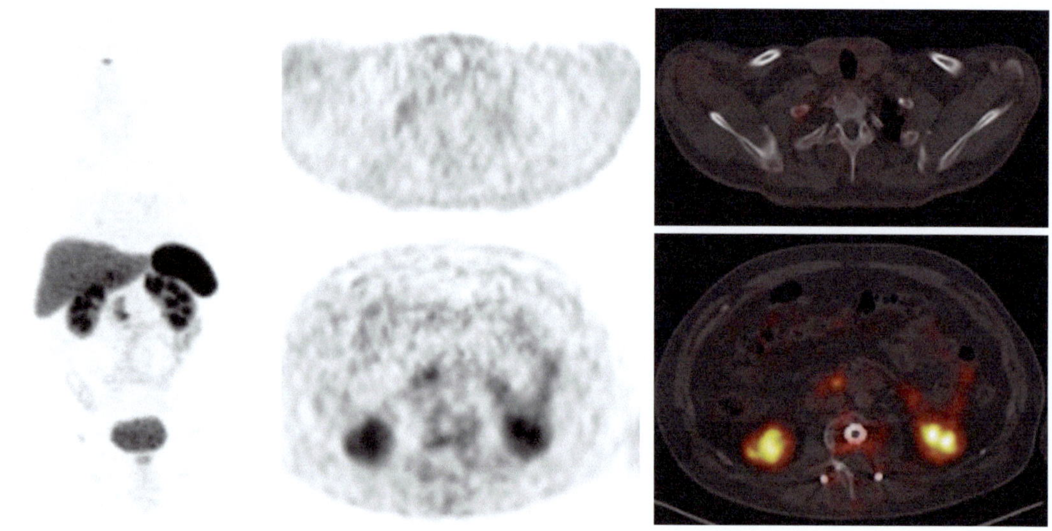

Fig. 55.4 ^{68}Ga-DOTATOC PET/CT. Mild uptake in right first rib and L2 vertebral body

In many recent studies, the possible contribution of SSTR imaging in DTC for evaluation of peptide receptor radionuclide therapy (PRRT) has been reported [9–12]. In a study investigating the role of ^{68}Ga-DOTATATE PET/CT in non-iodine-concentrating DTC, it was shown that in patients having intense SSTR-expressing tumor serum, chromogranin A levels were elevated suggesting a possible neuroendocrine differentiation [9]. Tumor heterogeneity is reported to be a predictor of response to PRRT, and textural parameters are recommended to assess the patient selection rather than SUV measurements [10]. In radioiodine-negative and FDG-negative patients, SSTR imaging with PET/CT is suggested to be beneficial for assessment of therapy with PRRT [11, 12].

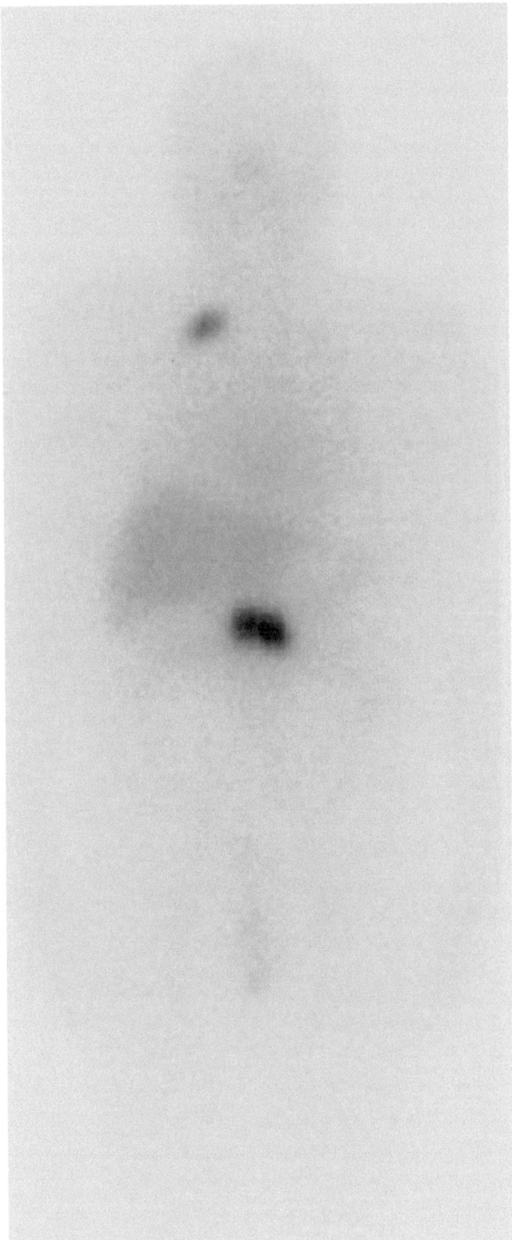

Fig. 55.5 Whole-body scan after second cure of 200 mCi radioiodine therapy. High uptake in right upper ribs and L2 vertebra

55.3 Follow-Up and Outcome

Three months after the second cure of radioiodine therapy, Tg level decreased from 2764 to 123 ng/ml. In 6-month follow-up period, Tg level decreased gradually to 67.8 ng/ml. A third cure of 200 mCi I-131 was planned because of a still high Tg level.

What Can We Learn from This Case?

- In DTC patients, radioiodine scintigraphy should take place in first-line diagnostic tool for initial staging and management of the disease. ^{18}F-FDG PET or SSTR imaging should be considered in case of a radioiodine-negative disease.
- In well-differentiated disease, the tumor cells may not express somatostatin receptors even in FDG-negative condition.
- Radioiodine therapy is the preferred therapy in metastatic patients as long as iodine uptake is present in lesions.

References

1. Ito S, Kato K, Ikeda M, Iwano S, Makino N, Tadokoro M, et al. Comparison of 18F-FDG PET and bone scintigraphy in detection of bone metastases of thyroid cancer. J Nucl Med. 2007;48:889–95.
2. Nagamachi S, Wakamatsu H, Kiyohara S, Nishii R, Mizutani Y, Fujita S, et al. Comparison of diagnostic and prognostic capabilities of ^{18}F-FDG-PET/CT, ^{131}I-scintigraphy, and diffusion-weighted magnetic resonance imaging for postoperative thyroid cancer. Jpn J Radiol. 2011;29:413–22.
3. Qiu ZL, Xue HL, Song HJ, Luo QY. Comparison of the diagnostic and prognostic values of 99mTc-MDP-planar bone scintigraphy, 131I-SPECT/CT and 18F-FDG-PET/CT for the detection of bone metastases from differentiated thyroid cancer. Nucl Med Commun. 2012;33:1232–42.
4. Haugen BR, Alexander EK, Bible KC, Doherty GM, Mandel SJ, Nikiforov YE, et al. 2015 American Thyroid Association management guidelines for adult patients with thyroid nodules and differentiated thyroid cancer. Thyroid. 2016;26:1–133.
5. Weidinger T, Putzer D, Von Guggenberg E, Dobrozemsky G, Nilica B, Kendler D, et al. Multiparametric PET imaging in thyroid malignancy characterizing tumour heterogeneity: somatostatin receptors and glucose metabolism. Eur J Nucl Med Mol Imaging. 2015;42:1995–2001.
6. Nockel P, Millo C, Keutgen X, Klubo-Gwiezdzinska J, Shell J, Patel D, et al. Rate and clinical significance

of incidental thyroid uptake as detected by Gallium-68 DOTATATE positron emission tomography/computed tomography. Thyroid. 2016;26:831–5.

7. Ocak M, Demirci E, Kabasakal L, Aygun A, Tutar RO, Araman A, et al. Evaluation and comparison of Ga-68 DOTA-TATE and Ga-68 DOTA-NOC PET/CT imaging in well-differentiated thyroid cancer. Nucl Med Commun. 2013;34:1084–9.
8. Middendorp M, Selkinski I, Happel C, Kranert WT, Grünwald F. Comparison of positron emission tomography with [(18)F]FDG and [(68)Ga]DOTATOC in recurrent differentiated thyroid cancer: preliminary data. Q J Nucl Med Mol Imaging. 2010;54:76–83.
9. Jois B, Asopa R, Basu S. Somatostatin receptor imaging in non-(131)I-avid metastatic differentiated thyroid carcinoma for determining the feasibility of peptide receptor radionuclide therapy with (177) Lu-DOTATATE: low fraction of patients suitable for peptide receptor radionuclide therapy and evidence of chromogranin a level-positive neuroendocrine differentiation. Clin Nucl Med. 2014;3:505–10.
10. Lapa C, Werner RA, Schmid JS, Papp L, Zsótér N, Biko J, et al. Prognostic value of positron emission tomography-assessed tumor heterogeneity in patients with thyroid cancer undergoing treatment with radiopeptide therapy. Nucl Med Biol. 2015;42:349–54.
11. Binse I, Poeppel TD, Ruhlmann M, Ezziddin S, Görges R, Sabet A, et al. 68Ga-DOTATOC PET/CT in patients with iodine- and 18F-FDG-negative differentiated thyroid carcinoma and elevated serum thyroglobulin. J Nucl Med. 2016;57:1512–7.
12. Versari A, Sollini M, Frasoldati A, Fraternali A, Filice A, Froio A, et al. Differentiated thyroid cancer: a new perspective with radiolabeled somatostatin analogues for imaging and treatment of patients. Thyroid. 2014;24:715–26.

56 Somatostatin Receptor Imaging in Differentiated Thyroid Cancer

Levent Kabasakal and Onur Erdem Şahin

Abstract

Most of the thyroid cancers consist of differentiated thyroid cancers (DTCs). Generally having a good prognosis, with the surgery and radioactive iodine (RAI) treatment in selected patients, a good outcome can be obtained. In contrast, some DTC patients are resistant to RAI (RAI-R). Treatment options for RAI-R patients are restricted. On the other hand, local limited RAI-R DTC patients have a chance of surgical operation and external radiotherapy. In addition, early detection of lesions and initial surgery are critical points in the management of the disease. FDG-PET imaging is a modality used in high-risk patients with elevated Tg. However, FDG-PET imaging in some patients may fail to detect the lesion.

The monitoring of somatostatin receptor (SSTR) expression in DTC cells allows the use of somatostatin receptor scintigraphy in DTC patients. Somatostatin receptor scintigraphy demonstrated to be positive in FDG-negative DTC patients provided an effective imaging method for lesion detection in those patients. In addition, patients with positive Tc-99m-labeled somatostatin receptor imaging have an operative chance with an intraoperative gamma probe. This modality increases the chances of success in patients with a history of multiple operations. Also in patients with positive somatostatin receptor scintigraphy, Lu-177-labeled or Y-90-labeled somatostatin analogs constitute a new treatment option.

56.1 Case Presentations

Case A 69-year-old male patient with a history of subtotal thyroidectomy due to multinodular goiter in 1998 has been examined. He did not have the pathology report of this operation. After a complementary thyroidectomy operation and bilateral neck dissection in 2013, the patient's pathological inspection resulted as compatible with an extensive invasive follicular carcinoma. The obtained levels in first blood control were 82 μIU/ml for TSH, 1.53 ng/ml for Tg and 10 IU/ml for anti-Tg, the patient has been given a 100 mCi (3.7 GBq) radioactive iodine (RAI) treatment. In the posttreatment checkup, TSH result was 100 μIU/ml, and Tg was 0.1 ng/ml. Also, I-131 diagnostic whole-body scintigraphy (DxWBS) showed no pathological uptake, so he's been followed under TSH suppression. After 3 years of uneventful monitoring, a progression has been determined in the patient's Tg values, and a 50 mCi (9.25 GBq) RAI treatment has been performed. Posttreatment, no retention has been

L. Kabasakal (✉) · O. E. Şahin
Department of Nuclear Medicine, Cerrahpaşa Faculty of Medicine, İstanbul University, Istanbul, Turkey
e-mail: lkabasakal@tsnm.org

T. Özülker et al. (eds.), *Thyroid and Parathyroid Diseases*, https://doi.org/10.1007/978-3-319-78476-2_56

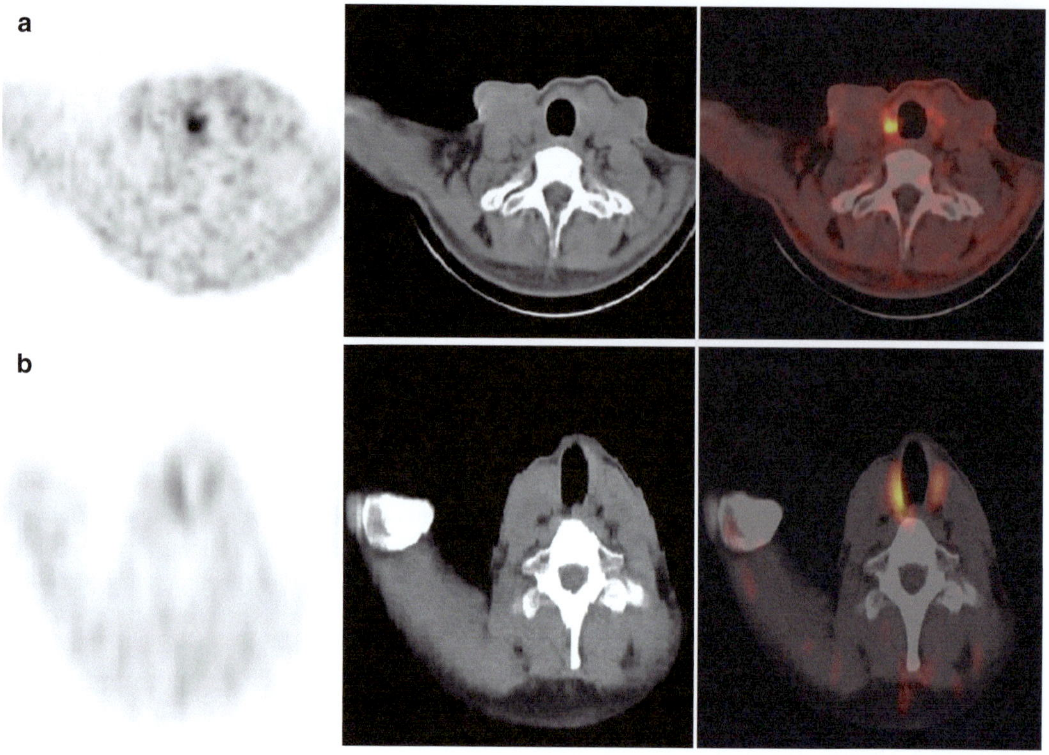

Fig. 56.1 68Ga-DOTATE PET/CT (row **a**) and 99mTc HYNIC-TATE SPECT/CT (row **b**) images of patient (PET/SPECT, CT, and fusion). Axial PET/CT and SPECT/CT images showed focal intense uptake in the right side of thyroid bed and lower uptake in in the left side of thyroid

observed in the I-131 whole-body scintigraphy (WBS) study. With the Tg progression ongoing and no suspicious lymph node determined in the neck USG, an FDG-PET/CT imaging was asked of the patient.

In the FDG-PET/CT imaging, two lesions in the neck consistent with the relapsed disease were detected. Afterward, a Ga-68 DOTA-TATE PET/CT imaging was asked of the patient, in which increased activity retention was observed consistent with the lesions observed in the FDG-PET/CT imaging (Fig. 56.1a). The decision was made to evaluate the patient in council with endocrine surgeons. Endocrine surgeons stated that because it would be the patient's third surgery, difficulty and the risk of complication would increase. In the somatostatin receptor scintigraphy, activity retention in the lesions has been observed, and the decision was made to conduct Tc-99m-HYNIC-TATE workup and, in the case of lesion positivity, to operate with the help of intraoperative gamma probe to increase the chance of success. In the Tc-99m-HYNIC-TATE scintigraphy, a lower density of activity retention has been observed than the Ga-68 DOTA-TATE PET/CT imaging, but it was still at a significant level. In response, the decision to operate with intraoperative gamma probe has been made. 5 mCi (185 MBq) 99mTc HYNIC-TATE has been intravenously injected into the patient on the morning of the operation. 1 h after the injection, local imaging has been taken from the neck area (Fig. 56.1b). Once it was confirmed that lesions displayed retention, the operation was immediately carried out.

56.2 Discussion

Differentiated thyroid cancer (DTC) makes up most of the thyroid cancers. DTC, which saw its diagnosis rate go up with the spread of radiologic imaging, generally has an excellent prognosis.

With appropriate surgery and, where necessary, RAI treatment and TSH suppression, most cases of DTC can be controlled. Maintaining the ability to concentrate iodine has made it possible to apply RAI treatment to DTC patients and has become the turning point in the treatment of the disease. Also, keeping the ability to synthesize thyroglobulin (Tg) in DTCs has made it possible to use serum Tg evaluation in following up and diagnosis. Regular neck USG workups and serum Tg evaluations are the basic components of the follow-up of the disease. Metastasis has been observed in approximately 10–15% of DTC patients, most frequently to lungs, and one-third of these patients lose their ability to concentrate iodine and become refractory to RAI treatment [1]. The disappearance of the RAI treatment option in radioiodine-refractory (RAI-R) DTC patients severely reduces the treatment options. Also, in DTCs that lose differentiation over time, the ability to synthesize Tg deteriorates and loses its importance in the follow-up. Although tyrosine kinase inhibitor treatment used in RAI-R DTCs has been proven to lengthen progression-free survival (PFS), no cure has been established, and the side effect profile makes the drug more difficult to use [2]. Systemic chemotherapies are also known not to produce satisfactory results. Instead, in RAI-R DTC patients with locally limited metastases, there is a chance of treatment with a surgical operation or external radiotherapy. Therefore, early detection and correctly localizing the tumor make up the most crucial aspect of disease management.

American Thyroid Association (ATA) guideline suggests FDG-PET/CT imaging for high-risk patients with elevated Tg values (usually >10 ng/ml) and negative RAI imaging. Also, it's been noticed that observing positivity in FDG-PET is a negative predictive factor in the RAI response [3]. On the other hand, it's also known that in some patients, FDG-PET/CT imaging fails in lesion detection. It's been observed that in DTCs, somatostatin receptor expression is displayed [4]. This, in turn, made it possible to use somatostatin analogs in lesion detection in DTC patients. Indium-111 labeled octreotide was first used for this purpose [5]. The 99mTc-labeled somatostatin analogs produced later provided more efficient imaging with advantages that 99mTc provided on gamma camera. Ga-68-labeled somatostatin receptor (SSTR) analogs (DOTATOC-, DOTANOC-, DOTA-TATE-) produced in recent years have further improved the imaging quality. In studies comparing SSTR PET/CT with F-18 FDG-PET/CT, the latter has been found to be more sensitive in identifying lesions in DTC patients. On the other hand, these studies show that some lesions can only be detected with SSTR PET/CT [6–9]. A relationship with criteria like imaging success and Tg value has not been clearly identified. Extensive and more detailed studies need to be carried out on this subject. On the other hand, somatostatin receptor imaging can be beneficial in patient managing, who has negative I-131WBS and FDG-PET/CT imaging [9].

For metastatic RAI-R DTC patients who have no chance of local treatment, treatment options are extremely limited. Systemic chemotherapeutics are known to be ineffective. In recent years, tyrosine kinase inhibitors (TKIs) used in systemic treatment of RAI-R DTC patients have been proven to contribute to progression-free survival (PFS) and formed an encouraging treatment option. However, the high side effect profile of these drugs causes difficulties in their use. The fact that somatostatin receptor (SSTR) analogs (DOTATOC-, DOTANOC-, DOTA-TATE-) developed for lesion detection in DTC patients can link with radionuclides like Lu-177 and Y-90 used in treatment has provided a new treatment option to RAI-R DTC patients [10]. Lesions that display significant retention in SSTR PET/CT imaging are candidates for peptide receptor radionuclide therapy (PRRT). In this regard, also, somatostatin receptor imaging contributes to DTC patient management.

Despite DTC patients having very good prognoses, the relapse rate is 5–30%. Each operation makes the next operation more difficult due to scarring, fibrosis development, and anatomical changes and increases the risk of complications secondary to the operation [11]. Reoperations with gamma probe provide a more minimal invasive attempt and the chance of a more target-specific intervention, providing fewer complications and more successful results [12, 13]. 99mTc-labeled somatostatin receptor imaging, along with lesion detection, also provides opportunity to operate with intraoperative gamma probe. This, in turn, increases the rate of success, especially in patients who previously had operations, and reduces complications related to the operation. In our case, it provided a target-specific and minimally invasive attempt to our patient who had metastatic lymph nodes and was having his third operation. This led to a successful operation by removing all metastatic lesions correctly from the patient, for whom lesion detection was more difficult due to his changed anatomy from the scar and fibrosis of the previous operation, and provided a complication-free operation in the case where, for the same reasons, the risk of complications was higher.

56.3 Follow-Up and Outcome

The patient who was operated on with gamma probe due to relapse had his third operation in total with no complications. The results for two mass materials removed in the operation came back consistent with follicular thyroid cancer infiltration. In the blood panel for control purposes, TSH: 80 μIU/ml and Tg: <2 ng/ml, the patient was put under observation, under TSH suppression.

56.4 Future

Prostate-specific membrane antigen (PSMA) is a transmembrane protein whose expression increases in prostate cancer. It's observed that PSMA molecule's expression, related to neovascularization, displays an increase in some other cancer types as well. In some case reports, activity retentions are observed in DTC's Ga-68 PSMA PET/CT imaging [14, 15]. Ga-68 PSMA PET/CT can provide a new and efficient imaging method, especially in high-risk RAI-R DTC patients whose FDG and SSTR-PET/CT imaging don't show lesion. Several more detailed studies are needed on this subject.

What Can We Learn from This Case?

- In metastatic RAI-R DTC patients who developed distant metastasis, treatment options are severely limited. In DTC patients who have the chance of operation or external RT in limited local disease, it's crucial that the lesion is detected early and correctly.
- For RAI-R DTC patients, FDG-PET/CT is an effective imaging method both in lesion detection and in giving an idea in terms of prognosis.
- In I-131 whole-body scan-negative, FDG-PET/CT-negative DTC patients, somatostatin receptor scintigraphy has created a new imaging modality.
- Lesions that go undetected in FDG-PET/CT can be detected in the somatostatin receptor imaging, which contributes to disease management.
- Besides, the fact that somatostatin receptor analogs can be labeled with radionuclides like Lu-177 and Y-90 used in treatment creates a new treatment alternative for metastatic RAI-R DTC patients who display activity retention in somatostatin receptor imaging
- Observing lesion positivity in 99mTc-labeled somatostatin receptor scintigraphy, especially in DTC patients with a history of operations, creates an opportunity to operate with intraoperative gamma probe. This, in turn, increases the chance of success for the operation and reduces the rate of complications.
- Ga-68 PSMA PET/CT, an effective imaging method in prostate cancer, shows promise in thyroid cancer imaging.

References

1. Durante C, Haddy N, Baudin E, Leboulleux S, Hartl D, Travagli JP, et al. Long-term outcome of 444 patients with distant metastases from papillary and follicular thyroid carcinoma: benefits and limits of radioiodine therapy. J Clin Endocrinol Metabol. 2006;91:2892–9. https://doi.org/10.1210/jc.2005-2838.

2. Lorusso L, Pieruzzi L, Biagini A, Sabini E, Valerio L, Giani C, et al. Lenvatinib and other tyrosine kinase inhibitors for the treatment of radioiodine refractory, advanced, and progressive thyroid cancer. Onco Targets Ther. 2016;9:6467–77. https://doi.org/10.2147/OTT.S84625.
3. Haugen BR, Alexander EK, Bible KC, Doherty GM, Mandel SJ, Nikiforov YE, et al. 2015 American Thyroid Association management guidelines for adult patients with thyroid nodules and differentiated thyroid cancer: the American Thyroid Association guidelines task force on thyroid nodules and differentiated thyroid cancer. Thyroid. 2016;26:1–133. https://doi.org/10.1089/thy.2015.0020.
4. Ain KB, Taylor KD, Tofiq S, Venkataraman G. Somatostatin receptor subtype expression in human thyroid and thyroid carcinoma cell lines. J Clin Endocrinol Metab. 1997;82:1857–62. https://doi.org/10.1210/jcem.82.6.4013.
5. Tenenbaum F, Lumbroso J, Schlumberger M, Caillou B, Fragu P, Parmentier C. Radiolabeled somatostatin analog scintigraphy in differentiated thyroid carcinoma. J Nucl Med. 1995;36:807–10.
6. Kundu P, Lata S, Sharma P, Singh H, Malhotra A, Bal C. Prospective evaluation of 68Ga-DOTANOC PET-CT in differentiated thyroid cancer patients with raised thyroglobulin and negative 131I-whole body scan: comparison with 18F-FDG PET-CT. Eur J Nucl Med Mol Imaging. 2014;41:1354–62. https://doi.org/10.1007/s00259-014-2723-9.
7. Middendorp M, Selkinski I, Happel C, Kranert WT, Grunwald F. Comparison of positron emission tomography with [(18)F]FDG and [(68)Ga]DOTATOC in recurrent differentiated thyroid cancer: preliminary data. Q J Nucl Med Mol Imaging. 2010;54:76–83.
8. Traub-Weidinger T, Putzer D, von Guggenberg E, Dobrozemsky G, Nilica B, Kendler D, et al. Multiparametric PET imaging in thyroid malignancy characterizing tumour heterogeneity: somatostatin receptors and glucose metabolism. Eur J Nucl Med Mol Imaging. 2015;42:1995–2001. https://doi.org/10.1007/s00259-015-3114-6.
9. Binse I, Poeppel TD, Ruhlmann M, Ezziddin S, Gorges R, Sabet A, et al. 68Ga-DOTATOC PET/CT in patients with iodine- and 18F-FDG-negative differentiated thyroid carcinoma and elevated serum thyroglobulin. J Nucl Med. 2016;57:1512–7. https://doi.org/10.2967/jnumed.115.171942.
10. Salavati A, Puranik A, Kulkarni HR, Budiawan H, Baum RP. Peptide receptor radionuclide therapy (PRRT) of medullary and nonmedullary thyroid cancer using radiolabeled somatostatin analogues. Semin Nucl Med. 2016;46:215–24. https://doi.org/10.1053/j.semnuclmed.2016.01.010.
11. Na'ara S, Amit M, Fridman E, Gil Z. Contemporary management of recurrent nodal disease in differentiated thyroid carcinoma. Rambam Maimonides Med J. 2016;7:e0006. https://doi.org/10.5041/RMMJ.10233.
12. Aras G, Gultekin SS, Kucuk NO, Demirer S, Tug T. Intraoperative gamma probe guidance with 99mTc-pertechnetate in the completion thyroidectomy. Ann Nucl Med. 2009;23:421–6. https://doi.org/10.1007/s12149-009-0251-7.
13. Terzioglu T, Senyurek YG, Tunca F, Turkmen C, Mudun A, Salmaslioglu A, et al. Excision efficiency of radioguided occult lesion localization in reoperative thyroid and parathyroid surgery. Thyroid. 2010;20:1271–8. https://doi.org/10.1089/thy.2009.0441.
14. Verburg FA, Krohn T, Heinzel A, Mottaghy FM, Behrendt FF. First evidence of PSMA expression in differentiated thyroid cancer using [(6)(8)Ga]PSMA-HBED-CC PET/CT. Eur J Nucl Med Mol Imaging. 2015;42:1622–3. https://doi.org/10.1007/s00259-015-3065-y.
15. Taywade SK, Damle NA, Bal C. PSMA expression in papillary thyroid carcinoma: opening a new horizon in management of thyroid cancer? Clin Nucl Med. 2016;41:e263–5. https://doi.org/10.1097/rlu.0000000000001148.

57 Anaplastic Thyroid Carcinoma

Abut Kebudi, Uğur Deveci, and Bülent Çitgez

Abstract

Anaplastic thyroid carcinoma (ATC) is a relatively uncommon highly malignant tumor originating from the follicular cells of the thyroid gland having a poor prognosis. It accounts for 2–5% of all thyroid carcinomas, and patients typically present with a rapidly growing anterior neck mass with aggressive symptoms. A 66-year-old male presented with dyspnea, neck pain, and voice changes. Ultrasonographic neck examination demonstrated an enlarged thyroid gland and substernal extension of the right thyroid lobe. Fine needle aspiration (FNA) from the thyroid nodule biopsy showed benign cytology. Because of symptomatic disease and radiologic malignancy doubt, operation has been done. Histopathologic examination with frozen section demonstrated anaplastic thyroid carcinoma. After total thyroidectomy, the patient is discharged. The patient died 20 days after the start of systemic treatment because of septic multiorgan failure derived from bronchopneumonic lung infection. In the evaluation of sudden growing neck masses in elderly patients, anaplastic thyroid cancer should be considered as a differential diagnosis, even if the needle biopsy is normal.

57.1 Case Presentation

A 66-year-old male patient was admitted to our clinic with 2 months history of dyspnea, neck pain, and voice changes. He had no operation and medical disorder in history. On physical examination, 5 cm diameter solid mass at the right neck was palpated and no palpable lymph node was determined. Laboratory examinations were within the normal ranges. Ultrasonographic neck examination demonstrated an enlarged thyroid gland and substernal extension of the right thyroid lobe. Thyroid fine needle aspiration biopsy showed benign colloidal goiter. To show tracheal pressure and margin of substernal mass, magnetic resonance imaging (MRI) was obtained (Fig. 57.1). There was a clear need for surgical intervention because of symptomatic disease. After preparation under general anesthesia with semi-fowler position, Kocher incision was made. In the course of intraoperative neck exploration, the strap muscle and trachea adhesions derived from the right

A. Kebudi (✉)
Division of Breast and Endocrine Surgery, General Surgery Department, Okan University, Istanbul, Turkey

U. Deveci
Division of Breast and Endocrine Surgery, General Surgery Department, Maltepe University, Istanbul, Turkey

B. Çitgez
Division of Breast and Endocrine Surgery, General Surgery Department, Şişli Hamidiye Etfal Training and Research Hospital, Istanbul, Turkey

T. Özülker et al. (eds.), *Thyroid and Parathyroid Diseases*, https://doi.org/10.1007/978-3-319-78476-2_57

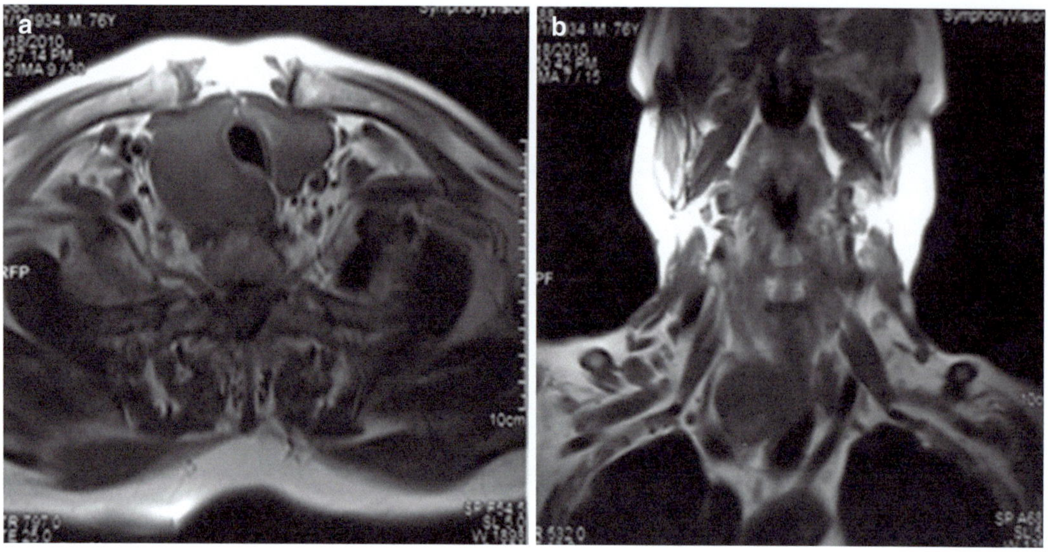

Fig. 57.1 MRI images of the neck, axial section (**a**), coronal section (**b**)

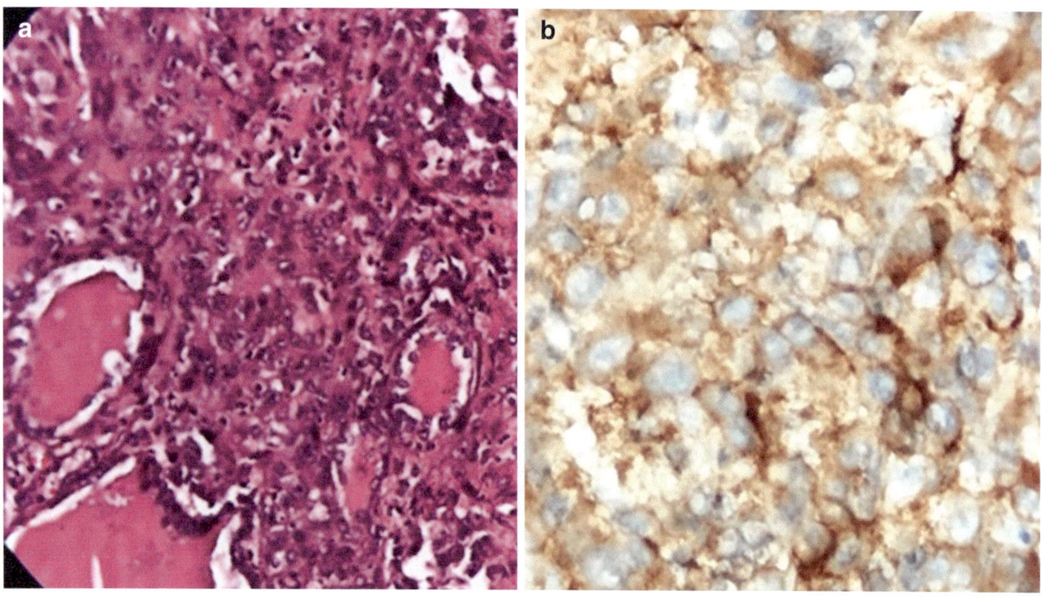

Fig. 57.2 H&E staining (×400) (**a**), immune-staining with thyroglobulin (×400) (**b**)

thyroid mass were determined. Histopathologic examination with frozen section demonstrated anaplastic thyroid carcinoma (ATC). Total thyroidectomy and partial strap muscles excision were performed. Histologic examination revealed anaplastic thyroid cancer with hyperchromatic, pleomorphic, atypical cells with narrow cytoplasm. Right lobe was 8 × 5 × 4 cm and left lobe was 5 × 3 × 2 cm diameter. The tumor was 5 cm diameter in the right lobe and showing invasion to thyroid capsule and adjacent structures. Lymphadenectomy was not performed because of no survival benefit for R1 resection. There were marked mitotic activity and necrosis. The immune-staining analysis was positive for TTF1, galectin, and thyroglobulin and negative for calcitonin, CK-19, HBME-1, chromogranin, and CEA (Fig. 57.2). According to TNM Staging

(7th ed., 2010) and the American Joint Committee on Cancer (AJCC) system, he was staged as pathological T4a N1b (stage IVA) and R1 indicating microscopic residual tumor cells. Thyroxine replacement therapy was started postoperatively. In the Endocrine Committee, combined chemoradiotherapy was planned for the patient.

57.2 Discussion

ATC is one of the most aggressive forms of cancer seen in humans. In marked contrast to differentiated thyroid cancers, anaplastic cancers are extremely aggressive, with disease-specific mortality approaching 100%. Despite a decrease in its incidence worldwide, it still accounts for 14–50% of mortality from thyroid cancer [1]. In an American and German prospective study which included 5583 cases of thyroid carcinoma, 67% of patients with ATC were over 70 years of age. In that study, females constituted 70% and males 30% of ATC patients [2]. In many series, patients were elderly women with a female to male ratio of 3:1 [3]. ATC is more common in areas with endemic goiter and low socioeconomic status. An overall analysis of 1771 published cases of ATC patients revealed median patient survival duration of only 5 months and a median 1-year survival rate of 20% [4]. Extensive local invasion and lymph node metastasis of the tumor with distant metastasis to lungs, bones, and other parts of the body are commonly seen at the diagnosis of ATC, leaving the disease incurable and deadly at the early stage after the diagnosis. Some experts have concluded that patients undergoing radical resection with negative margins have no survival benefit over those with positive microscopic or macroscopic margins [5]. Other authors have shown that complete resection is a positive prognostic factor [6].

57.3 Evaluation and Diagnosis

Most patients with ATC present with a rapidly enlarging neck mass. Clinicians should carry a high index of suspicion for ATC in all elderly patients with a symptomatic or rapidly enlarging neck mass. ATCs are generally large and cause local symptoms from their mass effect, including a sensation of pressure, dysphagia, and dysphonia. They also frequently cause respiratory problems because of their large size, including tracheal obstruction or recurrent or vagal nerve dysfunction.

The diagnosis of ATC is usually established by cytologic examination of cells obtained by fine needle aspiration biopsy or of tissue obtained by large needle or surgical biopsy. Large needle or surgical biopsy is typically performed when the fine needle aspiration shows necrotic or inflamed tissue without a specific diagnosis. Careful examination of aspirates by an experienced cytologist can correctly diagnose ATC in 84–90% of cases [7]. ATC can mimic the other malignancies that have significantly different treatments and prognoses. Evaluation of the biopsy material should include routine light microscopy and analysis with immunohistochemistry. Immune-staining is necessary to distinguish from the other malignancies such as melanoma, sarcoma, lymphoma, and medullary thyroid cancer. Macroscopically, ATC has a pale, white, or tan appearance on sectioning and is firm or hard on palpation. Extracapsular invasion of the tumor into surrounding structures is also commonly observed [8]. These tumors have mixed morphology. Most common mixed morphologic type is biphasic spindle and giant cell tumor [9]. ATC contains few if any cells that stain positively for thyroglobulin unlike more differentiated forms of thyroid cancer. Stains for keratin and vimentin are positive in up to 80 and 93% of cases, respectively, and confirm an epithelial origin of the tumor. Unlike differentiated thyroid cancer, ATC cells are much less likely to stain positive for thyroid transcription factor1 (TTF1) or PAX8 and do not stain positive for thyroglobulin in the anaplastic component of the tumor [9].

After FNA results, computed tomography (CT) and magnetic resonance imaging (MRI) of the neck can characterize the extent of locoregional disease and the presence of invasion into the esophagus, trachea, and soft tissues. Thyroid function tests (free T4 and TSH), complete blood count, electrolytes, blood urea nitrogen (BUN), creatinine, glucose, and liver function tests are measured. Calcium and phosphorus are measured to assess for hypercalcemia of malignancy or hypocalcemia due to compromise of the parathyroid glands secondary to invading ATC [9]. The evaluation should include direct laryngoscopy to determine if the tracheal invasion exists and to evaluate for vocal cord dysfunction from possible invasion of the recurrent laryngeal nerve. Esophagoscopy with or without endoscopic ultrasonography can evaluate for esophageal invasion. Although positron emission tomography (PET) may demonstrate increased [18F]2-fluoro-2-deoxyglucose (FDG) avidity from the primary site and distant metastases, not all ATCs are FDG avid [10].

57.4 Management

There is a nonuniform consensus about the standard treatment approach of ATC due to the very low incidence. American Thyroid Association (ATA) guidelines recommend that patients with stage IVA and IVB ATC be considered for radical surgical resection if gross negative margins (R0/R1) can be achieved with minimal morbidity and should not be attempted if there is a high chance of an incomplete resection (R2) [11]. Surgery aims to obtain a complete macroscopic resection, with microscopically clear resection margins. For intrathyroidal or local advanced disease, the surgical resection is recommended. After the intervention, combined chemotherapy and radiotherapy are given [12]. For patients who present with the locally advanced inoperable disease, combined chemotherapy and radiotherapy are recommended. Surgical resection of the residual tumor could be considered if the disease is responsive [12]. In patients with metastatic disease, palliative resection may be necessary for the treatment of tracheal or esophageal obstruction. In a randomized study of the Eastern Cooperative Oncology Group, Shimaoka et al. observed that combination chemotherapy based on doxorubicin and cisplatin was more effective than doxorubicin alone and provided a higher complete response rate [13]. In a prospective phase II clinical trial of paclitaxel, a remarkable response rate of 53% was obtained [14]. Hyman et al. demonstrated a 29% response rate in patients with *BRAF* mutant anaplastic thyroid cancer who were treated with the BRAF inhibitor, vemurafenib [15].

Many studies suggest that radiotherapy can provide very good locoregional control in patients with ATC, a disease often associated with significant local morbidity, in either the definitive or palliative setting [16]. ATA guideline recommends that radiation therapy should be started as soon as the patient is sufficiently recovered from neck surgery, usually within 2–3 weeks after surgery [11]. Definitive/adjuvant treatment was recommended for patients with good performance status and either stage IVA/IVB disease. Palliative radiotherapy to the primary was considered in younger patients with metastatic disease (stage IVC) or elderly patients (>70 years) who were predicted to have sufficiently long-life expectancy to derive benefit from radiotherapy taking into consideration their symptoms, tempo, and extent of disease, performance status, and comorbidities [16]. The most appropriate radiation volumes remain uncertain and require further investigation.

57.5 Follow-Up and Outcome

After the postoperative second week, doxorubicin/cisplatin-based chemotherapy was started. But the patient died 20 days after the start of systemic treatment because of septic multiorgan failure derived from bronchopneumonic lung infection.

Unfortunately, the prognosis of patients with ATC remains poor despite improvements in diagnosis, surgical technique, and the development of chemoradiotherapy protocols. Complications of disseminated metastatic disease are frequently the cause of death and limit survival even where effective local control can be achieved with aggressive surgical resection and radiotherapy.

57.6 The Future

The molecular investigation may contribute to treatment ATC when the targeted therapies are at the forefront, and early diagnostic methods are developed. By detecting genetic markers of well-differentiated thyroid cancers, cases with predisposing findings for ATC can be identified, and perhaps redifferentiation of the tumor can be achieved.

What Can We Learn from This Case?

- In the evaluation of sudden growing neck masses in elderly patients, anaplastic thyroid cancer should be considered as a differential diagnosis, even if the needle biopsy is normal.

References

1. Ursino S, Fiorica F, Stafenelli A, Pedriali M, Colosimo C, Cocuzza P, et al. Anaplastic thyroid cancer: a case report of a long term survival patient and review of literature data. Eur Rev Med Pharmacol Sci. 2014;18:1368–72.
2. Hundahl SA, Cady B, Cunningham MP, Mazzaferri E, McKee RF, Rosai J, et al. Initial results from a prospective cohort study of 5583 cases of thyroid carcinoma treated in the United States during 1996. U.S. and German thyroid cancer study group. An American College of Surgeons Commission on cancer patient care evaluation study. Cancer. 2000;89:202–17.
3. Xing JC, Bishop JA, Mathioudakis N, Agrawal N, Tufano RP. A large nonmetastatic anaplastic thyroid cancer with complete thyroidal confinement. Case Rep Med. 2011;2011:1–4. https://doi.org/10.1155/2011/58397.
4. Smallridge RJ, Copland JA. Anaplastic thyroid carcinoma: pathogenesis and emerging therapies. Clin Oncol. 2010;22:486–7.
5. Goffredo P, Thomas SM, Adam MA, Sosa JA, Roman SA. Impact of timeliness of resection and thyroidectomy margin status on survival for patients with anaplastic thyroid cancer: an analysis of 335 cases. Ann Surg Oncol. 2015;22:4166–74. https://doi.org/10.1245/s10434-015-47472-6.
6. Brown RF, Ducic Y. Aggressive surgical resection of anaplastic thyroid carcinoma may provide long-term survival in selected patients. Otolaryngol Head Neck Surg. 2013;148:564–71.
7. Us-Krasovec M, Golouh R, Auersperg M, Besic N, Ruparcic-Oblak L. Anaplastic thyroid carcinoma in fine needle aspirates. Acta Cytol. 1996;40:953–8.
8. Chambers AJ, Pasieka JL. Poorly differentiated and undifferentiated thyroid cancer. In: Johnathan H, William BI, Chung-Yau L, editors. Endocrine surgery principles and practice. London: Springer; 2009. p. 121–36.
9. Michael Tuttle R, Sherman EJ, Cooper DS, Ross DS, Mulder JE. Uptodate Knowledgebase. Massachusetts, US; 2017. http://www.uptodate.com/contents/anaplastic-thyroid-cancer. Accessed Mar 2017.
10. Ruan DT, Clark OH. Anaplastic thyroid carcinoma, metastases to the thyroid gland, and thyroid lymphoma. In: Morita SY, Dackiw APB, Zeiger MA, editors. Endocrine surgery. New York: McGraw-Hill; 2010. p. 110–24.
11. Smallridge RC, Ain KB, Asa SL, Bible KC, Brierley JD, Burman KD, et al. American Thyroid Association guidelines for Management of Patients with anaplastic thyroid cancer. Thyroid. 2012;22:1104–39. https://doi.org/10.1089/thy.2012.0302.
12. De Crevoisier R, Baudin E, Bachelot A, Leboulleux S, Travagli JP, Caillou B, et al. Combined treatment of anaplastic thyroid carcinoma with surgery, chemotherapy, and hyperfractionated accelerated external radiotherapy. Int J Radiat Oncol Biol Phys. 2004;60:1137–43. https://doi.org/10.1016/j.ijrobp.2004.05.032.
13. Shimaoka K, Schoenfeld DA, DeWys WD, Creech RH, DeConti R. A randomized trial of doxorubicin versus doxorubicin plus cisplatin in patients with advanced thyroid carcinoma. Cancer. 1985;56:2155–216.
14. Voigt W, Kegel T, Weiss M, Mueller T, Simon H, Schmoll HJ, et al. Potential activity of paclitaxel, vinorelbine and gemcitabine in anaplastic thyroid carcinoma. J Cancer Res Clin Oncol. 2005;131:585–90. https://doi.org/10.1007/s00432-005-0673-0.
15. Hyman DM, Puzanov I, Subbiah V, Faris JE, Chau I, Blay JY, et al. Vemurafenib in multiple nonmelanoma cancers with BRAF V600 mutations. N Engl J Med. 2015;373:726–36. https://doi.org/10.1056/NEJMoa1502309.
16. So K, Smith RE, Davis SR. Radiotherapy in anaplastic thyroid carcinoma: an Australian experience. J Med Imaging Radiat Oncol. 2017;61:279–87.

58 The Clinical Management of a Patient with Insular Thyroid Carcinoma

Gülin Uçmak and B. Büşra Demirel

Abstract

Insular carcinoma is a rare tumor that was first described as a unique histological subtype of thyroid cancer, in 1984. The World Health Organization (WHO) classified insular carcinoma as a separate existence and as a larger group of poorly differentiated thyroid carcinomas, in 2004. It was described as a thyroglobulin producing non-papillary non-follicular thyroid carcinoma, and it possesses an intermediate behavior between well-differentiated (papillary and follicular carcinoma) and anaplastic thyroid carcinomas with regard to both histological features and biologic aggressiveness. Insular carcinomas represent 0.4–6.2% of all thyroid carcinomas. Despite its rarity, it represents the main cause of death from non-anaplastic follicular cell-derived thyroid cancers. Distant metastasis and lymph node metastasis are most frequent, and moreover, 20% of patients with insular carcinoma have distant metastasis at the time of diagnosis. In patients with insular carcinoma, radioiodine uptake ability of primary tumor and distant metastasis is more than 80%. The current approach of management is total thyroidectomy followed by radioiodine therapy and close follow-up. In the view of the fact that worse prognosis, multidisciplinary approach combining surgery, bone-directed agents, and external radiation therapy concomitant with radioiodine therapy may provide treatment success and significant improvement in progression-free survival.

58.1 Case Presentation

A 55-year-old male patient was admitted to hospital with low back pain. On radiological imaging, a metastatic lesion was detected on his lumbar vertebra. The core biopsy was consistent with insular thyroid carcinoma metastasis. After total thyroidectomy, he was referred to our department for further treatment. Pathological examination determined poorly differentiated insular carcinoma with vascular and capsular invasion and areas showing well differentiation in the right lobe of the thyroid gland. At this time thyroglobulin (Tg) level was 4968 ng/ml and TSH level was 26 μIU/ml. On magnetic resonance imaging (MRI) which was performed after thyroidectomy, a mass lesion approximately

G. Uçmak (✉) · B. B. Demirel
Department of Nuclear Medicine, University of Health Sciences (SBÜ) Dr. Abdurrahman Yurtaslan Ankara Oncology Training and Research Hospital, Ankara, Turkey

T. Özülker et al. (eds.), *Thyroid and Parathyroid Diseases*, https://doi.org/10.1007/978-3-319-78476-2_58

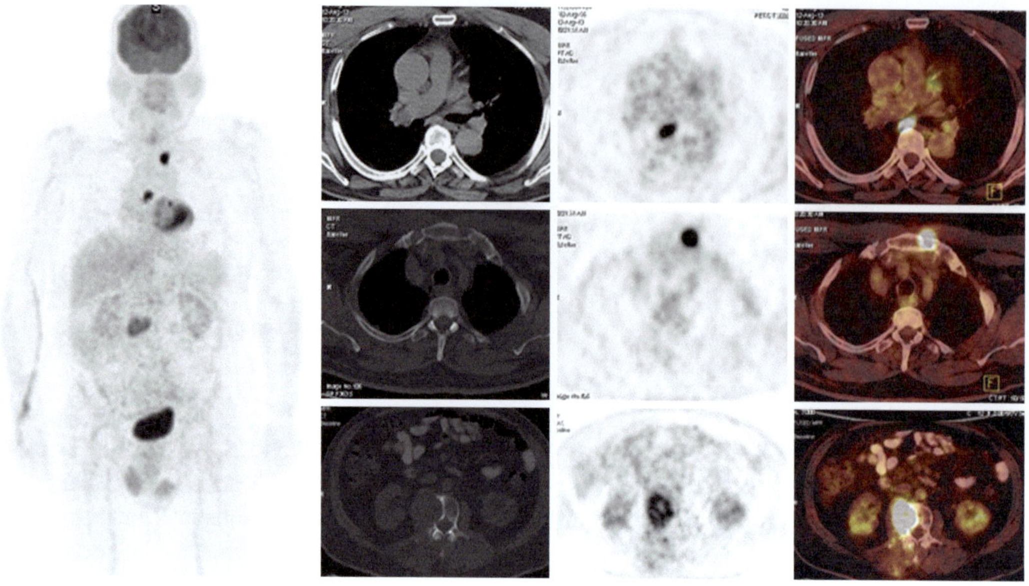

Fig. 58.1 Left column demonstrates MIP (maximal intensity projection) image, and the right column shows axial slices of patient's first FDG PET/CT scan. Intense FDG uptakes were seen in mediastinal lymph node (upper row), lytic and destructive lesions in sternum (middle row), and lumbar vertebra (lower row)

5 × 6 cm in diameter at L2 vertebra with intense contrast enhancement was seen. F-18 fluorodeoxyglucose (FDG) positron emission tomography/computed tomography (PET/CT) was performed to evaluate the extent of disease. FDG PET/CT revealed increased FDG uptake in lytic-destructive metastatic bone lesions with soft tissue component at the sternum and L-2 vertebra (Fig. 58.1). In addition, metastatic mediastinal lymph nodes and lung metastasis were observed on PET/CT.

The patient underwent surgery for his lumbar vertebra, and the metastatic lesion at L2 vertebra was partially resected. 30 Gy external beam radiation therapy (EBRT) was administered with palliative intent postoperatively. Following radiation therapy, 200 mCi (7.4 GBq) radioiodine therapy was given while serum TSH was 46 μIU/ml and Tg was 3416 ng/ml. Recombinant TSH stimulation was not used, and TSH elevation was achieved by thyroid hormone withdrawal prior to adjuvant treatment as recommended by the current ATA 2015 guideline. Premedication with oral corticosteroids, antiemetics, and careful hydration was given before radioiodine therapy. Post-therapy whole-body scan (WBS) performed 4 days after therapy demonstrated radioiodine uptake in thyroid bed and several uptakes related to bone metastasis at sternum, lumbar vertebra, and focal uptake in bilateral lung zones that may be prominently related to lung metastasis (Fig. 58.2).

On routine follow-up visits, serum Tg level remained significantly elevated (517 ng/ml on L-thyroxine therapy), and a second radioiodine therapy with dose of 250 mCi (9.2 GBq) I-131 was planned. Also, bisphosphonate treatment was started for bone metastasis. The patient was hospitalized for radioiodine therapy, and following proper premedication procedures, 250 mCi I-131 was administered orally. Simultaneous TSH and Tg levels were > 150 μIU/ml and 3033 ng/ml, respectively. Although serum Tg level was slightly decreased compared to the initial therapy, it was considered as a biochemical response as TSH stimulation was significantly stronger during the last therapy (46 μIU/ml vs. >150 μIU/ml).

Besides, on posttreatment WBS, parallel to biochemical response, we observed a significant regression on the intensity of radioiodine uptake, and also the size and the number of metastatic sites. In addition, no uptake was seen in thyroid bed (Fig. 58.2).

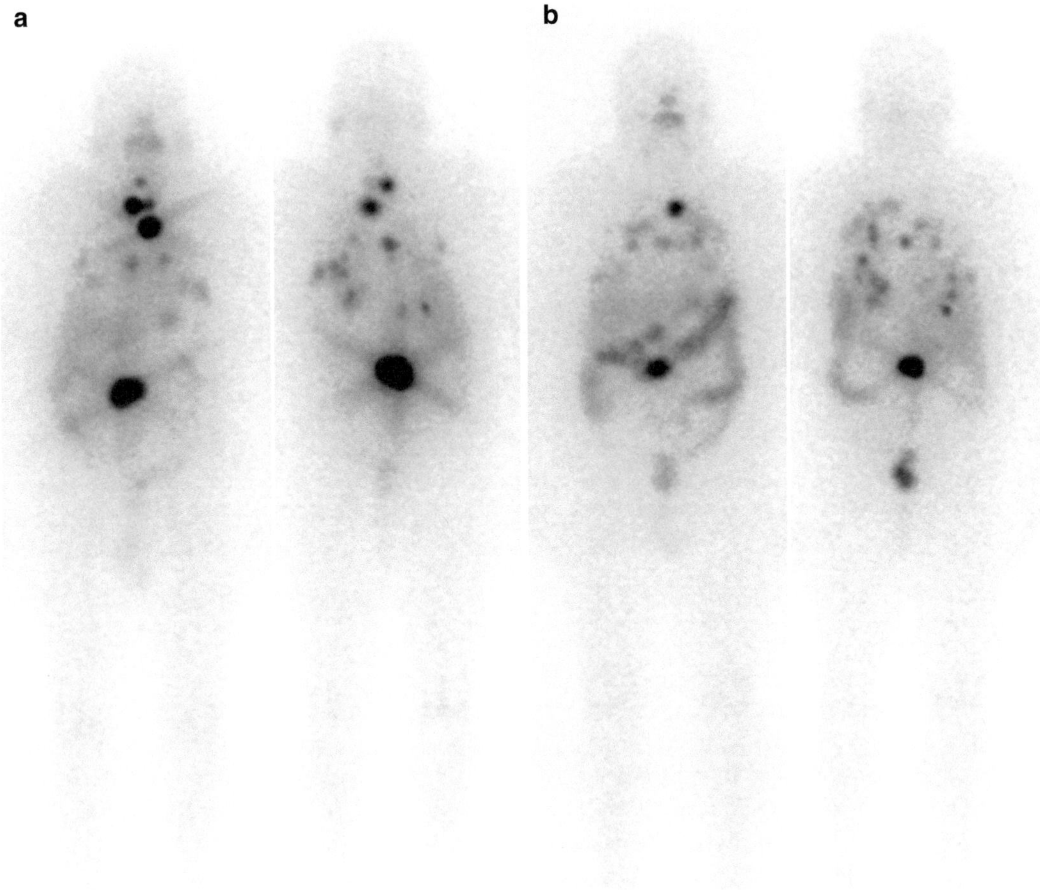

Fig. 58.2 Anterior and posterior images of WBS after initial radioiodine therapy of 200 mCi demonstrate distinct radioiodine uptake in thyroid bed, metastatic sites of bones, and heterogeneous uptake in thorax (**a**). Anterior and posterior WBS images acquired after the second radioiodine therapy with 250 mCi demonstrate decreased radioiodine uptake in all sites, compared to the prior treatment (**b**)

On follow-up, we observed that Tg levels on L-thyroxine therapy was decreased from 517 ng/dl to 228 ng/dl. A follow-up PET/CT study demonstrated a significant decrease in FDG uptake at mediastinal lymph nodes, pulmonary nodules, and bone metastasis sites (Fig. 58.3).

The clinical management of our patient was continued with annual radioiodine treatments that reached to a cumulative dose of 1100 mCi (40.7 GBq) supported by careful clinical and laboratory control for bone marrow reserve. Radioiodine uptake can still be seen in the final post-therapy WBS.

58.2 Discussion

Insular carcinoma is a rare tumor that was first described as a unique histological subtype of thyroid cancer by Carcangiu et al. [1]. The World Health Organization (WHO) classified insular carcinoma as a separate existence and as a larger group of poorly differentiated thyroid carcinomas, in 2004 [2]. Histologically, this tumor is characterized by partial loss of the features of thyroid differentiation, well-defined nests (insulae) that are comprised of relatively small, uniform cells and are associated sometimes with

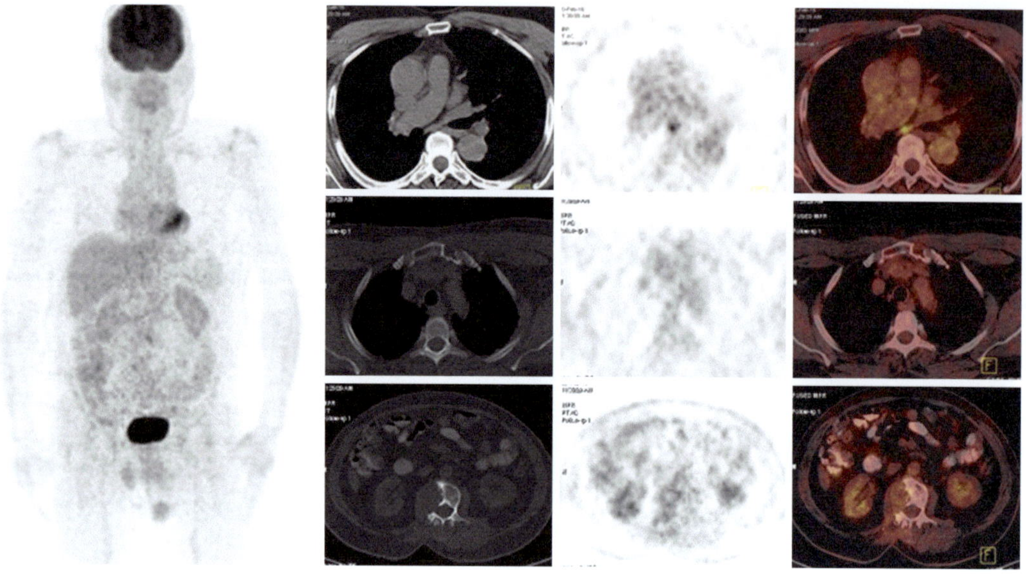

Fig. 58.3 MIP image (left column) and axial slices (right column) of final FDG PET/CT scan demonstrated significant decrease in FDG uptake of mediastinal lymph nodes and bone metastasis

small, thyroglobulin-containing follicles [3]. It was described as a thyroglobulin producing non-papillary non-follicular thyroid carcinoma, consistently with high-grade features such as invasive growth, high mitotic index, and necrosis. It possesses an intermediate behavior between well-differentiated (papillary and follicular carcinoma) and anaplastic thyroid carcinomas with regard to both histologic features and biologic aggressiveness [2].

Insular carcinomas represent 0.4–6.2% of all thyroid carcinomas [4]. Despite its rarity, it represents the main cause of death from non-anaplastic follicular cell-derived thyroid cancers [5], and rates of disease-specific mortality that related to distant metastasis and progression of disease in the neck and/or mediastinum ranges from 9% to 75% [3, 4]. Patients with older age (>45 y), larger tumor size, the presence of necrosis, and high mitotic activity are factors that may influence a more unfavorable outcome in patients with poorly differentiated thyroid cancer [6, 7]. Besides, advanced tumor stage, extrathyroidal extension, the presence of distant metastasis, and the absence of radioiodine therapy administration are associated with worse prognosis [8]. Poorly differentiated carcinomas have significantly worse prognosis as compared to well-differentiated thyroid cancers. The 5-year survival rate for patients with poorly differentiated cancer is 25.1–80.4%, and a 10-year survival is about 50% depending on treatment and the presence of independent prognostic factors [1, 6, 9]. The frequency of lymph node metastasis range was 50–84.6%, and distant metastasis rate was 36.4–84.6%. Distant metastases present 20% of patients at the time of diagnosis and most commonly present in lungs and bones. However, distant spread of disease was reported in unusual sites such as liver, skin, ovary, retroperitoneum, and intraocular [4, 10].

Insular carcinoma has a better prognosis than anaplastic cancers, and aggressive treatment is beneficial for the patients. The current approach of management is total thyroidectomy followed by radioiodine therapy and close follow-up. In a study of large series, it was reported that patients who received radioactive iodine had an improved overall survival compared to others [11]. In case of distant metastasis, although most patients have radioiodine uptake, some of them rapidly progress despite repeated radioiodine treatments. In these cases, an aggressive therapeutic approach with combined treatment modalities, which include high doses of radioiodine therapy, cytoreductive surgery, external radiation therapy, chemotherapy, and targeted agents, should be evaluated. And also bone-directed agents such as bisphosphonates should be used for patients with bone metastasis who are radioiodine-refractory, either alone or concomitantly with other systemic therapies. We considered that multidisciplinary approach combining surgery, bone-directed agents, and external radiation therapy concomitant with radioiodine therapy provided treatment success and significant improvement in the quality of life for our patient.

Genetic mutations in RET, p53, and RAS are important in many thyroid carcinomas. Mutations in p53 and RAS were noted in insular carcinoma, and more than 20% of poorly differentiated carcinomas showed p53 alteration [12]. Similarly, BRAF mutations were determined in poorly differentiated thyroid carcinomas which had papillary carcinoma foci [8]. A recent study reported that BRAF mutations have been associated with FDG avidity in radioiodine-refractory thyroid cancers [13]. FDG PET/CT is suggested by guidelines, in initial staging in poorly differentiated thyroid cancers, especially those with other evidence of disease on imaging or because of elevated serum Tg levels [14]. Also, PET/CT is considered as a significant prognostic tool to determine patients at highest risk for rapid disease progression, a sensitive method to detect surgically resectable disease for the selection of patients who may benefit from curative surgery select, and finally a reliable indicator of posttreatment response following therapy [14–16].

In patients with insular carcinoma, radioiodine uptake ability of primary tumor and distant metastasis is more than 80%. The impact of radioiodine treatment on the prognosis of patients with insular carcinoma is not well established. It was denoted that radioiodine therapy was effective in many patients, including those who had metastases at the time of diagnosis. Iodine uptake was much higher in patients who were treated shortly after thyroidectomy compared to uptake in patients who were treated at the time of local recurrence or distant disease [9]. As mentioned in our case, clear radioiodine uptake in metastatic deposits was observed on first post-therapy WBS. In a recent study, a definite clinical benefit from radioiodine therapy was observed only in patients who did not have TSH-R gene mutation and an unusually high radioiodine uptake [3]. It was suggested that the radioiodine uptake is related with efficiency of therapy response and a significant prognostic factor for survival [3, 6], but, some authors did not share this opinion. They suggest that geographical differences regarding different disease stages at the time of radioiodine therapy and/or different timing and dosage of radioiodine administration may reflect the success of therapy [17]. Aggressive surgery modalities may be suitable due to poorer prognosis and advanced clinical stage. It was shown that wide resection is associated with low recurrence and low mortality rates, previously [18].

In conclusion, considering the worse prognosis of insular carcinoma compared to well-differentiated thyroid cancers, optimal initial treatment should be determined by a multidisciplinary approach. Aggressive surgery with curative intent when available is the mainstay of treatment. Even in patients with widespread metastatic disease, maximum cytoreduction can provide success for radioiodine treatment and may decrease disease-specific mortality. In cases with radioiodine avid tumors, high dose sequential radioiodine treatments with dosimetric studies, where applicable, should be applied concomitant with other treatment modalities. For iodine-refractory tumors, risk-adapted personalized molecular targeted therapies should be considered. In the presented case, we aimed to discuss the multidisciplinary management in a patient with metastatic, poorly differentiated insular carcinoma, which provided a relatively long progression-free survival.

58.3 Follow-Up

During the 5 years of follow-up, we reached a significant biochemical and anatomical therapy response. At the time of the last follow-up, the patient is free of symptoms, and the patient's current Tg level is 98 ng/ml under TSH suppression.

What Can We Learn from This Case?

- Insular carcinoma is a rare type of thyroid carcinoma with an intermediate behavior between well-differentiated and anaplastic thyroid carcinomas.
- Up to 80% of patients are radioiodine positive. The current treatment approach is radioiodine therapy after total thyroidectomy.
- A multidisciplinary approach combining surgery, bone-directed agents, external radiation therapy concomitant with radioiodine therapy may provide treatment success and significant improvement in progression-free survival.

References

1. Carcangiu ML, Zampi G, Rosai J. Poorly differentiated ("insular") thyroid carcinoma: a reinterpretation of Langhans' "wucherndestruma.". Am J Surg Pathol. 1984;8:655–8.
2. DeLellis RA, LLoyd R, Heitz PU, editors. WHO classification of tumors, pathology and genetics—tumors of endocrine organs. Lyon: IARC Press; 2004.
3. Pellegriti G, Giuffrida D, Scollo C, Vigneri R, Regalbuto C, Squatrito S, et al. Long-term outcome of patients with insular carcinoma of the thyroid: the insular histotype is an independent predictor of poor prognosis. Cancer. 2002;15(95):2076–85. https://doi.org/10.1002/cncr.10947.
4. Chao TC, Lin JD, Chen MF. Insular carcinoma: infrequent subtype of thyroid cancer with aggressive clinical course. World J Surg. 2004;28:393–6. https://doi.org/10.1007/s00268-003-7264-5.
5. Ibrahimpasic T, Ghossein R, Carlson DL, Nixon I, Palmer FL, Shaha AR, et al. Outcomes in patients with poorly differentiated thyroid carcinoma. J Clin Endocrinol Metab. 2014;99:1245–52. https://doi.org/10.1210/jc.2013-3842.
6. Volante M, Landolfi S, Chiusa L, Palestini N, Motta M, Codegone A, et al. Poorly differentiated carcinomas of the thyroid with trabecular, insular, and solid patterns: a clinicopathologic study of 183 patients. Cancer. 2004;100:950–7. https://doi.org/10.1002/cncr.20087.
7. Pulcrano M, Boukheris H, Talbot M, Caillou B, Dupuy C, Virion A, et al. Poorly differentiated follicular thyroid carcinoma: prognostic factors and relevance of histological classification. Thyroid. 2007;17:639–46. https://doi.org/10.1089/thy.2007.0029.
8. Volante M, Papotti M. Poorly differentiated thyroid carcinoma: 5 years after the 2004 WHO classification of endocrine tumours. Endocr Pathol. 2010;21:1–6. https://doi.org/10.1007/s12022-009-9100-4.
9. Papotti M, BottoMicca F, Favero A, Palestini N, Bussolati G. Poorly differentiated thyroid carcinomas with primordial cell component. A group of aggressive lesions sharing insular, trabecular, and solid patterns. Am J Surg Pathol. 1993;17:291–301.
10. Ozpacaci T, Mulazimoglu M, Tamam MO, Leblebici C, Yildiz K, Uyanik E, et al. Intraocular and orbital metastasis as a rare form of clinical presentation of insular thyroid cancer. Ann Endocrinol (Paris). 2012;73:222–4. https://doi.org/10.1016/j.ando.2012.02.002.
11. Pezzi TA, Sandulache VC, Pezzi CM, Turkeltaub AE, Feng L, Cabanillas ME, et al. Treatment and survival of patients with insular thyroid carcinoma: 508 cases from the National Cancer Data Base. Head Neck. 2016;38:906–12. https://doi.org/10.1002/hed.24342.
12. Lam KY, Lo CY, Chan KW, Wan KY. Insular and anaplastic carcinoma of the thyroid: a 45-year comparative study at a single institution and a review of the significance of p53 and p21. Ann Surg. 2000;231:329–38.
13. Ricarte-Filho JC, Ryder M, Chitale DA, Rivera M, Heguy A, Ladanyi M, et al. Mutational profile of advanced primary and metastatic radioactive iodine-refractory thyroid cancers reveals distinct pathogenetic roles for BRAF, PIK3CA, and AKT1. Cancer Res. 2009;69:4885–93. https://doi.org/10.1158/0008-5472.CAN-09-0727.
14. Haugen BR, Alexander EK, Bible KC, Doherty GM, Mandel SJ, Nikiforov YE, et al. 2015 American Thyroid Association management guidelines for adult patients with thyroid nodules and differentiated thyroid cancer: the American Thyroid Association guidelines task force on thyroid nodules and differentiated thyroid cancer. Thyroid. 2016;26:1–133. https://doi.org/10.1089/thy.2015.0020.
15. Akkaş BE, Demirel BB, Vural GU. Prognostic factors affecting disease specific survival in patients with recurrent and/or metastatic differentiated thyroid carcinoma detected by PET/CT. Thyroid. 2014;24:287–95. https://doi.org/10.1089/thy.2013.0195.
16. Vural GU, Akkas BE, Ercakmak N, Basu S, Alavi A. Prognostic significance of FDG PET/CT on the follow-up of patients of differentiated thyroid carcinoma with negative 131I whole-body scan and elevated thyroglobulin levels: correlation with clinical and histopathologic characteristics and long-term follow-up data. Clin Nucl Med. 2012;37:953–9. https://doi.org/10.1097/RLU.0b013e31825b2057.
17. Lai HW, Lee CH, Chen JY, Tseng LM, Yang AH. Insular thyroid carcinoma: collective analysis of clinicohistologic prognostic factors and treatment effect with radioiodine or radiation therapy. J Am Coll Surg. 2006;203:715–22. https://doi.org/10.1016/j.jamcollsurg.2006.07.008.
18. Sakamoto A, Kasai N, Kitagawa T, Sugano H. Postoperative recurrence and death rates of poorly differentiated carcinoma of the thyroid. Gan No Rinsho. 1986;32:955–7.

59 Prophylactic and Therapeutic Surgery in Familial Medullary Thyroid Cancer

Atakan Sezer and Mehmet Çelik

Abstract

Medullary thyroid cancer (MTC) is a neuroendocrine malignancy, which originates from C cells (parafollicular) of the gland. MTC is inherited in autosomal dominant pattern in 20–25% of patients with MEN syndromes. Familial MTC (FMTC) is the most frequent type of MEN syndromes.

The most accepted approach for deciding surgical treatment of the disease based on the precise polymer mutation within the douse factor occurring within the family and blood serum calcitonin levels.

RET mutations may be classified as highest, high, and moderate risk, concerning the potential risk for native and distant MTC metastases at an early age. The advised temporal order of excision relies upon proof of age-dependent and codon-specific progression of early MTC.

In conclusion, patients with inherited MTC ought to experience age-suitable thyroidectomy in view of RET mutational status to evade recurrences.

A. Sezer (✉)
Department of Surgery, Trakya University Medical Faculty, Edirne, Turkey

M. Çelik
Department of Endocrinology, Trakya University Medical Faculty, Edirne, Turkey

59.1 Case Presentation

A 44-year-old woman was referred to general surgery department with swelling on the neck. Physical examination revealed a 15-mm thyroid nodule in the thyroid gland. Neck ultrasonography (USG) examination demonstrated a 11 × 18 × 26 mm sized hypoechogenic nodule with irregular margins and microcalcifications in the left thyroid lobe and 13 × 14 × 15 mm sized nodule in the right thyroid lobe (Fig. 59.1a and b). The patient had no history of radiation exposure and no family history of thyroid cancer. Laboratory examination reports were as follows: calcitonin (Ct), 419 pg/ml (n, 0–10); fT3, 3.6 pg/ml (n, 1.71–3.81); fT4, 1.41 ng/dl (n, 0.7–1.48); and TSH, 0.53 mlU/ml (n, 0.35–4.94). Calcium, parathyroid hormone (PTH), urinary 24-h catecholamine levels were within normal ranges, which were confirmed twice. The patient underwent a fine needle aspiration biopsy (FNAB) in right thyroid nodule, which was reported as suspicious for follicular neoplasia. Total thyroidectomy (TTx) and central lymph node dissection (CLND) were performed due to high preoperative Ct levels (Fig. 59.1c). Pathologic examination of the specimen revealed 26 mm sized medullary thyroid carcinoma (MTC) on the left thyroid lobe and 15 mm sized MTC on the right thyroid lobe. The specimen margins were free of tumor

T. Özülker et al. (eds.), *Thyroid and Parathyroid Diseases*, https://doi.org/10.1007/978-3-319-78476-2_59

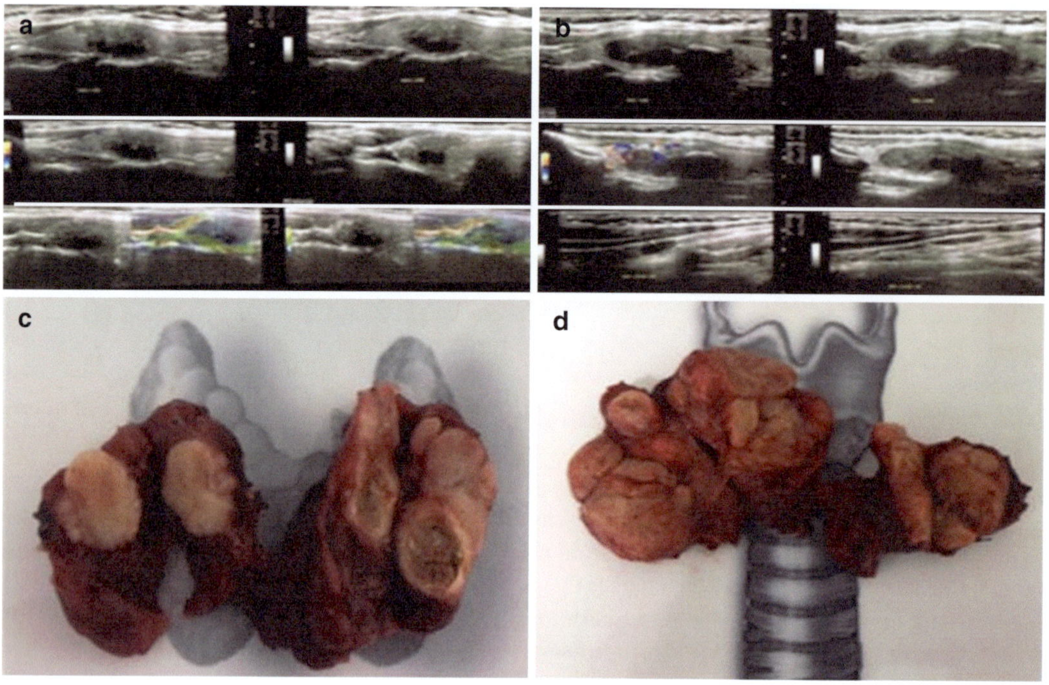

Fig. 59.1 Thyroid USG of the index case (**a** and **b**), macroscopic appearance of total thyroidectomy specimens of the index case (**c**), macroscopic appearance of total thyroidectomy specimens of index case's elderly brother (**d**)

involvement and lymph node metastasis (pT2pN0pMx). Codon 634 of exon 11 for RET gene was detected. The patient's family, the mother, son, brothers, and two sisters were clinically evaluated and also underwent FNAB. The elder brother (55-year-old) has the same RET gene mutation, and a hypoechogenic, 15 × 18 × 25 mm-sized nodule in the left thyroid lobe and 15 × 18 × 25 mm-sized nodule in the right thyroid lobe were detected on USG examination. Thyroid hormone levels and urinary 24-h catecholamine and derivatives were within normal ranges. Serum Ct was measured as 4496 pg/ml (n, 0–10). The elder brother underwent TTx and CLND (Fig. 59.1d). Pathologic examination of the specimen revealed two tumors in 1 cm on the right lobe as multifocal MTC and four tumors in 1.5 cm size in the left lobe also as MTC. The patients were discharged uneventfully, and the patients and pedigrees were in clinical follow-up for new events.

59.2 Discussion

59.2.1 Evaluation and Diagnosis

MTC is a rare form of thyroid carcinomas, which originates from calcitonin secreting C cells (parafollicular cells) of the thyroid gland. The rare thyroid cancer constitutes 3–5% of all thyroid cancers and shows autosomal dominant inheritance pattern in 20–25% of patients (MEN syndromes) [1, 2]. "Germ line" activating mutations in proto-oncogene are thought to be responsible for familial inheritance. Familial MTC (FMTC) is the most common component of MEN two syndromes, or it can be seen as sporadic FMTC.

Sporadic MTC is generally observed in fourth and sixth decades. Tumor location is usually unilateral (80%) and rarely bilateral (20%). MTC has no specific feature on thyroid USG. FNAB is the most useful and safe method for diagnosis. The other option for confirming MTC diagnosis is immunolocalization of chromogranin, CEA or Ct, negative staining with thyroglobulin, and detecting the elevation of serum calcitonin levels [3, 4]. Basal Ct levels in 7% of familial MTC cases were measured in normal ranges [5–7]. Calcium, pentagastrin, gastrin, glucagon, pancreozymin, glucocorticoids, Ct gene-related peptide, and beta-adrenergic agents increase calcitonin secretion. Thus, calcium infusion is recently the most commonly used calcitonin stimulation test for verifying MTC diagnosis in suspicious cases. The test results are in close relation to the amount of calcium applied, time of infusion, and sampling time. The basic protocol of the test is 2.5 mg/kg calcium gluconate infusion during 30 s and collecting blood samples before infusion (basal), 2nd and 5th min. Test results are accepted to be positive if peak Ct level is three times of basal value or basal level is ≥300 ng/l. False-negative results may be obtained in micro MTC or C cell hyperplasia [8]. In patients diagnosed with MTC, RET proto-oncogene must be examined for "germ line" mutations even in the absence of positive family history. In case of positive result, all first-degree relatives of the patient with MTC should undergo RET gene mutation analysis. Depending on the degree of risk of mutation, prophylactic thyroidectomy (PTx) or CLND is indicated. In patients suspected to have hereditary MTC or detected to have RET proto-oncogene mutations, primary hyperparathyroidism (PHP) and pheochromocytoma should be excluded prior to surgery of MTC. In all cases with clinical findings suggesting regional and distant metastasis or patients who have serum Ct level > 500 pg/ml, in addition to preoperative neck USG, contrast-enhanced neck and thoracic computerized tomography (CT), three-phase dynamic liver CT or contrast-enhanced liver magnetic resonance imaging (MRI), and bone scintigraphy are recommended [4].

59.2.2 Management

In patients with no neck lymph node metastasis or distant metastasis on preoperative clinical evaluation, TTx is recommended. In subjects with cervical lymph node metastasis, CLND and dissection for ipsilateral neck compartments must be carried out in addition to TTx. In case of basal Ct level > 200 pg/ml, contralateral neck dissection may be performed in addition to ipsilateral lymph node dissection [4]. When distant metastasis is present, less aggressive neck surgery is preferred to preserve phonation, airway, and swallowing and parathyroid functions, prevent central neck morbidity, and provide regional disease control. Since MTC is bilateral and multicentric in all MEN2 syndromes, TTx is preferred treatment modality. Since some cases that seem to have the sporadic form of the disease may turn to have a hereditary type of the disease, TTx is also recommended for these subjects. Presence of pheochromocytoma must be evaluated prior to thyroidectomy, and if present, it should first be treated. During thyroidectomy, CLND is also performed, and suspicious nodules in the neck and anterior-upper mediastinum are excised. Surgery may be curative even in the presence of nodal involvement. However, MTC in MEN2B is more aggressive than in MEN2A and FMTC, and surgery is mostly not curative treatment. The timing of prophylactic thyroidectomy (PTx) is very important in children in whom screening reveals RET mutation. All patients should be referred to academic centers experienced in MEN2 management [4].

American Thyroid Association (ATA) recommends PTx to be performed during the first year and even during first months of life in children who are found to be in very high-risk category (M918T) according to risk classification given in Table 59.1 [4, 9–14]. Children in high-risk category (C634F/G/R/S/W/Y, A883F) should undergo PTx at the age of 5 years, or it may be performed earlier in case of increased levels of basal or stimulated CT. CLND may be applied to children with Ct >40 pg/ml or lymph node metastasis detected by imaging methods. In this case, the surgical experience of the operator is very important. Surgical morbidity is high during childhood, and experienced pediatric or endocrine surgeons should operate these children. For children in moderate-risk category according to ATA, periodic physical examination and follow-up with

Table 59.1 Relationship of common RET mutations to risk of aggressive MTC in MEN2A and MEN2B

RET mutation	MTC risk level	Exon
G533C	MOD	8
C609F/G/R/S/Y	MOD	10
C611F/G/S/Y/W	MOD	10
C618F/R/S	MOD	10
C620F/R/S	MOD	10
C630R/Y	MOD	11
D631Y	MOD	11
C634F/G/R/S/W/Y	*H*	*11*
K666E	MOD	11
E768D	MOD	13
L790F	MOD	13
V804L	MOD	14
V804M	MOD	14
A883F	*H*	*15*
S891A	MOD	15
R912P	MOD	16
M918T	*HST*	*16*

MOD moderate, *H* high, *HST* highest

neck USG and serum Ct level are recommended, and thyroidectomy may be delayed until the age of 5 years. If the family is concerned about long-term follow-up programs and prefers early thyroidectomy, it may be performed around the age of 5 years. In adult subjects with germ line mutation, serum calcitonin level is measured if neck USG is normal. Annual follow-up is recommended in case of normal calcitonin level. If Ct level is elevated, total thyroidectomy is applied after exclusion of pheochromocytoma [4].

59.2.3 Follow-Up of Patients

Postoperative thyroid hormone replacement is given to ensure euthyroid state. Since C cells are not TSH sensitive, suppressive doses are not required. Follow-up schedule is different for familial and sporadic cases. The most important postoperative follow-up parameters in patients with MTC are TNM classification, lymph node metastasis, and postoperative Ct levels. Serum Ct and CEA levels should be measured in postoperative 3rd month. If CT and CEA levels are found to be undetectable or within the normal range, follow-up examinations should be carried out at 6-month intervals for the first year and, then, annually. If postoperative Ct level is found to be high but lower than 150 pg/ml, neck USG should be done. In case of normal neck USG findings, physical examination, neck USG, and Ct and CEA level measurements should be performed at 6-month intervals. In cases which are found to have postoperative Ct levels ≥150 pg/ml and normal neck USG, thoracic, and mediastinal CT findings, the metastatic focus may be investigated by contrast-enhanced MRI or three-phase contrast-enhanced CT of the liver, bone scintigraphy, and MR imaging for the pelvic-axial skeleton. If high Ct levels persist during the postoperative period, a second surgery may be performed if the causative focus is operable and can be localized by imaging modalities. In case of undetectable focus, the patient is scheduled for close follow-up (wait and see) if basal and/or stimulated CT levels are high [4].

In persistent postoperative disease, serial CT and CEA measurements and doubling time of these parameters may be calculated. Ct doubling time is an important predictive parameter for prognosis. Patients with short doubling time (<6 months) have low 5–10-year survival rates, and they need aggressive treatment approach. In subjects with low risk and doubling time > 2 years, follow-up with Ct and CEA measurements with 6-month intervals may be enough, and these patients have long survival time. In cases with doubling time of 6 months to 2 years, additional treatment regimens may be necessary considering 5–10-year survival rates. Systemic treatment is not recommended in patients with elevated serum Ct and CEA levels but undetectable metastatic focus, stable metastatic disease with low tumoral load, and subjects with Ct and CEA doubling time > 2 years. Liet biopsy is recommended before difficult and recurrent neck operations to reveal occult liver metastasis in patients in whom disease persists or recurs after TTx. MTC follow-up and treatment are similar for MEN2 and sporadic cases. It should be known that 50% of individuals of the MEN2 family carrying this genotype will develop pheochromocytoma, and 5–10% will have PHP at some time during their lives. Therefore, annual measurements for corrected Ca or ionized Ca, phosphorus, plasma-free metanephrine, and normetanephrine or 24-h urine metanephrine and normetanephrine and biyearly adrenal CT examinations are required. Unilateral adrenalectomy does not eliminate the need for follow-up. In these families, the incidence of bilateral pheochromocytoma is higher than 60%, which may not be concurrent [4].

59.2.4 The Future

Not long ago, an agent named arylidene-2-indolinone (RPI-1) has been shown to prevent autonomic tyrosine phosphorylation related to RET mutation in codon 634 in patients with MEN2A, which is promising for the future [15].

What Can We Learn from This Case?

- MEN2 accounts for about 25% of medullary thyroid cancer.
- The current standard of care for MEN2 includes genetic testing of all potentially affected family members for the RET proto-oncogene, and patients should be evaluated in terms of risk grade.
- Select among the surgical treatment options for prophylactic surgery in genetic carriers.

References

1. Cancer of the Thyroid Invasive: Trends in SEER Incidence and U.S. Mortality Using the Joinpoint Regression Program, 1975–2011(SEER) Stat version 8.1.2 Rate Session. Access the SEER 18 database at www.seer.cancer.gov). Incidence - SEER 18 Regs Research Data + Hurricane Katrina Impacted Louisiana Cases, Nov 2012 Sub (2000–2010) - Linked To County Attributes - Total U.S., 1969–2011 Counties, National Cancer Institute, DCCPS, Surveillance Research Program, Surveillance Systems Branch, released April 2013, based on the November 2012 submission.
2. Hadoux J, Pacini F, Tuttle RM, Schlumberger M. Management of advanced medullary thyroid cancer. Lancet Diabetes Endocrinol. 2016;4:64–71.
3. Leboulleux S, Baudin E, Travagli J, Schlumberger M. Medullary thyroid carcinoma. Clin Endocrinol. 2004;61:299–310.
4. Wells S, Asa S, Dralle H, Elisei R, Evans D, Gagel R, et al. Revised American Thyroid Association guidelines for the Management of Medullary Thyroid Carcinoma. Thyroid. 2015;25:567–610.
5. Bockhorn M, Frilling A, Rewerk S, Liedke M, Dirsch O, Schmid K, et al. Lack of elevated serum Carcinoembryonic antigen and calcitonin in medullary thyroid carcinoma. Thyroid. 2004;14:468–70.
6. Redding A, Levine S, Fowler M. Normal preoperative calcitonin levels do not always exclude medullary thyroid carcinoma in patients with large palpable thyroid masses. Thyroid. 2000;10:919–22.
7. Diez JJ, Iglesias P. Lack of elevated serum carcinoembryonic antigen and calcitonin in medullary thyroid carcinoma. Thyroid. 2004;14:984–5.
8. Heshmati HM, Hofbauer LC. Multiple endocrine neoplasia type 2: recent progress in diagnosis and management. Eur J Endocrinol. 1997;137:572–8.
9. Schilling T, Burck J, Sinn HP, Clemens A, Otto HF, Hoppner W, et al. Prognostic value of codon 918 (ATG-->ACG) RET proto-oncogene mutations in sporadic medullary thyroid carcinoma. Int J Cancer. 2001;95:62–6.
10. Elisei R, Cosci B, Romei C, Bottici V, Renzini G, Molinaro E, et al. Prognostic significance of somatic RET oncogene mutations in sporadic medullary thyroid cancer: a 10-year follow-up study. J Clin Endocrinol Metab. 2008;93:682–7.
11. Raue F, Frank-Raue K. Genotype-phenotype correlation in multiple endocrine neoplasia type 2. Clinics (Sao Paulo). 2012;67(Suppl 1):69–75.
12. Imai T, Uchino S, Okamoto T, Suzuki S, Kosugi S, Kikumori T, et al. High penetrance of pheochromocytoma in multiple endocrine neoplasia 2 caused by germ line RET codon 634 mutation in Japanese patients. Eur J Endocrinol. 2013;168:683–7.
13. Jasim S, Ying AK, Waguespack SG, Rich TA, Grubbs EG, Jimenez C, et al. Multiple endocrine neoplasia type 2B with a RET proto-oncogene A883F mutation displays a more indolent form of medullary thyroid carcinoma compared with a RET M918T mutation. Thyroid. 2011;21:189–92.
14. Frank-Raue K, Rybicki LA, Erlic Z, Schweizer H, Winter A, Milos I, et al. Risk profiles and penetrance estimations in multiple endocrine neoplasia type 2A caused by germline RET mutations located in exon 10. Hum Mutat. 2011;32:51–8.
15. Cuccuru G, Lanzi C, Cassinelli G, Pratesi G, Tortoreto M, Petrangolini G, et al. Cellular effects and antitumor activity of RET inhibitor RPI-1 on MEN2A-associated medullary thyroid carcinoma. J Natl Cancer Inst. 2004;96:1006–14.

Sporadic Medullary Thyroid Cancer

60

Nuh Zafer Cantürk, Sertaç Ata Güler, and Turgay Şimşek

Abstract

Medullary thyroid cancer (MTC) is a neuroendocrine tumor of the parafollicular or C cells of the thyroid gland. It accounts for approximately 1–2% of thyroid cancers. The production of calcitonin is a characteristic feature of this tumor. Most of the MTCs are sporadic whereas 25% of cases are familial as part of the multiple endocrine neoplasia type 2 (MEN2) syndrome. For sporadic MTCs, there are no germline RET mutations. The most common presentation of sporadic MTC is a solitary thyroid nodule. Systemic symptoms may occur due to hormonal secretion by the tumor. Most sporadic MTCs also secrete carcinoembryonic antigen (CEA). The diagnosis of sporadic MTC is usually made after fine needle aspiration (FNAB) biopsy in a patient who has a solitary thyroid nodule. Patients with sporadic MTC can be cured only by complete resection of the thyroid tumor with bilateral central neck lymph node dissection. For patients with the residual or recurrent disease after primary surgery or for those with distant metastases, the most appropriate treatment is less clear and still debatable.

In this case presentation, we discussed a patient with an MTC, its evaluation, diagnosis, management and the future of the MTC according to the literature.

N. Z. Cantürk · S. A. Güler (✉) · T. Şimşek
Division of Breast and Endocrin Surgery, Kocaeli University, Kocaeli, Turkey
e-mail: drsataguler@me.com

60.1 Case Presentation

A 63-year-old female patient was admitted to the clinic with the findings of a nodule in her right thyroid gland with a history of 3 months. After admission, ultrasonographic (USG) examination of the thyroid gland was performed, and a 10 × 6 mm iso-hypoechoic nodular lesion at the right thyroid gland without any pathological lympadenomegalies or any vascular abnormalities was detected (Fig. 60.1). The nodule was hypoactive on ^{99m}Tc pertechnetate scintigraphy. Thyroid fine needle aspiration biopsy (FNAB) was performed, and histopathological examination of the nodule was reported as suspicious for medullary thyroid cancer (MTC). Thyroid function tests of the patient were in normal range. For further evaluation of disorder, calcitonin and carcinoembryonic antigen (CEA) were measured in which calcitonin was 69.58 pg/mL (normal range 0.07–12.97 pg/mL) and CEA was 5.43 ng/mL (normal range 0.00–5.00 ng/mL nonsmoker). It is remarkable that the calcitonin levels were above normal laboratory range. In her medical history, there was not any family history of any syndrome.

T. Özülker et al. (eds.), *Thyroid and Parathyroid Diseases*, https://doi.org/10.1007/978-3-319-78476-2_60

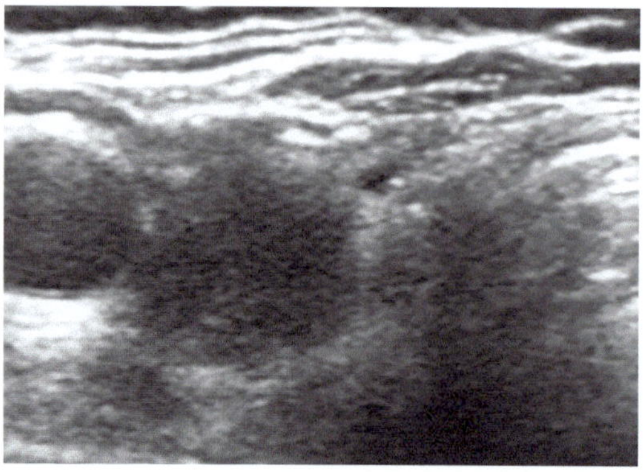

Fig. 60.1 Ultrasonography of the thyroid gland showing a 10 × 6 mm iso-hypoechoic nodular lesion at the right lobe

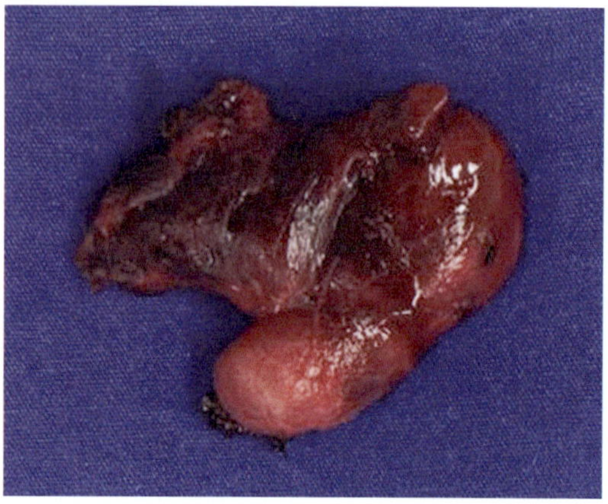

Fig. 60.2 Specimen view of the sporadic medullary thyroid cancer

Germline RET tests were studied, but no mutations were reported. After discussion at the multidisciplinary endocrine meeting, bilateral total thyroidectomy and central neck lymph node dissection were performed. Specimen view of the medullary thyroid cancer is seen in Fig. 60.2. The postoperative pathological evaluation showed that the nodule was 0.9 cm in diameter, located in the right thyroid lobe as MTC. The tumor was in the thyroid gland but invaded its capsule without any lymphovascular invasion. By immunohistochemical evaluation, the tissue was dyed negative with HMBE-1, nonspecifically positive with Galactin-3, positive with calcitonin, positive with chromogranin and focally positive with thyroglobulin (Tg). All the right and left sided central neck lymph nodes came out as reactive lymphoid hyperplasia and there were no metastatic lymph nodes. Whole body bone scintigraphy, chest computed tomography (CT) and total abdominal ultrasonography (USG) did not show any pathological findings. The postoperative neck USG was performed in every 6 months, and until today any relapses or residual thyroid tissues and pathological cervical lymph nodes have not been reported yet. Early postoperative calcitonin level was 3.08 pg/mL and preoperatively high calcitonin levels normalized after the surgery. Calcitonin and CEA levels were measured in every 3 months for 3 years and afterward both of them were measured annually. And in all of the measurements of both markers were within normal ranges.

60.2 Discussion

Medullary thyroid cancer (MTC) is a neuroendocrine tumor derived from the parafollicular or C cells of the thyroid gland. Approximately 1–2% of thyroid cancers are MTC [1]. The calcitonin production is a characteristic feature of this disease. The C cells come from the embryonic neural crest. For this reason, they often show the clinical and histological features of other neuroendocrine tumors like islet-cell tumors and carcinoids. The 75% of MTC cases are sporadic. Whereas, approximately 25% of MTC cases are familial as part of the multiple endocrine neoplasia type 2 (MEN2) syndrome. Sporadic cases have no germline RET mutations whereas germline RET mutations are seen in hereditary type [1].

60.2.1 Evaluation and Diagnosis

The fourth and sixth decades of life are the typical age of MTCs are seen [1]. In our case, our patient was in her 60's as the average age of the disease in the literature.

Sporadic MTC is commonly presented with a solitary thyroid nodule, that is seen approximately in 75–95% of patients [2–5] as presented in our case. The C cells are located in the upper part of each thyroid lobe; thus, most tumors are found in this part of the thyroid gland. The disease has already metastasized at the time of diagnosis in most sporadic MTC cases. Approximately 70% of cases have clinically detectable cervical lymph node involvement. Totally 15% of cases have symptoms of the upper digestive tract and tracheal compression or invasions. In those patients symptoms such as dysphagia or hoarseness are reported. Approximately 5–10% of MTCs have the distant metastatic disease [1–6]. Distant metastases may include liver, lung, bones, and in fewer percentages brain and skin. Patients with the multifocal disease have commonly nodal metastases [7]. But, as calcitonin screening tests are improved in the identification of more "micro" MTCs, the number of patients with metastases at presentation appears to be decreasing [8–10]. Calcitonin screening for sporadic MTC is controversial in patients who have thyroid nodules.

Hormonal secretion by the tumor such as calcitonin, calcitonin gene-related peptide, or other substances causes systemic symptoms of the disease. In advanced disease, diarrhea or facial flushing might be the symptoms. MTCs also may secrete corticotropin (ACTH), resulting in ectopic Cushing's syndrome. Our case did not present any symptoms results of those secreted hormones [6].

Basal serum calcitonin concentrations usually correlate with the volume of the tumor mass. They also reflect differentiation of the tumor. Patients with palpable tumor usually have a high amount of basal serum calcitonin levels [6]. Most sporadic MTC cases also secrete carcinoembryonic antigen (CEA). Similarly, as calcitonin, CEA may be used as a tumor marker in the diagnosis of the MTCs [11, 12]. Also, the expression of CEA may be used as anti-CEA antibodies for immunotherapy in MTCs cases. As laboratory tests especially the thyroid function tests might be normal. In our case, the patient had normal thyroid function tests. The Calcitonin was calculated as 69.58 pg/mL (normal range 0.07–12.97 pg/mL) and CEA was 5.43 ng/mL (normal range 0.00–5.00 ng/mL nonsmoker). As seen CEA was normal, but elevated calcitonin level was consistent with the diagnosis of MTC.

In the radiological evaluation, there are several ultrasonic features of thyroid nodules like hypoechogenicity, microcalcifications which may present thyroid cancer. However, there are no pathognomonic ultrasound features that are related to thyroid cancer. Most of the studies show ultrasound characteristics of thyroid nodules focused on papillary subtype [13]. Rarely, the presence of dense calcifications on radiographs and anterior neck images may point out sporadic MTC. In our case, the ultrasonography was reported as the iso-hypoechoic nodule, and the features of the sporadic MTC was not able to be differentiated.

Fine needle aspiration biopsy (FNAB) is the major diagnostic tool for sporadic MTC which has a solitary thyroid nodule. The sensitivity of FNAB is 50–80%, but higher sensitivities can be obtained by the addition of immunohistochemical staining techniques used for calcitonin [14]. In most sporadic MTCs with high clinical suspicion, calcitonin measurement may be performed by the washout of the FNAB biopsy. But this technique may not be readily available in most laboratories [14]. In our case, the histopathological report was suspicious for MTC, but calcitonin measurement in the washout of the FNAB biopsy could not be studied because of the laboratory restrictions.

The diagnosis of sporadic MTC is performed just after thyroid lobectomy although FNAB of the nodule is suspicious or indeterminate in some of the cases. Sporadic MTC surgical specimens show spindle-shaped and frequently pleomorphic cells without follicle development because these cells come from the calcitonin-secreting parafollicular C cells of the gland [14].

For the routine diagnosis of the thyroid nodule, the use of serum calcitonin measurement with complement to USG and FNAB is controversial. For the patients with thyroid nodules measurement of serum, calcitonin is not a part of the routine evaluation tests [15]. The high frequency of false high serum calcitonin levels, the inability to confirm the high calcitonin by pentagastrin stimulation, and the accuracy of FNAB would argue against a change in this recommendation. Patients with locoregional metastases or locally invasive sporadic MTC will have normal levels of serum calcitonin concentrations without any stimulation [2, 15].

The differential diagnosis in a patient with a neck mass varies with age. The majority of masses are benign thyroid nodules or cysts. Neck masses may be congenital, inflammatory, or neoplastic disorders, instead of thyroidal origin [16].

In the differential diagnosis of sporadic MTC hypercalcemia, hypergastrinemia, neuroendocrine tumors, renal insufficiency, papillary and follicular thyroid carcinomas, goiter, and chronic autoimmune thyroiditis must be taken into consideration. In all of them, elevated calcitonin levels might be represented [16, 17]. Use of omeprazole longer than 2–4 months, beta blockers, and glucocorticoids have been associated with hypercalcitoninemia. In addition, heterophilic antibodies to calcitonin can falsely elevate serum calcitonin levels [17]. Gastrointestinal tract inflammatory disease, benign lung disease, and nonthyroidal malignancies and cigarette smoking may also cause high CEA levels [1]. Our case was a non-smoker, and her CEA values were normal in range.

Calcitonin and CEA levels also show the capability of the hormones hypersecretion and, if so, the results can be compared with postoperative values. Calcitonin and CEA levels may provide a prognostic factor postoperatively. Also, they indicate the biochemical cure for the MTC [18]. Assessment of calcitonin and CEA doubling times postoperatively provides sensitive markers for progression and aggressiveness of the disease [19]. Following the FNAB of the nodule, we looked for calcitonin and CEA values soon after the FNAB result to evaluate any metastasis of the disease. And according to the results, we eliminated the metastasis.

Sporadic MTC can spread locally, invade the neck lymph nodes or can metastasize to distant sites [4, 6]. Neck USG is used to detect for cervical lymph node involvement just after the diagnosis by FNAB. In our case, cervical lymph nodes were reported as reactive by neck USG which had been performed just after the diagnosis by FNAB.

If local lymph node metastasis detected by the USG and/or high serum calcitonin levels are reported, additional radiological techniques must be performed to detect for the probable metastasis [20]. Cross-sectional imaging techniques like chest CT, neck CT, three-phase contrast-enhanced liver CT or contrast-enhanced liver magnetic resonance imaging (MRI), axial MRI, and bone scintigraphy are the suggested ones. For the suspect of skeletal metastases, MRI may be superior to other imaging modalities [20].

18-fluoro-2-deoxyglucose positron emission tomography (^{18}F-FDG-PET) imaging or somatostatin receptor imaging is not recommended for routine initial screening for metastatic disease seeing that the sensitivity of ^{18}F-FDG-PET scanning for detection of metastases may be variable [21]. But imaging with ^{111}In-octreotide or [99mTc]-Pentavalent dimercaptosuccinic acid (V)-DMSA) is not currently recommended as routine screening tests [20]. Type of scanning may be more useful in localizing residual or recurrent disease after primary therapy.

Diagnosis of sporadic MTC with cytologic evaluation of a thyroid nodule should be supported with measurements of serum calcitonin and carcinoembryonic antigen (CEA), USG of the neck and also genetic testing of germline RET mutations, and biochemical evaluation for coexisting tumors, especially to exclude pheochromocytoma [18]. Somatic mutations at RET, HRAS, KRAS and NRAS genes can be determined for patients with sporadic MTC [1]. For germline RET mutations genetic tests with the sequencing of exons 10, 11, and 13 through 16 for all patients with newly diagnosed C cell hyperplasia or apparently sporadic MTC are suggested. Sequencing of the remaining exons should be considered for patients whom hereditary medullary cancer is suggested clinically or with the family history [22]. In our case germline RET mutation genetic tests were studied and seeing that no mutations were reported, we excluded MEN 2, and sporadic MTC diagnosis gained in strength.

It is important that what proportion of patients with apparently sporadic MTC have unsuspected germline mutations in the RET proto-oncogene which has the underlying defect in MEN2 and, therefore, have the heritable disease. The familial medullary cases in 75% had no prior family history. 60% of the patients with sporadic MTC have somatic or acquired mutations in the RET gene within the tumor cells [23]. These mutations are present only in the tumor cells. They are not detected by standard genetic tests such as using leukocyte DNA detection. In MTCs the presence of somatic RET mutations may point persistent disease, lymph node metastases and may decrease the survival period [23].

Generally, biochemical evaluation for particularly pheochromocytoma and hyperparathyroidism is required before thyroidectomy. The results may rarely be known before surgery though genetic screening tests are preoperatively studied. With no family history of MEN2 syndrome and negative RET proto-oncogene test result, biochemical tests are not always needed [23].

The pathological tumor-node-metastasis (pTNM) staging adopted by the Union International Contre le Cancer (UICC) and the American Joint Committee on Cancer (AJCC) are tumor size, lymph node metastases and distant metastases [24] (Table 60.1). In the present case, the nodule was nearly 1 cm in diameter, and there was no evidence of disease outside the thyroid gland without any node invasion. So, it is reported as a Stage I disease.

Table 60.1 The pathological tumor-node-metastasis (pTNM) staging adopted by the Union International Contre le Cancer (UICC) and the American Joint Committee on Cancer (AJCC)

Stages	Features
Stage I	Medullary thyroid cancers that are less than 2 cm in diameter without evidence of disease outside of the thyroid gland
Stage II	Any tumor between 2 and 4 cm without evidence of extrathyroidal disease
Stage III	Any tumor greater than 4 cm, or level VI nodal metastases or microscopic extrathyroidal invasion regardless of tumor size
Stage IV	Any distant metastases, or lymph node involvement outside of level VI, or gross soft tissue extension

60.2.2 Management

Sporadic MTC can only be treated by complete resection of the thyroid tumor and any local and regional metastases for complete cure. If there is residual or recurrent disease after primary resection or for those with distant metastases, the most appropriate treatment is not clear. There are debates for the treatment approaches in the literature.

For patients with sporadic MTC confined to the neck and no evidence of involved cervical lymph nodes on preoperative USG, total thyroidectomy with prophylactic bilateral dissection of the central lymph nodes is the suggested treatment [1]. But prophylactic central neck lymph node dissection is not required if the tumor is small and intrathyroidal with a preoperative calcitonin level less than 20 pg/mL. Metastatic lymph nodes are exceedingly rare in this circumstance [20]. In the absence of clinically or ultrasonographically identifiable lymph node metastases, performing lateral neck dissections with the primary surgery remains controversial. The American Thyroid Association (ATA) guidelines committee could not achieve a consensus agreement on this topic but did recommend that prophylactic lateral neck dissections may be considered according to serum calcitonin levels [1]. Routine prophylactic lateral neck dissections if there was no evidence of disease on preoperative neck USG might be recommended or the decision according to the utilized preoperative calcitonin values is recommended. Prophylactic ipsilateral central and ipsilateral lateral neck dissection might be recommended for the patients with basal serum calcitonin values over 20 pg/mL. But if serum calcitonin levels are more over 200 pg/mL prophylactic dissection of uninvolved contralateral lateral neck compartments is recommended [1]. For sporadic MTC with the thyroid and cervical lymph nodal involvement diagnosed preoperatively, total thyroidectomy with bilateral central neck dissection and dissection of the involved lateral neck is the recommended treatment. If there is no suspect of distant metastases, dissection of the clinically involved ipsilateral neck with prophylactic neck dissection of uninvolved contralateral neck compartments should also be considered in patients with a basal calcitonin level more than 200 pg/mL [1]. All patients with inherited MTC and 10% of sporadic MTC have the bilateral or multifocal disease [1].And they have premalignant diffuse C cell hyperplasia. Thus, total thyroidectomy is the preferred surgical treatment.

The dissection of the adjacent nodal tissue in the central compartment is recommended to be performed from the hyoid bone to the innominate veins and medial to the jugular veins [25]. The lateral jugular and mediastinal lymph nodes should be carefully evaluated. If there are positive lymph nodes modified neck and/or mediastinal dissections are also recommended [25].

Prophylactic neck dissection of the lateral neck with the absence of structurally identifiable disease is not routinely recommended. It should be considered if extensive lymph node metastases are identified in the adjacent central neck, or the preoperative serum calcitonin is more over 200 pg/mL [1]. In our case, preoperative calcitonin level was 69.58 pg/mL. It was over the given average value of 20 pg/mL and below 200 pg/mL. According to these results, we decided to perform only bilateral central neck lymph node dissection without any lateral neck lymph node dissection.

For locally advanced or metastatic disease, total thyroidectomy with central and/or lateral neck dissection is recommended treatment. In this situation surgery is mostly palliative, so a less aggressive surgical approach to the thyroid and lymph nodes is recommended in order not to impair speech, swallowing, parathyroid function, and shoulder mobility [1]. For invasive disease, more extended procedures containing resection of the involved neck with function-preserving approaches for speech, swallowing must be preferred. Radical neck dissections do not improve prognosis, so they are not indicated. The surgical treatment should be individualized according to the patient's life expectancy, wishes and other medical conditions [1].

If sporadic MTC is diagnosed after a unilateral lobectomy, the approach is not certain. There is not enough data for management of this situation [1]. The incidence of bilateral disease in patients with sporadic MTC is low, ranging from 0% to 9%. Therefore, completion thyroidectomy is not routinely indicated for patients if germline RET mutation is also negative. However, it is recommended to perform thyroidectomy for the other lob if the postoperative calcitonin level is elevated, or if there is imaging evidence of persistent disease in the thyroid or regional lymph nodes [1].

For short-term follow up, the development of hypoparathyroidism or injury to either the recurrent or superior laryngeal nerves should be detected [1].

Thyroxine (T4) therapy should be started just after the surgery. The initial dose is 1.6 mcg/kg daily. The adequacy of treatment should be clinically evaluated and by measurement of serum thyroid-stimulating hormone (TSH) level in 6 weeks period after the surgery. The goal of T4 treatment is to restore and maintain a euthyroid state. Suppression of TSH is not recommended seeing that C cells are not TSH responsive [26]. Radioiodine treatment is also contraindicated because the tumor cells do not concentrate iodine [26].

After the surgery, evaluating if surgery was curative is important. Serum calcitonin and CEA must be measured for this purpose. Serum calcitonin and CEA should be measured within 2–3 months after surgery to detect the presence of residual disease. Patients who have normal serum CEA and undetectable serum calcitonin values are considered biochemically cured. Those patient groups have the best prognosis [27]. For this group of patients, subsequent follow-up may be performed by physical examination twice yearly for 2 years and then yearly thereafter with measurement of serum calcitonin and CEA levels twice yearly for 2 years and then yearly thereafter including neck ultrasound 3–12 months postoperatively. Additional imaging is not recommended if calcitonin or CEA values do not increase during follow-up [1].

A high basal serum calcitonin level in three or more months after surgery is presumptive evidence of residual disease. The prognosis for this group of patients depends on primarily the patient's age and the extent of disease at the time of initial surgery [1].

As parallel to the literature for our case, we followed up with calcitonin and CEA levels including physical examination and neck USG imaging. Up to recent time, no elevation in the levels of both tests was reported with no findings of physical examination and neck USG. So our patient is in the first group known as biologically cure.

For patients with recurrent/residual disease observation/active surveillance, surgical resection, external beam radiation therapy (EBRT), and other directed therapies such as radiofrequency ablation, cryoablation, embolization, or systemic therapies are the treatment modalities [28]. Identifiable residual or recurrent MTC patients were being operated on routinely in the past time. But despite routine lymphadenectomy or excision of the palpable tumor, their serum calcitonin concentrations often did not normalize after the surgery [28]. For this reason treatment approach for persistent/recurrent disease depends upon a variety of clinical factors. Localisation of the disease, the volume of disease, the precise location of the metastatic disease, symptoms if any, the rate or likelihood of clinically significant structural disease progression are the factors for deciding the treatment approach [28].

Age and stage of disease at the time of diagnosis is an important factor for prognosis [1]. The 5- and 10-year disease-free survival rates are higher among patients 40 years old or less as compared with patients over age 40 years [2]. The 10-year survival rates for patients with stages I, II, III, and IV MTC are 100%, 93%, 71%, and 21%, respectively [29]. A nomogram that integrates age, gender, postoperative calcitonin, vascular invasion, tumor, node, and metastasis status has been developed that can be used to predict cause-specific mortality easily [30]. Calcitonin and CEA doubling times are sensitive markers for prediction of progression and aggressiveness of metastatic disease [30]. Calcitonin doubling times less than 6–12 months are associated with poor survival rates while doubling times more than 24 months are associated with a better prognosis [19]. Cellular heterogeneity, paucity of tumor immunostaining for calcitonin, prominent tissue immunostaining for galectin-3 or CEA associated with scant or absent tissue staining for calcitonin, high preoperative serum CEA, a less than tenfold increase in preoperative calcitonin levels after stimulation with pentagastrin, an elevated procalcitonin:calcitonin ratio, and a rising CEA level associated with a stable or declining calcitonin level are the other factors that effects the prognosis [11, 31–34].

60.2.3 The Future

For persistent or recurrent MTC patients clinical management strategies are still under debate. These patients either have long-term survival, because of an indolent course of the disease or develop rapidly progressing disease causing death from distant metastases. Today, it cannot be predicted what will happen in most individual MTCs. Biomarkers, indicators which can be measured objectively, can be helpful in MTC diagnosis, molecular imaging, and treatment, and/or identification of MTC progression. But most of the MTC biomarkers are already implemented in the daily management of those patients [35]. More researches are being studied to improve the molecular imaging techniques and to develop systemic molecular therapies. Recent discoveries, like the prognostic value of plasma calcitonin and CEA doubling-time and the presence of somatic RET mutations in MTC tissue, may be useful for treatment [35].

There is no single method to detect all MTC recurrences or metastases. Conventional radiological imaging methods like USG, CT, MRI and several methods of nuclear medicine are being used for this purpose. The main role of nuclear medicine imaging is the detection of the residual or recurrent tumor in the postoperative follow-up. The most used radiopharmaceuticals labeled with γ emitters are Metaiodobenzylguanidine (MIBG), labeled with ^{131}I or ^{123}I, ^{111}In-pentetreotide (Octreoscan), (^{99m}Tc(V)-DMSA), and ^{99m}Tc-EDDA/HYNIC-Tyr3-Octreotide (Tektrotyd) [36]. The radiopharmaceuticals labelled with a positron-emitting radionuclide (β+), suitable for positron emission tomography (PET) imaging are: ^{18}F-fluorodeoxyglucose ^{18}F-FDG), (^{18}F-fluorodihydroxyphenylalanine (^{18}F-DOPA), and ^{68}Ga-labelled somatostatin analogues (^{68}Ga-DOTATATE or DOTATOC). The usage of these radiopharmaceuticals in the diagnosis of MTC recurrence needs further studies to be routinely used [36].

Surgery is currently the only potentially curative treatment for sporadic MTC. Complete tumor resection and removal of suspicious lymph nodes are the most important initial treatment to avoid recurrence and metastasis. When recurrence or metastatic MTC develops, the decision for continued observation or systemic therapy is based on the degree of tumor aggressiveness. Lymph node involvement, calcitonin doubling time, types of RET mutation, and tumor stage are factors that are used determine the need for further treatment [37].

Therapeutic options for aggressive and inoperable MTC primarily include tyrosine kinase inhibitors, external beam radiation therapy (EBRT), or other medications. Among tyrosine kinase inhibitors, vandetanib is the first drug that is approved by FDA for treatment of MTC. Focused EBRT can be reconsidered for patients with cervical lymph node involvement. Although other targeted drug therapies have been tried, definitive clinical studies are not enough [37]. In recurrent or advanced MTC, when systemic therapy is planned to be used, vandetanib is available for treatment. But side effects of this drug can be problematic, and impact on overall survival is presently unknown [37].

Newer drugs and treatment alternatives are being studied for the control of tumor growth with maintaining the patient's quality of life [37].

What Can We Learn from This Case?

Medullary thyroid carcinoma (MTC) is a rare malignancy arising from parafollicular C cells of the thyroid gland. Approximately 1–2% of thyroid cancers are MTC. As discussed, it may have a poor prognosis unless appropriate management is performed.

- Most sporadic MTC cases secrete carcinoembryonic antigen (CEA) which is used as tumor marker for the diagnosis
- Fine needle aspiration biopsy (FNAB) is the major diagnostic tool for sporadic MTC which has a solitary thyroid nodule
- Somatic mutations at RET, HRAS, KRAS and NRAS genes can be determined for patients with sporadic MTC
- Sporadic MTC can only be treated by complete resection of the total thyroid gland with the tumor and any local and regional metastases for complete cure
- After the surgery, serum calcitonin and CEA must be measured for follow-up of the disease
- For patients with recurrent/residual disease observation/active surveillance, surgical resection, external beam radiation therapy (EBRT), and other directed therapies such as radiofrequency ablation, cryoablation, embolization, or systemic therapies are the treatment modalities
- Newer drugs and treatment alternatives are being studied for the control of tumor growth with maintaining the patient's quality of life

References

1. Wells SA Jr, Asa SL, Dralle H, Elisei R, Evans DB, Gagel RF, et al. Revised American Thyroid Association guidelines for the management of medullary thyroid carcinoma. Thyroid. 2015;25:567.

2. Saad MF, Ordonez NG, Rashid RK, Guido JJ, Hill CS Jr, Hickey RC, et al. Medullary carcinoma of the thyroid. A study of the clinical features and prognostic factors in 161 patients. Medicine (Baltimore). 1984;63:319.
3. Dottorini ME, Assi A, Sironi M, Sangalli G, Spreafico G, Colombo L, et al. Multivariate analysis of patients with medullary thyroid carcinoma. Prognostic significance and impact on treatment of clinical and pathologic variables. Cancer. 1996;77:1556.
4. Gagel RF, Hoff AO, Cote GJ. Medullary thyroid carcinoma. In: Braverman LE, Utiger RD, editors. Werner & Ingbar's the thyroid. 9th ed. Philadelphia: Lippincott Williams & Wilkins; 2005. p. 967.
5. Kebebew E, Ituarte PH, Siperstein AE, Duh QY, Clark OH, et al. Medullary thyroid carcinoma: clinical characteristics, treatment, prognostic factors, and a comparison of staging systems. Cancer. 2000;88:1139.
6. Pacini F, Castagna MG, Cipri C, Schlumberger M. Medullary thyroid carcinoma. Clin Oncol (R Coll Radiol). 2010;22:475.
7. Machens A, Hauptmann S, Dralle H. Increased risk of lymph node metastasis in multifocal hereditary and sporadic medullary thyroid cancer. World J Surg. 2007;31:1960.
8. Scheuba C, Kaserer K, Bieglmayer C, Asari R, Riss P, Drosten R, et al. Medullary thyroid microcarcinoma recommendations for treatment—a single-center experience. Surgery. 2007;142:1003.
9. Machens A, Dralle H. Surgical cure rates of sporadic medullary thyroid cancer in the era of calcitonin screening. Eur J Endocrinol. 2016;175:219.
10. Kwon H, Kim WG, Sung TY, Jeon MJ, Song DE, Lee YM, et al. Changing trends in the clinicopathological features and clinical outcomes of medullary thyroid carcinoma. J Surg Oncol. 2016;113:152.
11. Machens A, Ukkat J, Hauptmann S, Dralle H. Abnormal carcinoembryonic antigen levels and medullary thyroid cancer progression: a multivariate analysis. Arch Surg. 2007;142:289.
12. Busnardo B, Girelli ME, Simioni N, Nacamulli D, Busetto E. Nonparallel patterns of calcitonin and carcinoembryonic antigen levels in the follow-up of medullary thyroid carcinoma. Cancer. 1984;53:278.
13. Trimboli P, Nasrollah N, Amendola S, Rossi F, Ramacciato G, Romanelli F, et al. Should we use ultrasound features associated with papillary thyroid cancer in diagnosing medullary thyroid cancer? Endocr J. 2012;59:503.
14. Bugalho MJ, Santos JR, Sobrinho L. Preoperative diagnosis of medullary thyroid carcinoma: fine needle aspiration cytology as compared with serum calcitonin measurement. J Surg Oncol. 2005;91:56.
15. Costante G, Filetti S. Early diagnosis of medullary thyroid carcinoma: is systematic calcitonin screening appropriate in patients with nodular thyroid disease? Oncologist. 2011;16:49.
16. Toledo SP, Lourenço DM Jr, Santos MA, Tavares MR, Toledo RA, Correia-Deur JE. Hypercalcitoninemia is not pathognomonic of medullary thyroid carcinoma. Clinics (Sao Paulo). 2009;64:699.
17. Castro MR, Gharib H. Continuing controversies in the management of thyroid nodules. Ann Intern Med. 2005;142:926.
18. http://www.nccn.org/professionals/physician_gls/f_guidelines.asp. Accessed 20 Aug 2012.
19. Barbet J, Campion L, Kraeber-Bodéré F, Chatal JF, GTE Study Group. Prognostic impact of serum calcitonin and carcinoembryonic antigen doubling-times in patients with medullary thyroid carcinoma. J Clin Endocrinol Metab. 2005;90:6077.
20. Machens A, Dralle H. Biomarker-based risk stratification for previously untreated medullary thyroid cancer. J Clin Endocrinol Metab. 2010;95:2655.
21. Oudoux A, Salaun PY, Bournaud C, Campion L, Ansquer C, Rousseau C, et al. Sensitivity and prognostic value of positron emission tomography with F-18-fluorodeoxyglucose and sensitivity of immunoscintigraphy in patients with medullary thyroid carcinoma treated with anticarcinoembryonic antigen-targeted radioimmunotherapy. J Clin Endocrinol Metab. 2007;92:4590.
22. Moline J, Eng C. Multiple endocrine neoplasia type 2: an overview. Genet Med. 2011;13:755.
23. Romei C, Elisei R, Pinchera A, Ceccherini I, Molinaro E, Mancusi F, et al. Somatic mutations of the ret proto-oncogene in sporadic medullary thyroid carcinoma are not restricted to exon 16 and are associated with tumor recurrence. J Clin Endocrinol Metab. 1996;81:1619.
24. American Joint Committee on Cancer (AJCC). In: Edge SB, Byrd DR, Compton CC, et al., editors. Cancer staging manual. 7th ed. New York: Springer; 2010.
25. Fleming JB, Lee JE, Bouvet M, et al. Surgical strategy for the treatment of medullary thyroid carcinoma. Ann Surg. 1999;230:697.
26. Saad MF, Guido JJ, Samaan NA. Radioactive iodine in the treatment of medullary carcinoma of the thyroid. J Clin Endocrinol Metab. 1983;57:124.
27. Engelbach M, Görges R, Forst T, Pfützner A, Dawood R, Heerdt S, et al. Improved diagnostic methods in the follow-up of medullary thyroid carcinoma by highly specific calcitonin measurements. J Clin Endocrinol Metab. 2000;85:1890.
28. van Heerden JA, Grant CS, Gharib H, Hay ID, Ilstrup DM. Long-term course of patients with persistent hypercalcitoninemia after apparent curative primary surgery for medullary thyroid carcinoma. Ann Surg. 1990;212:395.
29. Modigliani E, Cohen R, Campos JM, Franc B, Niccoli-Sire P, Conte-Devolx B, et al. Prognostic factors for survival and for biochemical cure in medullary thyroid carcinoma: results in 899 patients. The GETC Study Group. Groupe d'étude des tumeurs à calcitonine. Clin Endocrinol (Oxf). 1998;48:265.
30. Ho AS, Wang L, Palmer FL, Yu C, Toset A, Patel S, et al. Postoperative nomogram for predicting cancer-specific mortality in medullary thyroid Cancer. Ann Surg Oncol. 2015;22:2700.

31. Faggiano A, Talbot M, Lacroix L, Bidart JM, Baudin E, Schlumberger M, et al. Differential expression of galectin-3 in medullary thyroid carcinoma and C-cell hyperplasia. Clin Endocrinol (Oxf). 2002;57:813.
32. Mendelsohn G, Wells SA Jr, Baylin SB. Relationship of tissue carcinoembryonic antigen and calcitonin to tumor virulence in medullary thyroid carcinoma. An immunohistochemical study in early, localized, and virulent disseminated stages of disease. Cancer. 1984;54:657.
33. Machens A, Hauptmann S, Dralle H. Medullary thyroid cancer responsiveness to pentagastrin stimulation: an early surrogate parameter of tumor dissemination? J Clin Endocrinol Metab. 2008;93:2234.
34. Walter MA, Meier C, Radimerski T, Iten F, Kränzlin M, Müller-Brand J, et al. Procalcitonin levels predict clinical course and progression-free survival in patients with medullary thyroid cancer. Cancer. 2010;116:31.
35. Azar FK, Lee SL, Rosen JE. Medullary thyroid cancer: an update for surgeons. Am Surg. 2015;81:1–8.
36. Skoura E. Depicting medullary thyroid cancer recurrence: the past and the future of nuclear medicine imaging. Int J Endocrinol Metab. 2013;11:8156. https://doi.org/10.5812/ijem.8156.
37. Sugawara M, Ly T, Hershman JM. Medullary thyroid cancer--current treatment strategy, novel therapies, and perspectives for the future. Horm Cancer. 2012;3:218–26. https://doi.org/10.1007/s12672-012-0119-5.

61 Concurrent Papillary Thyroid Cancer and Medullary Thyroid Cancer

Neslihan Kurtulmuş

Abstract

Concurrent occurrence of medullary thyroid carcinoma (MTC) and papillary thyroid carcinoma (PTC) in a single patient is uncommon. The cell origin, histopathologic features, and prognosis of these two carcinomas are considered completely different. A 40-year-old man was diagnosed MTC after fine needle aspiration biopsy of the right thyroid nodule and the lymph node on the right side. The patient underwent total thyroidectomy with unilateral central compartment and right lateral neck dissection. Histopathological evaluation was identified as MTC in the nodule of the right lobe and the MTC metastasis in the lymph nodes. Besides, papillary microcarcinoma foci were determined on the same thyroid lobe. He had c.1585 > A (p.Glu529Lys) heterozygous variant mutation of RET proto-oncogene. Sixteen months after the operation, his serum calcitonin, carcinoembryonic antigen (CEA), and thyroglobulin levels are undetectable.

N. Kurtulmuş
Department of Endocrinology, Acibadem University, Istanbul, Turkey

61.1 Case Presentation

A 40-year-old man was referred to our thyroid disease clinic with an autoimmune thyroid disease which had been under monitoring for a few years. It was grade 1b in thyroid palpation, and there was no palpable cervical lymph node. On ultrasonography (USG), a nodule with an irregular border, 13.2 × 6.9 mm in size, was observed in the right lobe of the thyroid. And nodules which were 8.6 × 5.7 mm and 5.3 × 4.1 mm in size were detected in the right lobe. A hypoechoic nodule which was 3.8 × 2.1 mm in size was observed in the left lobe. Also, a lymph node with a pathological appearance which is 16.7 × 6.3 mm in size was detected in the neck on the right, next to the arteria carotis communis bifurcation (level III). A fine needle aspiration biopsy (FNAB) was performed on the dominant nodule in the right lobe and on the suspicious lymph node at level III. The pathological and immunohistochemical evaluation showed the medullar thyroid carcinoma (MTC) in the nodule in the right lobe and the MTC metastasis in the lymph node. Therefore, serum calcitonin was measured, and its value was 235 pg/ml (N:0–8.4), and carcinoembryonic antigen (CEA) was 0.8 ng/ml (N:0–2.5). Before thyroid surgery, the patient underwent laboratory and clinical investigations in order to diagnose the multiple endocrine neoplasia (MEN). Serum calcium and

T. Özülker et al. (eds.), *Thyroid and Parathyroid Diseases*, https://doi.org/10.1007/978-3-319-78476-2_61

parathormone tests were measured for primary hyperparathyroidism. Pheochromocytoma was evaluated with the measurement of 24 h urinary excretion rate of catecholamines. We could not identify any pathologic findings suggesting MEN. The patient underwent total thyroidectomy with unilateral central compartment and right lateral neck dissection. In the postoperative pathological evaluation, the medullary cancer focus with 8 mm in diameter and with lymphovascular invasion was detected in the right lobe of the thyroid (Fig. 61.1). MTC cells showed positive immunostaining for calcitonin (Fig. 61.2). Thyroid papillary cancer classical type tumor foci with diameters of 4 mm and 2 mm were detected in the right lobe of the thyroid (Fig. 61.3). In the non-tumor tissue in the right lobe, C-cell hyperplasia and chronic lymphocytic thyroiditis were observed (Figs. 61.1, 61.3, and 61.4). And in the left lobe of the thyroid, there were only the findings of chronic lymphocytic thyroiditis. Metastasis of MTC was detected in 18 lymph nodes out of 41 in total. The tumor was evaluated T1, N1b, and M0 (stage 4A) [1]. The level of serum calcitonin, which was observed after the operation, was <2.0 pg/ml (N:0–8.4) and CEA:<0.58 ng/ml (N:0–2.5). After the operation, the mutation analysis of the RET proto-oncogene in the chromosome region 10q11.2 in the peripheral blood of the patient was evaluated, and c.1585 > A(p.Glu529Lys) heterozygous variant was identified on exon 8. This is a variant that has not previously been defined in the literature, as far as we know.

Because there was not any indication, radioactive iodine treatment was not applied [2]. L-Thyroxin treatment started and it has still been under close monitoring.

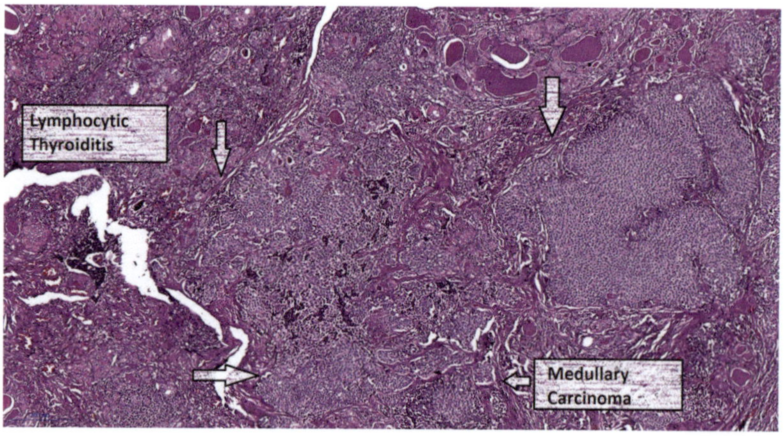

Fig. 61.1 The tumor cells of MTC component (arrows) and lymphocytic thyroiditis around the tumor

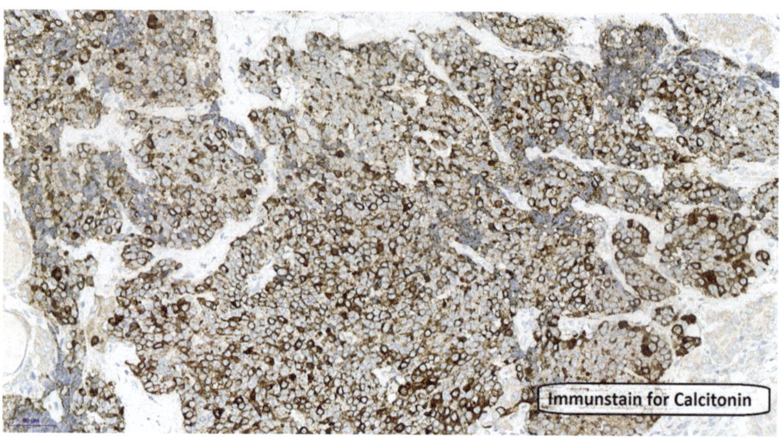

Fig. 61.2 The positive immunostaining with calcitonin in MTC cells

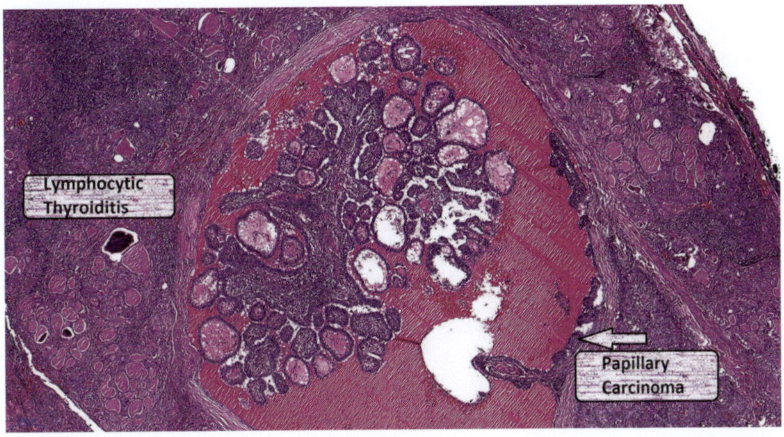

Fig. 61.3 The tumor cells of PTC component (arrows) and lymphocytic thyroiditis around the tumor

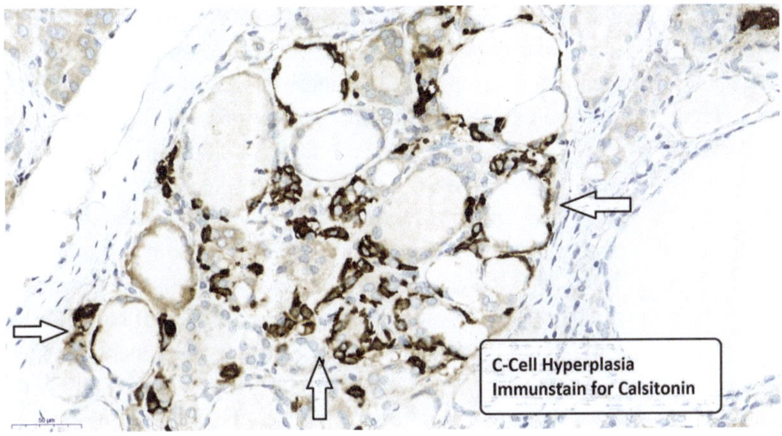

Fig. 61.4 C-cell hyperplasia with calcitonin immunostaining

61.2 Discussion

Thyroid cancers are the most common endocrine cancers [3]. The number of the cases of thyroid cancers has increased around three to four times over the last 30 years [3]. More than 94% of these cancers are differentiated thyroid cancers of papillary and follicular type, which derive from follicular epithelial cells [4]. The increase in the incidence of thyroid cancers is observed mainly in differentiated thyroid cancers. Poorly differentiated and anaplastic thyroid cancers represent around 1–2%. MTC is a malignancy of parafollicular C cells that derive from neural crest, and it constitutes 3–4% of thyroid malignancies. Seventy-five percent of MTC is sporadic. There is a known genetic predisposition to these tumors. The missense mutations on exon 10 and 11 of the rearranged during transfection (RET) proto-oncogene lead to MTC [5]. Forty to sixty percent of sporadic MTC cases have somatic RET mutations. H and K-Ras mutations were also reported in the RET-negative MTC cases [5–7]. Twenty-five percent of MTC cases are hereditary. The hereditary ones present as MEN type 2 or familial medullary cancer. Hereditary MTC has the RET mutation with autosomal dominant inheritance.

The activation of various pathways is started by the various genetic and epigenetic factors which play a role in thyroid tumorigenesis [4, 8]. The basic pathway is the mitogen-associated protein kinase (MAPK)/extracellular signal-regulated kinase (ERK). The MAP kinase/ERK pathway functions in cell division, proliferation, differentiation, adhesion, migration, and apoptosis are also serving as the primary mechanism in PTC tumorigenesis. The somatic point mutation of BRAF, which encodes the serine/threonine kinase functioning in this cascade, is quite important in PTC [9]. The BRAF ^{V600E} is the most common mutation, and there are studies that suggest that its presence is a poorly prognostic factor [9, 10]. Apart from the mutations in the BRAF, the mutations in the RET/PTC and RAS genes also play a role in the pathogenesis of thyroid cancers. The RET proto-oncogene encodes cell membrane tyrosine kinase. Concomitant RET/PTC and BRAF mutations are reported in papillary thyroid cancer (PTC) [8]. Epigenetic mechanisms are essential for normal cell development and tissue-specific gene expression. In case of a change in these mechanisms, activity or inhibition of various signal ways occurs, which leads to tumorigenesis. The epigenetic patterns include the modifications on chromatin, DNA cytosine methylation, noncoding RNA expression, and nucleosome remodeling [11, 12, 13]. Gene expression is observed in aberrant DNA methylation, and it plays an important role in tumorigenesis, whereas in hypomethylation gene decrease occurs, and cancer develops as a result of genomic instability and activation of proto-oncogenes [12]. Epigenetic regulations might also be related to microRNA. Transcriptional regulation regulates many genes related to cell proliferation and apoptosis, and changes in these genes may promote tumorigenesis. MicroRNA may function as either tumor suppressors or oncogenes depending on the affected gene. The aberrant DNA methylation of tumor suppressor genes and proto-oncogenes is often observed in thyroid cancers. Certain specific tumor suppressor genes in the thyroid cancer are PTEN, RASSF1A, TIMP3, SLC5A8, DAPK, RAPβ2, and RAP1GAP. PTEN negatively regulates the AKT/PKB signal way and is involved in the regulation of cell cycle [13]. In PTC and FTC, it is reported that there is aberrant methylation in the PTEN gene. The RASSF1A gene encodes a gene which is similar to the RAS effector protein. The inactivation of this gene with aberrant DNA methylation leads to the development of cancer. This mechanism may play a role to some extent in PTC development. In spite of the differences in cell origins and pathogenesis of PTC and MTC, they may rarely coincide in the same tumor or may be located in the same thyroid tissue. This concurrence does not have a clear relation with the mechanisms defined in thyroid tumorigenesis, and it is also considered that there might be other factors playing a role in that.

PTC and MTC coincidence was first reported by Lamberg [14]. If PTC and MTC are in the same tumor foci, it is called "mixed medullary and papillary thyroid carcinoma" (MMPTC). It is very rare with a prevalence of around 0.11%. The coincidence of PTC and MTC on the same thyroid tissue, as in our case, is an entity which is different from MMPTC, which is also rare [15, 16]. And it is true prevalence that is not known. In a study, it was evaluated to be 2.6%. It has been observed that the patients with PTC and MTC coincidence often had micro papillary cancer [17]. One of the hypotheses about this coincidence suggests that both the papillary and medullary tumor cells might have had the RET proto-oncogene mutations. In PTC, around 20–40% of the cases have the point mutations and rearrangements of the tyrosine kinase receptors RET (ret/PTC). There are some opinions about the pathogenesis of the PTC and MTC coincidence [15, 16, 18, 19]. One of them is the "common stem cell" theory. Stem cell derives from the ultimobranchial body and turns into follicular epithelial cell (endoderm-derived) or parafollicular C cell (ectoderm-derived), which is why both tumors carry the same receptors and the immunochemical markers in spite of their different embryological developments. A more accepted opinion is the "field effect theory," which suggests a shared neoplastic stimulation simultaneously transforms the follicle cell and the parafollicular C cell. Another theory is the "collision theory," which suggests that two independent tumors are located on the same lesion by a simple coincidence. In other words, papillary micro cancer has already been a frequently encountered situation. Thus it may coincide with MTC. The fourth is the "hostage theory," where nonneoplastic follicular cells are trapped by the MTC and are proliferated by the stimulation of trophic factors.

The coincidence of PTC and MTC might be seen in the form of single focus or multicentric in the same lobe or the different lobes of the thyroid gland [17–21]. There is not any factor known to determine this distribution. The treatment of PTC and MTC is different, just like the cells where they derive from, and their histopathological findings are. In PTC, lobectomy or total thyroidectomy is applied. If there is an indication, radioactive iodine is given. The mainstay of treatment in hereditary and sporadic MTC is surgery according to ATA guideline. The patients with MTC who have no evidence of neck lymph node metastases in preoperative USG examination and no evidence of distant metastases should have a total thyroidectomy and dissection of the lymph nodes in the central compartment [1]. If calcitonin level is high in these patients, dissection of lymph nodes in the lateral compartments (levels II–V) may be considered. Patients with MTC confined to the neck and cervical lymph nodes should have a total thyroidectomy, dissection of the central lymph node compartment (level VI), and resection of the involved lateral neck compartments (level II–V). When preoperative imaging is positive in the ipsilateral lateral neck compartment but negative in the contralateral neck compartment, contralateral neck dissection should be considered if the basal calcitonin level is greater than 200 pg/ml.

PTC and MTC coincidence is generally noticed during post-thyroidectomy pathological diagnosis, which is why the post-operation treatment is planned according to the tumor of higher clinical importance. Because the number of these patients is not high, the prognosis is unclear. Case reports from various centers would help shape a treatment and a monitoring plan.

61.3 Outcome

Sixteen months after the operation, the patient is alive. His serum calcitonin, CEA, and thyroglobulin levels are undetectable. There is no recurrent cancer or metastasis.

What Can We Learn from This Case?

- The simultaneous occurrence of PTC and MTC in the same thyroid gland is very rare.
- The pathogenesis of this association is unclear.
- MEN should be evaluated clinically and biologically if MTC is known before thyroidectomy.
- Treatment and follow-up should be planned separately for PTC and MTC.

References

1. Wells SA Jr, Asa SL, Dralle H, Elisei R, Evans DB, Gagel RF, et al. Revised American Thyroid Association guidelines for the Management of Medullary Thyroid Carcinoma: the American Thyroid Association guidelines task force on medullary thyroid carcinoma. Thyroid. 2015;25:567–610. https://doi.org/10.1089/thy.2014.0335.
2. Haugen BR, Alexander EK, Bible KC, Doherty GM, Mandel SJ, Nikiforov YE, et al. 2015 American Thyroid Association management guidelines for adult patients with thyroid nodules and differentiated thyroid cancer. The American Thyroid Association guidelines task force on thyroid nodules and differentiated thyroid cancer. Thyroid. 2016;26:1–133. https://doi.org/10.1089/thy.2015.0020.
3. Siegel R, Ma J, Zou Z, Jemal A. Cancer statistics. Cancer J Clin. 2014;64:9–29. https://doi.org/10.3322/caac.21208.
4. Xing M. Molecular pathogenesis and mechanisms of thyroid cancer. Nat Rev Cancer. 2013;13:184–99. https://doi.org/10.1038/nrc3431.
5. Accardo G, Conzo G, Esposito D, Gambardella C, Mazzella M, Castaldo F, et al. Genetics of medullary thyroid cancer: an overview. Int J Surg. 2017;41(Suppl 1):2–6.
6. Lian EY, Maritan SM, Cockburn JG, Kasaian K, Crupi MJ, Hurlbut D, et al. Differential roles of RET isoforms in medullary and papillary thyroid carcinomas. Endocr Relat Cancer. 2017;24:53–69. https://doi.org/10.1530/erc-16-0393.
7. Moura MM, Cavaco BM, Pinto AE, Leite V. High prevalence of RAS mutations in RET-negative sporadic medullary thyroid carcinomas. J Clin Endocrinol Metab. 2011;96:E863–8. https://doi.org/10.1210/jc.2010-1921.
8. Faam B, Ghaffari MA, Ghadiri A, Azizi F. Epigenetic modifications in human thyroid cancer (review).

Biomed Rep. 2015;3:3–8. https://doi.org/10.3892/br.2014.375.

9. Tufano RP, Teixeira GV, Bishop J, Carson KA, Xing M. BRAF mutation in papillary thyroid cancer and its value in tailoring initial treatment: a systematic review and meta-analysis. Medicine (Baltimore). 2012;91:274–86. https://doi.org/10.1097/MD.0b013e31826a9c71.
10. Kurtulmus N, Duren M, Ince U, Yakicier CM, Peker O, Aydın O, et al. BRAF(V600E) mutation in Turkish patients with papillary thyroid cancer: strong correlation with indicators of tumor aggressiveness. Endocrine. 2012;42:404–10. https://doi.org/10.1007/s12020-012-9651-x.
11. Kondo T, Nakazawa T, Ma D, Niu D, Mochizuki K, Kawasaki T, et al. Epigenetic silencing of TTF-1/NKX2,1 through DNA hypermethylation and histon H3 modification in thyroid carcinoma. Lab Investig. 2009;89:791–9. https://doi.org/10.1038/labinvest.2009.50.
12. Eden A, Gaudet F, Waghmare A, Jaenisch R. Chromosomal instability and tumors promoted by DNA hypomethylation. Science. 2003;300:455. https://doi.org/10.1126/science.1083557.
13. Alvarez-Nuñez F, Bussaglia E, Mauricio D, Ybarra J, Vilar M, Lerma E, et al. Thyroid Neoplasia study group: PTEN promoter methylation in sporadic thyroid carcinomas. Thyroid. 2006;16:17–23. https://doi.org/10.1089/thy.2006.16.17.
14. Lamberg BA, Reissel P, Stenman S, Koivuniemi A, Ekbolm M, Mäkinen J, et al. Concurrent medullary and papillary thyroid carcinoma in the same thyroid lobe and in siblings. Acta Med Scand. 1981;209:421–4.
15. Machens A, Dralle H. Simultaneous medullary and papillary thyroid cancer: a novel entity? Ann Surg Oncol. 2012;19:37–44. https://doi.org/10.1245/s10434-011-1795-z.
16. Ljungberg O, Ericsson UB, Bondeson L, Thorell J. A compound follicular parafollicular cell carcinoma of the thyroid: a new tumor entity? Cancer. 1983;52:1053–61.
17. Adnan Z, Arad E, Dana J, Shendler Y, Baron E. Simultaneous occurrence of medullary and papillary thyroid microcarcinomas: a case series and review of the literature. J Med Case Rep. 2013;21:7–26. https://doi.org/10.1186/1752-1947-7-26.
18. Kim WG, Gong G, Kim EY. Concurrent occurrence of medullary thyroid carcinoma and papillary thyroid carcinoma in the same thyroid should be considered as coincidental. Clin Endocrinol. 2010;72:256–63. https://doi.org/10.1111/j.1365-2265.2009.03622.x.
19. Lax SF, Beham A, Kronberger-Schönecker D, Langsteger W, Denk H. Coexistence of papillary and medullary carcinoma of the thyroid gland mixed or collision tumour? Clinicopathological analysis of three cases. Virchows Arch. 1994;424:441–7.
20. Seki T, Kameyama K, Hayashi H, Nagahama M, Masudo K, Fukunari N, et al. Composite metastatic carcinoma in lymph nodes of patients with concurrent medullary and papillary thyroid carcinoma: a report of two cases. Endocr Pathol. 2004;15:83–8.
21. Nangue C, Bron L, Portmann L, Volante M, Ris HB, Monnier P, et al. Mixed medullary-papillary carcinoma of the thyroid: report of a case and review of the literature. Head Neck. 2009;31:968–74. https://doi.org/10.1002/hed.20984.

Medullary Thyroid Carcinoma

62

Ülkem Yararbaş and Zehra Özcan

Abstract

Medullary thyroid carcinoma is a part of "multiple endocrine neoplasia" syndromes in 25% of the cases. Surgery is the primary curative treatment modality in the management of medullary thyroid carcinoma. Detection of the presence and the extent of the metastatic disease is important for the appropriate therapy planning. The contribution of two nuclear medicine procedures ^{18}F-FDG PET/CT' and ^{68}Ga-DOTATATE PET/CT to the management of medullary thyroid carcinoma is presented in this section.

62.1 Case Presentation

A 22-year-old male patient with symptoms of cough and hoarseness during the last 5 months underwent diagnostic evaluation. Thorax computerized tomography (CT) showed a mass of 4 cm in diameter at the right lobe of the thyroid gland which narrows the airway and a 4.5 × 4.0 cm consolidation with irregular margins in the left lung. Neck ultrasound (USG) revealed bilateral hypoechoic thyroid nodules that have anarchic vascular architecture and bilateral cervical lymphadenopathies in levels II, III, IV, and V. Fine needle aspiration biopsy (FNAB) of the thyroid nodule was interpreted as "suspicious," and the patient was referred for further evaluation. He underwent ^{18}F-FDG PET/CT scanning which showed multiple FDG avid lesions in addition to bilateral hypermetabolic thyroid nodules and lymph nodes in the jugular chain. There were hypermetabolic lesions in the liver, nodular uptake in both adrenal glands, and multiple hypermetabolic foci in bones (Fig. 62.1). Pulmonary findings were considered as infectious due to the regression between thorax CT and PET/CT. Detailed medical history of the patient also revealed chronic diarrhea starting from 2 years old. On physical examination, papular tongue lesions were detected. The family history of the patient showed no existence of medullary thyroid carcinoma (MTC) but papillary thyroid carcinoma in the father and two paternal aunts.

Repeated FNABs from the thyroid and also lymph nodes revealed "medullary thyroid carcinoma." Biochemical analyses showed abnormalities in serum calcitonin (>2000 pg/ml; normal range, 0–10), carcinoembryonic antigen (411 ng/ml; normal range, 0–5) and LDH (529 U/l; normal range, 240–480) levels. According to abdominal magnetic resonance imaging (MRI) performed following ^{18}F-FDG PET/CT, bilateral surrenal gland lesions were interpreted as "pheochromocytoma" due to the hyperintense appearance on

Ü. Yararbaş (✉) · Z. Özcan
Ege University School of Medicine, Department of Nuclear Medicine, Izmir, Turkey

T. Özülker et al. (eds.), *Thyroid and Parathyroid Diseases*, https://doi.org/10.1007/978-3-319-78476-2_62

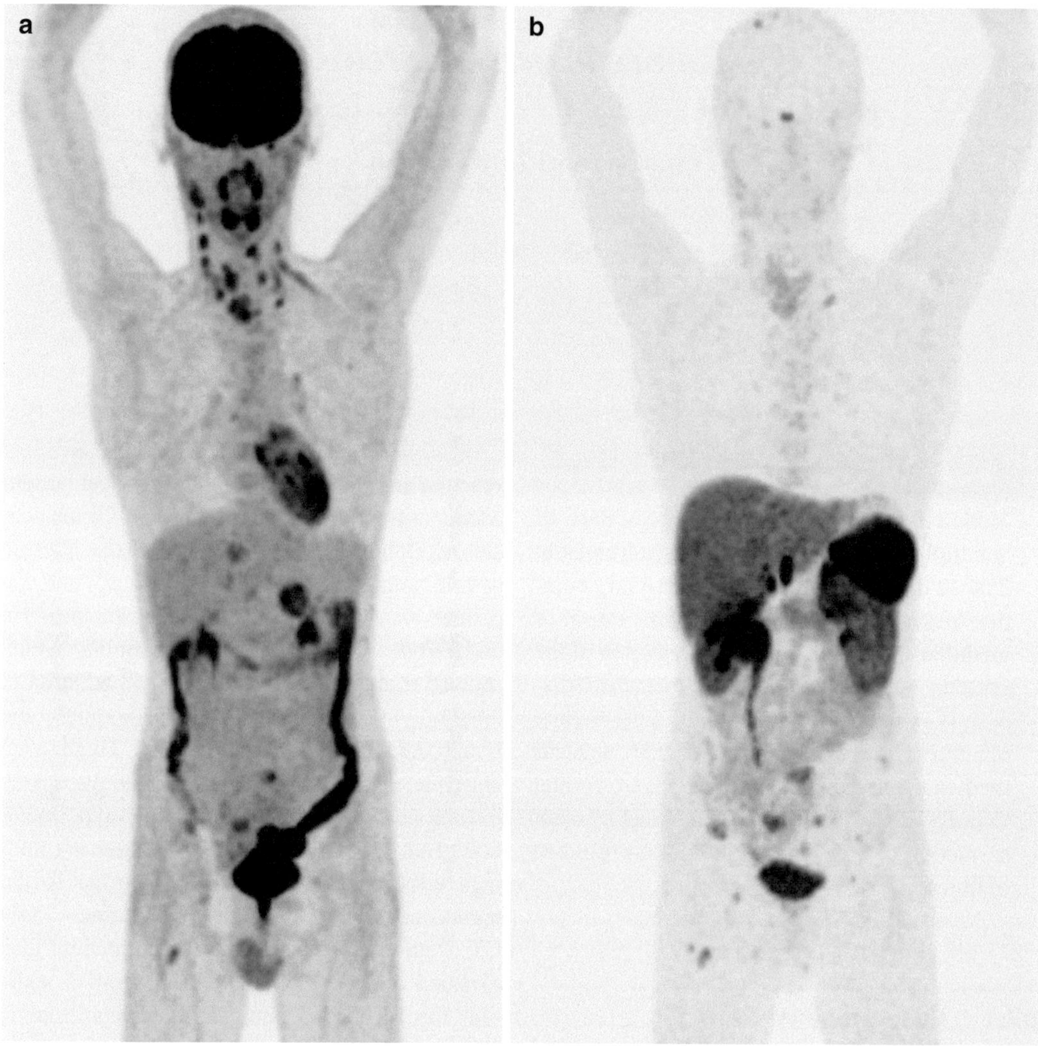

Fig. 62.1 Maximum intensity projection (MIP) images of F-18 FDG (**a**) and Ga-68 DOTATATE (**b**) are shown. F-18 FDG study reveals increased metabolic activity in thyroid nodules, jugular chain lymph nodes, liver, adrenal glands, and bones. In the Ga-68 DOTATATE study, thyroid lesion and jugular chain lymph nodes have faint uptake, and bone lesions have prominent peptide uptake. The number of bone lesions detected on Ga-68 DOTATATE was higher when compared with F-18 FDG PET/CT. The liver lesion did not show Ga-68 DOTATATE avidity

T2-weighted images and no evidence of lipid content in-phase/out-of-phase imaging. MRI also showed additional multiple metastatic liver lesions apart from those lesions detected on ^{18}F-FDG PET/CT.

The patient was considered inoperable due to multiple metastatic involvement, and chemotherapy was started by medical oncology.

During the follow-up period, the patient underwent a ^{68}Ga-DOTATATE PET/CT. Liver lesions detected on ^{18}F-FDG PET/CT and/or on MRI and thyroid lesions did not show increased ^{68}Ga-DOTATATE uptake. Bilateral lymph nodes in the jugular chain had moderately and bone lesions had significantly increased ^{68}Ga-DOTATE uptake. In the retroperitoneal area, a lymph node with low metabolic activity on ^{18}F-FDG FDG PET/CT is found to have high ^{68}Ga-DOTATATE avidity (Figs. 62.1 and 62.2).

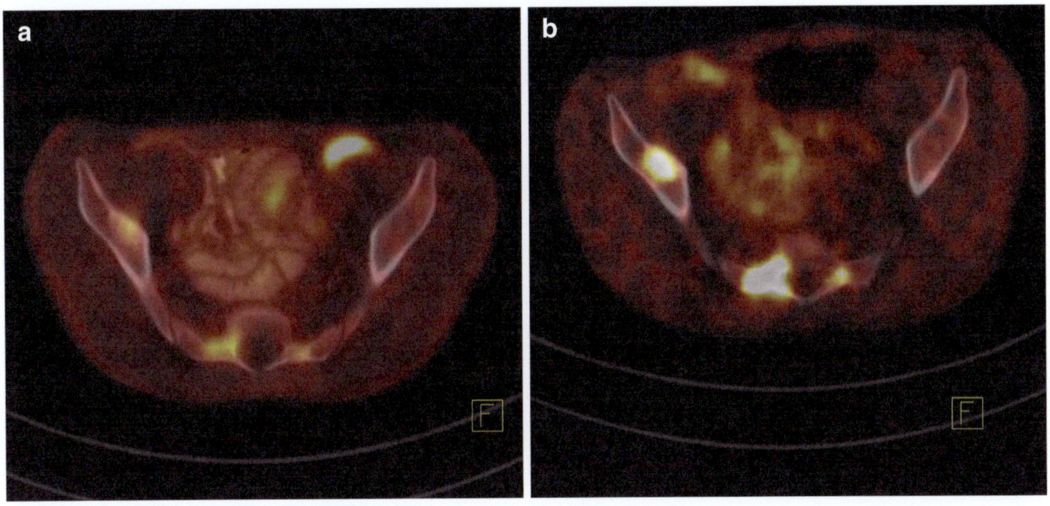

Fig. 62.2 Among metastatic involvements, bone lesions had more prominent Ga-68 DOTATATE uptake. It shows uptake patterns of F-18 FDG (**a**) and Ga-68 DOTATATE (**b**) in right iliac and sacral metastatic lesions

62.2 Discussion

62.2.1 Evaluation and Diagnosis

Medullary thyroid carcinoma (MTC) accounts for 3–5% of thyroid cancers. It is a neuroendocrine tumor originating from parafollicular C-cells of the thyroid gland [1]. MTC is a component of multiple endocrine neoplasia (MEN) type 2 syndromes in 25% of the cases [2]. MEN 2 syndromes consist of three main subtypes. While the co-occurrence of MTC, pheochromocytoma, and parathyroid hyperplasia or adenoma is the characteristic of MEN 2A, the presence of pheochromocytoma, mucosal neuromas, intestinal autonomic ganglion dysfunction, medullated corneal fibers, and marfanoid habitus with MTC is typical for MEN 2B. In "familial MTC," the third form of MEN syndromes, MTC is not associated with additional pathology [3]. Both MEN 2A and MEN 2B have autosomal dominant inheritance pattern which activates germline mutations of the ret proto-oncogene [4]. Most of the diagnosed cases (75%) have de novo mutations [5].

In the current case having the diagnosis of MTC according to thyroid and lymph node biopsies, with the contribution of ^{18}F-FDG FDG PET/CT findings and histopathological analysis of the papular tongue lesion that revealed "mucosal neuroma," diagnosis of MEN 2B syndrome is supported. Being a component of MEN 2B syndrome, mucosal neuromas are usually located on the lips, tongue, or buccal mucosa. Mucosal neuromas when detected especially in early childhood may allow early diagnosis of the MEN 2B, and therefore MTC which is a life-threatening malignancy can be prevented by total thyroidectomy [6].

Most patients with MEN 2B have gastrointestinal symptoms that precede the development of MTC. Symptoms usually start in the infancy period. Gastrointestinal ganglioneuromatosis which is defined as hyperplasia of the myenteric plexus and hypertrophy of ganglion cells is the main etiological factor for most of the gastrointestinal symptoms in patients with MEN 2B and may occur anywhere along the gastrointestinal tract [7]. On the other hand, biopsy specimens obtained from different sites of the colon and rectum at the time of diagnosis in our case did not reveal ganglioneuromatosis that might indicate chronic diarrhea. However, 6 months after the diagnosis, the patient developed sigmoid colon perforation. Sigmoid colon resection and colostomy operations were performed. Histopathological evaluation showed neuronal plexus hypertrophy, and ganglia cells increased in number.

In the initial staging of a patient with MTC, lymph node involvement is a frequent finding reaching an incidence of 80%. Bone, liver, and lung metastases are less frequent with an incidence of 10–15%. The surgical approach including total thyroidectomy and neck dissection is the standard approach in patients without metastatic disease and elevated basal serum calcitonin, and carcinoembryonic antigen levels following surgery suggest residual tumor tissue [8]. The American Thyroid Association (ATA) recommends neck USG if serum calcitonin is below 150 pg/ml. If calcitonin is greater than 150 pg/ml, imaging modalities including CT, MRI, and nuclear medicine procedures should be considered [9]. Among nuclear medicine procedures, newer techniques including PET/CT using ^{18}F-FDG and ^{68}Ga-labeled somatostatin analogs are preferred over previously used technetium-99m pentavalent dimercaptosuccinic acid (Tc-99m DMSA-V), iodine-123-labeled metaiodobenzylguanidine (I-123 MIBG), and ^{111}indium-octreotide (^{111}In-octreotide) scans with advantages of higher sensitivity and superior imaging characteristics.

^{18}F-FDG PET/CT has become widely available in the last decade and is currently a mainstay in oncology practice. Although the sensitivity of ^{18}F-FDG PET/CT in MTC is lower when compared with other malignancies, it is still reasonable (64–72%) especially when calcitonin doubling time is short [10].

Somatostatin, an endogenous peptide, is secreted by a group of cells including neuroendocrine, activated immune, and inflammatory cells [11]. Somatostatin binds to one of five types of somatostatin receptors (SSTR1–SSTR5). Like other neuroendocrine tumors, MTC expresses somatostatin receptors (SSTR) on the cell membrane. SSTR2 is the most commonly expressed receptor type [12]. Therefore, radiolabeled somatostatin analogs can be used in the imaging of MTC. Two main radionuclide somatostatin receptor imaging modalities are available in current practice. In-111 octreotide is introduced earlier and is used in SPECT in SPECT/CT systems. More recently, ^{68}Ga-labeled somatostatin analogs are popularized with the advantages of high-affinity SSTR2 and superior imaging properties of PET over SPECT imaging. Another yield of the radiolabeled peptide imaging is to reveal the suitability for the radionuclide therapy in inoperable cases [13]. The case presented had multiple thyroid medullary carcinoma lesions having increased F-18 FDG uptake and a hypermetabolic liver lesion that did not show ^{68}Ga-DOTATATE uptake. On the other hand, ^{68}Ga-DOTATATE scan revealed the existence of somatostatin receptors in jugular lymph nodes, in bone lesions, and also in a retroperitoneal lymph node which is not hypermetabolic on ^{18}F-FDG FDG PET/CT. The review of the relevant literature, in accordance with the case presented here, shows that neither ^{18}F-FDG PET/CT nor Ga-68-labeled somatostatin analogs perfectly detect the extent of the disease. When two modalities are compared, a clear superiority was not found between ^{18}F-FDG and Ga-68 peptide PET/CT in terms of sensitivity [8, 14].

62.3 Follow-Up and Clinical Course

Currently, the patient is in follow-up for 5 years. Having multiple metastatic lesions, he is considered inoperable and treated with chemotherapeutic agents. ^{18}F-FDG PET/CT scans obtained during this period showed stable disease. Radionuclide therapy using Lu-177-labeled somatostatin analog remains as an option.

What Can We Learn from This Case?

- Surgery is the primary curative modality in the management of MTC. However, patients with metastatic disease are considered inoperable. Detection of mucosal neuromas on physical examination or detection of gastrointestinal ganglioneuromatosis in patients having gastrointestinal symptoms especially in infancy period may provide early diagnosis and therefore the cure for the disease.
- ^{18}F-FDG PET/CT and Ga-68-labeled somatostatin receptor imaging studies should be considered as complementary in the detection of the extent of the disease.
- Inoperable patients having increased radiolabeled somatostatin analog uptake are candidates for radionuclide therapy.

References

1. Geller G, Laskin J, Cheung WY, Ho C. A retrospective review of the multidisciplinary management of medullary thyroid cancer: eligibility for systemic therapy. Thyroid Res. 2017;10:6. https://doi.org/10.1186/s13044-017-0041-6.
2. Fagin JA, Wells SA Jr. Biologic and clinical perspectives on thyroid cancer. N Engl J Med. 2016;375:1054–67. https://doi.org/10.1056/NEJMra1501993.
3. Accardo G, Conzo G, Esposito D, Gambardella C, Mazzella M, Castaldo F, et al. Genetics of medullary thyroid cancer: an overview. Int J Surg. 2017;41(Suppl 1):S2–6. https://doi.org/10.1016/j.ijsu.2017.02.064.
4. Carlson KM, Dou S, Chi D, Scavarda N, Toshima K, Jackson CE, et al. Single missense mutation in the tyrosine kinase catalytic domain of the RET protooncogene is associated with multiple endocrine neoplasia type 2B. Proc Natl Acad Sci U S A. 1994;91:1579–83.
5. Wells SA Jr, Asa SL, Dralle H, Elisei R, Evans DB, Gagel RF, et al. Revised American Thyroid Association guidelines for the management of medullary thyroid carcinoma. Thyroid. 2015;25:567–610. https://doi.org/10.1007/s00259-016-3404-7.
6. Qualia CM, Brown MR, Ryan CK, Rossi TM. Oral mucosal neuromas leading to the diagnosis of multiple endocrine Neoplasia type 2B in a child with intestinal pseudo-obstruction. Gastroenterol Hepatol (N Y). 2007;3:208–11.
7. Cohen MS, Phay JE, Albinson C, DeBenedetti MK, Skinner MA, Lairmore TC, et al. Gastrointestinal manifestations of multiple endocrine neoplasia type 2. Ann Surg. 2002;235:648–54.
8. Naswa N, Sharma P, Suman Kc S, Lata S, Kumar R, Malhotra A, et al. Prospective evaluation of 68Ga-DOTA-NOC PET-CT in patients with recurrent medullary thyroid carcinoma: comparison with 18F-FDG PET-CT. Nucl Med Commun. 2012;33:766–74. https://doi.org/10.1097/MNM.0b013e3283541157.
9. American Thyroid Association Guidelines Task Force, Kloos RT, Eng C, Evans DB, Francis GL, Gagel RF, et al. Medullary thyroid cancer: management guidelines of the American Thyroid Association. Thyroid. 2009;19:565–612. https://doi.org/10.1089/thy.2008.0403.
10. Cheng X, Bao L, Xu Z, Li D, Wang J, Li Y. ^{18}F-FDG-PET and ^{18}F-FDG-PET/CT in the detection of recurrent or metastatic medullary thyroid carcinoma: a systematic review and meta-analysis. J Med Imaging Radiat Oncol. 2012;56:136–42. https://doi.org/10.1111/j.1754-9485.2012.02344.x.
11. Patel YC. Somatostatin and its receptor family. Front Neuroendocrinol. 1999;20:157–98.
12. Papotti M, Kumar U, Volante M, Pecchioni C, Patel YC. Immunohistochemical detec- tion of somatostation receptor types 1-5 in medullary carcinoma of the thyroid. Clin Endocrinol. 2001;54:641–9.
13. Kwekkeboom DJ, Bakker WH, Kam BL, Teunissen JJ, Kooij PP, de Herder WW, et al. Treatment of patients with gastro-entero-pancreatic (GEP) tumors with the novel radiolabelled somatostatin analog [177Lu-DOTA(0), Tyr3]octreotate. Eur J Nucl Med Mol Imaging. 2003;30:417–22.
14. Conry BG, Papathanasiou ND, Prakash V, Kayani I, Caplin M, Mahmood S, et al. Comparison of (68) Ga-DOTATATE and (18)F-fluorodeoxyglucose PET/CT in the detection of recurrent medullary thyroid carcinoma. Eur J Nucl Med Mol Imaging. 2010;37:49–57. https://doi.org/10.1007/s00259-009-1204-z.

Hurthle Cell Carcinoma

63

Elgin Özkan and Çiğdem Soydal

Abstract

Hurthle cell carcinoma (HCC) is a histopathologic variant of follicular thyroid carcinoma. HCC is more aggressive than follicular tumors. It causes more nodal metastases than follicular cancer, and it has the highest metastatic frequency among the differentiated thyroid cancers. In this report, we describe a 50-year-old female patient who presented with an enlarging palpable mass in the left thyroid lobe for 3 years. Neck ultrasonography (USG) demonstrated a 4 × 2.5 × 4 cm heterogeneous isoechoic nodule in the left thyroid lobe. There was no pathologic lymph node on USG. The patient underwent a left hemithyroidectomy, and histopathological examination of the surgical specimen revealed a Hurthle cell carcinoma with a maximum diameter of 4.2 cm. Radioiodine ablation treatment (RAT) with 3700 MBq (100 mCi) iodine-131 (^{131}I) was applied approximately 2 months after the operation. Six months after the RAT, diagnostic whole-body scintigraphy with 185 MBq (5 mCi) ^{131}I was performed. The serum-stimulated Tg level and the ^{131}I whole-body scintigraphy were entirely normal. There has been no evidence of disease, on the 8-year follow-up period. Despite of good response to therapy, due to high risk of HCC, the patient is still under close follow-up.

E. Özkan (✉)
Department of Nuclear Medicine, Medical Faculty of Ankara University, Ankara, Turkey

Ç. Soydal
Department of Nuclear Medicine, Ankara University School of Medicine, Ankara, Turkey

63.1 Case Presentation

In this report, we describe a 50-year-old female patient who presented with an enlarging palpable mass in the left thyroid lobe for 3 years. A 4.5 × 4.5 cm mobile mass was palpated in the left thyroid lobe upon physical examination. Neck ultrasonography (USG) demonstrated a 4 × 2.5 × 4 cm heterogeneous isoechoic nodule in the left thyroid lobe. Additionally, a 0.7 cm isoechoic nodule with a hypoechoic outer halo was observed in the right thyroid lobe. There was no pathologic lymph node on USG. Serum thyroid function tests were compatible with euthyroidism. Thyroid fine needle aspiration biopsy (FNAB) revealed a Hurthle cell neoplasm. The patient underwent a left hemithyroidectomy, and histopathological examination of the surgical specimen revealed a Hurthle cell carcinoma (HCC) in the left thyroid lobe with a maximum diameter of 4.2 cm. Additionally, capsular and vascular invasion was detected during the

T. Özülker et al. (eds.), *Thyroid and Parathyroid Diseases*, https://doi.org/10.1007/978-3-319-78476-2_63

histopathological examination. Following lobectomy, a completion thyroidectomy was performed. Histopathological analysis revealed no tumor in the right thyroid lobe. Radioiodine ablation treatment (RAT) with 3700 MBq (100 mCi) iodine-131 (^{131}I) was applied approximately 2 months after the operation. The serum thyroid-stimulating hormone (TSH) and thyroglobulin (Tg) levels were measured as 32 IU/ml and <0.5 ng/ml, respectively. Radioiodine uptake limited to the thyroid bed was observed on postablative whole-body scintigraphy. Six months after RAT, a diagnostic whole-body scintigraphy with 185 MBq (5 mCi) ^{131}I was performed to evaluate the success of the ablation. The serum-stimulated Tg level and the ^{131}I whole-body scintigraphy were normal. There has been no evidence of disease over an 8-year follow-up period.

63.2 Evaluation and Diagnosis

Hurthle cell carcinoma of the thyroid gland accounts for approximately 2–10% of all differentiated thyroid cancers [1, 2]. HCC, which is also known as oncocytic or oxyphilic carcinoma, is classified as a variant of follicular thyroid carcinoma [3]. HCC contains at least 75% Hurthle cells, or oxyphilic cells, which have abundant granular cytoplasm because of an extreme number of mitochondria and a large nucleus [4]. Hurthle cells are also observed in nonneoplastic conditions of the thyroid gland, such as thyroiditis and nodular and toxic goiters. The cytological features of Hurthle cell neoplasms are hypercellularity of the Hurthle cells (usually >75%), few or no lymphocytes, and insufficient or absent colloid. A benign neoplasm cannot be distinguished from a malignant neoplasm based on cytological analysis of FNAB samples. The definitive differentiation of Hurthle cell carcinoma from Hurthle cell adenoma is based on histopathological analysis and the presence of capsular and/or vascular invasion [5]. The incidence of malignancy in Hurthle cell neoplasms varies between 13% and 67%. Hurthle cell tumors are more aggressive than follicular tumors. HCC has the potential to cause more nodal metastases than follicular cancer, although not as many as papillary cancer. Additionally, HCC has the highest metastatic frequency among the differentiated thyroid cancers [6–8].

A palpable mass in the thyroid is the most common clinical sign of Hurthle cell neoplasms. In certain cases, pressure symptoms, such as dysphagia, dyspnea, and coughing, can accompany HCC. If the mass rapidly enlarges, pain and other compressive symptoms may be more obvious. In our case, the patient had a growing palpable mass for the last 3 years, and she did not have local pressure symptoms.

Hurthle cell carcinoma can be multifocal and bilateral, and regional lymph node metastasis may occasionally also be felt in the neck. Careful collection of the patient's history and an attentive neck examination can provide clues regarding Hurthle cell carcinomas. In particular, the presence of a family history of thyroid cancer and the history of head and neck external beam irradiation should be questioned. Vocal cord paralysis may also indicate a carcinoma. The presence of pathological bone fractures and physical findings of metastases are essential for the diagnosis of a carcinoma.

In most cases, thyroid function test results are concordant with euthyroidism. Accordingly, in our case, the thyroid function tests were normal. However, in rare instances, thyrotoxicosis due to functional metastases may be observed.

Neck USG is a vital imaging modality for the evaluation of the nature of thyroid nodules and the neck lymph nodes. Computed tomography (CT) and magnetic resonance imaging (MRI) also provide more detailed information regarding the tumor and adjacent neck structures.

According to the 2015 ATA guideline, diagnostic FNAB is recommended, especially in the presence of a nodule $\geq$1 cm in the greatest dimension with a sonographic pattern of high or intermediate suspicion and in the presence of a nodule $\geq$1.5 cm in the greatest dimension with a sonographic pattern of low suspicion [9]. However, FNAB cannot differentiate an adenoma from a carcinoma in Hurthle cell lesions. Definitive differentiation is based on histopathological analysis and the presence of capsular and/or vascular invasion.

63.3 Management

The surgical approach is the primary treatment modality for patients with Hurthle cell carcinomas. According to the 2015 ATA guideline, all patients with differentiated thyroid carcinomas should undergo total or near-total thyroidectomy [9]. The ATA recommendation 35 states that, in the presence of a thyroid tumor >1 and <4 cm without extrathyroidal extension and without the clinical manifestations of any lymph node metastases, a unilateral procedure can be selected. In our case, a histopathological examination of the surgical specimen revealed a Hurthle cell carcinoma, i.e., a high-risk tumor, with a diameter of 4.2 cm in the left thyroid lobe. Additionally, the patient was older than 45 years. Completion thyroidectomy was applied to enable RAI therapy. No tumor was detected in the surgical specimen. Approximately 2 months after the last operation, a treatment dose of ^{131}I (3700 MBq) was administered, and a total body scan was obtained 6 days later. Radioiodine uptake limited to the thyroid bed was observed on the postablative whole-body scintigraphy. Postoperative ^{131}I or ^{123}I scanning can also be performed 4–6 weeks after surgery. In our department, we do not use routine postoperative iodine scintigraphy because of stunning effect of ^{131}I. Low-dose (37–111 MBq) ^{131}I or alternative isotopes, such as ^{123}I, can be used to avoid or prevent this effect.

Because the ^{131}I avidity of Hurthle cell carcinomas is lower than those of other well-differentiated thyroid carcinomas, the efficacy of radioiodine treatment is limited. Therefore, therapy for recurrent or metastatic Hurthle cell carcinoma may be difficult. However, radioiodine treatment is used as a first-choice treatment for most patients with HCC after thyroidectomy and in the treatment of recurrent and metastatic HCC patients. In a recent study involving 1909 cases, the authors reported that radioactive iodine therapy improved the survival of patients with HCC [10]. According to the findings of this study, the 5- and 10-year survival rates of patients who received ^{131}I and those who did not were statistically significant (88.9% vs. 83.1% and 74.4% vs. 65%, respectively, $p < 0.001$).

63.4 Follow-Up and Outcome

Although HCC is a histopathologic variant of follicular carcinoma, it exhibits differences in biological behavior compared to the conventional type of follicular carcinoma. Because of the ability of HCC to metastasize to the lymph nodes and possibly higher rates of recurrence and tumor-related mortality, close follow-up is most critical for HCC patients. Specifically, neck USG can identify small-volume metastatic cervical lymph nodes. In cases of suspected lymph nodes, serum Tg measurements in the washout of fine needle aspirates and/or cytological evaluations may be applied. The surgical approach is the first choice for the management of recurrent HCC. However, in cases of metastatic disease, due to low avidity for ^{131}I, other methods, such as tyrosine kinase inhibitors, can be selected for multiple progressive metastatic diseases [11]. Chemotherapy is generally ineffective for metastatic thyroid carcinomas. The 2015 ATA guideline indicates a weak recommendation for the use of cytotoxic chemotherapy. Cytotoxic chemotherapy may provide a selective benefit to patients who do not respond to kinase inhibitors and, perhaps, to patients with poorly differentiated thyroid cancers [12]. External radiotherapy may be applicable to symptomatic metastatic disease and iodine-negative tumors and can also be used to control recurrent tumors [13].

Although HCC is more aggressive than follicular carcinoma, our patient's clinical course was excellent. The good clinical outcome may be associated with the absence of local recurrence and/or metastatic disease in the follow-up.

63.5 Future

Hurthle cell carcinomas have low avidity for ^{131}I. Non-radioiodine avid metastatic thyroid carcinomas create a particularly challenging patient group. Surgical resection can be performed in cases with a limited number of metastases. In addition to tyrosine kinase inhibitors, new targeted treatments should be developed. Regarding radionuclides, Lu-177 DOTA-peptide treatment has been reported to be an alternative option for somatostatin receptor-expressing tumors. However, large prospective studies with large numbers of patients should be designed to reveal the effectiveness of Lu-177 DOTA-peptide treatment.

What Can We Learn from This Case?

- Hurthle—oncocytic or oxyphilic—cell carcinoma is a histopathologic variant of follicular thyroid carcinoma.
- It contains hypercellularity of Hurthle cells (usually >75%).
- Definitive diagnosis is based on histopathological analysis, with a presence of capsular and/or vascular invasion.
- Hurthle cell carcinoma is more aggressive than follicular tumors. It causes more nodal metastases than follicular cancer, and it has the highest metastatic frequency among the differentiated thyroid cancers.
- Hurthle cell carcinoma has lower ^{131}I avidity than the other well-differentiated thyroid carcinomas.

References

1. Masood S, Auguste LJ, Westerband A, Belluco C, Valderama E, Attie J. Differential oncogenic expression in thyroid follicular and Hürthle cell carcinomas. Am J Surg. 1993;166:366–8.
2. McDonald MP, Sanders LE, Silverman ML, Chan HS, Buyske J. Hürthle cell carcinoma: prognostic factors and results of surgical treatment. Surgery. 1996;120:1000–4.
3. De Lellis RA, Lloyd RV, Heitz PU, Eng C. Pathology and genetics of tumours of endocrine organs in WHO classification of tumours. 1st ed. Lyon: World Health Organization; 2004.
4. Ahmed M, Bin Yousef H, Greer W, Faraz H, Al Sobhi S, Al Zahrani A, et al. Hurthle cell neoplasm of the thyroid gland. ANZ J Surg. 2008;78:139–43.
5. Mills SC, Haq M, Smellie WJ, Harmer C. Hurthle cell carcinoma of the thyroid: retrospective review of 62 patients treated at the Royal Marsden Hospital between 1946 and 2003. Eur J Surg Oncol. 2009;35:230–4.
6. Hundahl SA, Fleming ID, Fremgen AM, Menck HR. A National Cancer Data Base report on 53,856 cases of thyroid carcinoma treated in the U.S., 1985–1995. Cancer. 1998;83:2638–48.
7. Haigh PI, Urbach DR. The treatment and prognosis of Hurthle cell follicular thyroid carcinoma compared with its non-Hurthle cell counterpart. Surgery. 2005;138:1152–7.
8. Shaha AR, Loree TR, Shah JP. Prognostic factors and risk group analysis in follicular carcinoma of the thyroid. Surgery. 1995;118:1131–6.
9. Haugen BR, Alexander EK, Bible KC, Doherty GM, Mandel SJ, Nikiforov YE, et al. American thyroid association management guidelines for adult patients with thyroid nodules and differentiated thyroid cancer. Thyroid. 2015;26:1–133.
10. Jillard C, Youngwirth L, Scheri R, Roman S, Sosa JA. Radioactive iodine treatment is associated with improved survival for patients with hurthle cell carcinoma. Thyroid. 2016;26:959–64.
11. Anderson RT, Linnehan JE, Tongbram V, Keating K, Wirth LJ. Clinical safety and economic evidence in radioactive iodine-refractory differentiated thyroid cancer: a systematic literature review. Thyroid. 2013;23:392–407.
12. Spano JP, Vano Y, Vignot S, De La Motte RT, Hassani L, Mouawad R, et al. GEMOX regimen in the treatment of metastatic differentiated refractory thyroid carcinoma. Med Oncol. 2012;29:1421–8.
13. Foote RL, Brown PD, Garces YI, McIver B, Kasperbauer JL. Is there a role for radiation therapy in the management of Hurthle cell carcinoma? Int J Radiat Oncol Biol Phys. 2003;56:1067–72.

Thyroid Lymphoma

64

Dilek Yazıcı

Abstract

Thyroid lymphomas typically present as rapidly growing masses in the thyroid gland, with or without causing compression symptoms. They are usually of B-cell origin and are seen as mucosa-associated lymphoid tissue (MALT) lymphoma. The patients are mostly euthyroid. The best method to diagnose thyroid lymphoma is through incisional or core biopsy. These tumors respond well to combination of chemotherapy (mostly commonly CHOP regimen) and radiotherapy. Rituximab may be added in diffuse large cell lymphomas to increase the efficacy of therapy.

64.1 Case Presentation

A 38-year-old woman presented with the complaint of swelling on the right side of her neck. She did not have any pain, tenderness, hoarseness, or dysphagia. She also did not have any symptoms of thyrotoxicosis, like palpitations, tremor, sweating, or weight loss. She did not have a personal history of radiotherapy to the neck region. She had no one in the family with thyroid disease. In her laboratory findings, while the TSH was normal, antithyroglobulin antibody level was elevated (806.7 IU/mL; normal <115 IU/mL). The thyroid ultrasonography (USG) revealed a heterogeneous thyroid parenchyma, revealing thyroiditis. There was a heterogeneous, hypoechoic region that is 26 × 16 × 29 mm in the right lobe next to the isthmus. The fine needle aspiration biopsy (FNAB) performed revealed benign thyrocytes and also lymphoid cells.

The patient was very bothered about the swelling and went to another center within a month's time, while again her only symptom was swelling. The new TSH level was 5.74 mU/L and the new USG performed showed three nodules in the right lobe [16 × 12 mm hypoechoic solid nodule, 22 × 12 mm well-contoured hypoechoic solid nodule, and three areas (26 × 17 mm, 23 × 12 mm, and 17 × 11 mm) that cannot be differentiated between focal thyroiditis regions and nodule]. There was no nodule in the left lobe. An FNAB was repeated from the largest hypoactive nodule in the right lobe. "The aspirate contained degenerated lymphoid tissue, which might be indicative of lymphocytic thyroiditis," was the result of the cytological examination.

A few days after the biopsy, there appeared a fast enlarging mass in the isthmic region. The mass was initially rubbery but became hard within a few days' time (Fig. 64.1). The cervical

D. Yazıcı
Koç University Medical School,
Section of Endocrinology and Metabolism,
Istanbul, Turkey

T. Özülker et al. (eds.), *Thyroid and Parathyroid Diseases*, https://doi.org/10.1007/978-3-319-78476-2_64

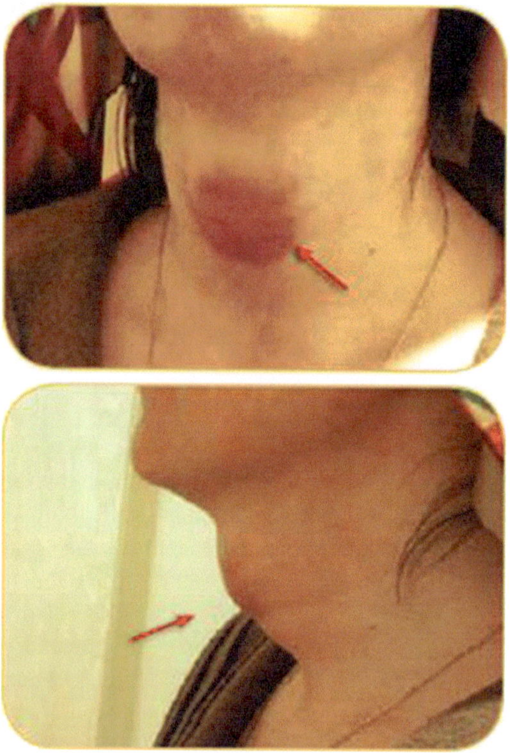

Fig. 64.1 Mass in the neck

magnetic resonance imaging study (MRI) revealed multiple nodules in the right lobe. The margins of the nodules cannot be differentiated from each other. There was a lobulated mass in the midline starting from the isthmus, extending to the vocal cords and anteriorly to the skin beyond the hyoid. The mass had similar signal properties as the nodules in the thyroid gland and was considered as a nodule, originating from thyroid tissue, possibly from a remnant in the thyroglossal duct. The surrounding fat planes were spared, and there was no invasion. There was also no lymphadenopathy (Fig. 64.2).

The FNAB of the new mass had lymphoid series cells and histiocytic cells. There were no thyroid follicular cells or Hurthle cells in the aspirate. Then excisional biopsy was performed. There was a 14 × 10 mm mass in the midline extending from the hyoid bone to the thyroid gland. The mass was fixed to the surrounding tissues. There were nodules of similar characteristics in both thyroid glands.

The pathology was consistent with high-grade B-cell lymphoma, consisting of undetermined

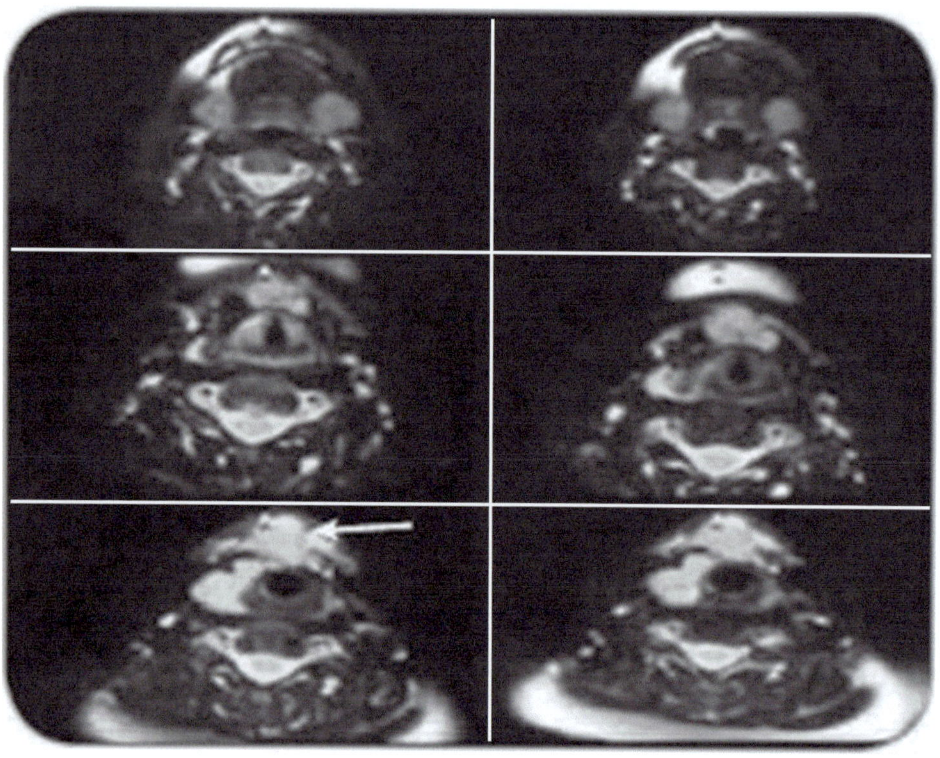

Fig. 64.2 Axial slices of MRI images showing lobulated mass in the midline of the neck (arrow)

follicular pattern that is infiltrating the fat and muscle planes. Immunocytochemistry was consistent with CD20 +;Bcl6 +;Bcl2 +; Pax5 +; CD5 −;CD3 −;cyclin D1 −. F-18 FDG position emission tomography/computed tomography (PET/CT) revealed highly hypermetabolic, lobulated mass lesion or conglomerated multiple lymph nodes in the right thyroid lobe that is extending to the upper cervical region and the skin, beyond the hyoid bone. There were also medium to highly hypermetabolic lymph nodes at the left cervical level VI (Fig. 64.3).

64.2 Discussion

Primary thyroid lymphoma (PTL) is defined as a lymphoma involving only the thyroid gland or the thyroid gland and regional lymph nodes without contiguity or metastasis of other areas at the time of diagnosis [1]. The secondary thyroid lymphoma originates from a non-thyroidal region and metastasizes to the thyroid gland. It is important to differentiate between the two tumors as the approach differ significantly [2]. Thyroid lymphomas constitute 2.5% of all non-Hodgkin lymphomas and 2–8% of thyroid malignancies [3]. It is of B-cell origin and is usually seen as mucosa-associated lymphoid tissue (MALT) lymphoma [3]. Diffuse large B-cell lymphoma (DLBCL) is the other type that may be observed. The pathology of our patient was consistent with high-grade B-cell lymphoma. The presence of other types of lymphoma, such as follicular lymphoma or small B-cell lymphoma, is less frequent, and T- cell lymphoma, Burkitt lymphoma, and Hodgkin lymphoma are extremely rare [4]. It is mostly seen in female patients and in the seventh decade of life [5]. The suggested mechanism explaining the occurrence of these neoplasms in elderly patients may be that the development of these neoplasms takes many years before they become clinically evident [6]. Our patient was younger compared to the literature. Most

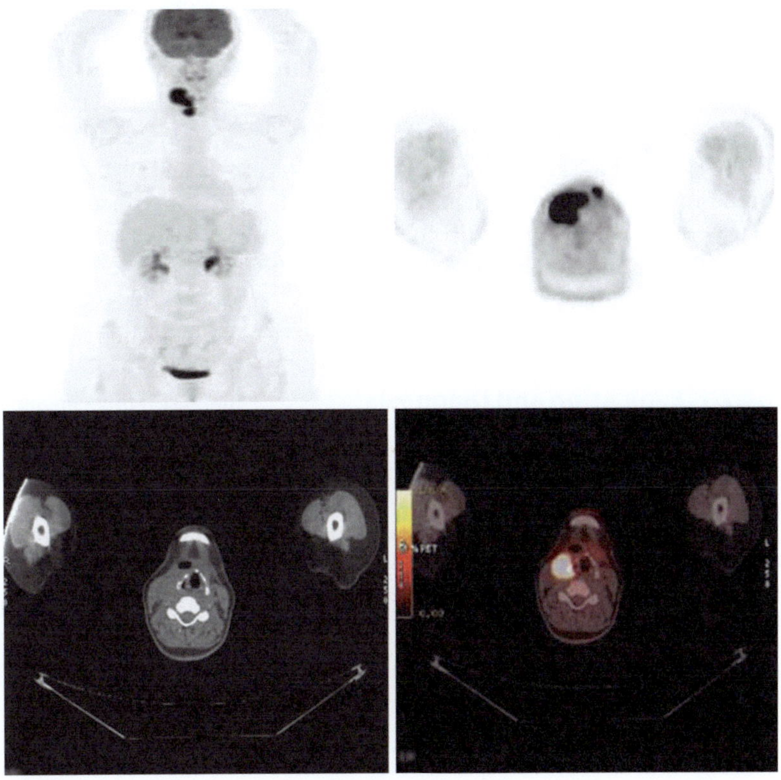

Fig. 64.3 MIP and axial slices of PET, CT, and fusion images showing hypermetabolic, lobulated mass lesion or conglomerated multiple lymph nodes in the right thyroid lobe

individuals are euthyroid at presentation, but 10% may be hypothyroid [7]. They are usually diagnosed in stage IE (according to the Ann Arbor staging system), with the disease being confined to the thyroid gland, or stage IIE characterized by the involvement of the lymph nodes on the ipsilateral side of the diaphragm. Stages IIIE and IVE are rarely reported [6]. The staging of the presented patient was Stage IIE, with metastatic lymph nodes in the neck region.

It is generally observed in patients with a background history of chronic thyroiditis. Hashimoto's disease is associated with more than 90% of the PTL in some reports [7]. There is increased risk of MALT lymphoma in patients having autoimmune thyroid disease. The pathophysiology is suggested to be originating of the lymphoma from intrathyroidal lymphoid tissue during the course of chronic inflammation or an autoimmune process. Chronic antigenic stimulation and proliferation of lymphoid tissue are proposed to increase the susceptibility to neoplastic transformation in the lymphoid tissue [8]. Presence of MALT lymphoma in the organs that physiologically do not contain lymphoid tissue has suggested lymphocytic proliferation of inflammatory origin [9]. DLBCL is usually seen as a result of MALT transformation. The presence of mixed lymphomas (MALT/DLBCL) in the same patient confirms this transformation [9]. Our patient, being DLBLC in the presence of lymphocytic thyroiditis, may be consistent with a possible transformation from MALT lymphoma.

64.2.1 Evaluation and Diagnosis

Primary thyroid lymphomas usually present as a rapidly enlarging anterior cervical mass that may or may not be associated with lymphadenopathy. The patient may experience symptoms of compression such as hoarseness, dyspnea, and dysphagia [9]. Compression from rapidly growing mass results in narrowing of the trachea leading to stridor and, in some cases, unilateral or bilateral right laryngeal nerve palsy leading to hoarseness. Dysphagia and superior vena cava syndrome are rare in these tumors [10]. There is even a case reported that has presented with severe respiratory dyspnea [9]. Some patients may present with B-symptoms: fever, nocturnal sweating, weight loss, and enlarged cervical lymph nodes [10]. On the other hand, the patient may be asymptomatic, and the diagnosis may be established incidentally during FNAB or surgery. In the index case, the tumor presented as a very rapidly enlarging mass that even invaded the skin in about 10 days' time. Preoperative diagnosis can be established using USG and FNAB along with immunochemistry and flow cytometry [9]. FNAB has low sensitivity and specificity in the diagnosis of MALT lymphomas, so core biopsy or excisional biopsy may be required for definitive diagnosis [11]. Especially differentiating between thyroid lymphoma, lymphocytic thyroiditis, and anaplastic carcinoma may be difficult in some cases [12]. There are several small retrospective studies that have demonstrated increased sensitivity and specificity with the introduction of other techniques such as flow cytometry and immunohistochemical studies or molecular techniques such as polymerase chain reaction (PCR) [12]. No correlation has been shown between the Ki-67 index and the extent of the tumor [9]. In our patient, the FNAB of the mass had lymphoid series cells and histiocytic cells, but there were no thyroid follicular cells or Hurthle cells in the aspirate. Thus the diagnosis could be determined through an excisional biopsy. Immunocytochemistry was performed on this material.

USG usually reveals a diffuse mass, with marked hypoechogenicity. There is again a diffuse homogeneous enhancement pattern in contrast-enhanced USG, which is helpful for detecting necrotic areas of PTL [13]. The ultrasonography in our patient was not very helpful since there was not a diffuse infiltration, but there were a few hypoechoic thyroid nodules. Computed tomography (CT) enables visualization of the tumor size as well as its relationship to vital structures of the neck and their possible infiltration. MRI does not have an advantage over CT and is used mostly in the planning of radiation therapy [9]. F-18 FDG PET/CT can be used to determine the stage or extent of thyroid lymphoma and also for follow-up after treatment. No typical features have been suggested for these lesions on CT, MRI, or PET scan [9].

Determining the extent of the disease is important for estimating the prognosis and the therapeutic strategies. MALT thyroid lymphoma cases are staged on the basis of the international prognosis index (Table 64.1) [14].

64.2.2 Management

MALT lymphomas have a slow progression and better prognosis (survival of 75–100%), whereas diffuse large B-cell lymphomas have a more aggressive course [3]. The therapy depends on the histologic type, invasion, and prognostic factors. There are controversies regarding the optimal management of thyroid lymphomas. The usual management approach is combined chemotherapy with locoregional radiotherapy. Surgery alone is only recommended for intrathyroidal MALT lymphoma [15]. Surgery may also be used as palliative therapy for the compressive symptoms associated with the tumor [16]. It is especially emphasized that tracheostomy can preferentially be avoided; instead, endoscopic stenting of tracheal stenosis may be performed, as the results of medical treatment may be awaited [9]. Debulking and cytoreductive operations are not recommended since they increase the risk of postoperative complications, and they affect the course of the radiation therapy and evaluation of response in the follow-up imaging. Corticosteroids may be used to alleviate the compressive symptoms associated with the tumor [9].

Table 64.1 International prognosis index

International prognosis index for MALT-omas
MALT-oma located within the thyroid (1E)
MALT-oma located within the thyroid and regional lymph nodes (2E)
MALT-oma located at both sides of the diaphragm (3E)
Disseminated MALT-oma

Radiotherapy alone is the only suggested therapy for localized stage IE tumors usually achieving remarkable local control in most of the cases. It may also be used as consolidation after systemic therapy or palliation. Site radiotherapy, involved-node radiotherapy, and irradiation of residual tissue after full-course therapy are the usual modes of radiotherapy that are used in the management of thyroid lymphomas [17].

The conventional chemotherapeutic regimen for all PTL includes cyclophosphamide, doxorubicin, vincristine, and prednisone (CHOP). Rituximab may be added in more aggressive cases. The therapeutic response is rapid with these regimens. However, the addition of radiotherapy to chemotherapy has increased the complete response rates and overall survival rates, along with the reduction of relapse [18]. The 5-year survival rate for primary thyroid lymphomas is 50–70% ranging to 90% in lesions confined to the gland (IE) and 20–50% for those with extracapsular invasion. For stages IIIE and IVE, these rates go down to 15–35% [19]. The prognosis depends on the histological classification of the tumor and the stage of the disease. MALT lymphomas have a better prognosis than DLBCL. They are more indolent and have a favorable therapeutic response. Clinical factors that predict a worse prognosis include tumor size over 10 cm, advanced stage (greater than stage IE), presence of local obstructive symptoms, rapid tumor growth, mediastinal involvement, age > 60 years, and elevated LDH and b2 microglobulin levels [12].

64.3 Follow-Up and Outcome

Our patient was then given six cycles of R-CHOP (rituximab-CHOP) therapy. The PET/CT performed revealed no hypermetabolic foci in the follow-up after the chemotherapy ended.

64.4 The Future

Combination of chemotherapy and radiotherapy has been shown to provide the best regimen for thyroid lymphomas, both the MALT lymphomas and the diffuse B-cell lymphoma. The chemotherapy protocol that is most commonly used is the CHOP scheme. The addition of rituximab, a monoclonal antibody anti-CD20, to the treatment protocol has improved disease-free and overall survival in DLBCL. Perhaps different molecular disease-specific agents may be developed in the future for these kinds of lymphomas.

What Can We Learn from This Case?

- Primary thyroid lymphomas should be considered in the differential diagnosis of a fast enlarging nodule of the thyroid.
- The best diagnostic workup method for thyroid lymphomas is excisional or core biopsy.
- Most commonly observed thyroid lymphoma is MALT lymphoma, but DLBCL may also be observed.
- These tumors respond to chemotherapy (CHOP regimen) combined with radiotherapy successfully. Rituximab may be added in diffuse large cell lymphomas to improve disease-free and overall survival.

References

1. Ansell SM, Grant CS, Habermann TM. Primary thyroid lymphoma. Sem Oncol. 1999;26:316–23.
2. Takashima S, Takayama F, Momose M, Shingu K, Sone S. Secondary malignant lymphoma which simulated primary thyroid cancer. J Clin Imaging. 2000;24:162–5.
3. Diaconescu MR, Costea I, Glod M, Diaconescu S. An unwonted clinicopathological subtype of thyroid primary lymphoma. Chirurgia (Bucur). 2016;111:428–31.
4. Thieblemont C, Mayer A, Dumontet C, Barbier Y, Callet-Bauchu E, Felman P, et al. Primary thyroid lymphoma is a heterogeneous disease. J Clin Endocrinol Metab. 2002;87:105–11.
5. Sangalli G, Serio G, Zampatti C, Lomuscio G, Colombo L. Fine-needle aspiration cytology of primary lymphoma of the thyroid: a report of 17 cases. Cytopathology. 2001;12:257–63.
6. Niitsu N, Okamoto M, Nakamura N, Nakamine H, Bessho M, Hirano M. Clinicopathological correlations of stage IE/IIE primary thyroid diffuse large B-cell lymphoma. Ann Oncol. 2007;18:1203–8.
7. Katna R, Shet T, Sengar M, Menon H, Laskar S, Prabhash K. Clinicopathologic study and outcome analysis of thyroid lymphomas: experience from a tertiary cancer center. Head Neck. 2013;35:165–71.
8. Graff-Baker A, Roman SA, Thomas DC, Udelsman R, Sosa JA. Prognosis of primary thyroid lymphoma: demographic, clinical and pathologic predictors of survival in 1,408 cases. Surgery. 2009;146:1105–15.
9. Czopnik P, Aporowicz M, Niepokój-Czopnik A, Wojtczak B, Domosławski P, Bolanowski M. Primary thyroid lymphoma: a rare but challenging diagnosis. Pol Arch Intern Med. 2017;127:361–4.
10. Mack LA, Pasieka JL. An evidence-based approach to the treatment of thyroid lymphoma. World J Surg. 2007;31:978–86.
11. Kaba S, Hirokawa M, Higuchi M, Suzuki A, Kojima M, Miyauchi A. Cytological findings for the diagnosis of primary thyroid mucosa-associated lymphoid tissue lymphoma by fine needle aspiration. Acta Cytol. 2015;59:26–36.
12. Peixoto R, Correia Pinto J, Soares V, Koch P, Taveira, et al. Primary thyroid lymphoma: a case report and review of the literature. Ann Med Surg (Lond). 2016;13:29–33.
13. Wei X, Li Y, Zhang S, Li X, Gao M. Evaluation of primary thyroid lymphoma by ultrasonography combined with contrast-enhanced ultrasonography: a pilot study. Indian J Cancer. 2015;52:546–50.
14. Jaffe ES, Harris NL, Diebold J, Muller-Hemmelink HK. World Health Organization classification of neoplastic diseases of the hematopoietic and lymphoid tissues. A progress report. Am J Clin Pathol. 1999;111(1 Suppl 1):S8–12.
15. Latheef N, Shenoy V, Kamath MP, Hegde MC, Rao AR. Maltoma of thyroid: a rare thyroid tumour. Case Rep Otolaryngol. 2013;2013:740241.
16. Meyer-Rochow GY, Sywak MS, Reeve TS, Delbridge LW, Sidhu SB. Surgical trends in the management of thyroid lymphoma. Eur J Surg Oncol. 2008;34:576–80.
17. Witkowska M, Majchrzak A, Smolewski P. The role of radiotherapy in Hodgkin's lymphoma: what has been achieved in the last 50 years? Biomed Res Int. 2015;2015:485071.
18. Horning SJ, Weller E, Kim K, Earle JD, O'Conell MJ, Habermann TM, et al. Chemotherapy with or without radiotherapy in limited-stage diffuse aggressive non-Hodgkin's lymphoma: eastern cooperative oncology group study 1484. Clin Oncol. 2004;22:3032–8.
19. Chai YJ, Hong JH, Koo do H, Yu HW, Lee JH, Kwon H, et al. Clinicopathological characteristics and treatment outcomes of 38 cases of primary thyroid lymphoma: a multicenter study. Ann Surg Treat Res. 2015;89:295–9.

65 Radioiodine Therapy During Breastfeeding

Hakan Demir

Abstract

In a 34-year-old female patient, 1.2 cm thyroid nodule was detected in the right lobe of the thyroid in neck ultrasound. Classical type of thyroid papillary carcinoma was confirmed after histopathological examination of thyroidectomy specimens.

Radioiodine ablation had been planned. However, the patient had been breastfeeding. Since radioiodine is contraindicated, breastfeeding had been ceased. In order to expedite of delectation period, cabergoline was used. Tc-99m (technetium) pertechnetate scintigraphy was performed to demonstrate any mammary uptake of the patient before ablation. There was no Tc-99m pertechnetate uptake in mammary glands. The patient had been given 100 mCi I-131 for ablation. At post-ablative whole-body I-131 scintigraphy, there was no pathological uptake both in the neck region and in mammary glands.

In summary in women who are breastfeeding, lactating must be stopped before radioiodine treatment (ablation or metastasis). Some lactation inhibition medications could be used in order to quicken the procedure. In order to control any mammary gland uptake, I-123 or Tc-99m pertechnetate scintigraphy could be used.

H. Demir
Department of Nuclear Medicine, School of Medicine, Kocaeli University, Kocaeli, Turkey

65.1 Case Presentation

In a 34-year-old female patient, 1.2 cm thyroid nodule was detected in the right lobe of the thyroid in neck ultrasound (USG). Classical type of thyroid papillary carcinoma was determined according to the histopathological examination of fine needle aspiration biopsy (FNAB) of the nodule. For treatment bilateral total thyroidectomy was performed. Classical type of thyroid papillary carcinoma was confirmed after histopathological examination of thyroidectomy specimens. The tumor had no capsule. Perineural invasion, multicentricity, and lymphovascular invasion were not detected. Radioiodine ablation had been planned after the operation. However, the patient had been breastfeeding her baby, at 6 months age. Since radioiodine could be secreted to milk, it might be hazardous for the baby and mammary of the patient. For these reasons, breastfeeding had been ceased. In order to expedite of delactation, cabergoline 0.5 mg every other day for 6 weeks was used. No adverse effect was observed due to medication. Lactation had stopped 2 months later. In hypothyroid state, whole-body, Tc-99m (technetium) pertechnetate scintigraphy was performed to demonstrate any mammary uptake of the patient. There was no Tc-99m pertechnetate uptake in mammary glands of the patient (Fig. 65.1). In hypothyroid state (TSH = 71.6 mIU/l), thyroglobulin (Tg) and anti-thyroglobulin (anti-Tg) values were normal

T. Özülker et al. (eds.), *Thyroid and Parathyroid Diseases*, https://doi.org/10.1007/978-3-319-78476-2_65

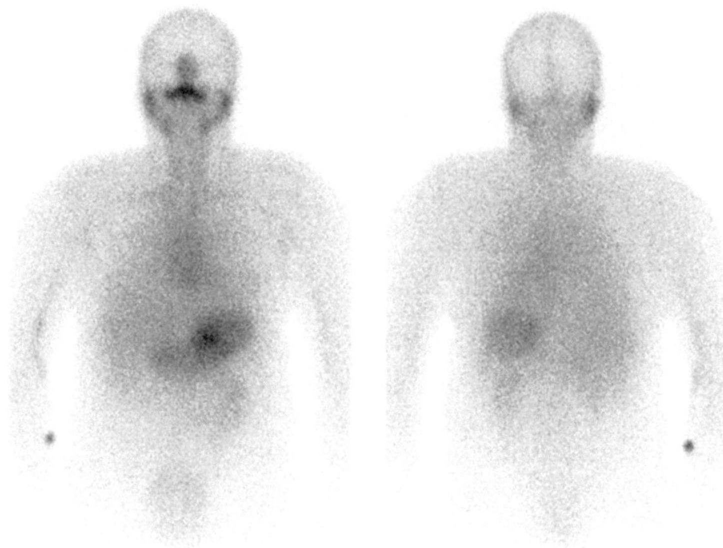

Fig. 65.1 Whole-body Tc-99m pertechnetate scintigraphy. Ten mCi Tc-99m pertechnetate was injected intravenously. Twenty minutes later anterior whole-body images were obtained using a double-head SPECT system (Infinia, GE Medical Systems, Milwaukee, WI, USA). There was no Tc-99m pertechnetate uptake in the mammary glands of the patient

(0.20 ng/ml and 21.1 IU/ml, respectively). One week later, 3700 MBq (100 mCi) I-131 (radioiodine) was given orally to the patient for remnant ablation. At the seventh day of ablation, post-ablative whole-body I-131 scintigraphy was performed (Fig. 65.2). There was no pathological uptake both in the neck region and in the mammary glands of the patient. After 9 months five mCi I-131 was given to the patient for control whole-body scintigraphy when the patient's TSH, Tg, and anti-Tg were 92 mIU/l, <0.2 ng/ml, and <2.2 IU/ml, respectively. There was no pathological uptake in that scintigraphy (Fig. 65.3).

65.2 Discussion

Primary curative treatment of well-differentiated thyroid carcinoma is known for that surgery. On the other hand, radioiodine (I-131) has been used efficiently not only for thyroid remnant ablation but also for metastasis of well-differentiated thyroid carcinoma. According to practice guidelines, ablation with I-131 is effective for preventing local recurrence of well-differentiated thyroid carcinoma [1–3]. Although there are some conflicts between procedure guidelines for indications of radioiodine ablation, usually it is recommended for thyroid cancer patients with high-risk factors (1–3). Tg is considered as a very useful tumor marker of well-differentiated thyroid cancer. After successful ablation of thyroid remnants, Tg is not detectable. This circumstance simplifies the follow-up of thyroid cancer patients, because any rise in Tg means that local recurrence or metastasis is present. Remnant ablation of thyroid cancer patients with radioiodine at least provides enhancement of sensitivity of Tg results. At the same time, ablation of the thyroid increases the sensitivity and specificity of whole-body I-131 scintigraphy in follow-up period [1].

Since I-131 could cross the placenta and be secreted to milk, radioiodine is contraindicated in pregnant and breastfeeding patients [1–3]. In a lactating patient, usage of I-131 exposes the patients' mammary and baby to unnecessary radiation. This radiation could cause radiation damage to baby's thyroid and other organs. Also, it is theoretically carcinogenic for the baby and patients' mammary.

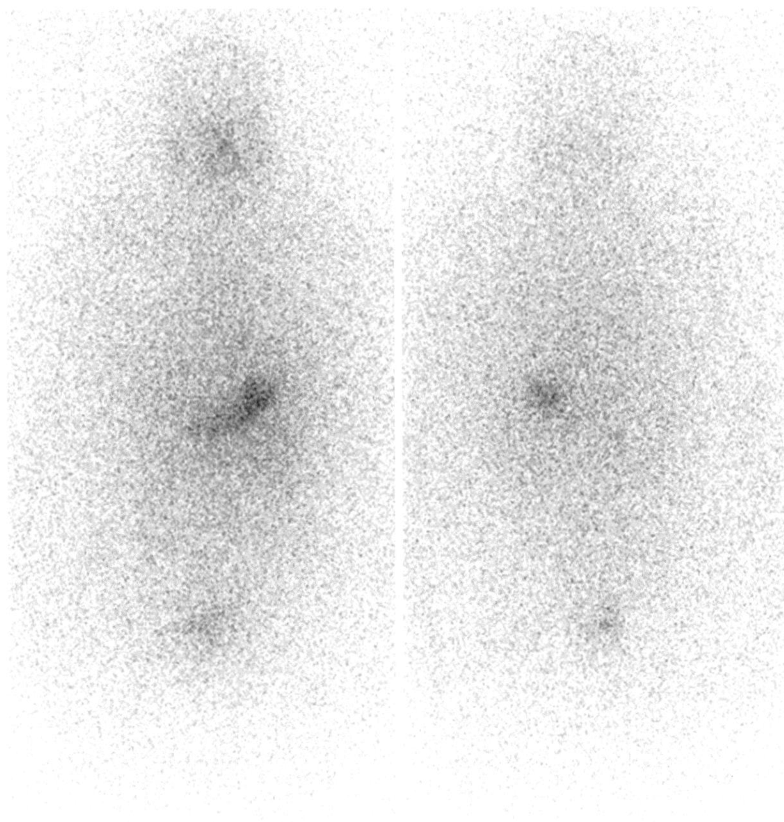

Fig. 65.2 Post-ablative whole-body I-131 scintigraphy. At the 7th day of ablation, post-ablative whole-body I-131 scintigraphy was performed by the same gamma camera. There was no pathological uptake both in the neck region and in the mammary glands of the patient

Therefore, breastfeeding must be ceased in patients who are a candidate for radioiodine remnant ablation or treatment of metastasis of well-differentiated thyroid carcinoma. Lactation could be disappeared spontaneously after stopping of breastfeeding. However, sometimes it may prolong and cause delaying of radioiodine treatment. In this situation, lactation inhibition medications such as bromocriptine and cabergoline may be used for acceleration of delactation [3]. Therefore, we preferred to use cabergoline in the present case. It provided ceasing of lactation quickly and efficiently. In order to be sure that there was no mammary gland uptake, ^{123}I or Tc-99m pertechnetate scintigraphy could be performed as a guidance of radioiodine ablation timing. Cellular uptake of ^{123}I is the same for I-131. I-131 has beta and gamma energy, whereas ^{123}I has only gamma radiation. Therefore, ^{123}I has no destructive effects. However, ^{123}I is expensive and has availability problems because it is produced in the cyclotron. In spite of that, ^{99m} Tc pertechnetate is a pure gamma emitter agent, cheap, and routinely available in any nuclear medicine department since it is produced from the generator. At the same time, uptake of ^{99m}Tc pertechnetate in the epithelial cells of the breast, like that of iodide, depends on the transmembrane sodium/iodide symporter (NIS). Therefore, ^{99m}Tc pertechnetate is a good alternative radiopharmaceutical for control of mammary uptake. In the present case, we performed ^{99m}Tc pertechnetate scintigraphy after ceasing of lactation to control mammary uptake.

Cellular uptake of radioiodine to follicular thyroid cell is done via sodium iodide symporter (NIS) located in the basal membrane of follicular cells [4]. Expression of NIS in salivary and lacrimal glands, stomach, choroid plexus, ciliary

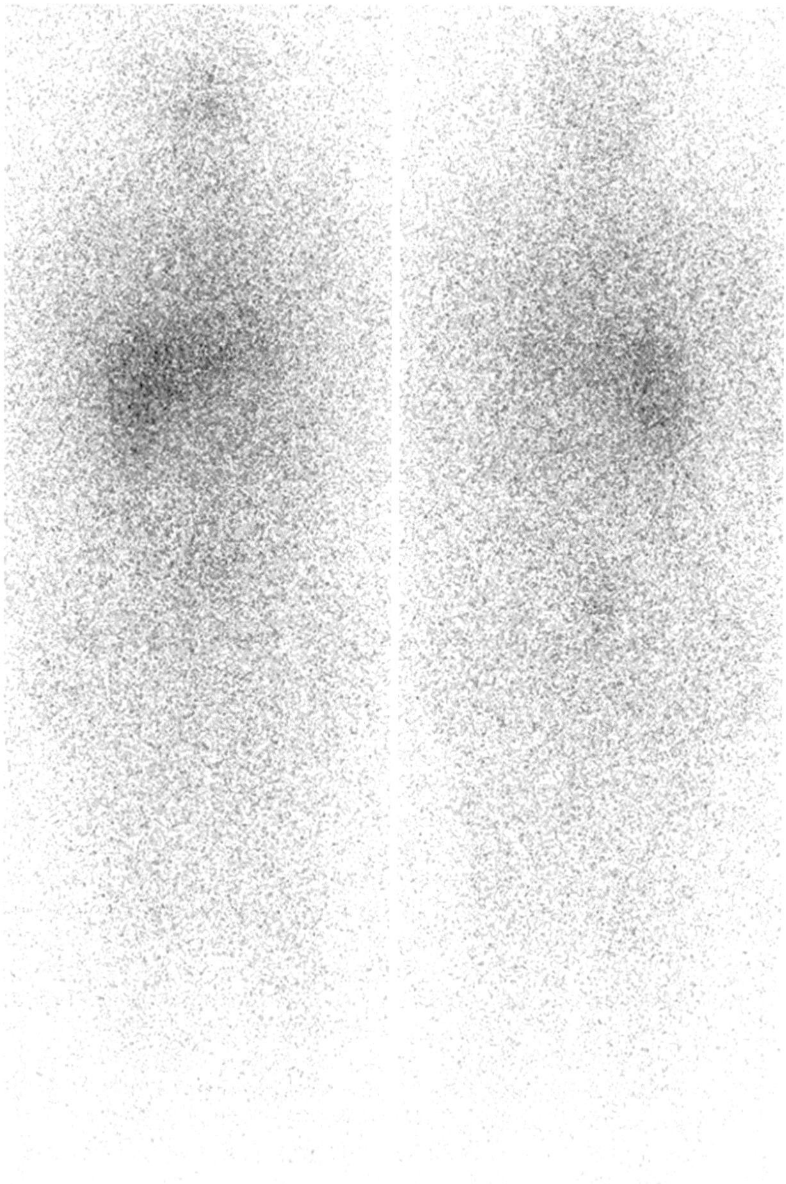

Fig. 65.3 Control whole-body I-131 scintigraphy at the 9th month of radioiodine ablation. Images were obtained by the same gamma camera after 72 h of oral intake of 5 mCi I-131. Also, there was no pathological I-131 uptake

body of the eye, skin, placenta, lactating mammary gland, thymus, and, to a lesser extent, the prostate, ovary, adrenal gland, lung, and heart has been demonstrated [4–6]. Therefore physiologic radioiodine uptake in lactating mammary gland could be explained by these mechanisms.

Although in the present case there was no breast uptake of I-131, it may be observed depending on several reasons. Lactation and breastfeeding are the main causatives of mammary uptake of radioiodine [4, 7–9]. Also, some drugs, breast stimulation, hypothyroidism, prolactinemia, galactorrhea, fat necrosis, gynecomastia, benign fibroadenoma, breast metastasis, breast carcinoma, and breast cyst can cause mammary uptake [10–16]. Sometimes, breast uptake in diagnostic or post-ablative I-131 scintigraphy may be misinterpreted as lung metastasis. Lateral images and SPECT and/or SPECT-CT images prevent this misdiagnosis.

In summary in women who are breastfeeding, lactating must be stopped before radioiodine treatment (ablation or metastasis). Some lactation inhibition medications could be used in order to quicken the procedure. In order to control any mammary gland uptake, I-123 or Tc-99m pertechnetate scintigraphy could be used.

What Can We Learn from This Case?

- Since I-131 could cross to the placenta and be secreted to milk, radioiodine is contraindicated in pregnant and breastfeeding patients.
- Cellular uptake of radioiodine to follicular thyroid cell is done via sodium iodide symporter (NIS) located in the basal membrane of follicular cells.
- In women who are breastfeeding, lactating must be stopped before radioiodine treatment.
- Some lactation inhibition medications could be used in order to quicken delectating procedure.
- ^{99m}Tc pertechnetate is a good alternative radiopharmaceutical for control of mammary uptake in well-differentiated thyroid carcinoma patients who are candidates for radioiodine treatment.

References

1. Luster M, Clarke SE, Dietlein M, Lassmann M, Lind P, Oyen WJ, European Association of Nuclear Medicine (EANM), et al. Guidelines for radioiodine therapy of differentiated thyroid cancer. Eur J Nucl Med Mol Imaging. 2008;35:1941–59. https://doi.org/10.1007/s00259-008-0883-1.
2. Silberstein EB, Alavi A, Balon HR, Clarke SE, Divgi C, Gelfand MJ, et al. The SNMMI practice guideline for therapy of thyroid disease with I-131 3.0. J Nucl Med. 2012;53:1633–51.
3. Haugen BR, Alexander EK, Bible KC, Doherty GM, Mandel SJ, Nikiforov YE, et al. American Thyroid Association management guidelines for adult patients with thyroid nodules and differentiated thyroid Cancer: the American Thyroid Association guidelines task force on thyroid nodules and differentiated thyroid Cancer. Thyroid. 2015;26:1–133.
4. Oh JR, Ahn BC. False-positive uptake on radioiodine whole-body scintigraphy: physiologic and pathologic variants unrelated to thyroid cancer. Am J Nucl Med Mol Imaging. 2012;2:362–85.
5. Simon SL, Luckyanov N, Bouville A, VanMiddlesworth L, Weinstock RM. Transfer of I-131 into human breast milk and transfer coefficients for radiological dose assessments. Health Phys. 2002;82:796–806.
6. Bruno R, Giannasio P, Ronga G, Baudin E, Travagli JP, Russo D, et al. Sodium iodide symporter expression and radioiodine distribution in extrathyroidal tissues. J Endocrinol Investig. 2004;27:1010–4.
7. Hsiao E, Huynh T, Mansberg R, Bautovich G, Roach P. Diagnostic I-123 scintigraphy to assess potential breast uptake of I-131 before radioiodine therapy in a postpartum woman with thyroid cancer. Clin Nucl Med. 2004;29:498–501.
8. Bakheet SM, Hammami MM. Patterns of radioiodine uptake by the lactating breast. Eur J Nucl Med. 1994;21:604–8.
9. Hammami MM, Bakheet S. Radioiodine breast uptake in nonbreastfeeding women: clinical and scintigraphic characteristics. J Nucl Med. 1996;37:26–31.
10. Itani M, Lewis DH. I-131 uptake in fat necrosis of the breast. Radiol Case Rep. 2016;23:161–7.
11. Uslu L, Ozbayrak M, Vatankulu B, Sonmezoglu K. Bilateral breast uptake of radioiodine in a male patient with gynecomastia: a case report. Indian J Nucl Med. 2015;30:345–6.
12. Ronga G, Bruno R, Puxeddu E, Calcinaro F, Montesano T, Travascio L, et al. Radioiodine uptake in non-lactating mammary glands: evidence for a causative role of hyperprolactinemia. Thyroid. 2007;17:363–6.
13. Berger F, Unterholzner S, Diebold J, Knesewitsch P, Hahn K, Spitzweg C. Mammary radioiodine accumulation due to functional sodium iodide symporter expression in a benign fibroadenoma. Biochem Biophys Res Commun. 2006;349:1258–63.
14. Tutal E, Tütüncü NB, Akçaer N, Bilezikçi B, Güvener N, Arican A. Unusual case of metastatic thyroid nodule: nonpalpable breast mass as origin. Endocr Pract. 2001;7:379–82.
15. Serafini A, Sfakianakis G, Georgiou M, Morris J. Breast cyst simulating metastases on iodine-131 imaging in thyroid carcinoma. J Nucl Med. 1998;39:1910–2.
16. Kim MH, Kim HS, Park SA. Extrathyroidal radioiodine accumulation in a Fibroadenoma of the breast. Clin Nucl Med. 2017;42:123–5.

A Child with Papillary Thyroid Carcinoma: Role of Radioactive Iodine Therapy in Pediatric Patients

66

Çiğdem Soydal and Elgin Özkan

Abstract

A 13-year-old girl with a family history of thyroid carcinoma underwent thyroid ultrasound. A hypoechoic thyroid nodule with a 4 cm diameter was detected on the right thyroid lobe accompanying enlarged central compartment lymph nodes. Thus, the patient underwent total thyroidectomy and bilaterally central compartment lymph node dissection. Pathological examination revealed a conventional subtype papillary thyroid carcinoma located on the right thyroid lobe with a 4 cm diameter. Contrast-enhanced tomography of the thorax showed multiple metastatic nodules in both lungs. The patient was referred for radioiodine treatment (RAT) with a T3N1aM1 tumor. During radioiodine treatment, serum thyroglobulin (Tg) levels were measured as >472 ng/ml. Posttreatment I-131 whole-body scintigraphy showed multiple radioactivity accumulations in the neck and both hemithoraces.

Ç. Soydal (✉)
Department of Nuclear Medicine, Ankara University School of Medicine, Ankara, Turkey

E. Özkan
Department of Nuclear Medicine, Medical Faculty of Ankara University, Ankara, Turkey

66.1 Case Presentation

A 13-year-old girl with a family history of thyroid carcinoma underwent thyroid ultrasound (USG). A hypoechoic thyroid nodule with a 4 cm diameter was detected on the right thyroid lobe accompanying enlarged central compartment lymph nodes. Thus, the patient underwent total thyroidectomy and bilaterally central compartment lymph node dissection. Pathological examination revealed a conventional subtype papillary thyroid carcinoma located on the right thyroid lobe with a 4 cm diameter. Additionally, multiple metastatic lymph nodes were detected in the central compartment with the largest being 2 cm in diameter. Contrast-enhanced tomography (CT) of the thorax revealed multiple metastatic nodules in both lungs. The patient was referred for radioiodine treatment (RAT) with a T3N1aM1 tumor. During radioiodine treatment, serum thyroglobulin (Tg) levels were measured as >472 ng/ml. An empiric does of 3700 Mbq (100 mCi) I-131 was administered orally. Posttreatment I-131 whole-body scintigraphy showed multiple foci of radioiodine in the neck and both hemithoraces (Fig. 66.1).

Although differentiated thyroid carcinomas (DTC) are rare in children and adolescents, it is the most common endocrine neoplasia [1–3].

T. Özülker et al. (eds.), *Thyroid and Parathyroid Diseases*, https://doi.org/10.1007/978-3-319-78476-2_66

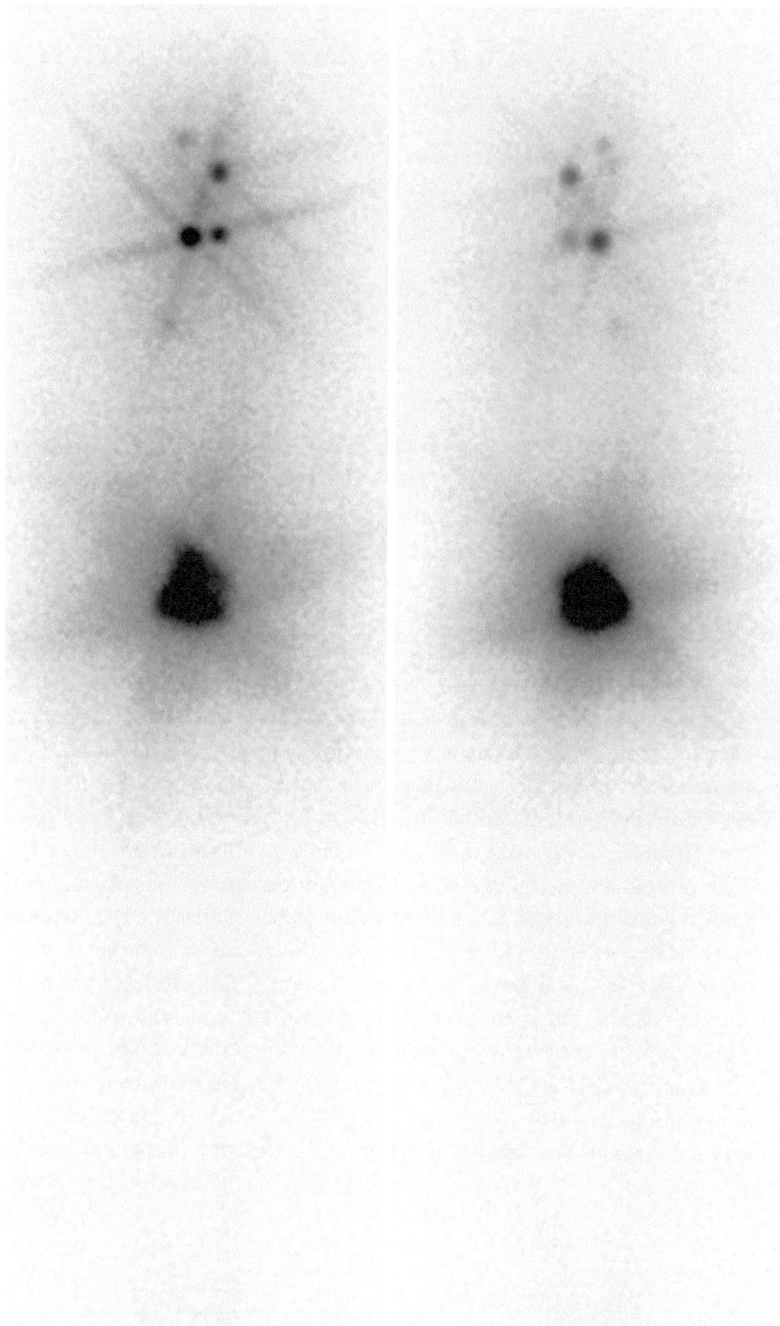

Fig. 66.1 Posttreatment I-131 whole-body scintigraphy demonstrated multiple accumulations of radioactivity in the neck and both hemithoraces

Moreover, its incidence has been rising [4–6]. As observed in our patient, DTCs in childhood are more often manifested as lymph node or lung metastases as compared to adults. For this reason, detailed ultrasonographic evaluation of thyroid gland and lymph nodes by an experienced hand is necessary during the preoperative stage. In patients with suspected lymph nodes, central compartment lymph node dissection is recommended [7]. This group of patients also has a high risk of developing lung metastases. A chest X-ray and/or chest CT may be considered for evaluation of possible lung metastases [8, 9]. Routine chest CT is not recommended for patients with minimal neck disease because lung metastases are likely to be identified when the patient is staged with stimulated Tg measurement and diagnostic whole-body scintigraphy. Differently from our patient, lung metastases tend to be in the miliary pattern [7]. In this case, they could be apparent after RAI treatment but are not usually visible using chest X-ray or CT. Regardless of the stage of the metastases at the diagnosis, the prognosis can be excellent when appropriately treated [1, 10, 11, 12]. Because pediatric DTCs are rare, treatment concepts for this population are derived from experience in treating the adult population. From diagnosis to treatment to long-term follow-up, several issues need to be addressed. In radioiodine avid patients, lung metastases are especially affected by radioiodine treatment. However, in regard to life expectancy, a benefit-loss ratio should be considered for repeated treatments [9].

The patient received a suppressive dose of LT4 after RAIT, and a sixth-month diagnostic whole-body scintigraphy was performed with 185 MBq (5 mCi) I-131. Stimulated Tg levels were measured at 38.2 ng/ml, and scintigraphy was normal. Because lung metastases were radioiodine avid, the second dose of RAIT was administered with 5550 MBq (150 mCi) I-131. Posttreatment, whole-body scintigraphy revealed faint radioactivity accumulation on both hemithoraces. Distant metastases of children are more amenable and responsive to RAT. Serial administrations of RAT can result in a complete response in many patients. However, the vast majority of patients will have stable metastatic disease [8, 9]. Moreover, studies have demonstrated a continuous improvement in serum Tg levels for years without repeated treatment with RAI. In regard to low complete response rates, a full response can take several years, so undetectable Tg levels should not be the goal of the treatment [7].

66.2 Follow-Up and Outcome

Following the second dose of RAI, Tg levels dropped dramatically to undetectable levels. Thorax CT was normal and stimulated Tg levels were within acceptable levels (<5 ng/ml). The patient was followed up with indeterminate biochemical response 5 years after. During this period, pulmonary fibrosis of secondary malignancies was not observed. There are acute and chronic side effects of RAI treatment. The acute side effects are generally transient. However, the chronic side effects on life expectancy may be an important consideration in regard to treating children [7]. Development of secondary malignancies should also be considered in children. Previous reports have found that children treated with radiation (external beam radiation, radium implants, and RAIT) developed secondary malignancies, such as leukemia and cancers of the stomach, bladder, colon, salivary gland, and breast [8, 9]. Unfortunately, it is difficult to determine a safe cumulative dose for pediatric patients. Different safe cumulative dose limits have previously been described [10, 12]. Another important concern in patients with lung metastases is that pulmonary fibrosis can develop when retained RAT dose exceeded 80 mCi [10, 11]. In summary, the risks and benefits of RAT treatment should be taken into greater consideration when treating children.

66.2.1 The Future

The nature of childhood DTCs is different from adults in the timing of its presentation at diagnosis and response to treatment. Children-specific management guidelines should be prepared to guide long-term follow-up protocols. Another issue that needs to be addressed is the lack of data on the usage of other systemic treatment options, such as tyrosine kinase inhibitors (TKI), for non-avid radioiodine child patients.

What Can We Learn from This Case?

- DTCs are the most common endocrine neoplasia in childhood.
- DTCs in children manifest as lymph node or lung metastases more often than adults.
- Lung metastases exhibit mostly miliary patterns in children.
- Regardless of the disease stage at diagnosis, the prognosis is excellent when appropriately treated.

References

1. Verburg FA, Van Santen HM, Luster M. Pediatric papillary thyroid cancer: current management challenges. Onco Targets Ther. 2016;28:165–75. https://doi.org/10.2147/OTT.S100512.
2. Rapkin L, Pashankar FD. Management of thyroid carcinoma in children and young adults. J Pediatr Hematol Oncol. 2012;34:39–46. https://doi.org/10.1097/MPH.0b013e31824e37a6.
3. Hung W, Sarlis NJ. Current controversies in the management of pediatric patients with well-differentiated nonmedullary thyroid cancer: a review. Thyroid. 2002;12:683–702. https://doi.org/10.1089/105072502760258668.
4. Ying AK, Huh W, Bottomley S, Evans DB, Waguespack SG. Thyroid cancer in young adults. Semin Oncol. 2009;36:258–74. https://doi.org/10.1053/j.seminoncol.2009.03.009.
5. Hogan AR, Zhuge Y, Perez EA, Koniaris LG, Lew JI, Sola JE. Pediatric thyroid carcinoma: incidence and outcomes in 1753 patients. J Surg Res. 2009;156:167–72. https://doi.org/10.1016/j.jss.2009.03.098.
6. Shapiro NL, Bhattacharyya N. Population-based outcomes for pediatric thyroid carcinoma. Laryngoscope. 2005;115:337–40. https://doi.org/10.1097/01.mlg.0000154743.71184.09.
7. Francis GL, Waguespack SG, Bauer AJ, Angelos P, Benvenga S, Cerutti JM, et al. Management guidelines for children with thyroid nodules and differentiated thyroid cancer.; American Thyroid Association guidelines task force. Thyroid. 2015;25:716–59. https://doi.org/10.1089/thy.2014.0460.
8. Brink JS, van Heerden JA, McIver B, Salomao DR, Farley DR, Grant CS, et al. Papillary thyroid cancer with pulmonary metastases in children: long-term prognosis. Surgery. 2000;128(6):881. https://doi.org/10.1067/msy.2000.109728.
9. Jarzab B, Handkiewicz-Junak D. Differentiated thyroid cancer in children and adults: same or distinct disease? Hormones (Athens). 2007;6:200–9.
10. Rachmiel M, Charron M, Gupta A, Hamilton J, Wherrett D, Forte V, et al. Evidence-based review of treatment and follow up of pediatric patients with differentiated thyroid carcinoma. J Pediatr Endocrinol Metab. 2006;19:1377–93.
11. Thompson GB, Hay ID. Current strategies for surgical management and adjuvant treatment of childhood papillary thyroid carcinoma. World J Surg. 2004;28:1187–98. https://doi.org/10.1007/s00268-004-7605-z.
12. Rubino C, de Vathaire F, Dottorini ME, Hall P, Schvartz C, Couette JE, et al. Second primary malignancies in thyroid cancer patients. Br J Cancer. 2003;89:1638–44. https://doi.org/10.1038/sj.bjc.6601319.

67 Pediatric PTC with Diffuse Lung Metastases: Pulmonary Function Testing and Steroid Therapy Prior to RAI

Zehra Özcan and Ülkem Yararbaş

Abstract

Thyroid carcinoma is an uncommon malignancy in children, and metastatic involvement at initial presentation is much more common than adults. The clinical course of the disease is favorable; however, management is challenging due to differences in biologic behavior of the tumor and potential side effects of I-131 in the long-term follow-up. The current pediatric case highlights the possible pulmonary fibrosis after radioiodine treatment and indicates the importance of dose optimization particularly in children with diffuse lung metastases.

67.1 Case Presentation

The represented case is a child with differentiated thyroid carcinoma under clinical follow-up since 1998. He was initially presented with a neck mass when he was 8 years old. Excisional biopsy showed lymph node metastasis of papillary thyroid carcinoma. He underwent total thyroidectomy and completion surgery after that. Surgical specimen showed papillary carcinoma 2 cm in size with a follicular histologic variant with microscopic involvement on both lobes. There were capsular invasion and a metastatic lymph node in left cervical level IV with the largest diameter of 15 mm. He received a fixed dose of 80 mCi (2.96 GBq) radioactive iodine (RAI) adjusted according to the body weight (7.4 MBq/kg) [1, 2]. Posttreatment scan revealed remnant tissue and iodine uptake in the right lateral cervical region and in both lungs more prominently in the basal regions (Fig. 67.1). At the time of RAI therapy, serum Tg was 64.5 ng/ml, and anti-Tg antibodies were normal. He was T4a, N1b, M1, and stage II according to the AJCC/UICC TNM system as noted in ATA guidelines on pediatric thyroid cancer [2]. CT scan detected multiple tiny parenchymal nodules supporting lung involvement. He received three additional therapeutic doses of I-131 for locoregional disease and metastatic lung involvement with the spread over a period of 11 years. The total cumulative activity was 430 mCi (15.9 GBq). These repeated doses were applied using a fixed-dose approach according to the body weight. After the first RAI treatment, he presented with pulmonary problems such as a cough and exertional dyspnea and referred to a pediatric pulmonologist. Respiratory function test showed subnormal diffusing capacity. It was stated that this might be related to both micrometastatic lung disease and radiation-induced changes, and follow-up is recommended. Twelve months after the first treatment second dose, I-131 was given 100 mCi (3.7 GBq).

Z. Özcan (✉) · Ü. Yararbaş
Department of Nuclear Medicine, Ege University School of Medicine, Izmir, Turkey

T. Özülker et al. (eds.), *Thyroid and Parathyroid Diseases*, https://doi.org/10.1007/978-3-319-78476-2_67

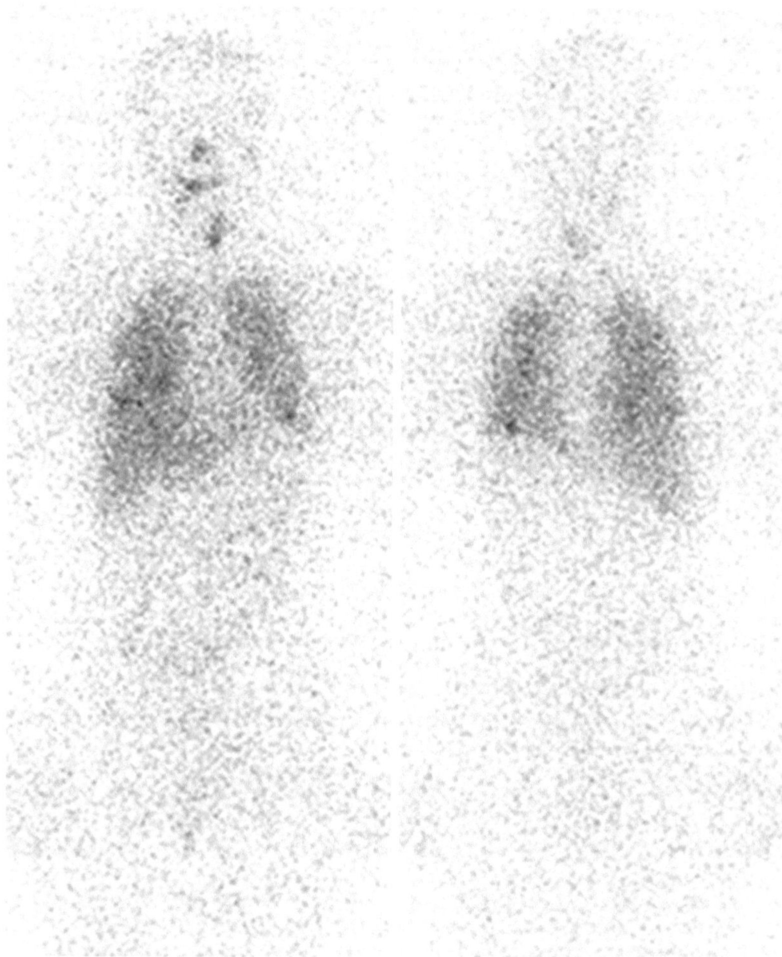

Fig. 67.1 Posttreatment I-131 scan shows diffuse bilateral involvement and uptake in the left cervical region

Posttreatment scan revealed iodine accumulation in both lungs in a diffuse pattern. Pulmonary function tests indicated by FEV1 and VC suggested restrictive changes. Pediatric pulmonologists recommended that oral corticosteroid treatment can be given for a week (during the hospitalization period of RAI treatment and slowly stopping after hospital discharge) to avoid pulmonary edema and to control the consequences of absorbed radiation dose in the bronchoalveolar system.

67.2 Discussion

Pediatric thyroid carcinoma generally has favorable clinical course despite the locoregional disease or distant metastatic involvement at the initial presentation [1, 3]. On the other hand, therapeutic approach is thought-provoking due to the increased risk for secondary tumors and late-term radiation-induced complications, particularly in young children. As defined in ATA guideline, there is a consensus that the goal of therapy in children is to decrease disease-specific mortality and reduce possible side effects [1]. I-131 treatment is mostly given by the simplest method, empiric fixed-dose administration. Additionally, as there is no standard dose for pediatric ages, the adult fixed dose is modified according to the child's age, body weight, or surface area [2]. On the other hand, pulmonary involvement is usually in a micronodular pattern spread diffusely over both lungs, and there is a concern about treatment-inducd pulmonary fibrosis [4–7]. Reduced dose or dosimetric approach is suggeted to protect healthy lung tissue and to reduce the risk of radiation-induced changes [6, 7]. It is widely accepted that the absorbed dose should not exceed 200 cGy, and the whole-body retention should not be more than 80 mCi (2.96 GBq) and 120 mCi (4.44 GBq) in the absence or presence of pulmonary metastases, respectively [8]. It is also stated that the intervals between the subsequent doses should be extended, and cumulated activity should be disseminated over a long time (4). In the current case, unfortunately, we were not able to perform whole-body dosimetry; however, as the initial treatment dose was 2.96 GBq, it can be postulated that the safety limit defined as 80 mCi (2.96 GBq) whole-body retention at 48 h after RAI administration is hardly surpassed. Interestingly, we have observed mild pulmonary functional impairment after the first radioiodine treatment. As there is no data about the previous lung functioning tests or thorax CT, it is problematic to comment on the causal relationship of radiation-induced pulmonary fibrosis. But there was no prior radiation exposure to the thorax or concomitant use of a chemotherapeutic agent that might accentuate pulmonary fibrotic changes. Nevertheless, it is postulated radiation-induced lung injury may either happen as an early (<6 months) or late event (>6 months) [9]. Within the days to weeks after radiation exposure, destruction of alveolar epithelium leads to accumulation of inflammatory cells and induces cytokine release. In the second stage of this process, oxidative damage, an influx of fibroblasts, and their conversion to myofibroblasts result in lung fibrosis. Although there is no defined standard regimen for the management of radiation-induced pulmonary fibrosis, anti-inflammatory drugs including corticosteroids and supportive measures can be effective [10].

Pulmonary fibrosis due to radioiodine is reported as an infrequent sequel. Hebestreit et al. documented seven cases of pulmonary fibrosis in his series covering 69 children with juvenile thyroid carcinoma [7]. However, the authors stated that the development of pulmonary fibrosis poses a significant problem in patient management. Moreover, young age at the time of the iodine treatment and the use of concomitant chemotherapeutic agents may increase the risk for fibrotic pulmonary changes. It is therefore recommended to perform pulmonary function test in young children with diffuse high iodine avid lung involvement particularly when subsequent treatments are planned [1, 6]. Therefore, pretherapeutic dosimetry seems to be a valuable approach for nuclear medicine physicians to estimate the effective dose within safe limits in children with lung metastases [11, 12].

67.3 Follow-Up and Clinical Course

This case had received the first RAI treatment at the age of 10 and the last one when he was 21 years old. The total cumulative activity (15.9 GBq) was distributed over a very long time with intervals exceeding 12 months. He is currently stable with the disease under TSH suppression, and his Tg level is 0.3 ng/dl. There is a restrictive pattern of functional impairment and CT findings suggesting pulmonary fibrosis (Fig. 67.2) which did not show significant changes throughout the clinical course.

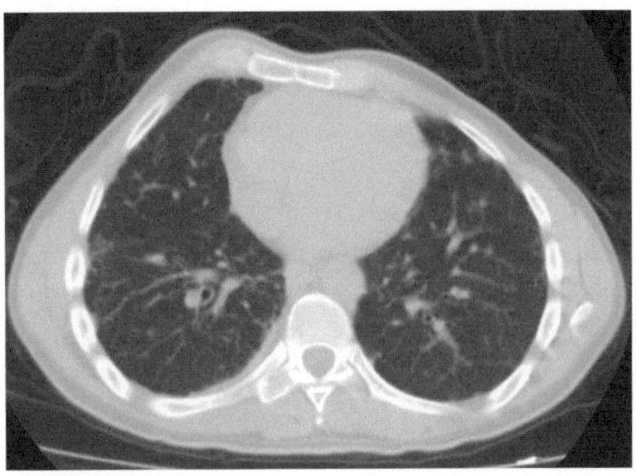

Fig. 67.2 Transaxial CT scan shows bilateral diffuse septal thickening and pleural irregularities suggesting pulmonary fibrosis

What Can We Learn from This Case?

- It is not uncommon to come across with diffuse micrometastatic lung involvement in children with DTC even at the initial presentation.
- RAI treatment is the current choice as long as the metastatic foci are iodine avid implying that good response is possible.
- However, regarding the radiosensitivity of children and expected life-span, it is essential to focus on the possible side effects.
- When available, the dosimetric approach might be reasonable to provide the safe therapeutic dose that would not do more harm than good.
- Moreover, it is suggested that those patients should be kept under clinical follow-up within the collaboration of a medical team to manage the late-term side effects.

References

1. Francis GL, Waguespack SG, Bauer AJ, Angelos P, Benvenga S, Cerutti JM, et al. Management guidelines for children with thyroid nodules and differentiated thyroid Cancer. Thyroid. 2015;25:716–59. https://doi.org/10.1089/thy.2014.0460.
2. Luster M, Clarke SE, Dietlein M, Lassmann M, Lind P, Oyen WJ, et al. Guidelines for radioiodine therapy of differentiated thyroid cancer. Eur J Nucl Med Mol Imaging. 2008;35:1941–59. https://doi.org/10.1007/s00259-008-0883-1.
3. Luster M, Pfestroff A, Hänscheid H, Verburg FA. Radioiodine therapy. Semin Nucl Med. 2017;47:126–34. https://doi.org/10.1053/j.semnuclmed.2016.10.002.
4. Verburg FA, Van Santen HM, Luster M. Pediatric papillary thyroid cancer: current management challenges. Onco Targets Ther. 2016;28:165–75. https://doi.org/10.2147/OTT.S100512.
5. Albano D, Bertagna F, Panarotto MB, Giubbini R. Early and late adverse effects of radioiodine for pediatric differentiated thyroid cancer. Pediatr Blood Cancer. 2017;64:1–7. https://doi.org/10.1002/pbc.26595.
6. Samuel AM, Rajashekharrao B, Shah DH. Pulmonary metastases in children and adolescents with well-differentiated thyroid cancer. J Nucl Med. 1998;39:1531–6.
7. Hebestreit H, Biko J, Drozd V, Demidchik Y, Burkhardt A, Trusen A. Pulmonary fibrosis in youth treated with radioiodine for juvenile thyroid cancer and lung metastases after Chernobyl. Eur J Nucl Med Mol Imaging. 2011;38:1683–90. https://doi.org/10.1007/s00259-011-1841-x.
8. Benua RS, Leeper RD. A method and rationale for treating metastatic thyroid carcinoma with the largest safe dose of 131I. In: Mederios-Neta G, Gaitan E, editors. Frontiers in thyridology. New York: Plenum Medical; 1986. p. 1317–21.
9. Tsoutsou PG, Koukourakis MI. Radiation pneumonitis and fibrosis: mechanisms underlying its pathogenesis and implications for future research. Int J Radiat Oncol Biol Phys. 2006;66:1281–93.
10. Giridhar P, Mallick S, Rath GK, Julka PK. Radiation induced lung injury: prediction, assessment and management. Asian Pac J Cancer Prev. 2015;16(7):2613.
11. Song H, He B, Prideaux A, Du Y, Frey E, Kasecamp W, Ladenson PW, et al. Lung dosimetry for radioiodine treatment planning in the case of diffuse lung metastases. J Nucl Med. 2006;47:1985–94.
12. Verburg FA, Biko J, Diessl S, Demidchik Y, Drozd V, Rivkees SA, et al. I-131 activities as high as safely administrable (AHASA) for the treatment of children and adolescents with advanced differentiated thyroid cancer. J Clin Endocrinol Metab. 2011;96:E1268–71. https://doi.org/10.1210/jc.2011-0520.

Part III

Parathyroid Diseases

68 Ectopic Parathyroid Adenoma

Hakan Demir

Abstract

Elevated serum calcium and parathyroid hormone (PTH) values were determined in routine laboratory examinations of a 66-year-old female patient. Parathyroid scintigraphy (PS) and neck ultrasonography (USG) were performed for diagnosis of primary hyperparathyroidism.

PS revealed an ectopic parathyroid gland in the mediastinum. Fused SPECT/CT images were generated from PS SPECT and CT images using the co-registration software. Exact localization of ectopic parathyroid adenoma could be performed by fused SPECT/CT images. With the help of gamma probe, a soft tissue mass 1 cm in size was excised from anterior mediastinum in mediastinoscopy. Histopathological examinations were consistent with parathyroid adenoma. The patient was discharged from hospital after dropping of serum calcium value to the normal level.

In conclusion preoperative localization of abnormal ectopic parathyroid gland was done easily and more precisely by PS SPECT/CT in this case. And also, using gamma probe in parathyroidectomy helped to surgeons to find ectopic parathyroid adenoma quickly and precisely.

68.1 Case Presentation

Elevated serum calcium (11 mg/dl) and parathyroid hormone (PTH) (311.9 pg/ml) values were determined in routine laboratory examinations of a 66-year-old female patient. Parathyroid scintigraphy (PS) and neck ultrasonography (USG) were performed for diagnosis of primary hyperparathyroidism.

After intravenous injection of 15 mCi ^{99m}Tc-MIBI (technetium-99m-sestamibi), planar and single photon emission computerized tomography (SPECT) images were obtained using a dual-head SPECT system (Infinia, GE Medical Systems, Milwaukee, WI, USA) at 15 (early) and 120 min (late) of injection (Figs. 68.1 and 68.2).

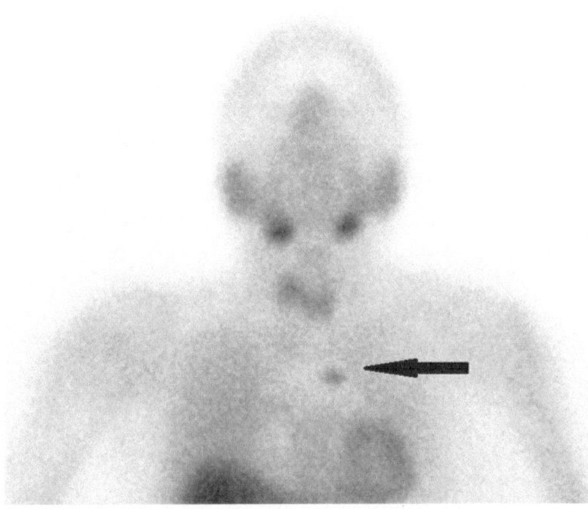

Fig. 68.1 Early (15 min) planar images of PS. Faint focal uptake was seen near to myocardium (arrow)

H. Demir
Department of Nuclear Medicine, School of Medicine, Kocaeli University, Kocaeli, Turkey

T. Özülker et al. (eds.), *Thyroid and Parathyroid Diseases*, https://doi.org/10.1007/978-3-319-78476-2_68

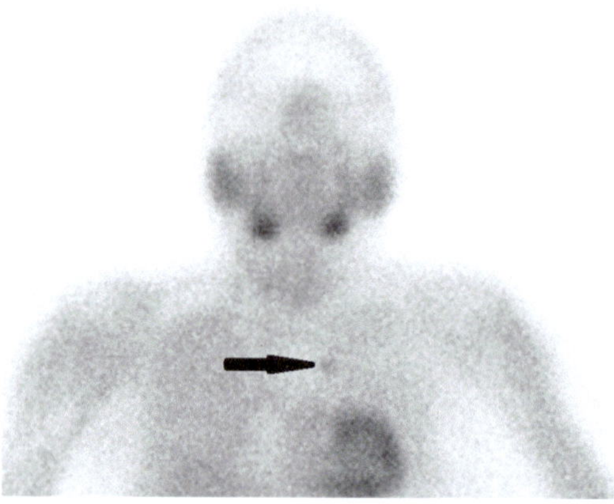

Fig. 68.2 Late (120 min) planar images of PS. Abnormal focal uptake near to myocardium was increased and could be distinguished more easily (arrow)

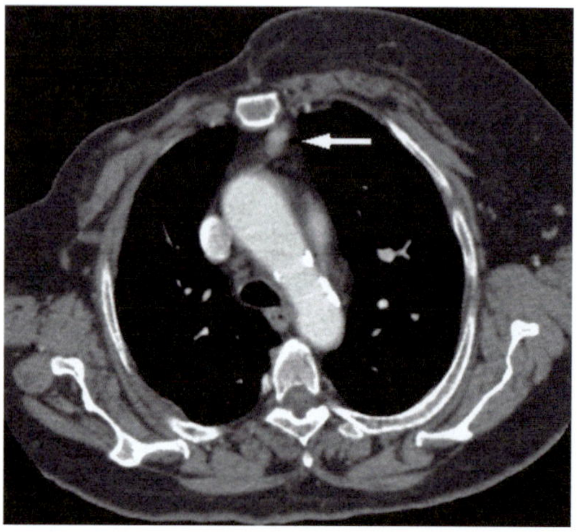

Fig. 68.3 Thorax CT images. A soft tissue mass (arrow) 15 × 9.5 mm. was seen in anterior mediastinum between sternum and arcus aorta

Focal pathological high uptake was found in early and late images of PS in the left part of anterior mediastinum, near to myocardium (Figs. 68.1 and 68.2). A soft tissue mass 15 × 9.5 mm. was detected in thorax computerized tomography images (CT) (Fig. 68.3). Fused SPECT/CT images were generated from PS SPECT and CT images using co-registration software (Integrated Registration, Xeleris 1.0, GE) (Fig. 68.4). Neck USG of the patient was normal.

According to these findings in PS ectopic parathyroid gland pathology was determined for the reason of primary hyperparathyroidism. Mediastinoscopy was planned for exact histopathological diagnosis and also treatment. A soft tissue mass 1 cm in size was excised from anterior mediastinum in mediastinoscopy with the help of gamma probe. Both frozen and final sections in histopathological examinations were consistent with parathyroid adenoma. The patient was discharged from hospital after dropping of serum calcium value to the normal level.

68.2 Discussion

There are usually two pairs (superior and inferior) of parathyroid glands in the neck region. They are located behind the thyroid gland. Occasionally the fifth gland may be present. In the embryologic period, the parathyroid glands develop at 6 weeks and migrate caudally at 8 weeks, and they reach their eutopic region [1, 2]. However, some migration

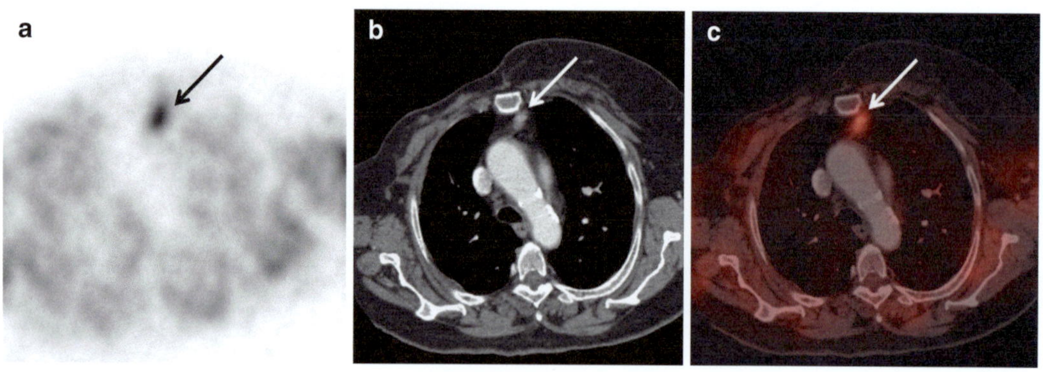

Fig. 68.4 Co-registered SPECT/CT images. Abnormal focal uptake of MIBI (arrows) in the soft tissue mass could be determined in transaxial SPECT (**a**), CT (**b**), and fused SPECT/CT images (**c**)

problems can cause ectopic parathyroid glands. Ectopic parathyroid glands may be present in mediastinum, thyroid gland, cervical region, thymus, carotid sheath, retropharynx, and retro- or paraesophageal space [1, 2].

Parathyroid glands are responsible for serum calcium and phosphorus ions' concentrations via secretion of parathyroid hormone (PTH). The secretion of PTH is regulated directly by the plasma concentration of ionized calcium [3]. Hyperparathyroidism is caused by factors that increase the production of PTH. It is usually subdivided into primary, secondary, and tertiary hyperparathyroidism. Hyperparathyroidism may occur because of a problem with the parathyroid glands themselves (primary hyperparathyroidism) or because of another disease that affects the glands' function (secondary hyperparathyroidism). Tertiary hyperparathyroidism is a state of excessive secretion of PTH after long-standing secondary hyperparathyroidism. It is characterized by the development of autonomous hypersecretion of PTH [4]. Sign and symptoms of hyperparathyroidism may be mild and nonspecific. Some of the most frequent signs and symptoms of hyperparathyroidism are nausea, vomiting, loss of appetite, weakness, excessive urination, abdominal pain, bone and joint pain, depression, forgetfulness, osteoporosis, kidney stones, and hypertension [5].

Primary hyperparathyroidism is frequently caused by (75–85%) solitary adenoma. Double adenomas are seen in 12%, three glands adenoma in <1–2%, and four or more adenomas in <1–15% of cases. Parathyroid carcinoma is responsible approximately 1% of cases with primary hyperparathyroidism [6].

The only curative treatment option is surgery for primary hyperparathyroidism. Four-gland exploration was gold standard procedure until recently. Nowadays, minimally invasive techniques are preferred after the rapid development of successful preoperative imaging methods such as PS for localization of pathological parathyroid gland. USG, CT, 4-D CT, and magnetic resonance imaging (MRI) are the other modalities for preoperative imaging for hyperparathyroidism. PS is preferred more than the others because of high-sensitivity values. According to a meta-analysis, published by Wong KK, CT sensitivity values of PS were 0.61–0.80, 0.74, and 0.86 for planar, SPECT, and SPECT/CT, respectively [7]. Preoperative imaging of pathological parathyroid glands offers several benefits to surgeons and patients. With the help of PS, length and complications of operation and anesthesia could be decreased meaningfully. Using minimally invasive technique reduces the size of the surgical incision. Patient's comfort could be increased. And also, cosmetic complaints of the patient's after surgery due to scar tissue may be reduced easily [8–10].

A few different radiopharmaceutical and imaging techniques could be used for PS. Dual-phase or tracer methods using single or combination of ^{201}Tl, ^{99m}Tc-MIBI, ^{99m}Tc- pertechnetate, and ^{123}I are the choices for PS. Coakley AJ and his colleagues used firstly ^{99m}Tc-MIBI as a radiopharmaceutical for PS, in 1989 [11]. Since then, usage of ^{99m}Tc-MIBI as a single agent (dual phase) or with other radiopharmaceutical (dual tracer) has gradually been increased. Nowadays, dual-phase ^{99m}Tc-MIBI imaging is the most preferred method for PS due to easy availability, high image quality, low cost, and easy practice [12, 13].

In the past planar and single photon emission tomography (SPECT) imaging procedures were performed, usually. Recently, the hybrid technique of SPECT/CT could be used after wide availability of new generation hybrid gamma cameras. With the help of SPECT/CT, precise localization of pathological parathyroid glands, especially ectopic, could be done more easily and correctly. Because of the high cost of modern hybrid gamma cameras, availability of this technique may be limited in some nuclear medicine departments. Nevertheless, a fusion of SPECT and CT images obtained in separate devices could be performed easily and effectively using the certain co-registration software. On the other hand, routine use of SPECT/CT for PS is not recommended in procedure guidelines [14, 15]. Sensitivity and specificity values of SPECT are higher than planar images [16]. Conversely, the superiority of SPECT/CT method over SPECT alone is controversial. Some authors did not find any significant difference between two methods [1]. They also emphasized some disadvantages of SPECT/CT: increasing cost, radiation dose, and total examination time because of CT [1, 17–20]. On the other hand, according to some recent literature, SPECT/CT has higher detection rates for parathyroid pathologies comparing only SPECT or planar images. Also, SPECT/CT provides more precise anatomic localization of ectopic parathyroid adenomas [7, 16, 21].

In the present case we performed planar, SPECT and fused SPECT/CT images for PS. We used ^{99m} Tc-MIBI and dual-phase method. Abnormal uptake in mediastinum due to pathological parathyroid tissue could be easily determined with not only planar but also SPECT images. However, exact anatomic localization of pathological uptake had been defined by fused SPECT/CT images. After precise localization of pathological ectopic parathyroid gland by PS with the help of gamma probe, a soft tissue mass was excised from anterior mediastinum of the present patient in mediastinoscopy. Gamma probe is a useful device for detecting sentinel lymph nodes in malignant melanoma and breast cancer patients [22, 23]. At the same time, gamma probe has been used for parathyroidectomy [24]. Firstly, Bonjer HJ and his colleagues used gamma probe for parathyroidectomy. They suggested using gamma probe in patients with persistent or recurrent hyperparathyroidism [24]. Recently usage rate of gamma probe in parathyroidectomy has been increasing. Since this technique shortens the total operation time. And also, it helps surgeons to be sure that excised tissue is related parathyroid gland because of high radioactivity [25–27]. Especially in ectopic parathyroid adenomas, gamma probe is very helpful [28–30].

In summary preoperative localization of abnormal ectopic parathyroid gland was done easily and more precisely by PS SPECT/CT in this case. And also, using gamma probe in parathyroidectomy helped surgeons to find ectopic parathyroid gland quickly and precisely.

What Can We Learn from This Case?

- An ectopic parathyroid adenoma could be responsible for primary hyperparathyroidism.
- PS is known as the most useful imaging modality for preoperative localization of pathological parathyroid glands.
- SPECT/CT has higher detection rates for parathyroid pathologies comparing only SPECT or planar images.
- SPECT/CT provides more precise anatomic localization of ectopic parathyroid adenomas.
- Surgeons can find ectopic parathyroid glands quickly and precisely in parathyroidectomy operations with the help of gamma probe.

References

1. Dasgupta DJ, Navalkissoor S, Ganatra R, Buscombe J. The role of single-photon emission computed tomography/computed tomography in localizing parathyroid adenoma. Nucl Med Commun. 2013;34:621–6.
2. Roy M, Mazeh H, Chen H, Sippel RS. Incidence and localization of ectopic parathyroid adenomas in previously unexplored patients. World J Surg. 2013;37:102–6.
3. Smith JR, Oates ME. Radionuclide imaging of the parathyroid glands: patterns, pearls, and pitfalls. Radiographics. 2004;24:1101–15.
4. Vestergaard P, Thomsen SV. Medical treatment of primary, secondary, and tertiary hyperparathyroidism. Curr Drug Saf. 2011;6:108–13.
5. Campbell MJ. The definitive management of primary hyperparathyroidism: who needs an operation? JAMA. 2017;317:1167–8.
6. Fraser WD. Hyperparathyroidism. Lancet. 2009;374:145–58.
7. Wong KK, Fig LM, Gross MD, Dwamena BA. Parathyroid adenoma localization with 99mTc-sestamibi SPECT/CT: a meta-analysis. Nucl Med Commun. 2015;36:363–75.
8. Desiato V, Melis M, Amato B, Bianco T, Rocca A, Amato M, et al. Minimally invasive radioguided parathyroid surgery: a literature review. Int J Surg. 2016;28(Suppl 1):S84–93.
9. Rubello D, Casara D, Giannini S, Piotto A, De Carlo E, Muzzio PC, et al. Importance of radio-guided

minimally invasive parathyroidectomy using hand-held gamma probe and low (99m)Tc-MIBI dose. Technical considerations and long-term clinical results. Q J Nucl Med. 2003;47:129–38.
10. Ikeda Y, Takayama J, Takami H. Minimally invasive radioguided parathyroidectomy for hyperparathyroidism. Ann Nucl Med. 2010;24:233–40.
11. Coakley AJ, Kettle AG, Wells CP, O'Doherty MJ, Collins RE. 99Tcm sestamibi—a new agent for parathyroid imaging. Nucl Med Commun. 1989;10:791–4.
12. Treglia G, Trimboli P, Huellner M, Giovanella L. Imaging in primary hyperparathyroidism: focus on the evidence-based diagnostic performance of different methods. Minerva Endocrinol. 2017. https://doi.org/10.23736/S0391-1977.17.02685-2.
13. Geatti O, Shapiro B, Orsolon PG, Proto G, Guerra UP, Antonucci F, et al. Localization of parathyroid enlargement: experience with technetium-99m methoxyisobutylisonitrile and thallium-201 scintigraphy, ultrasonography and computed tomography. Eur J Nucl Med. 1994;21:17–22.
14. Hindié E, Ugur O, Fuster D, O'Doherty M, Grassetto G, Ureña P, et al. Parathyroid task group of the EANM. 2009 EANM parathyroid guidelines. Eur J Nucl Med Mol Imaging. 2009;36:1201–16.
15. Greenspan BS, Dillehay G, Intenzo C, Lavely WC, O'Doherty M, Palestro CJ, et al. SNM practice guideline for parathyroid scintigraphy 4.0. J Nucl Med Technol. 2012;40:111–8.
16. Serra A, Bolasco P, Satta L, Nicolosi A, Uccheddu A, Piga M. Role of SPECT/CT in the preoperative assessment of hyperparathyroid patients. Radiol Med. 2006;111:999–1008.
17. Setabutr D, Vakharia K, Nogan SJ, Kamel GN, Allen T, Saunders BD, et al. Comparison of SPECT/CT and planar MIBI in terms of operating time and cost in the surgical management of primary hyperparathyroidism. Ear Nose Throat J. 2015;94:448–52.
18. Papathanassiou D, Flament JB, Pochart JM, Patey M, Marty H, Liehn JC, et al. SPECT/CT in localization of parathyroid adenoma or hyperplasia in patients with previous neck surgery. Clin Nucl Med. 2008;33:394–7.
19. Gayed IW, Kim EE, Broussard WF, Evans D, Lee J, Broemeling LD, et al. The value of 99mTc-sestamibi SPECT/CT over conventional SPECT in the evaluation of parathyroid adenomas or hyperplasia. J Nucl Med. 2005;46:248–52.
20. Treglia G, Sadeghi R, Schalin-Jäntti C, Caldarella C, Ceriani L, Giovanella L, et al. Detection rate of (99m)Tc-MIBI single photon emission computed tomography (SPECT)/CT in preoperative planning for patients with primary hyperparathyroidism: a meta-analysis. Head Neck. 2016;38(Suppl 1):E2159–72.
21. Lavely WC, Goetze S, Friedman KP, Leal JP, Zhang Z, Garret-Mayer E, et al. Comparison of SPECT/CT, SPECT, and planar imaging with single- and dual-phase (99m)Tc-sestamibi parathyroid scintigraphy. J Nucl Med. 2007;48:1084–9.
22. Tardelli E, Mazzarri S, Rubello D, Gennaro M, Fantechi L, Duce V, et al. Sentinel lymph node biopsy in cutaneous melanoma: standard and new technical procedures and clinical advances. A systematic review of the literature. Clin Nucl Med. 2016;41:498–507.
23. Manca G, Tardelli E, Rubello D, Gennaro M, Marzola MC, Cook GJ, et al. Sentinel lymph node biopsy in breast cancer: a technical and clinical appraisal. Nucl Med Commun. 2016;37(6):570.
24. Bonjer HJ, Bruining HA, Pols HA, de Herder WW, van Eijck CH, Breeman WA, et al. Intraoperative nuclear guidance in benign hyperparathyroidism and parathyroid cancer. Eur J Nucl Med. 1997;24:246–51.
25. Mehrabibahar M, Mousavi Z, Sadeghi R, Layegh P, Nouri M, Asadi M. Feasibility and safety of minimally invasive radioguided parathyroidectomy using very low intraoperative dose of Tc-99m MIBI. Int J Surg. 2017;39:229–33.
26. Onoda N, Ishikawa T, Nishiyama N, Kawabe J, Takashima T, Hirakawa K. Focused approach to ectopic mediastinal parathyroid surgery assisted by radioguided navigation. Surg Today. 2014;44:533–9.
27. Rubello D, Kapse N, Grassetto G, Massaro A, Al-Nahhas A. Minimally invasive radio-guided surgery for primary hyperparathyroidism: from preoperative to intraoperative localization imaging. Ann Endocrinol (Paris). 2010;71:511–8.
28. Minamiya Y, Saito H, Ito M, Motoyama S, Katayose Y, Ogawa J. Radio-guided thoracoscopic surgery with (99m)Tc-methoxy-isobutylisonitrile for treating an ectopic mediastinal parathyroid adenoma in an adolescent girl. Gen Thorac Cardiovasc Surg. 2009;57:657–9.
29. García-Talavera P, González-Selma ML, Ruiz M, Gamazo C, Sainz-Esteban A, Villanueva JG, Olmos R. The value of early SPECT/CT and hand-held γ-camera in radio-guided surgery: a case of a hard-to-locate parathyroid adenoma. Clin Nucl Med. 2014;39:1009–11.
30. Jorna FH, Jager PL, Lemstra C, Wiggers T, Stegeman CA, Plukker JT. Utility of an intraoperative gamma probe in the surgical management of secondary or tertiary hyperparathyroidism. Am J Surg. 2008;196:13–8.

Parathyroid Adenoma Which Was Negative on Tc99m-MIBI Scintigraphy and Considered as Paratracheal Lymphadenopathy on Other Imaging Studies

69

Meral Mert

Abstract

Surgery is the most important treatment method in patients with primary hyperparathyroidism. Imaging studies for localization of parathyroid adenoma should be performed in all patients with hyperparathyroidism before surgical intervention. Tc99m scintigraphy, neck ultrasonography, and neck magnetic resonance imaging (MRI) are the most common imaging modalities used for the localization of a parathyroid adenoma. Atypical localization of parathyroid adenoma and multiple gland disease are the most important causes of persistent disease and redo surgery. We aimed to introduce a case of primary hyperparathyroidism with the presence of double adenoma. In our case, the second adenoma was mistakenly interpreted as lymphadenopathy in the preoperative imaging studies. The lesion has been confirmed as parathyroid adenoma in the final histopathologic examination.

Therefore, multiple or atypical localized parathyroid adenoma should be considered in all patients to be operated.

M. Mert
Department of Endocrinology and Metabolism, Bakirkoy Dr. Sadi Konuk Training and Research Hospital, Health Sciences University (SBÜ), İstanbul, Turkey

69.1 Case

A 56-year-old woman visited the outpatient clinic because of hypothyroidism. Her routine laboratory studies revealed a high serum calcium level of 12.3 mg/dl. Her main complaints were skeletal pain and weakness. Laboratory results at admission are shown in Table 1.

The patient underwent 99mTc-MIBI scintigraphy and conventional radiologic imaging studies for the localization of parathyroid adenoma.

Technetium-99m-methoxyisobutylisonitrile (99mTc-MIBI) scintigraphy of the patient showed focal accumulation in the right inferior lobe which is consistent with parathyroid adenoma detection (Fig. 69.1). Neck ultrasonography (USG) revealed findings in thyroid gland consistent with thyroiditis and cervical lymph nodes which were considered as benign reactive in terms of sonographic characteristics. There was no lesion consistent with a parathyroid adenoma in her initial USG examination.

Consequently, a magnetic resonance imaging (MRI) of the neck revealed a lesion suspicious for parathyroid adenoma in the inferior site of the right thyroid gland and 1.3 × 1.7 cm lymphadenopathy at right paratracheal level VI (Figs. 69.2 and 69.3).

The patient underwent surgery for the removal of the parathyroid gland. The quick parathyroid

T. Özülker et al. (eds.), *Thyroid and Parathyroid Diseases*, https://doi.org/10.1007/978-3-319-78476-2_69

Table 1 Laboratory results of the patients

Ca	P	Creatinine	Albumin	PTH	Hgb	Hct	Sedimentation	25OH vit D
12.3 mg/dl	1.56 mg/dl	0.54 mg/dl	4.33 g/dl	310 pg/ml	13.4 g/dl	40.2%	8 mm/h	26.2 ng/ml

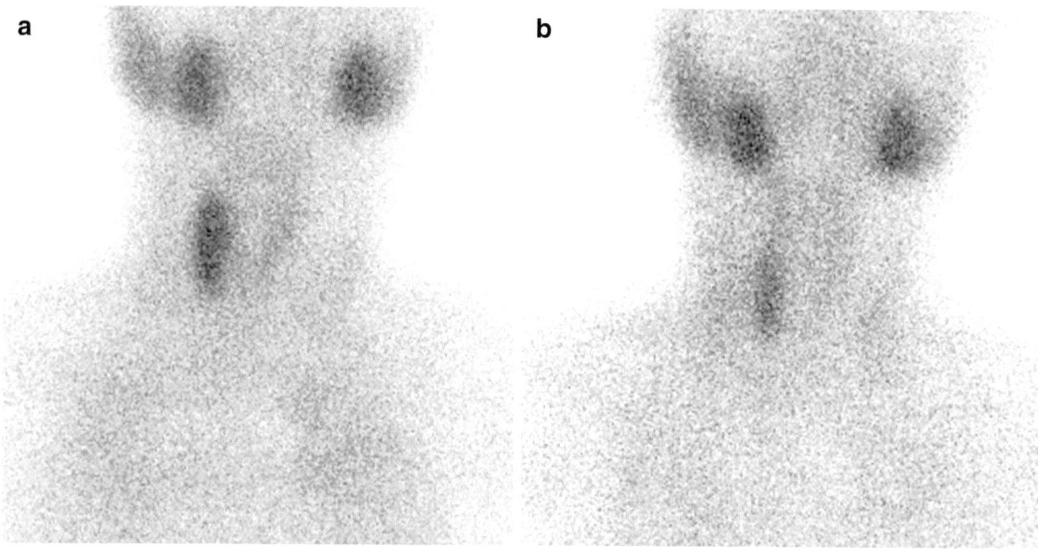

Fig. 69.1 Dual-phase Tc99m-MIBI parathyroid scintigraphy shows an asymmetrical diffuse MIBI uptake in right thyroid lobe (**a**), persistent uptake at the inferior pole of the right lobe in the delayed phase image (**b**)

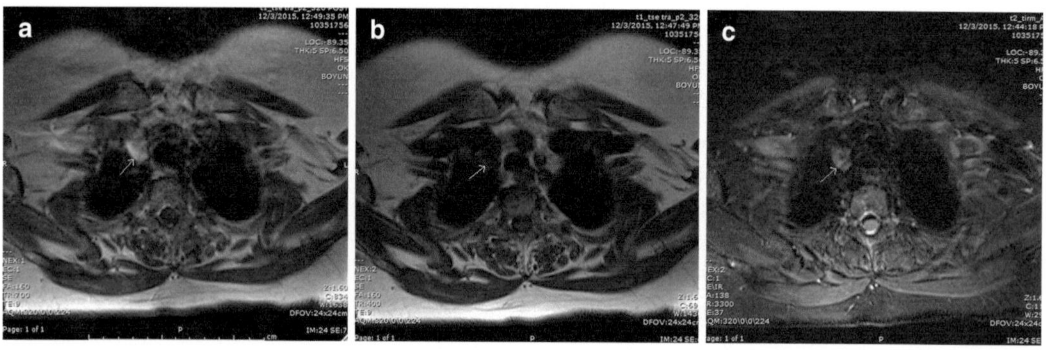

Fig. 69.2 Diffuse contrast-enhanced lesion suggesting lymphadenomegaly was seen right inferior paratracheal area 17 × 10mm (**a**), hypointense in T1 weighted (**b**), hyperintense in T2-weighted images (**c**)

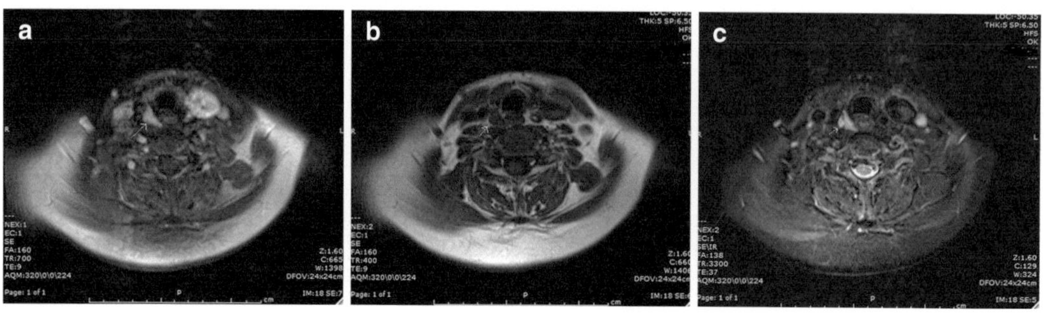

Fig. 69.3 Diffuse contrast-enhanced 26 × 15 × 10-mm-sized lesion compatible with parathyroid adenoma at the right thyroid gland infero-postero-medial area (**a**), hypointense in T1 weighted (**b**), hyperintense in T2-weighted images (**c**)

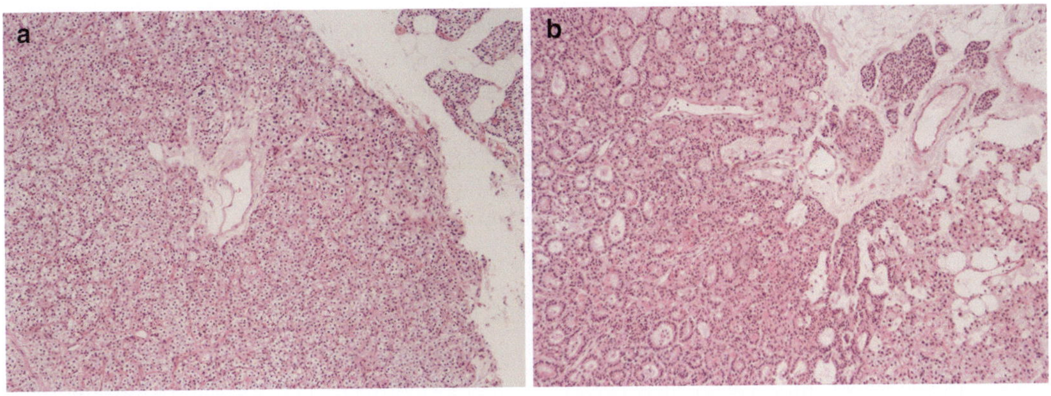

Fig. 69.4 Histopathology of the parathyroid adenoma located at the right inferior thyroid lobe (**a**), hematoxylin eosin stain ×40 (**a**), second parathyroid adenoma which was thought to be a lymph node macroscopically. Hematoxylin eosin stain ×40 (**b**)

hormone measurement was not available in the laboratory. During the operation, the lesions which were suspicious for parathyroid adenomas and lymphadenopathy were both resected. The resected lesion suspicious for parathyroid adenoma was confirmed as parathyroid adenoma in histopathologic assessment. However, the resected lesion which had been assumed to be a lymph node turned out to be a second parathyroid adenoma unexpectedly (Fig. 69.4).

Encapsulated and nodular-shaped, 3.2 × 1.7 × 0.6 cm-sized hemorrhagic lesion was seen at the inferior site of the right thyroid gland, and 1.7 × 0.7 × 0.5 cm encapsulated nodular tissue with surrounding fat tissue was seen at right paratracheal region macroscopically.

The adenoma-like lesion at the right inferior site and the lymphadenopathy-like lesion at paratracheal region were both identified as double parathyroid adenomas. Microscopically, adenomas showed diffuse nodular growth pattern. They contain stroma rich in vascularity and combinations of chief cells and clear cells. These parathyroid tumors were surrounded by an atrophic rim-shaped parathyroid tissue.

69.2 Discussion

The etiologies of primary hyperparathyroidism include benign adenoma (80–85%), diffuse or nodular hyperplasia (10–15%), double adenoma (2–5%), and parathyroid carcinoma (<1%) [1]. In the preoperative workup, the imaging studies which are crucial for the selection of operative approach should be performed after biochemical confirmation of primary hyperparathyroidism. In terms of location of a parathyroid adenoma, about 75% involve one of the inferior glands, 15% involve one of the superior glands, and 10% may be present in abnormal localizations. Approximately 30% of reoperated patients had hyperparathyroidism with multiple gland disease. Therefore, multiple or atypically localized parathyroid adenoma should be considered in all patients who will undergo surgery [2, 3].

Technetium-99m-methoxyisobutylisonitrile (99mTc-sestamibi or MIBI) scintigraphy, neck USG, MRI, and invasive studies can be used for the localization of parathyroid adenomas. A single-focus positive imaging result does not reliably exclude the presence of multiglandular parathyroid disease [4–6]. A negative 99mTc-sestamibi scan can be seen in 12–25% of patients with primary hyperparathyroidism [7, 8]. Parathyroid hyperplasia, multiple parathyroid adenomas, calcium-channel blockers, small size, superior position, and the paucity of oxyphil cells may cause false-negative results. Coexisting thyroid disease requiring surgery significantly increases both the false-positive and false-negative rate of sestamibi scanning [7, 8]. Single-photon emission computed tomography (SPECT-CT) adds the ability to discriminate parathyroid adenomas from other anatomic locations, which may affect the surgical procedure [9, 10]. CT alone has low sensitivity for parathyroid adenoma localization.

Neck USG is one of the most common imaging techniques for hyperparathyroidism, but the accuracy of USG is operator-dependent. Normal-sized parathyroid glands are not usually visualized with USG. The sensitivity of USG in detecting parathyroid adenomas has been reported from 49 to 85%. Obesity, previous neck surgery, small size, mediastinal glands, and localization behind the clavicles may cause false-negative results in USG. Conversely, extrathyroidal artery, thyroid nodules, enlarged lymph nodes, the esophagus, and longus colli muscles may cause false-positive result [11]. Discrimination of lymph node and parathyroid adenoma is crucial. Parathyroid lesions are usually very vascular, typically showing a peripheral vascular arc and a prominent polar feeding vessel that arises from the branches of the inferior thyroidal artery. The identification of a polar feeding artery can distinguish parathyroid glands from lymph nodes, which usually have a hilar blood supply. Other features include asymmetrically increased vascularity in the thyroid gland on the side of the lesion and the hyperechoic capsule [12].

One of the other imaging modality is MRI of the neck, and it is also performed in most of the patients for the localization of parathyroid adenomas. Normal parathyroid glands usually are not seen on MRI. The characteristics of parathyroid adenoma and cervical lymph nodes are similar to MRI [13, 14]. The reported sensitivity of MRI for abnormal parathyroid tissue ranges from 40% to 85%. There are few data supporting advanced MRI techniques such as perfusion or dynamic contrast-enhanced MRI. Enlarged lymph nodes, thyroid nodules, and other neck masses such as sarcoid nodules and ganglia may cause false-positive results.

Enlarged lymph nodes have similar characteristics of signal intensity to those of abnormal parathyroid glands. Abnormal parathyroid glands are expected to be medial to the carotid sheath, whereas lymph nodes are most frequently situated around or lateral to the sheath [12]. But these features are not enough for the differential diagnosis. Clinicians should be aware of a contingency of multiple parathyroid adenomas as in our case. Otherwise persistent disease or recurrence may be an unintentional issue after surgery.

In our case, double adenomas were present, and secondary adenoma was considered as lymphadenopathy in the preoperative imaging methods. The use of intraoperative gamma probe prevented failure of the first operation. During the postoperative follow-up period, the patient was clinically well, and laboratory results were normal.

In the future four-dimensional CT (4D-CT) as a promising modality which is particularly useful in the reoperative setting when initial imaging with sestamibi is negative. Mahajan et al. found that 4D-CT is a superior preoperative imaging modality for the localization of parathyroid tumors. However, 4D-CT should be used wisely in younger patients due to its higher radiation dose [15].

Another option is the combination of 11C-methionine positron emission tomography and computed tomography (MET-PET-CT). Weber et al. found that MET-PET-CT scan correctly located a single gland adenoma in 83 of 97 patients (86%), with a positive predictive value of 93% in 102 patients [16]. One of the new imaging modalities is ^{18}F-fluorocholine (FCH), which can be delivered as easily as ^{18}F-fluorodeoxyglucose (FDG) and might be superior for localizing parathyroid adenomas and enabling minimal invasive parathyroidectomy when conventional imaging fails to do. Clinicians should consider its use as a second-line modality for optimal patient care [17].

If localization cannot be performed despite all noninvasive procedures, then invasive studies such as arteriography or selective venous sampling can be performed. Selective venous sampling is the most common invasive modality used for parathyroid localization. Another invasive technique is selective arteriography, which is performed by combining selective trans-arterial hypocalcemic stimulation with nonselective venous sampling [15].

69.3 Management

Imaging studies for localization of adenoma should be performed in all patients before surgery. Moreover, careful examination of the locations where atypical localization may be present, and preference of gamma probe-guided minimally invasive parathyroidectomy (GP-MIP) with quick parathyroid hormone measurement will reduce the probability of failure.

What Can We Learn from This Case?

As if it were our case, multigland parathyroid disease should be kept in mind and atypical localizations should be carefully assessed in all patients before surgery.

Acknowledgment We would like to thank Dr. Deniz Guzey and Cevher Akarsu for their valuable contribution to the surgical management of the patient.

References

1. Kaplan EL, Yashiro T, Salti G. Primary hyperparathyroidism in the 1990s. Choice of surgical procedures for this disease. Ann Surg. 1992;215:300.
2. Udelsman R, Pasieka JL, Sturgeon C, Young JE, Clark OH. Surgery for asymptomatic primary hyperparathyroidism: proceedings of the third international workshop. Clin Endocrinol Metab. 2009;94:366. https://doi.org/10.1210/jc.2008-1761.
3. Bilezikian JP, Brandi ML, Eastell R, Silverberg SJ, Udelsman R, Marcocci C, et al. Guidelines for the management of asymptomatic primary hyperparathyroidism: summary statement from the Fourth International Workshop. J Clin Endocrinol Metab. 2014;99:3561. https://doi.org/10.1210/jc.2014-1413.
4. Civelek AC, Ozalp E, Donovan P, Udelsman R. Prospective evaluation of delayed technetium-99m sestamibi SPECT scintigraphy for preoperative localization of primary hyperparathyroidism. Surgery. 2002;131:149.
5. Siperstein A, Berber E, Barbosa GF, Tsinberg M, Greene AB, Mitchell J, et al. Predicting the success of limited exploration for primary hyperparathyroidism using ultrasound, sestamibi, and intraoperative parathyroid hormone: analysis of 1158 cases. Ann Surg. 2008;248:420. https://doi.org/10.1097/SLA.0b013e3181859f71.
6. Chiu B, Sturgeon C, Angelos P. What is the link between nonlocalizing sestamibi scans, multigland disease, and persistent hypercalcemia? A study of 401 consecutive patients undergoing parathyroidectomy. Surgery. 2006;140:418. https://doi.org/10.1016/j.surg.2006.03.021.
7. Stephen AE, Roth SI, Fardo DW, Finkelstein DM, Randolph GW, Gaz RD, et al. Predictors of an accurate preoperative sestamibi scan for single-gland parathyroid adenomas. Arch Surg. 2007;142:381. https://doi.org/10.1001/archsurg.142.4.381.
8. Friedman K, Somervell H, Patel P, Melton GB, Garrett-Mayer E, Dackiw AP, et al. Effect of calcium channel blockers on the sensitivity of preoperative 99mTc-MIBI SPECT for hyperparathyroidism. Surgery. 2004;136:1199. https://doi.org/10.1016/j.surg.2004.06.047.
9. Lavely WC, Goetze S, Friedman KP, Leal JP, Zhang Z, Garret-Mayer E, et al. Comparison of SPECT/CT, SPECT, and planar imaging with single- and dual-phase (99m)Tc-sestamibi parathyroid scintigraphy. J Nucl Med. 2007;48:1084. https://doi.org/10.2967/jnumed.107.040428.
10. Spanu A, Falchi A, Manca A, Marongiu P, Cossu A, Pisu N, et al. The usefulness of neck pinhole SPECT as a complementary tool to planar scintigraphy in primary and secondary hyperparathyroidism. J Nucl Med. 2004;45:40.
11. Kobylecka M, Płazińska MT, Chudziński W, Fronczewska-Wieniawska K, Mączewska J, Bajera A, et al. Comparison of scintigraphy and ultrasound imaging in patients with primary, secondary and tertiary hyperparathyroidism - own experience. J Ultrason. 2017;17:17–22. https://doi.org/10.15557/JoU.2017.0002.
12. Sung JY. Parathyroid ultrasonography: the evolving role of the radiologist. Ultrasonography. 2015;34:268–74. https://doi.org/10.14366/usg.14071.
13. Wakamatsu H, Noguchi S, Yamashita H, Yamashita H, Tamura S, Jinnouchi S, et al. Parathyroid scintigraphy with 99mTc-MIBI and 123I subtraction: a comparison with magnetic resonance imaging and ultrasonography. Nucl Med Commun. 2003;24:755–62.
14. Kluijfhout WP, Vriens MR, Valk GD, Barth RE, Borel Rinkes IH, de Keizer B. 18F-Fluorocholine PET–CT enables minimal invasive parathyroidectomy in patients with negative sestamibi SPECT–CT and ultrasound: a case report. Int J Surg Case Rep. 2015;13:73–5. https://doi.org/10.1016/j.ijscr.2015.06.012.
15. Lebastchi AH, Aruny JE, Donovan PI, Quinn CE, Callender GG, Carling T, et al. Real-time super selective venous sampling in remedial parathyroid surgery. J Am Coll Surg. 2015;220:994. https://doi.org/10.1016/j.jamcollsurg.2015.01.004.
16. Gawrychowski J, Buła G. Imaging diagnostics for primary hyperparathyroidism. Endokrynol Pol. 2013;64:404–8. https://doi.org/10.5603/EP.2013.0024.
17. Kluijfhout WP, Pasternak JD, Gosnell JE, Shen WT, Duh QY, Vriens MR, et al. 18F fluorocholine PET/MR imaging in patients with primary hyperparathyroidism and inconclusive conventional imaging: a prospective pilot study. Radiology. 2017;284(2):460–7. https://doi.org/10.1148/radiol.2016160768.

70 Brown Tumor Due to Primary Hyperparathyroidism Disguised as Lung Cancer in a Patient with Rib Lesions

Betül Uğur Altun and Gülşah Yenidünya Yalın

Abstract

Primary hyperparathyroidism (PHPT) is the most common cause of hypercalcemia and is characterized with high (or in the upper limit of normal) parathyroid hormone levels despite the presence of hypercalcemia. PHPT diagnosis is becoming more common in the recent years due to frequent measurement of serum calcium levels in routine biochemical screening. The most common clinical presentation of PHPT is asymptomatic hypercalcemia. However, a broad range of clinical manifestations such as osteoporosis, skeletal manifestations, or nephrolithiasis may be seen as the disease sets on.

70.1 Case Report

A 42-year-old female patient was admitted to the outpatient clinic with symptoms of fatigue, generalized musculoskeletal pain, arthralgia and myalgia, constipation, depressive mood, and anxiety. Because the patient also complained of mild cough symptoms, a chest radiography was also performed during the initial evaluation. Suspicious nodular lesions were detected on the chest X-ray (Fig. 70.1), and the patient was referred to the pulmonary diseases outpatient clinic for further evaluation. She had no history of smoking and denied presence of lung disease in family history. On physical examination, her BMI was 28.6 kg/m^2 without a history of recent weight loss. Blood pressure was 160/100 mmHg and heart rate 90/min/R with the presence of mild abdominal discomfort and generalized bone ache. Examination of cardiovascular and respiratory systems was normal. Painful nodular lesions were palpated on ribs. In laboratory evaluation, fasting blood glucose was 87 mg/dl; BUN, 27 mg/dl; creatinine, 1.7 mg/dl; calcium (Ca) 12 mg/dl, and albumin 3.5 gr/dl, and complete blood count revealed presence of normochromic anemia with Hgb 11 gr/dl. Liver enzymes, TSH level, and electrolytes were normal. Urinalysis revealed the presence of hematuria and eGFR was 40 ml/min.

Thorax computerized tomography (CT) revealed the presence of multiple nodular lesions on the ribs (Fig. 70.2), and bone biopsy was performed for the differential diagnosis of metastasis and primary bone disease. Histopathological evaluation revealed increased osteoblastic and osteolytic activity which was compatible with

B. U. Altun
Department of Endocrinology, Başkent University Medical School, Ankara, Turkey

G. Y. Yalın (✉)
Department of Endocrinology, Başkent University Istanbul Hospital, Istanbul, Turkey

T. Özülker et al. (eds.), *Thyroid and Parathyroid Diseases*, https://doi.org/10.1007/978-3-319-78476-2_70

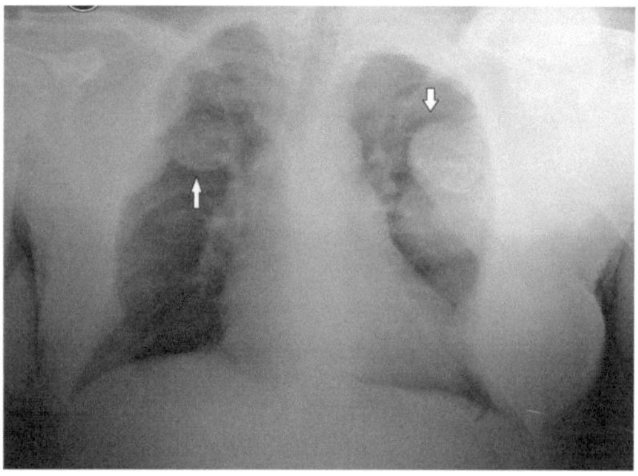

Fig. 70.1 Bilateral nodular lesions on Chest X-ray

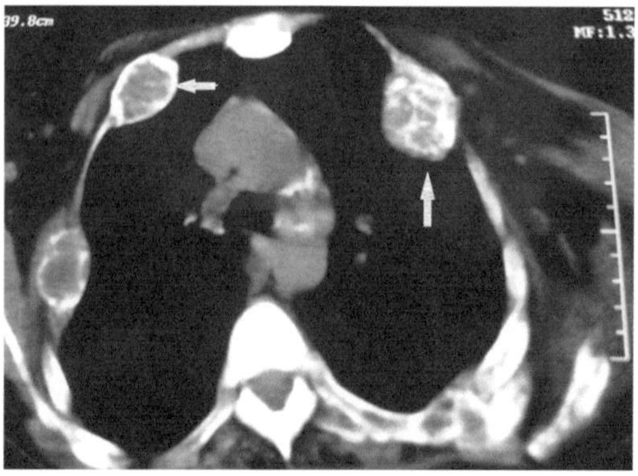

Fig. 70.2 Multiple nodular lesions on the ribs on Thorax CT

metabolic bone disease, and presence of malignancy was excluded. After the high plasma Ca level was confirmed with a repeat laboratory testing, serum PTH, alkaline phosphatase (ALP), phosphorus (P), and vitamin D levels were measured as 1200 pg/dl, 133 mg/dl, 1.6 mg/dl, and 10 ng/ml, respectively. Ca excretion in 24-h urine was measured as 460 mg/day. Urinary ultrasonography (USG) demonstrated the presence of bilateral nephrocalcinosis and renal pelvic nephrolithiasis on the left kidney.

The patient was diagnosed with symptomatic primary hyperparathyroidism (PHPT). Localization of parathyroid adenoma was determined with neck USG demonstrating the presence of left inferior parathyroid adenoma which was also confirmed with Tc-99 m sestamibi parathyroid scintigraphy, and the patient was referred for parathyroid surgery.

70.2 Discussion

When the PHPT was defined for the first time in the 1930s, the majority of the patients had symptoms of nephrolithiasis, bone lesions, and/or peptic ulcer [1]. Today, early diagnosis is possible due to the measurement of serum Ca in the routine clinical practice. In the presented case, the delay of diagnosis resulted in the manifestation of all the clinical complications at the time of admission. The prevalence of PHPT is 0.8–0.9% and 0.3–0.5% in North America for females and males, respectively. In Asian countries hypercalcemia and clinical complications are more frequent. However, the exact prevalence is not clear [1].

When hypercalcemia is detected, work-up for the differential diagnosis of hypercalcemia should be performed. High or inappropriately normal parathyroid hormone (PTH) levels (normal range: 10–65 pg/ml [ng/l]) in the presence of hypercalcemia indicates that the pathology is primarily related with parathyroid glands. PHPT, tertiary hyperparathyroidism, lithium ingestion, and familial hypocalciuric hypercalcemia are categorized under this section. Presence of low or low-normal PTH with hypercalcemia indicates that the pathology is primarily related to high calcium levels which may be due to malignancy, vitamin D intoxication, milk-alkali syndrome, thyrotoxicosis, and granulomatous diseases. The first step of evaluation should always begin with the confirmation of high serum Ca levels corrected accordingly with serum albumin levels. Calcium is transported in plasma largely as albumin-bound Ca; therefore every 1 gr/dl change in albumin above or below reference range (4 gr/dl) results with 0.8 mg/dl decrease or increase in the serum Ca levels, respectively. After the confirmation of hypercalcemia, PTH levels are the most valuable information in the differential diagnosis. Also, the measurement techniques are important for the establishment of an accurate diagnosis. The generation of PTH assay and the transfer of blood specimen under optimal circumstances are essential in the measurement of PTH levels. Second- and third-generation PTH measurements are more accurate in the evaluation of PHPT than the first-generation measurement methods [1–3].

In the case presented above, plasma PTH levels were high in the presence of hypercalcemia which indicated that the primary pathology was related to PTH over secretion. Other etiologies in the differential diagnosis were excluded with clinical and laboratory findings. The patient was not receiving lithium therapy, 24-h urinary Ca excretion was high, and she did not have an end-stage renal disease which may have caused tertiary HPT. In the evaluation of these patients obtaining a detailed medical history (related with exposure of previous head and neck radiotherapy, the presence of medications such as lithium, thiazide diuretics, calcium and vitamin D supplements, anticonvulsants) with careful physical examination is very important [4].

PHPT is defined with persistently high PTH levels (despite the presence of hypercalcemia), hypophosphatemia, and increased $1.25(OH)_2D_3$. Characteristic clinical findings are not present in asymptomatic PHPT. Normocalcemic PHPT is characterized by normal Ca, normal or low P levels, and high PTH levels when the presence of secondary hyperparathyroidism is excluded [5].

PHPT is the most common cause of hypercalcemia. The etiology is dependent on the presence of solitary parathyroid adenoma (80%), parathyroid hyperplasia (15–20%), multiple parathyroid adenomas (2–4%), or parathyroid carcinoma (0.5–1%) [6]. PHPT diagnosis is more frequent in the recent years due to the routine measurement of serum Ca levels with more sensitive laboratory methods, and the complications are less commonly detected as the rates of early diagnosis are increasing. PHPT is rarely seen under 15 years old, and the prevalence increases after the age of 45 reaching its highest at the age of 60. It is nearly three times more frequent in female patients (female to male ratio is 3:1) [6]. There are no clinical findings in the majority of these patients, and the patients are classified into two groups as symptomatic or asymptomatic (Table 70.1).

Typical bone lesions are presented as osteitis fibrosa cystica in PHPT, and the characteristical radiological features are "salt and pepper" appearance in the skull, subperiosteal resorption in phalangeal bones, and formation of cysts and brown tumors [6, 7]. Bone lesions occur due to increased osteoclastic bone resorption, fibrovas-

Table 70.1 Signs and symptoms of hypercalcemia [7, 8, 12, 13]

Nonspecific	*Gastrointestinal system*	*Renal system*
• Fatigue • Muscle weakness • Malaise • Anorexia • Depression • Hypertension	• Blunt abdominal pain • Constipation • Anorexia • Acute pancreatitis	• Polyuria • Nephrolithiasis • Renal tubular dysfunction • Concentration difficulties • Acute or chronic renal failure • Hypercalciuria • Chronic hypercalcemia nephropathy • Interstitial nephritis • Salt waste • Nephrogenic diabetes insipidus • Renal tubular acidosis (type 1)
Neuropsychiatric disorders	*Cardiovascular disorders*	*Rheumatological disorders*
• Anxiety • Depression • Cognitive dysfunctions • Organic brain syndrome • Personality changes • Behavioral disorders • Confusion • Organic psychosis • Hallucinations • Somnolence • Coma	• Valvular calcifications • Arterial calcification • Myocardial calcification, myocardial short action potentials • Short QT • Arrhythmia • Hypertension • Vasoconstriction	• Gout • Pseudogout • Chondrocalcinosis • Arthralgia • Myalgia

cular bone marrow, increased osteoblastic activity, diffuse bone demineralization, coarsened trabecular pattern, and subperiosteal resorption. The resorption of the endosteal bone primarily takes place in the cortical compartment [6, 7], whereas mineralization is prominent in the trabecular compartment. Therefore, the vertebral bone which predominantly consists of the trabecular bone compartment may not be significantly affected in asymptomatic PHPT, and vertebral fractures are not common in these patients. Because the cortical bone tissue is mostly present in the 1/3 distal compartment of radius, bone densitometry of this bone site should be evaluated during the initial work-up. However, it is known that both vertebral and nonvertebral fracture risk is increased in PHPT [3]. Bone cysts may present with multiple cystic lesions containing brown serous or mucoid liquid accumulation. These lesions tend to appear in the metacarpals, ribs, and central medullar region of the pelvis and may cause deterioration in the cortical bone structure with further invasion of the cortical compartment. Osteoclastoma (brown tumor) (Figs. 70.1 and 70.2) is a lesion characterized by stromal cells and giant osteoclasts. These are mostly located in the long bones and trabecular compartment of the jaw and ribs.

Recurrent nephrolithiasis and nephrocalcinosis may be detected in the kidneys. Polyuria and polydipsia due to diminished renal concentration capacity, end-stage renal disease, and renal colic pain are common renal symptoms. Hypercalciuria is common in PHPT patients, and PHPT is also one of the reasons for the development of renal calcium stones. However, other contributing factors are also held responsible in the etiopathogenesis. Hyperparathyroidism may also be secondary to renal failure. In time, secondary HPT may gain autonomous function which may lead to tertiary HPT and hypercalcemia.

Renal failure is an indication for surgical intervention in PHPT. Risk of nephrolithiasis decreases after parathyroid surgery. However, nephrocalcinosis remains unchanged [8]. In the presented case, eGFR was decreased (40 ml/min), but it was not as low as end-stage renal disease. Renal failure was due to hypercalcemia, but decreased eGFR level also had an additional effect on the further increase of plasma PTH levels.

Fatigue, myopathy, apathy, concentration difficulties, depression, dementia, psychosis, irritability, amnesia, emotional lability, and coma may present as neuropsychiatric signs and symptoms [9]. In our case, the patient had significant depression, agitation, and personality changes. Neuromuscular symptoms may present with symmetrical proximal muscle weakness, diffuse muscle atrophy, gait abnormalities, generalized hyperreflexia, and fasciculations of the tongue [6]. Cardiovascular signs and symptoms are hypertension, left ventricular hypertrophy, and arrhythmia. Quality of life is low even in patients who are asymptomatic. Nonspecific symptoms such as fatigue, irritability, weakness, malaise, somatization, lack of mental clarity, sleep disturbance, anxiety, and depression may be reversed after treatment of PHPT [1]. Other rare complications are listed as conjunctival calcification, band keratopathy, peptic ulcer, and acute or chronic pancreatitis.

Vitamin D deficiency is common in PHPT. Therefore, serum 25OH vitamin D should be measured routinely. 25OH vitamin D level over 30 ng/ml (some guidelines refer to 20 ng/ml as a threshold) indicates sufficient vitamin D levels especially in patients with normocalcemic PHPT. Routine measurement of 1.25 OH vitamin D level is not recommended [3]. Laboratory findings are the presence of hypercalcemia (high levels of corrected Ca and ionized Ca), hypophosphatemia or low-normal serum P level, mild hyperchloremic acidosis, high alkaline phosphatase level, and elevated urinary Ca excretion. eGFR is measured in the differential diagnosis of renal osteodystrophy and the decision of treatment. eGFR level lower than 60 ml/min/1.73 m^2 is the threshold for the onset of chronic renal failure. Genetic screening may be performed in the suspicion of hereditary diseases, but it is not routinely tested in clinical practice.

Routine imaging is not recommended for diagnosis and should only be used for preoperative localization of the parathyroid lesion [4]. Neck

USG is effective in the detection of cervical parathyroid lesions; however, its sensitivity is lower in mediastinal parathyroid lesions (75–85%). Magnetic resonance imaging, ^{18}F-FDG PET CT, or venous sampling may be useful for the detection of these lesions. Tc99m sestamibi imaging also has a high sensitivity (90%) [10]; however, it may be difficult to detect small parathyroid adenoma and hyperplasia.

The primary treatment of PHPT is surgery, especially in symptomatic patients. In patients for whom surgery is not feasible, medical treatment should be initiated to lower plasma calcium levels, to preserve bone and kidney health, and to prevent complications. Bisphosphonates, calcimimetics, or estrogen-targeted therapies are used in the medical treatment to maintain normal plasma Ca and vitamin D levels [11].

Familial hypocalciuric hypercalcemia should also be considered in the differential diagnosis of PHPT. This disorder is characterized by an autosomal dominant (AD) inheritance pattern. The mutation is located in the calcium-sensing receptors (CaSR), both in the kidneys and the parathyroid glands resulting in decreased calcium sensitivity in these receptors. Decreased calcium sensitivity in these receptors leads to increased PTH levels and increased renal tubular Ca reabsorption. Laboratory findings are mild hypercalcemia, hypophosphatemia, hypermagnesemia, normal or mildly elevated PTH levels, and hypocalciuria (Ca excretion less than 50 mg/day). Ca/creatinine clearance is lower than 0.01 (Calcium clearance = [urinary calcium/urinary creatinine] × [plasma creatinine/plasma calcium]) (4,6). Hypocalciuria is due to renal dysfunction and parathyroidectomy would not be beneficial in these patients. Diagnosis of this etiology is therefore important in order to eliminate unnecessary surgical interventions.

In patients who are younger than 30 years old and who have a family history of thyroid, adrenal gland, pancreas, or pituitary tumor, rare hereditary PHPT etiologies (multiple endocrine neoplasia (MEN) syndrome, hyperparathyroidism-jaw tumor syndrome, heterozygous Ca-sensing receptor gene mutations, familial hypocalciuric hypercalcemia) should also be considered. PHPT is present in 95% of MEN type 1 and is generally characterized with the involvement of multiple parathyroid glands. PHPT frequency is 90% in patients with MEN 1 who are over 40 years old. Loss of function mutation in tumor suppressor gene MENIN (located on 11q12-13) is held responsible in the etiopathogenesis. MENIN is a nuclear protein which interacts with AP1 transcription factor JunD [1, 2, 4]. PHPT is less common (5–20%) in multiple endocrine neoplasia type 2A (MEN 2A) and is seen in later decades. Asymptomatic PHPT, adenoma, or hyperplasia may be observed during thyroid surgery. The treatment approach is similar with PHPT. Mutation of RET proto-oncogene is held responsible for the development of MEN 2A. Presence of abnormal RET expression may be responsible for tumorigenesis. PHPT is not present in MEN 2B [2, 4]. Hereditary isolated PHPT is characterized by parathyroid tumors which may be multiple or malign without any concurrent endocrine gland abnormalities or MEN1 and MEN 2A mutations.

Hypercalcemia due to lithium treatment is associated with hypercalcemia, high PTH levels, and hypocalciuria. Mild hyperplasia may also be present in parathyroid glands. The clinical presentation is similar to familial benign hypocalciuric hypercalcemia. The laboratory results return to normal after the cessation of lithium therapy. The onset of nephrogenic diabetes insipidus and dehydration due to lithium therapy may also exacerbate hypercalcemia and high PTH levels via increasing the threshold limit of Ca-PTH suppression axis [2, 4].

In asymptomatic PHPT patients, surgical intervention is indicated due to the presence of certain clinical criteria, and patients are evaluated according to the National Institutes of Health (NIH) 2013 criteria [3]. Parathyroid surgery indications are listed as:

(A) Patients with significant findings of PHPT
   (1) Nephrolithiasis
   (2) Low creatinine clearance levels (GFR) which cannot be explained with other etiologies

(3) Radiological findings of PHPT-related bone lesions
(4) Presence of neuromuscular disease findings
(5) Symptoms related with hypercalcemia
(6) Presence of severe hypercalcemia

(B) Asymptomatic PHPT patients
(1) Serum Ca concentration over 1 mg/dl above the upper limit of normal
(2) Bone density at the lumbar spine, hip, or distal radius that is more than 2.5 standard deviations below peak bone mass (T-score < −2.5)
(3) Presence of previous vertebral fracture by X-ray, computed tomography, and magnetic resonance imaging or during vertebral fracture assessment
(4) GFR < 60 ml/min
(5) Twenty-four-hour urinary calcium >400 mg/day and demonstration of high urinary stone risk in the biochemical urine analysis
(6) Nephrolithiasis or nephrocalcinosis by X-ray, USG, or CT
(7) Age less than 50 years

In patients who are not candidates for parathyroid surgery, plasma Ca and PTH levels should be measured once a year, and bone densitometry should be performed with 1–2-year intervals. The intervals may be longer in clinically stable patients. One of the important complications after surgery is “hungry bone syndrome.” This syndrome is transient and generally recovers in a couple of weeks. It is due to the rapid replacement of previously increased osteoclastic activity with the osteoblastic process and is characterized with hypocalcemia, hypophosphatemia, and hypomagnesemia. Hypocalcemia is transient in most of the cases and rarely reaches to critically low levels. Bone disease is generally mild. Because the remaining parathyroid glands recover in a couple of weeks, it is recommended to plan the replacement treatment with close monitoring of plasma Ca levels [14].

What Can We Learn from This Case?

- Hypercalcemia should be assessed with total and corrected plasma Ca levels in blood samples which are obtained and transferred in optimal circumstances.
- Plasma Ca level should always be evaluated in accordance with plasma PTH levels which should also be measured under optimal conditions.
- Advanced clinical complications such as severe osteoporosis may be present when the diagnosis of PHPT is delayed.
- The primary treatment of PHPT is surgical intervention, and careful management is essential in pre- and postoperative period.

References

1. Bilezikian JP, Cusano NE, Khan AA, Liu JM, Marcocci C, Bandeira F. Primary hyperparathyroidism. Nat Rev Dis Primers. 2016;2:160–3.
2. Eastell R, Brandi ML, Costa AG, D’Amour P, Shoback DM, Thakker RV. Diagnosis of asymptomatic primary hyperparathyroidism: proceedings of the fourth international workshop. J Clin Endocrinol Metab. 2014;99:3570–9.
3. Bilezikian JP, Brandi ML, Eastell R, Silverberg SJ, Udelsman R, Marcocci C, Potts JT Jr. Guidelines for the management of asymptomatic primary hyperparathyroidism: summary statement from the fourth international workshop. J Clin Endocrinol Metab. 2014;99:3561–9.
4. Udelsman R, Åkerström G, Biagini C, Duh QY, Miccoli P, Niederle B, Tonelli F. The surgical management of asymptomatic primary hyperparathyroidism: proceedings of the fourth international workshop. J Clin Endocrinol Metab. 2014;99:3595–606.
5. Macfarlane DP, Yu N, Leese GP. Subclinical and asymptomatic parathyroid disease: implications of emerging data. Lancet Diabetes Endocrinol. 2013;1:329–40.
6. Bandeira L, Bilezikian J. Primary hyperparathyroidism. F1000Res. 2016;5:1–11.
7. Bandeira F, Cusano NE, Silva BC, Cassibba S, Almeida CB, Machado VC, Bilezikian JP. Bone disease in primary hyperparathyroidism. Arq Bras Endocrinol Metabol. 2014;58:553–61.

8. Hendrickson CD, Castro Pereira DJ, Comi RJ. Renal impairment as a surgical indication in primary hyperparathyroidism: do the data support this recommendation? J Clin Endocrinol Metab. 2014;99:2646–50.
9. Silverberg SJ, Clarke BL, Peacock M, Bandeira F, Boutroy S, Cusano NE, et al. Current issues in the presentation of asymptomatic primary hyperparathyroidism: proceedings of the fourth international workshop. J Clin Endocrinol Metab. 2014;99:3580–94.
10. Khan AA, Hanley DA, Rizzoli R, Bollerslev J, Young JE, Rejnmark L, et al. Primary hyperparathyroidism: review and recommendations on evaluation, diagnosis, and management. A Canadian and international consensus. Osteoporos Int. 2017;28:1–19.
11. Marcocci C, Bollerslev J, Khan AA, Shoback DM. Medical management of primary hyperparathyroidism: proceedings of the fourth international workshop on the Management of Asymptomatic Primary Hyperparathyroidism. J Clin Endocrinol Metab. 2014;99:3607–18.
12. Inzucchi SE. Understanding hypercalcemia. Its metabolic basis, signs, and symptoms. Postgrad Med. 2004;115:69–76.
13. Pappu R, Jabbour SA, Regianto AM, Reginato AJ. Musculoskeletal manifestations of primary hyperparathyroidism. Clin Rheumatol. 2016;35:3081–7.
14. Witteveen JE, van Thiel S, Romijn JA, Hamdy NA. Hungry bone syndrome: still a challenge in the post-operative management of primary hyperparathyroidism: a systematic review of the literature. Eur J Endocrinol. 2013;168:45–53.

71 Radiofrequency Ablation in a Patient with Primary Hyperparathyroidism

Ayşe Kubat Üzüm, Gülşah Yenidünya Yalın, and Arzu Poyanlı

Abstract

The most common cause of hypercalcemia and high plasma PTH levels is primary hyperparathyroidism (PHPT). Clinical features are associated with recurrent urolithiasis and osteoporosis. However, most of the patients are generally asymptomatic or have nonspecific complaints. Biochemical diagnosis is based on elevated plasma calcium and parathormone levels and high 24-h urine calcium excretion. The definitive treatment of PHPT is performing parathyroidectomy after the localization of parathyroid adenoma. In patients who are ineligible for surgery (due to comorbidities or surgical risk), management of hypercalcemia can be very challenging, and several medical agents such as bisphosphonates, calcitonin, or cinacalcet are being applied periodically to control high plasma calcium levels. Radiofrequency ablation is a minimally invasive ablation method which is generally used in the management of benign thyroid nodules for volume reduction and improvement of associated symptoms. Lately, this method has also been used in the management of PHPT patients when surgery is not eligible either because of contraindication due to high surgical risk or patient refusal. We hereby present our experience with radiofrequency ablation therapy in the management of hyperparathyroidism in a 59-year-old female patient.

71.1 Case Presentation

A 59-year-old female patient was referred to our endocrinology and metabolism disorders department due to the presence of hypercalcemia and high plasma PTH levels. On admission, she had symptoms of fatigue, nausea, and occasional abdominal discomfort. She had been hospitalized with the diagnosis of deep vein thrombosis and massive bilateral pulmonary embolism 2 months ago after an acute episode of dyspnea and chest pain. Her medical history revealed the presence of hypertension for 10 years which was under treatment with amlodipine 10 mg once daily. She had also been receiving warfarin 5 mg/day for 2 months. On examination, her blood pressure was 145/95 mm Hg, and heart rate was 88 beats per minute. Her cardiopulmonary and abdominal examination was unremarkable. Laboratory

A. K. Üzüm
Division of Endocrinology and Metabolism, Department of Internal Medicine, Istanbul Faculty of Medicine, Istanbul University, Istanbul, Turkey

G. Y. Yalın (✉)
Department of Endocrinology, Baskent University Istanbul Hospital, Istanbul, Turkey

A. Poyanlı
Radiology and Interventional Radiology, Istanbul Medical Faculty, Istanbul, Turkey
e-mail: apoyanli@istanbul.edu.tr

T. Özülker et al. (eds.), *Thyroid and Parathyroid Diseases*, https://doi.org/10.1007/978-3-319-78476-2_71

results were as follows: Ca, 14.3 mg/dL (8.5–10.5 mg/dL); P, 3.1 mg/dL (3.5–5.5 mg/dL); albumin, 4.1 g/dL; PTH, 351 pg/mL (15–65 pg/mL); ALP, 106 U/L (35–105 U/L); 25-OH vitamin D, 12 ng/mL; creatinine, 1.7 mg/dL (0.7–1.4 mg/dL); BUN, 26 mg/dL (0–20 mg/dL); ALT, 28 U/L (5–25 U/L); INR, 2.6; and eGFR, 31 mL/min/1.73m^2. Urinary ultrasonography (USG) revealed the presence of bilateral nephrolithiasis with dilated ureters and pelvicalyceal systems. Bone densitometry demonstrated the presence of low BMD in distal radius region (mid-radius T score, −2.6). Neck ultrasonography (USG) revealed 24 mm fusiform hypoechoic lesion on the left superior parathyroid region which was suspicious for parathyroid adenoma. MIBI scintigraphy also confirmed the presence of parathyroid adenoma at the same location. Due to the presence of hypercalcemia, nephrolithiasis, and osteoporosis, surgical intervention was planned for the definitive treatment of primary hyperparathyroidism. However, the surgical intervention had to be postponed until 3 months due to recent deep vein thrombosis and pulmonary embolism which was demonstrated to be secondary to the presence of heterozygous factor V Leiden mutation. In order to control high plasma calcium levels in this period, medical treatment with adequate hydration (200 mL/h), calcitonin 100 IU SC (bid), and ibandronic acid 2 mg IV (with dose adjustment according to low eGFR level) was performed. Three weeks later plasma calcium levels began to rise again (Ca:12.1 mg/dL) and bisphosphonate injection was repeated with IV zoledronate 4 mg as the eGFR levels were normalized. Due to recurrent high plasma calcium levels despite bisphosphonate treatment and unavailability of surgery, cinacalcet 30 mg PO bid was initiated 4 weeks later to control hypercalcemia, and the dose was gradually titrated up to 60 mg bid. Plasma calcium levels were barely maintained between 10.8 and 11.3 mg/dL with hydration and cinacalcet treatment. After 3 months of pulmonary embolism treatment, parathyroid adenoma surgery was planned. However, due to present comorbidities, the patient was reluctant to receive surgical treatment, and she refused invasive intervention. After a council meeting with divisions of endocrine surgery and nuclear medicine, the patient was referred for percutaneous radiofrequency ablation (RFA) therapy for the treatment of parathyroid adenoma.

71.2 Discussion

71.2.1 Evaluation and Diagnosis

Differential diagnosis of the two most common etiologies is essential in the evaluation of hypercalcemia: (1) primary hyperparathyroidism and (2) malignancy. In this patient presence of severe hypercalcemia (Ca > 14 mg/dL) and history of recent thromboembolism elicit diagnosis of malignancy more likely. However, malignancy-related hypercalcemia is generally associated with low PTH levels, and hypercalcemia is often more symptomatic associated with higher calcium levels with more rapid increases [1]. Presence of malignancy, vitamin D intoxication, multiple myeloma, thyrotoxicosis, or immobilization should be considered for the differential diagnosis in the absence of high PTH levels. In this patient, frankly elevated PTH levels with concurrent hypercalcemia, presence of bilateral urolithiasis, and cortical bone resorption in distal radius indicating a longer duration of hypercalcemia rather than a sudden onset made primary hyperparathyroidism (HPT) more likely in the initial evaluation, and the diagnosis was supported with the imaging findings which both revealed parathyroid adenoma on the left superior side.

71.2.2 Management

The three main steps in the treatment of severe hypercalcemia (Ca > 14 mg/dL) are (1) volume expansion with isotonic saline (200–300 mL/h), (2) administration of calcitonin (4 international units/kg), and (3) concomitant IV bisphosphonate injection. Isotonic saline infusion corrects possible volume depletion due to hypercalcemia and prevents exacerbation of hypercalcemia. Calcitonin is a relatively weak agent which works rapidly within 4–6 h; however, the efficacy is limited to the first 48 h due to the development of tachyphylaxis [2]. Bisphosphonates are effective in treating hypercalcemia resulting from excessive bone resorption of any cause. Their maximum effect occurs in 2–4 days; therefore, they are usually used concomitantly with saline and calcitonin treatment. Bisphosphonates have potential nephrotoxicity related to dose and infusion time. Lower initial doses of bisphosphonates (zoledronate 3 mg, ibandronic acid 2 mg) with a longer duration for infusion are recommended for patients with preexisting renal impairment (CrCl <60 mL/min but ≥30 mL/min). Ibandronic acid has a relatively safe renal profile, and it is reported that it can be safely used in patients with a GFR value over 30 mL/min/1.73m^2 [3]. Therefore, it was preferred in the management of this patient until the renal functions returned to normal.

Cinacalcet is a calcimimetic agent which is primarily used in the presence of severe hypercalcemia due to parathyroid carcinoma and hemodialysis patients with an elevated calcium-phosphorus product and secondary hyperparathyroidism. Calcimimetics have also been evaluated in patients with primary hyperparathyroidism [4]. Cinacalcet can be used to normalize serum calcium in patients with severe hypercalcemia who are unable to undergo parathyroidectomy and with hypercalcemia that is refractory to bisphosphonates or in whom bisphosphonates are contraindicated due to severe renal impairment [4]. For patients who are unable to have surgery, cinacalcet may be used at a dose of 30 mg, twice daily. Calcimimetic agents activate the calcium-sensing receptor in the parathyroid gland, thereby inhibiting PTH secretion [5]. Serum calcium should be monitored within 1 week after initiation or after dose adjustment. Common side effects are nausea, vomiting, abdominal pain, and arthralgia. In this patient, cinacalcet was used in order to control high plasma calcium levels which were unresponsive to repeated administration of bisphosphonates, and the aim was to achieve normocalcemia until definitive treatment was available.

Although parathyroidectomy operation was determined to be the definitive treatment for this patient, surgical intervention was postponed for at least 3 months due to the presence of recent pulmonary embolism episode secondary to heterozygous factor 5 Leiden mutation. The perioperative risk of venous thromboembolism (VTE) is higher in individuals who experienced recent pulmonary embolism within the prior 3 months [6]. Therefore, patients who require surgery within the first 3 months following an episode of VTE are likely to benefit from delaying elective surgery [6]. Without anticoagulation, the early risk of recurrent VTE is approximately 50% [7]. On the other hand, RFA treatment was also considered among the treatment options given that there was a risk of pulmonary embolism recurrence in the postoperative period which could further deteriorate clinical status of the patient.

Radiofrequency ablation is a minimally invasive ablation method which is generally used in the management of benign thyroid nodules for volume reduction and improvement of associated symptoms [8]. Lately, this method has also been used in the management of HPT patients when surgery is not eligible either because of contraindication due to high surgical risk associated with comorbidities or patient refusal [9, 10]. Nonsurgical ablation of parathyroid adenoma is performed to maintain normal plasma calcium and PTH levels in these patients. Common complications are thermal injury to the surrounding structures (recurrent laryngeal nerve, esophagus, trachea, and vessels), hoarseness, brachial plexus injury, and skin burn at the electrode puncture site [9, 10]. The procedure is performed via insertion of an electrode to the related lesion under USG guidance and ablation of the parathyroid adenoma with 30 W of radiofrequency power. Dextrose 5% injection may be used before the intervention to create a safe zone between parathyroid adenoma and adjacent structures to prevent the risk of thermal injury [9].

Differential diagnosis of parathyroid cancer and parathyroid hyperplasia is required in patients for whom RFA treatment is planned. Parathyroid carcinoma is a rare cause for hyperparathyroidism, and it accounts for approximately 1% of patients with primary hyperparathyroidism [11]. A markedly elevated PTH level (five to tenfold higher than the upper limit of normal), severe hypercalcemia (>14 mg/dL), or a large-sized tumor (>3 cm) are predictive factors for parathyroid cancer [12]. Fine needle aspiration (FNA) prior to initial operation is not recommended due to technical difficulty in differentiating benign and malignant disease on cytology specimens and the possible associated risk of tumor seeding from the needle track [11]. In patients with suspicious parathyroid malignancy, surgical treatment is mandatory to remove the malignant lesion and to obtain a histopathological diagnosis. The diagnosis of parathyroid carcinoma is based on histopathological findings such as local invasion and lymph node or distant metastasis [11]. However, nonsurgical RFA therapy should be an option to reduce serum calcium levels in which surgery is not possible due to comorbidities. Multiple-gland hyperplasia is accounted for approximately 6% of cases of primary hyperparathyroidism, and it should also be ruled out with clinical and laboratory evaluation before RFA treatment [13]. In this patient, degree of PTH elevation and parathyroid adenoma size were not particularly suspicious for the presence of parathyroid carcinoma, and there was no sign of parathyroid hyperplasia during the clinical, laboratory, or imaging evaluation. Therefore, RFA was performed in order to control high plasma calcium levels when surgery was not feasible.

71.3 Follow-Up and Outcome

On the first day after RFA, patient's plasma calcium and PTH levels were 10.2 mg/dL and 40 pg/mL, respectively. Six months later the patient's symptoms were significantly improved with normal calcium, and PTH levels (9.5 mg/dL and 69 pg/mL, respectively) and the size of parathyroid gland decreased by USG evaluation.

71.3.1 The Future

Further studies with larger patient series are required to demonstrate safety and efficacy of RFA therapy with longer-term management.

What Can We Learn from This Case?

- RFA is a minimally invasive ablation technique which has been used as a safe procedure in the treatment of benign thyroid nodules for volume reduction.
- Although the only definitive treatment of primary hyperparathyroidism is parathyroidectomy performed by an experienced endocrine surgeon, RFA which is a nonsurgical procedure might be considered for the treatment of hypercalcemia in patients with high surgical risks or who refuse surgical intervention.
- RFA therapy should not be considered when there is suspicion of parathyroid carcinoma or hyperplasia.

References

1. Lafferty FW. Differential diagnosis of hypercalcemia. J Bone Miner Res. 1991;6:51–9.
2. Bilezikian JP. Clinical review: management of hypercalcemia. J Clin Endocrinol Metab. 1993;77:1445–9.
3. Perazella MA, Markowitz GS. Bisphosphonate nephrotoxicity. Kidney Int. 2008;74:1385–93.
4. Marcocci C, Bollerslev J, Khan AA, Shoback DM. Medical management of primary hyperparathyroidism: proceedings of the fourth international workshop on the management of asymptomatic primary hyperparathyroidism. J Clin Endocrinol Metab. 2014;99:3607–18.
5. Silverberg SJ, Bone HG, Marriott TB. Short-term inhibition of parathyroid hormone secretion by a calcium-receptor agonist in patients with primary hyperparathyroidism. N Engl J Med. 1997;337:1506–10.
6. Douketis JD, Foster GA, Crowther MA. Clinical risk factors and timing of recurrent venous thromboembolism during the initial 3 months of anticoagulant therapy. Arch Intern Med. 2000;160:3431–6.
7. Kearon C, Hirsh J. Management of anticoagulation before and after elective surgery. N Engl J Med. 1997;336:1506–11.

8. Fuller CW, Nguyen SA, Lohia S, et al. Radiofrequency ablation for treatment of benign thyroid nodules: systematic review. Laryngoscope. 2014;124:346–53.
9. Sormaz IC, Poyanlı A, Açar S, İşcan AY, Ozgur I, Tunca F, et al. The results of ultrasonography-guided percutaneous radiofrequency ablation in hyperparathyroid patients in whom surgery is not feasible. Cardiovasc Intervent Radiol. 2017;40:596–602.
10. Kim BS, Eom TI, Kang KH, et al. Radiofrequency ablation of parathyroid adenoma in primary hyperparathyroidism. J Med Ultrason. 2014;41:239–43.
11. Wei CH, Harari A. Parathyroid carcinoma: update and guidelines for management. Curr Treat Options Oncol. 2012;13:11–23.
12. Bae JH, Choi HJ, Lee Y. Preoperative predictive factors for parathyroid carcinoma in patients with primary hyperparathyroidism. J Korean Med Sci. 2012;27:890–5.
13. Ruda JM, Hollenbeak CS, Stack BC Jr. A systematic review of the diagnosis and treatment of primary hyperparathyroidism from 1995 to 2003. Otolaryngol Head Neck Surg. 2005;132:359–72.

72 Clinical Usefulness of an Intraoperative "Quick Parathyroid Hormone" Measurement in Primary Hyperparathyroidism Management

Serpil Salman and Fatih Tunca

Abstract

Hypercalcemia was detected in an elderly female presenting with psychological symptoms. Primary hyperparathyroidism was diagnosed according to laboratory results. Normal serum calcium (Ca) levels were restored following hydration and the administration of furosemide and zoledronic acid. However, parathyroidectomy was required. Because of poor health, minimally invasive parathyroidectomy was the preferred method, requiring adenoma localization. Neck ultrasonography (USG) revealed a suspicious mass in the inferoposterior region of the right thyroid lobe that can be a parathyroid adenoma. Scintigraphic imaging could not be performed to confirm the USG findings because of poor health. Intraoperative parathyroid hormone assay (quick PTH) was scheduled. During the operation, following the removal of the mass revealed on USG findings, PTH levels decreased from 579 to 50.8 pg/mL. On follow-up, serum Ca, phosphate, and PTH levels remained in the normal range, and cognitive impairment gradually improved.

72.1 Case Presentation

An 82-year-old female was admitted to the emergency department of the hospital because of confusion, disorientation, and dehydration for the previous 3 days. An endocrinology consultation was requested because the serum calcium (Ca) level was found to be 16 mg/dL at baseline evaluation. Her family reported that she had experienced fatigue, weakness, anorexia, weight loss (8 kg), insomnia, and depression for a few months, and a psychiatrist had prescribed escitalopram and olanzapine 2 months previously. Her general health gradually worsened, food and fluid consumption markedly decreased, and she had been immobile for 2 weeks. She presented with chronic atrial fibrillation and chronic obstructive pulmonary disease. No bone fracture or determined kidney stone was observed. The prescribed medication did not include drugs affecting Ca levels (i.e., thiazides, vitamin A, etc.).

On physical examination, she was unconscious and dehydrated. Bilaterally, an expiratory

S. Salman (✉)
Istinye University Medical Faculty,
Department of Internal Medicine, Istanbul, Turkey

F. Tunca
Istanbul University Medical Faculty,
Department of General Surgery, Istanbul, Turkey

T. Özülker et al. (eds.), *Thyroid and Parathyroid Diseases*, https://doi.org/10.1007/978-3-319-78476-2_72

wheeze could be heard on auscultation. Blood pressure was 140/70 mmHg, with an arrhythmic heart rate of 94 beats/min. On neck examination, no mass was revealed. An approximately 5 cm hard mass on the right scapula was palpated, which was probably a lipoma; however, the possibility of an osteitis fibrosa cystica was also considered.

The patient was hospitalized in the intensive care unit (ICU).

72.2 Discussion

72.2.1 Evaluation and Diagnosis

In cases of hyper- or hypocalcemia, the first step is to ensure that alterations in serum Ca levels are not due to abnormal albumin concentrations. Thus, albumin levels should be measured to correct serum Ca level [1]. However, in our patient, serum Ca levels were extremely high and could not be explained by a high serum albumin concentration. Indeed, her medical history record showed a serum Ca level of 13.2 mg/dL 1 month previously that had unfortunately been overlooked.

The second most important laboratory test in the diagnostic evaluation of hypercalcemia is parathyroid hormone (PTH) assay. PTH can be found at high levels or less frequently at low levels. Inappropriately normal PTH levels in spite of hypercalcemia should be investigated the same way as high PTH. Reasons for high PTH levels (i.e., excessive PTH production) include primary hyperparathyroidism (pHPT) (parathyroid adenoma, hyperplasia, and rarely carcinoma), tertiary hyperparathyroidism (long-term stimulation of PTH secretion in renal insufficiency), ectopic PTH secretion (very rare), inactivating calcium-sensing receptor (CaSR) or G protein [familial hypocalciuric hypercalcemia (FHH)] mutations, and CaSR function alterations (lithium therapy). The most common etiology of chronic hypercalcemia is pHPT. Malignancy is the second most common cause of hypercalcemia with a suppressed PTH level [1]. Other leading causes of hypercalcemia with a low PTH level include granulomatous diseases (sarcoidosis, tuberculosis, silicosis), vitamin D intoxication, hyperthyroidism, and excessive Ca intake. Thiazides and prolonged bed rest or inactivity can aggravate hypercalcemia.

In all cases, serum creatinine (Cr) levels should be measured to assess the renal function because hypercalcemia may impair renal function, and the renal clearance of PTH may be altered depending on the fragments detected by the assay. It is essential to confirm low phosphate levels, which are almost specific to pHPT along with urinary Ca levels to distinguish pHPT from FHH [1].

The results of the baseline laboratory evaluations of our patient were as follows: (1) serum Ca, 16.0 (8.8–10.2) mg/dL; (2) phosphate, 1.41 (2.5–4.5) mg/dL; (3) sodium, 135 (136–145) mmol/L; (4) potassium, 2.57 (3.5–5.1) mmol/L; (5) magnesium, 1.26 (1.6–2.4) mg/dL; (6) albumin, 3.9 (3.5–5.2) g/dL; (7) Cr, 1.05 (0.5–0.9) mg/dL; (8) alkaline phosphatase, 107 (35–105) U/L; (9) thyroid-stimulating hormone, 4.1 (0.27–4.20) uIU/mL; (10) PTH, 443 (15–65) pg/mL (605 pg/mL on second check); (11) 25-hydroxyvitamin D, 42 (20–50) ng/mL; and (12) 24 h urinary Ca, 428 (100–300) mg.

The diagnosis was pHPT based on high levels of serum Ca (corrected Ca, 16.1 mg/dL), PTH, and urinary Ca and low levels of serum phosphate. Volume depletion because of low fluid consumption and inactivity in the previous weeks was an important factor that provoked hypercalcemia.

72.2.2 Management

The emergent issue was to reduce the life-threatening high serum Ca to an acceptable level. In most cases, because hypercalcemia leads to dehydration, the initial therapy for significant hypercalcemia begins with volume expansion. Additionally, the use of loop diuretics is necessary to enhance sodium and Ca excretion. Diuretics should not be initiated until the volume status has been restored [1]. Considering the risk of heart failure in our patient, rehydration was accomplished relatively slowly [3 L i.v. (intravenous) saline in the first 24 h, followed by 2 L daily]. Decreased magnesium and potassium levels were also recovered. On the second day, i.v. furosemide was added. Antiresorptive agents are used as a supporting modality in hypercalcemia treatment [1] and bone loss improvement due to pHPT [2]. The onset of i.v. bisphosphonates action on serum calcium levels occurs within following 1–3 days, with normalization of serum Ca levels in the 60–90% of patients [1]. Zoledronic acid (4 mg i.v.) was used in our patient, and the serum Ca level was decreased to 9.5 mg/dL on the third day of administration (the fifth day of admission).

Patients with pHPT often present with neuropsychiatric symptoms and cognitive impairment, which are rarely isolated manifestations [3, 4]. Cognitive tests on the third day of hospitalization revealed severe global impairment suggesting dementia. Escitalopram and olanzapine were stopped on the admission day.

Parathyroidectomy is the fundamental therapy of symptomatic pHPT. In patients with severe hypercalcemia, who are unable to undergo parathyroidectomy, cinacalcet can be used to normalize serum Ca levels [5]. Cinacalcet is a calcimimetic agent that increases the sensitivity of CaSR activation by extracellular Ca. However, in the long-term, the drug has only a modest effect on serum PTH levels and no effect on bone mineral density (BMD). Currently, cinacalcet can be particularly useful as a short-term pretreatment prior to surgery, allowing the completion of diagnostic procedures and a safe waiting period [6]. Because acceptable Ca levels were shown, calcimimetic drugs were not administered.

Advanced age is associated with greater morbidity, intra- and postoperative complications, and higher mortality rate following parathyroidectomy [7]. Nonetheless, surgery is also recommended in older individuals meeting the criteria for parathyroidectomy when they are medically stable with no contraindications for an operation and/or when the benefits of surgery outweigh the associated risks [8]. Our patient presented with symptomatic pHPT. Even though she had certain health problems, there were no absolute contraindications for surgery.

Ultrasonographic (USG) evaluation intended to identify the complications of pHPT revealed no kidney stones and the mass on the scapula to be a lipoma and not a brown tumor (osteitis fibrosa cystica). The measurement of BMD was postponed until the patient's condition improved.

Several studies have recommended the use of either sestamibi (MIBI) scintigraphy or USG as a single imaging modality in preoperative localization in pHPT [9, 10]. The sensitivity of USG for the detection of single parathyroid adenomas ranges from 65% to 90%. Therefore, if USG and MIBI imaging were concordantly positive for the same localization(s), accurate localization was accomplished in 91% of the patients. The rate of localization was 96% in single-gland disease in the setting of concordant imaging results but decreased to 42% in multiglandular disease [11]. On USG evaluation, a 10.3 × 9.4 × 16.5 mm mass was detected in the inferoposterior region of the right thyroid lobe which could not be clearly defined as a parathyroid adenoma or thyroid nodule. For further evaluation, parathyroid scintigraphy could not be performed in this patient because of the poor health status during the treatment in the intensive care unit. In patients with pHPT, parathyroid imaging has become a standard preoperative procedure to locate abnormal parathyroid tissue, emphasizing the value of imaging tests to accurately identify abnormal parathyroid tissue to assist in planning the appropriate parathyroid surgery. However, no level of imaging substitutes for the expert parathyroid surgeon [12].

Conventional parathyroidectomy with four-gland exploration is mostly preferred when preoperative imaging modalities could not localize the adenoma or if they reveal a suspicion of multiglandular disease [13]. Minimally invasive parathyroidectomy (MIP) is another surgical option in patients with preoperative imaging modalities (MIBI and USG) that reveal the same localization. MIP also has various benefits, such as reduced operative time and fewer complications than conventional four-gland exploration [13]. Our patient underwent minimally invasive parathyroidectomy.

PTH has a mean circulating half-life of 3.5–4 min in patients with normal renal function. Rapid intraoperative PTH assays (quick PTH) have proven remarkably accurate in either confirming the adequacy of resection or predicting residual disease [13]. The most commonly employed algorithm utilizes the Miami criterion, requiring a PTH fall of 50% compared with the highest of either the premanipulation or preexcision sample [13, 14]. A quick PTH assay can also analyze the aspirate of a resected parathyroid gland to prove the parathyroid origin of the tissue, thereby replacing frozen-section analyses [13]. The indication of intraoperative PTH measurement in all MIP procedures is controversial. Some studies have reported no benefit when the adenoma is localized [15]; however, other studies have concluded that monitoring is essential to avoid a surgical failure in MIP [16, 17]. In every case, having an experienced surgeon is vital. Our patient's operation was performed by an experienced surgeon. Respective PTH levels were found to be 579, 114, and 50.8 pg/mL preoperatively at 5 min and at 15 min following the removal of the mass, respectively.

Postoperatively, Ca levels were stable, at approximately 9.3 mg/dL, and not complicated by the hungry bone syndrome. A lower incidence of transient postoperative hypocalcemia following MIP compared with that following a traditional bilateral cervical exploration remains unclear [18].

72.3 Follow-Up and Outcome

Histopathological examination revealed a 12 × 10 × 5 mm parathyroid adenoma. During the follow-up, serum Ca, phosphate, and PTH levels remained in the normal range. According to the literature, cognitive impairment observed for different reasons among the older population in the ICU, particularly women, is multifactorial and irreversible [19]. On the third and sixth months of the follow-up, the cognitive impairment of the patient gradually improved to the mild-middle levels, which was expected following pHPT treatment [3, 4]. This improvement was partly explained by the baseline tests being performed in unfavorable conditions (i.e., in the ICU when she was dehydrated just a few days previously) [20].

BMD was measured by dual-energy X-ray absorptiometry 1 month after parathyroidectomy, which revealed T scores of −2.9, −2.7, and −3.2 on the vertebra, femur total, and distal radius, respectively. On follow-up, 800 IU/day vitamin D was initiated considering the long-term benefits of adenoma resection and zoledronic acid on bone metabolism.

What Can We Learn from This Case?

- Presentation with cognitive impairment of primary hyperparathyroidism is possible in elderly patients.
- Successful treatment can improve declined mental status.
- MIP is a suitable therapeutic option and has several benefits, such as reduced operative time and fewer complications.
- An experienced surgeon is very important for parathyroid surgery.
- Intraoperative PTH assay (quick PTH) increases the success of the surgery.

References

1. Khosla S. Hypercalcemia and hypocalcemia. In: Jameson JL, editor. Harrison's endocrinology. New York: Mc Graw Hill Education; 2017. p. 442–5.
2. Sankaran S, Gamble G, Bolland M, Reid IR, Grey A. Skeletal effects of interventions in mild primary hyperparathyroidism: a meta-analysis. J Clin Endocrinol Metab. 2010;95:1653–62. https://doi.org/10.1210/jc.2009-384.
3. Trombetti A, Christ ER, Henzen C, Gold G, Brändle M, Herrmann FR, et al. Clinical presentation and management of patients with primary hyperparathyroidism of the Swiss primary hyperparathyroidism cohort: a focus on neuro-behavioral and cognitive symptoms. J Endocrinol Investig. 2016;39:567–76. https://doi.org/10.1007/s40618-015-0423-3.
4. Dotzenrath CM, Kaetsch AK, Pfingsten H, Cupisti K, Weyerbrock N, Vossough A, et al. Neuropsychiatric and cognitive changes after surgery for primary hyperparathyroidism. World J Surg. 2006;30(5):680. https://doi.org/10.1007/s00268-005-0444-8.

5. Marcocci C, Bollerslev J, Khan AA, Shoback DM. Medical management of primary hyperparathyroidism: proceedings of the fourth international workshop on the Management of Asymptomatic Primary Hyperparathyroidism. J Clin Endocrinol Metab. 2014;99:3607–18. https://doi.org/10.1210/jc.2014-417.
6. Misiorowski W, Zgliczyński W. Cinacalcet as symptomatic treatment of hypercalcaemia in primary hyperparathyroidism prior to surgery. Endokrynol Pol. 2017;68:306–10. https://doi.org/10.5603/EP.2017.0023.
7. Thomas DC, Roman SA, Sosa JA. Parathyroidectomy in the elderly: analysis of 7313 patients. J Surg Res. 2011;170:240–6. https://doi.org/10.1016/j.jss.2011.03.014.
8. Denizot A, Grino M, Oliver C. Surgical management of primary hyperparathyroidism in older adults. J Am Geriatr Soc. 2014;62:1759–63. https://doi.org/10.1111/jgs.12968.
9. Borley NR, Collins RE, O'Doherty M, Coakley A. Technetium-99m sestamibi parathyroid localization is accurate enough for scan-directed unilateral neck exploration. Br J Surg. 1996;83:989–91.
10. Van Husen R, Kim LT. Accuracy of surgeon-performed ultrasound in parathyroid localization. World J Surg. 2004;28:1122–6.
11. Lumachi F, Zucchetta P, Marzola MC, Boccagni P, Angelini F, Bui F, et al. Advantages of combined technetium-99m-sestamibi scintigraphy and high-resolution ultrasonography in parathyroid localization: comparative study in 91 patients with primary hyperparathyroidism. Eur J Endocrinol. 2000;143:755–60.
12. Khan AA, Hanley DA, Rizzoli R, Bollerslev J, Young JE, Rejnmark L, et al. Primary hyperparathyroidism: review and recommendations on evaluation, diagnosis, and management. A Canadian and international consensus. Osteoporos Int. 2017;28:1–19. https://doi.org/10.1007/s00198-016-3716-2.
13. Udelsman R, Akerström G, Biagini C, Duh QY, Miccoli P, Niederle B, et al. The surgical management of asymptomatic primary hyperparathyroidism: proceedings of the Fourth International Workshop. J Clin Endocrinol Metab. 2014;99:3595–606. https://doi.org/10.1210/jc.2014-2000.
14. Barczynski M, Konturek A, Hubalewska-Dydejczyk A, Cichon S, Nowak W. Evaluation of Halle, Miami, Rome, and Vienna intraoperative iPTH assay criteria in guiding minimally invasive parathyroidectomy. Langenbeck's Arch Surg. 2009;394:843–9. https://doi.org/10.1007/s00423-009-0510-z.
15. Nair CG, Babu MJ, Jacob P, Menon R, Mathew J. Is intraoperative parathyroid hormone monitoring necessary in symptomatic primary hyperparathyroidism with concordant imaging? Indian J Endocrinol Metab. 2016;20:512–6. https://doi.org/10.4103/2230-8210.183451.
16. Kim HG, Kim WY, Woo SU, Lee JB, Lee YM. Minimally invasive parathyroidectomy with or without intraoperative parathyroid hormone for primary hyperparathyroidism. Ann Surg Treat Res. 2015;89:111–6. https://doi.org/10.4174/astr.2015.89.3.111.
17. Bobanga ID, McHenry CR. Is intraoperative parathyroid hormone monitoring necessary for primary hyperparathyroidism with concordant preoperative imaging? Am J Surg. 2017;213:484–8. https://doi.org/10.1016/j.amjsurg.2016.11.035.
18. Bergenfelz A, Lindblom P, Tibblin S, Westerdahl J. Unilateral versus bilateral neck exploration for primary hyperparathyroidism: a prospective randomized controlled trial. Ann Surg. 2002;236:543–51.
19. Zhao J, Yao L, Wang C, Sun Y, Sun Z. The effects of cognitive intervention on cognitive impairments after intensive care unit admission. Neuropsychol Rehabil. 2017;27:301–17. https://doi.org/10.1080/09602011.2015.1078246.
20. Pross N. Effects of dehydration on brain functioning: a life-span perspective. Ann Nutr Metab. 2017;70:30–6. https://doi.org/10.1159/000463060.

Robot-Assisted Endoscopic Mediastinal Parathyroidectomy

73

Özer Makay and Murat Özdemir

Abstract

Case Report: A 45-year-old man admitted to an outside hospital with a history of nephrolithiasis, diffuse joint pain, and problems with walking, lasting for a year. The patient had normal findings on physical examination. Blood tests revealed elevated serum calcium, alkaline phosphatase, parathyroid hormone (PTH), and a decreased phosphate level. Ultrasound of the neck showed no evidence of parathyroid adenoma. Subsequently, a computed tomography scan of the thorax showed a hypervascular solitary nodule of 2 cm in the anterior mediastinum, at the level of the anterior aspect of the ascending aorta. ^{99m}Tc methoxyisobutylisonitrile (MIBI) scintigraphy confirmed the presence of an adenoma.

Surgery was performed thoracoscopically with the da Vinci *Si* robotic system. Four ports were used for the operation, three of them for the robotics arms and one for assistance. Post-excision PTH level was used for intraoperative confirmation of success. The total operative time was 119 min. Intraoperative blood loss was minimal, and no complications occurred during the operation. The patient was discharged without any complications on the fourth postoperative day.

The robotic technique provides excellent visualization with a three-dimensional view, better color resolution, better contrast, precision, and enhanced skills in order to ensure an effective, safe, and accurate operation. The robotic approach is our preferred method for mediastinal located parathyroid glands. Besides, accurate localization of the ectopic parathyroid gland(s) due to preoperative screening is an important aspect of the robotic approach.

Ö. Makay (✉) · M. Özdemir
Division of Endocrine Surgery, Ege University, İzmir, Turkey

73.1 Case Presentation

A 45-year-old man with a body mass index of 22 is presented to an outside hospital with a history of nephrolithiasis, diffuse joint pain, and problems with walking for 1 year. His serum calcium, parathyroid hormone (PTH), and alkaline phosphatase (ALP) levels were increased. A bone scintigraphy was performed, and the findings confirmed a metabolic bone disease. For which, the patient was presented to our institution for further evaluation.

The patient had normal findings on physical examination. However, blood tests revealed an elevated serum calcium (12.9 mg/dL; normal value, 8.5–10.2 mg/dL), elevated ALP (2540 U/L; normal value, 20–120 IU/L), decreased phosphate (1.7 mg/dL; normal value, 2.4–4.1 mg/dL),

T. Özülker et al. (eds.), *Thyroid and Parathyroid Diseases*, https://doi.org/10.1007/978-3-319-78476-2_73

and an elevated PTH level (1529.2 pg/mL; normal value, 13–54 pg/mL).

Ultrasound (USG) of the neck which is performed with regard to these findings showed no evidence of parathyroid adenoma.

73.2 Discussion

73.2.1 Evaluation and Diagnosis

The parathyroid glands are generally located in the cervical region, just behind the thyroid gland. These glands are involved in the production of PTH, which is important for the concentration of calcium and phosphate in the blood. In some cases, there is an excess of PTH in the bloodstream due to overactivity of one or more of the parathyroid glands, also called primary hyperparathyroidism. In addition, 15–20% of patients with abnormally functioning parathyroid glands have ectopic parathyroid glands due to abnormal migration during embryogenesis [1]. These glands can be located at any anatomical location from the base of the tongue to the mediastinum. An ectopic parathyroid tissue outside the neck region cannot be seen with USG. ^{99m}Tc-methoxyisobutylisonitrile (MIBI) scintigraphy and computed tomography (CT) can be used to detect a mediastinal ectopic parathyroid adenoma.

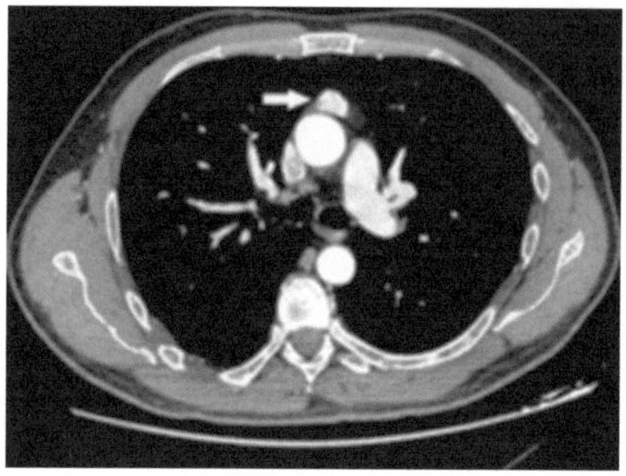

Fig. 73.1 Mediastinal parathyroid adenoma (CT image)

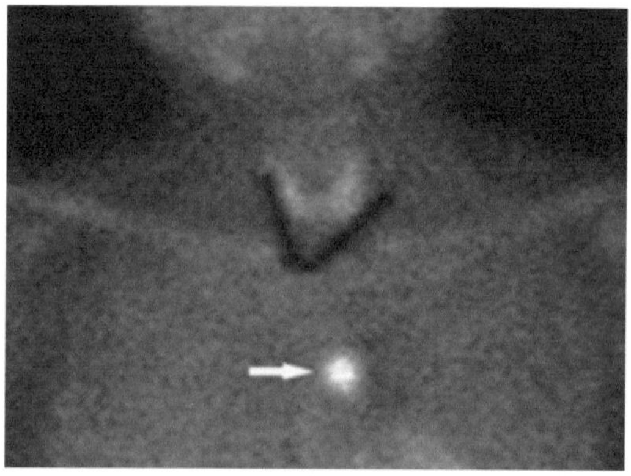

Fig. 73.2 Mediastinal parathyroid adenoma detected with MIBI scintigraphy

In this case, a CT scan of the thorax and abdomen showed a 2-cm hypervascular solitary nodule at the anterior mediastinum, at the level of the anterior aspect of the ascending aorta (Fig. 73.1). This was confirmed by a ^{99m}Tc-MIBI scintigraphy (Fig. 73.2). In addition, the CT scan identified the diffuse heterogeneous density of the bone structures and a well-defined lytic bone lesion of 2.2 cm at the level of the left femoral head, which may be associated with a brown tumor. With regard to this, a bone scintigraphy was performed which showed a diffusely increased bone activity. This finding could be consistent with the ectopic parathyroid adenoma. Primary hyperparathyroidism may occur as a part of multiple endocrine neoplasia type 1 (MEN-1) and type2A. Multiple endocrine neoplasia type 2A (MEN-2A) is a hereditary condition associated with three primary types of tumors: medullary thyroid cancer, parathyroid tumors, and pheochromocytoma. Multiple endocrine neoplasia (MEN-1) was originally known as Wermer's syndrome. The most common tumors seen in MEN-1 involve the parathyroid gland, islet cells of the pancreas, and pituitary gland. Therefore, a magnetic resonance imaging (MRI) of the pituitary gland was performed to exclude this option. The MRI scan showed no abnormalities, and therefore MEN-1 was ruled out. During the preoperative period, serum calcium level was determined daily due to hypercalcemia. High serum calcium level was tried to be corrected and treated with intravenous saline hydration, furosemide, and pamidronate. Nevertheless, the serum calcium levels remained high at two consequent measurements (>15.0 mg/dL); therefore, hemodialysis was carried out two times prior to surgery.

73.2.2 Management

Removal of these ectopic parathyroid glands depends on their size and location. In most cases, these glands are found in the superior mediastinum which can be successfully removed by a cervical approach [2]. One-third of the ectopic parathyroid glands migrate deep into the mediastinum which are not accessible with a low cervical incision [3]. The ectopic parathyroid glands were previously removed by performing a sternotomy or thoracotomy [4]. However, these open procedures were correlated with a higher morbidity risk, high complication rate, longer postoperative recovery, and poor cosmetic results [4]. In the past decades, video-assisted thoracoscopic surgery (VATS) was described to be safer, less invasive, effective, and a feasible procedure for resection of deep mediastinal parathyroid lesions [5]. However, randomized controlled trials should be carried out to support these findings.

Recently, another alternative minimally invasive technique was introduced to the surgical treatment of ectopic mediastinal parathyroid, namely, the da Vinci® robotic system. In a similar context, this technique has already made a significant contribution to, among others, thymectomies [6]. This technology revolutionized the field of minimally invasive surgery.

This patient was evaluated by the Multidisciplinary Endocrine Consultation Team. The team proposed to perform a thoracic resection of the MIBI-positive mediastinal solitary nodule using a robotic-assisted approach. Informed consent was obtained from the patient, and finally, the operation was performed totally thoracoscopically with the da Vinci *Si* robot system ® (Intuitive Surgical Sarl, Aubonne, Switzerland) with intraoperative intact PTH guidance.

The da Vinci robot consists of a manipulator unit with three arms (two instrument arms and a central arm to guide the endoscope) and a remote master console (optical control with three-dimensional vision and tele manipulators of the arms). A right-sided approach was chosen due to the location of the solitary ectopic gland. The patient was positioned in a supine position at the edge of the operating table by placing silicone gel behind his right shoulder/upper back. Finally, the patient was somewhat tilted to the left side. The right arm was positioned below the table level with flexion at the elbow. The procedure was performed under general anesthesia with double-lumen endotracheal tube intubation for left single-lung ventilation. The right parietal pleura was incised, and the right chest cavity was entered. A 12-mm port for the 30–*degree* upward stereo endoscope was placed in the fifth intercostal space at the mid-axillary line, where the incision was made previously for entering the right cavity. Subsequently, two 8-mm robotic operating ports were positioned, both at the anterior axillary line, in the third and sixth intercostal spaces. The three robotic arms of the da Vinci system were attached to these three ports. An accessory additional port was placed in the midclavicular line, just below the nipple of the breast (Fig. 73.3). The procedure was performed by two surgeons, one at the console and one surgeon assisting at the operating table using the additional port. The right lung was deflated, and CO_2 insufflation was set at 10 mm Hg through the camera port with careful hemodynamic monitoring. With this, there will be an improvement of the visualization of the operative field by washing out diathermy smoke. Fenestrated bipolar forceps and electrocautery hook with EndoWrist® action were used for dissection of the ectopic gland. Dissection was started toward the ectopic gland, which was marked previously on the skin. The mediastinal pleura was opened until the left parietal pleura was visible. Dissection proceeded toward the ascending aorta, and the ectopic gland was identified adjacent to this major blood vessel. The ectopic gland was manipulated and finally removed using the instruments (Fig. 73.4). The right nervus phrenicus and the esophagus were identified and preserved. After completion of the dissection, the ectopic gland was removed from the thoracic cavity using an Endo Catch™ bag. At the end of the operation, a chest tube was placed and directed toward the apex of the right hemithorax.

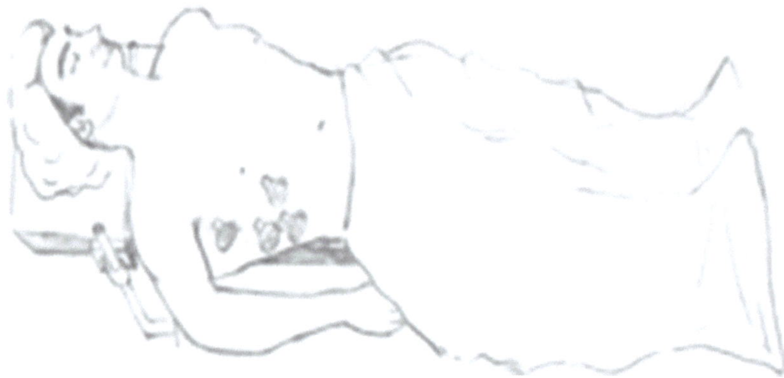

Fig. 73.3 Patient and port positioning for robotic transthoracic parathyroidectomy

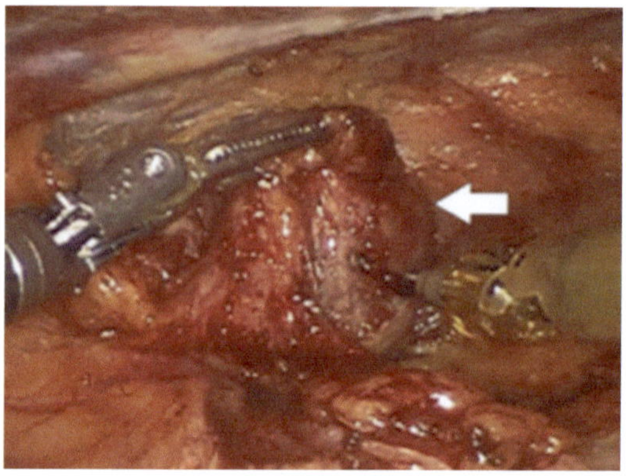

Fig. 73.4 Mediastinal parathyroid adenoma during transthoracic robotic surgery

The total operative time was 119 min; however, the robotic act took 35 min and the docking time lasted only 5 min. Intraoperative blood loss was minimal, and no complications occurred during the operation. There was no recorded bleeding. Serum PTH and calcium levels were determined 20 min post-excision. PTA level showed an appropriate decrease after removal of the ectopic gland (31.6 pg/mL), and calcium level also showed a decrease (9.1 mg/dL). The patient recovered from the post-anesthesia recovery unit and was transferred to the regular nursing unit on the same day. A chest X-ray was performed and did not show any signs of a pneumothorax. The chest tube was removed on day one, postoperatively.

With regard to hungry bone syndrome, serum PTH and calcium levels were assessed daily during the postoperative period. During the early postoperative period, calcium levels dropped slightly below normal levels. Hereby, the patient received calcium and vitamin D3 supplements. There were no postoperative complications. Finally, the patient was discharged with calcium and vitamin D3 supplements and the tissue was histopathologically confirmed as a parathyroid adenoma.

Parathyroid glands, which are often removed through sternotomy or thoracotomy, are rarely located in the mediastinum (<1–3%) [3]. In this article, we described the robotic approach of the ectopic mediastinal parathyroid gland. This method of the management of mediastinal adenomas has more significant advantages when compared to conventional and maybe even the VATS procedure. Compared with the conventional open approach, the robotic technique seems to have significant benefits in quality of life and morbidity [7]. Likewise, in the current literature, multiple case reports have described the robotic technique with similarly promising results like the VATS procedure [8, 9]. In addition, the da Vinci® robotic system gives the opportunity for a more comfortable approach of the tissue compared with the disadvantages of the VATS procedure (e.g., two-dimensional view, unstable camera platform, and poor ergonomic position of the surgeon). The robotic technique provides excellent visualization with a three-dimensional view, better color resolution, better contrast, precision, and enhanced skills in order to ensure an affective, safe, and accurate operation [8–10]. These potential advantages ensure the possibility for the differentiation of the ectopic parathyroid gland from surrounding tissue (e.g., adipose and thymus). Hereby, the technique is very useful to access small and remote surgical fields.

In the current literature, the robotic technique is increasingly described by other medical specialties. There are promising results in cardiac, gynecologic, urologic, transplantation, and general surgery. As aforementioned, there already have been several reports presenting the outcome of the robot-assisted mediastinal parathyroidectomy, which are promising [11, 12]. However, to date, there is a lack of studies with larger cohorts and randomized control trails to confirm these outcomes. Furthermore, almost all studies described robot-assisted mediastinal parathyroidectomy and have several limitations, such as small sample size and single-center experience, and most of them are case reports.

With the use of high sensitive radiographic modalities (e.g., MIBI scan, CT, MRI, and venous blood sampling), more ectopic parathyroid glands can be detected in patients with symptoms matching with hyperparathyroidism [13]. Due to the advances in preoperative screening, it provides the ability to determine the accurate localization of the ectopic parathyroid gland(s). This is one of the key concepts of endocrine and robotic surgery, which makes targeted minimally invasive approaches feasible. Inadequate diagnostic imaging could lead to wasted time and failed surgery procedure for a hyperactive ectopic parathyroid gland [14, 15]. At our center, localization begins with USG and a MIBI scan, involving the chest together with the neck.

Despite the potential advantages and promising results of the robotic technique, there are also some obstacles to perform this technique. First of all, there is a need for a specially trained surgical team to perform the robotic technique. All participants are closely involved with the operation, including the surgeon(s), assistants, anesthesiologist, and other personnel. The surgeons also have to undergo training to achieve the robotic surgery skills. These aspects are very important for a successful robotic procedure. Besides, the robotic technique ensures a high cost which is caused by the additional cost of the da Vinci® robotic system and the robotic instruments.

73.3 The Future

Robotic surgery will continue to evolve in parallel with people's imagination and technology. In the future, the robotic arms will feel human tissue as a real hand of a surgeon and provide tactile feedback. Also, we will see the single-incision port and snake-like arms in the future. These snake-like arms will be able to enter in a single incision and work in areas where human hands or other conventional tools cannot reach.

What Can We Learn from This Case?

- In patients with signs and symptoms of hypercalcemia, primary hyperparathyroidism should be the first diagnosis that comes to mind.
- The most common cause of primary hyperparathyroidism is solitary parathyroid adenomas.
- With the combined use of ultrasound and MIBI scintigraphy, 90% of solitary parathyroid adenomas can be localized.
- When parathyroid adenomas cannot be localized by USG and MIBI scintigraphy, advanced examinations such as CT, MRI, and endosonography can be performed.
- Endocrine surgeons have to know the anatomy and embryology of the parathyroid glands very well.
- Possible anatomical location of ectopic parathyroid adenomas should be known.
- Surgical planning should be performed in mediastinal parathyroid adenomas according to adenoma location.
- Minimally invasive thoracoscopic approach in deep mediastinal parathyroid adenomas is a good treatment option.
- The robotic technique provides excellent visualization with a three-dimensional view, better color resolution, better contrast, precision, and enhanced skills in order to ensure an effective, safe, and accurate operation.
- Therefore, the robotic approach is our preferred method for mediastinal located parathyroid glands.

References

1. Kaplan EL, Yashiro T, Salti G. Primary hyperparathyroidism in the 1990s. Choice of surgical procedures for this disease. Ann Surg. 1992;215:300–17.
2. Freeman JB, Sherman BM, Mason EE. Transcervical thymectomy: an integral part of neck exploration for hyperparathyroidism. Arch Surg. 1976;111:359–64.
3. Alesina PF, Moka D, Mahlstedt J, Walz MK. Thoracoscopic removal of mediastinal hyperfunctioning parathyroid glands: personal experience and review of the literature. World J Surg. 2008;32:224–31.
4. Russell CF, Edis AJ, Scholz DA, Sheedy PF, van Heerden JA. Mediastinal parathyroid tumors: experience with 38 tumors requiring mediastinotomy for removal. Ann Surg. 1981;193:805–9.
5. Iihara M, Suzuki R, Kawamata A, Horiuchi K, Okamoto T. Thoracoscopic removal of mediastinal parathyroid lesions: selection of surgical approach and pitfalls of preoperative and intraoperative localization. World J Surg. 2012;36:1327–34.
6. Rea F, Schiavon M, Di Chiara F, Marulli G. Single-institution experience on robot-assisted thoracoscopic operations for mediastinal diseases. Innovations (Phila). 2011;6:316–22.
7. Balduyck B, Hendriks JM, Lauwers P, Mercelis R, Ten Broecke P, Van Schil P. Quality of life after anterior mediastinal mass resection: a prospective study comparing open with robotic-assisted thoracoscopic resection. Eur J Cardiothorac Surg. 2011;39:543–8.
8. Ismail M, Maza S, Swierzy M, Tsilimparis N, Rogalla P, Sandrock D, et al. Resection of ectopic mediastinal parathyroid glands with the da Vinci robotic system. Br J Surg. 2010;97:337–43.
9. Chan AP, Wan IY, Wong RH, Hsin MK, Underwood MJ. Robot-assisted excision of ectopic mediastinal parathyroid adenoma. Asian Cardiovasc Thorac Ann. 2010;18:65–7.
10. Van Dessel E, Hendriks JM, Lauwers P, Ysebaert D, Ruyssers N Jr, Van Schil PE. Mediastinal parathyroidectomy with the da Vinci robot. Innovations (Phila). 2011;6(4):262.
11. Karagkounis G, Uzun DD, Mason DP, Murthy SC, Berber E. Robotic surgery for primary hyperparathyroidism. Surg Endosc. 2014;28:2702–7.
12. Brunaud L, Ayav A, Bresler L, Schjött B. Da Vinci robot-assisted thoracoscopy for primary hyperparathyroidism: a new application in endocrine surgery. Thoracoscopie robotique pour hyperparathyroidie primaire: nouvelle application en chirurgie endocrinienne. J Chir (Paris). 2008;145:165–7.
13. Johnson NA, Tublin ME, Ogilvie JB. Parathyroid imaging: technique and role in the preoperative evaluation of primary hyperparathyroidism. AJR Am J Roentgenol. 2007;188:1706–15.
14. Timmerman GL, Allard B, Lovrien F, Hickey D. Hyperparathyroidism: robotic-assisted thoracoscopic resection of a supernumary anterior mediastinal parathyroid tumor. J Laparoendosc Adv Surg Tech A. 2008;18:76–9.
15. Harvey A, Bohacek L, Neumann D, Mihaljevic T, Berber E. Robotic thoracoscopic mediastinal parathyroidectomy for persistent hyperparathyroidism: case report and review of the literature. Surg Laparosc Endosc Percutan Tech. 2011;21:24–7.

74 Focused Parathyroid Surgery: Minimally Invasive Parathyroidectomy via a Mini-incision

Orhan Yalçın and Semra Günay

Abstract

The most common cause of hypercalcemia is primary hyperparathyroidism (PHPT). Solitary adenoma is detected in 85% of cases, and it is possible to treat these cases with minimally invasive parathyroidectomy (MIP).

We present a 53-year-old female patient of PHPT diagnosed with asymptomatic hypercalcemia and single adenoma, who underwent open-focused MIP via a mini-incision.

In the event of a single adenomatous lesion, diagnosis is possible with the ultrasonography and Tc-99m-sestamibi scintigraphy. If necessary biochemical studies (parathormone washout, intraoperative parathormone monitoring (IPM)) and additional imaging (intraoperative USG) or radioguided approach can be used, which offers lower morbidity rates and similar success rates when compared to conventional methods, and this procedure yields good outcomes.

There are multiple MIP methods, and our clinic uses open mini-incision focused surgical technique. In this report, diagnosis and treatment methods of the disease are discussed.

The most critical factor regarding surgical success and treatment is the surgeon. If the appropriate surgical technique is selected according to the patient's condition, those surgeons experienced in endocrine surgery can safely apply open MIP.

74.1 Case Presentation

Hypercalcemia was detected on routine blood examination of a 53-year-old postmenopausal woman without any complaints. Physical examination was normal, and there were no remarkable findings other than a history of type 2 diabetes and hypertension. The patient had undergone surgery for ectopic pregnancy 20 years ago. Serum calcium level was 11.3 mg/dl (8.4–10.2 N), phosphor level 2.8 mg/dl (2.7–4.5), serum parathormone (PTH) level 154 mg/dl, and 24-h urinary calcium excretion 270 mg. Imaging studies were performed based on these data, and the preliminary diagnosis of primary hyperparathyroidism (pHPT) was made.

O. Yalçın · S. Günay (✉)
University of Health Sciences (SBÜ), Okmeydanı Training and Research Hospital, Division of Breast and Endocrin Surgery, Okmeydanı, Istanbul, Turkey

T. Özülker et al. (eds.), *Thyroid and Parathyroid Diseases*, https://doi.org/10.1007/978-3-319-78476-2_74

Head and neck ultrasonography (USG) of the thyroid gland showed an 18 × 13 × 10 mm mass in the inferior pole of the right lobe of the thyroid gland, and this was regarded as a parathyroid adenoma.

The abdominal USG showed normal findings, and no urinary stones were detected.

On bone mineral density, T-score of the spine was 1.5 (osteopenic). Tc-99m MIBI delayed-phase scans (120 min) showed an increased uptake in the inferior pole of the right thyroid lobe that may be compatible with an adenoma.

The case was discussed at the endocrinology council, and the patient became a candidate for focused surgery as the two imaging methods (USG and MIBI) consistently pointed to the same site. After preoperative procedures, a blood sample was withdrawn for PTH measurement before an incision was made to the marked surgical site under general anesthesia. A cutaneous and subcutaneous transverse incision of 2 cm was made parallel to the cleavage lines across the sternocleidomastoid (SCM) muscle on the side of the localized adenoma 2 cm above the sternal notch (Fig. 74.1) for preparing the mini flaps; platysma was split appropriately.

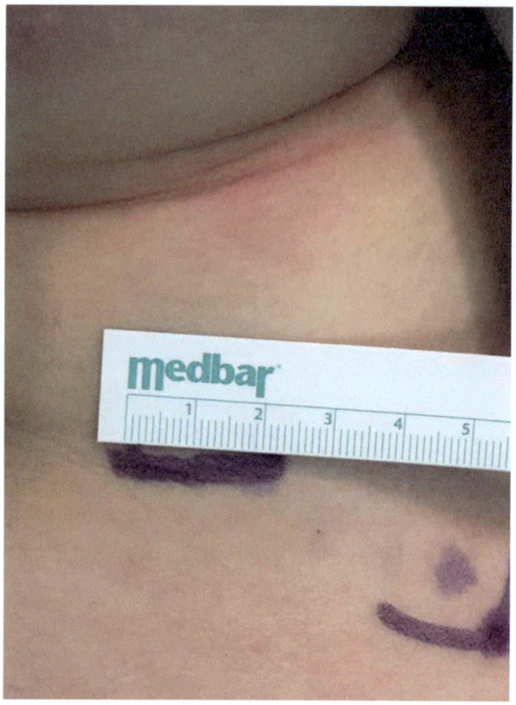

Fig. 74.1 Incision for MIP

The strap and sternocleidomastoid (SCM) muscles were separated to expose the thyroid gland, and the enlarged parathyroid gland was exposed posterior to the inferior pole of the thyroid gland by identifying the thyrothymic ligament (Fig. 74.2). The gland was handled with an atraumatic tool and separated from the median thyroid vein and thyrothymic ligament using hemostatic mini clips while preserving the surrounding tissue, particularly the carotid artery and internal jugular vein, and the adenoma was placed over the strap muscles and excised by preserving the capsule. After 10 min, blood was drawn for intraoperative PTH measurement. The baseline value (pre-incision PTH) was 148 mg/dl, and the second value was 28 mg/dl. The value was found to be sufficient, and the operation was terminated. Serum calcium at postoperative 2 h was 8.5 mg/dl. On the following day, the incision site was found to be intact. Calcium and PTH levels were within normal ranges, and the patient was discharged after she was provided with information about potential complications, particularly on the symptoms of hypocalcemia. Her serum calcium level was 8.9 mg/dl, and PTH level was 22 mg/dl at the 1-week follow-up. The pathologic examination revealed 18 mm diameter adenoma (Fig. 74.3).

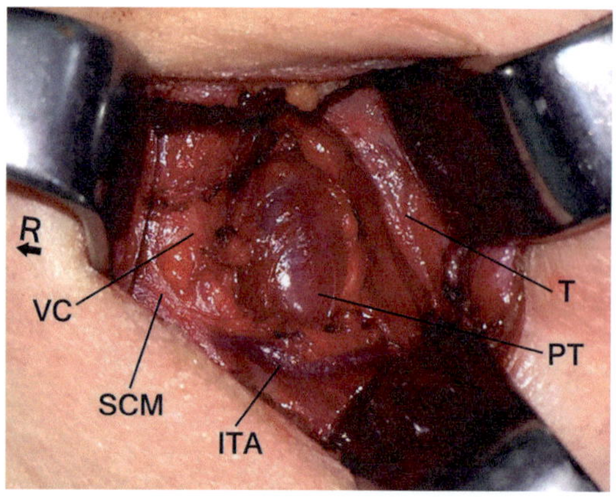

Fig. 74.2 Enlarged Parathyroid gland (*PT* parathyroid, *T* thyroid, *VC* vagina caroticum aroticum, *SCM* sternocleidomastoid muscle, *ITA* arteria thyroidea inferior)

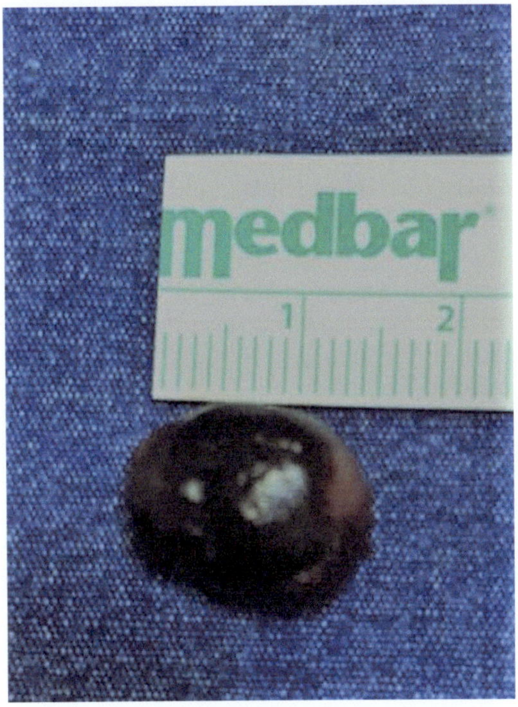

Fig. 74.3 Parathyroid adenoma

74.2 Discussion

74.2.1 Evaluation and Diagnosis

Hypercalcemia is defined as elevated plasma calcium levels above the upper limit of 1 mg/dl determined by the reference laboratory values, and the most common cause is pHPT. Adenomas or hyperplasia in multiple glands and parathyroid carcinoma are the responsible etiology. Solid adenoma is responsible for >85% of HPT cases; double adenoma is responsible for 7% of the cases and to a lesser extent intrathyroidal adenoma.

Elevated calcium levels are the characteristic feature of the disease, and it is a heterogeneous disorder manifesting with different symptoms in different age groups in clinical practice. The diagnosis is confirmed biochemically; therefore, in cases suspected to have pHPT, one should initially investigate the accuracy of the diagnosis. For this purpose, causes of secondary hyperparathyroidism (sHPT) and familial hypocalciuric hypercalcemia must be taken into consideration in differential diagnosis [1, 2]. In secondary HPT, calcium levels are normal or low, whereas in FHH, 24-h urinary calcium excretion is lower than 100 mg; therefore, repeated measurement of serum calcium and serum calcium corrected for albumin levels must be determined. Furthermore, 24-h urinary calcium excretion (<100 ml) and calcium/creatinine ratio (<0.01) favor the diagnosis of sHPT. These measurements have to be obtained because they are essential in confirming the diagnosis of pHPT and ruling out other possibilities.

In contrast to other etiologies, primary HPT is treated surgically [1] (Recommendation (Rec)-1-1). In cases diagnosed with primary HPT, the knowledge of bone mineral density is crucial for accurately estimating PTH and 25-hydroxyvitamin D levels [1] (Rec-1-5). Creatinine clearance and 24-h urinary calcium excretion as well as the urinary calcium/creatinine ratio play an essential role in the diagnosis and clinical judgment. Treatment must be planned for patients meeting diagnostic criteria for primary HPT by determining the location of pathological gland/glands as soon as possible [2, 3] (Table 74.1).

Parathyroidectomy is indicated in patients aged <50 years, those who are diagnosed with symptomatic or asymptomatic pHPT, those with a serum calcium level of >1 mg/dl above the upper limit, those with a T-score of 2.5 or existing fracture or fracture risk in the skeletal system, those with a creatinine clearance of <60 ml/min, and those with an existing or would have the risk of developing kidney stones [2, 3].

74.2.2 Management

Parathyroid surgery has shown important changes in the last 20 years; therefore, the decision to operate in cases diagnosed with pHPT should be followed by planning of surgical methods. Detection of pathological gland or glands is the most important factor that would guide this planning. Imaging methods are used for this purpose [4]. The results of the imaging studies are used for selecting the surgical technique and not for

Table 74.1 Indication for minimally invasive surgery in pHPT cases [2]

(1) Age < 50 years
(2) Serum calcium >1 mg/dl or > 0.25 mmol/l of the upper limit of the reference interval for total calcium and > 0.12 mmol/l for Ca^{2+}
(3) BMD T-score ≤ −2.5 at the lumbar spine, femoral neck, the total hip, or the 1/3 radius for postmenopausal women or males >50 years. A prevalent low-energy fracture (i.e., in the spine) is also considered an indication for surgery, which requires a routine X-ray of the thoracic and lumbar spine (or vertebral fracture assessment by DXA)
(4) Glomerular filtration rate (GFR) of <60 ml/min. Further evaluation of asymptomatic patients with renal imaging (X-ray, CT, or ultrasound) in order to detect silent kidney stones or nephrocalcinosis is advised [2]. A complete urinary stone risk profile should be performed in those individuals whose urinary calcium excretion is >400 mg/day. If stone(s), nephrocalcinosis, or high stone risk is determined, surgery should be recommended

confirming surgical indication or the diagnosis. The knowledge of concurrent thyroid pathologies requiring surgery is also necessary while evaluating the patients.

USG is the preferred imaging method among the other methods. The thyroid gland and lymphatic system have to be evaluated in detail with the parathyroid glands using head and neck USG. Abdominal USG must be performed for differential diagnosis of concurrent secondary HPT (to evaluate the urinary tract) [4].

Although USG performed by experienced radiologists is crucial, it may be inadequate for determining the localization of the pathological gland, but its diagnostic value can be significantly increased by performing scintigraphy together.

The most commonly used scintigraphy modality is Tc-99m MIBI. It was first introduced by O'Doherty and is still used [5]. It is not operator-dependent as USG. Furthermore, it is capable of visualizing ectopic and intrathoracic adenomas. Compared with USG, it was found to be more efficient particularly in cases with posteriorly located and ectopic parathyroid glands. The sensitivity of MIBI in detecting adenoma ranges from 60% to 93% [5, 6]. On the other hand, the sensitivity of USG varies between 53% and 90% in different series, and studies have reported that the rate of an accurate diagnosis increases up to 96% when Tc-99m MIBI is performed with USG together [5].

The two imaging methods being consistent in determining the location of the pathological gland would increase the success rate of focused surgery. It was also reported that false-negative results might lead to intraoperative switching to bilateral exploration in MIP and therefore to an increased cost of surgery [6].

In cases with suspicious USG findings, preoperative PTH analysis of ultrasound-guided fine needle aspiration (FNA) washout fluid contributes to confirming the localization [1, 2, 6]. We also have been using the same method in cases of discordant MIBI and US as well as in suspicious cases.

The result is considered positive if the PTH level in the washout fluid is higher than the serum PTH level [7]. In the present case, the diagnosis of pHPT was confirmed by serum calcium, PTH, and vitamin D levels; 24-h urinary calcium excretion; USG+ Tc-99m MIBI scintigraphy; and PTH analysis of preoperative FNA washout fluid.

For many years, bilateral exploration has been regarded as the standard of care in the treatment of primary HPT, and this method has been routinely performed until the end of the 1990s. In this method, all glands are explored through a classical KOCHER incision, and the pathological gland/glands are excised [8].

Improvements in the imaging methods have allowed the detection of the pathological glands as well as exploration and excision only of the involved gland. This is called MIP because it involves a small incision, and the procedure is termed as "focused" parathyroidectomy because a particular parathyroid gland is targeted. The focused surgery can be performed using an open (mini-incision), endoscopic, and even robot-assisted technique. Different from the open minimally invasive method, the minimally invasive video-assisted parathyroidectomy (MIVAP) method does not require flap preparation; the gland site is accessed by an endoscope through the layers after an incision has been made and the gland is dissected off as per the principles of endoscopic surgery [9].

Surgical planning prioritizes achieving normocalcemic level with minimum morbidity, but it also aims to minimize the rates of persistent or recurrent hyperparathyroidism. The open MIP approach allows better cosmetic results because of small incision, shorter operation time, and shorter duration of hospital stay; however, certain conditions constitute an absolute or relative contraindication for MIP. Cases with a thyroid volume of >30 ml and additional thyroid pathology, those with adenoma measuring ≥4 cm, a history of neck surgery and/or radiotherapy, suspected cancer, and familial or multiple gland involvements are absolute contraindications. Uncertainty regarding localization, coagulopathy, contralateral recurrent laryngeal nerve damage, and obesity are relative contraindications [2, 8, 9] (Table 74.2).

One of the limitations of the MIP technique in focused surgery is that not all glands can be explored via mini-incision. For this reason, intraoperative parathormone monitoring (IPM) was introduced to evaluate surgical success. For this purpose, PTH is measured before, and 10 min after the incision and determination of the sufficiency of surgery depends on more than 50% decrease in PTH level from baseline [10]. The exploration should be continued if the value does not decrease sufficiently. Open MIP is considered to be superior to MIVAP, as it allows extension of the incision to and exploration of other glands when necessary [11].

The majority of the publications indicate that IPM is required in focused surgery and it increases the success of surgery [11, 12]. Besides, the PTH test is recommended by clinical centers in which IPM is not in use; however, we prefer IPM recommended by contemporary guidelines [1] (Rec-6-1). Intraoperative use of USG by the surgeon is another approach for detecting the pathological gland during open MIP (surgeon-based ultrasound: SUS). This procedure is more accurate regarding localization than USG and USG + scintigraphy; moreover, SUS significantly contributes to cases where IPM is not possible [12].

Table 74.2 Contraindications to MIP [3]

Absolute	Relative
Neck irradiation therapy history	Neck surgery history
Suspected localization	Anticoagulation therapy
Suspected familiar history	Known contralateral nerve injury
Carcinoma	Chronic renal failure
Thyroid pathology	Morbid obesity
Giant adenoma	

Outcomes of focused surgery are similar to those of bilateral exploration. With regard to potential complications, focused surgery is distinctive and superior, and complications like hypocalcemia and nerve injury are few. The use of intraoperative nerve monitoring (IONM) has been evaluated during this procedure; however, it is not recommended during the first MIP, but it is recommended during the second intervention or bilateral exploration in case of recurrence [13].

Norman et al. examined 15,000 cases that underwent surgery because of pHPT by a single team to compare MIP and bilateral exploration, and they analyzed 10-year follow-up data. They used scanning instead of IPM and gamma meter during surgery and argued that it provided them to detect hyperplasia or adenoma in multiple glands and that bilateral exploration is superior to IPM. Furthermore, terminating the use of MIP was advocated on the grounds that <5% cases in which IPM was performed suffered from recurrence within 1–2 years and that they detected 25% more multiple gland disease in the other group [14]. Nevertheless, the results of the study were not confirmed during retrospective multicenter meta-analysis investigating the findings of the study, and they demonstrated that MIP would be the choice of method provided that it is used in accurately selected cases using an appropriate technique [15].

Today, robotic parathyroidectomy surgery is also performed. Although its extensive use is controversial because of the relatively prolonged learning curve and high costs, robotic parathyroidectomy is considered applicable in selected cases when it is performed by an experienced physician [16].

Open MIP intervention is performed on selected patients via local anesthesia and light sedation [17]. For the last 10 years, we have been performing open MIP at our clinic on appropriate cases, and we have used lateral mini-incision parathyroidectomy technique described by Agarwal [18]. We also have used local anesthesia on high-risk and elderly patients. Multicenter studies and meta-analysis comparing long-term outcomes did not find statistically significant differences between general and local anesthesia [17, 18]. Another advantage of this approach is that morbidity rates are lower because in case of recurrence after MIP, there is a chance for intervention on a site where no previous intervention has been performed.

First day and first 6 months postoperatively are termed as threshold periods. Hematoma or seroma may be observed on the first day in cases undergoing parathyroidectomy. The transient hypocalcemia rate is reported to range between 0.5% and 45%, whereas permanent hypoparathyroidism (persisting after 6 months) is said to range between 0% and 3.6%.

Although day surgery is possible in such cases, it is recommended that the patients stay overnight at the hospital. Operation notes must be written by the surgeon, and all details must be recorded [1] (-Rec-14-1). Monitoring for hematoma in the first few hours postoperatively [1] (Rec-14.2) and monitoring parathormone and calcium levels in the first 24 h would be appropriate [1] (Rec-14.3).

At the end of the first 6 months, the clinical condition of the patient must be evaluated with regard to recurrence, permanent hypoparathyroidism, nerve injury, and vitamin D levels (with the assistance of an endocrinologist) [1] (Rec-14-7).

If calcium and parathormone levels return to normal range at the end of the first 6 months, the patient may then be considered to be cured [1] (Rec-15.1a). The patient must be examined for sHPT if calcium levels return to normal levels, but PTH levels remain elevated, and if there is without any sign or symptoms, recurrence or rest should be considered [1] (Rec-15b).

In cases diagnosed with normocalcemic HPT, both calcium and PTH levels should return to normal levels for the patient to be considered to be cured.

In case of persistent hyperparathyroidism (ongoing hypercalcemia and HPT) during follow-up, initial findings should be carefully reviewed [1] (Rec-17.1).

Patients undergoing open MIP because of primary HPT are followed up with physical examination and blood calcium and PTH testing two or three times (1st week, 1st month, and 3rd month) in the first 6 months, and then with calcium, PTH, and vitamin D level testing at the end of 6 months; in case no problem is observed, we suggest that patients should be followed up at 1-year intervals.

74.3 Outcome

The patient was discharged from the hospital on the first postoperative day. Early controls at the 1st week and 1st month were normal. No pathology was found also on the control examinations on the late period (over the past 15 months).

74.4 Future

In the current practice, the principle of surgery is to solve the problem using a minimally invasive procedure as far as possible without compromising the patient's quality of life. Minimally invasive approaches during parathyroid surgery provide effective treatment with better life quality and lower costs. We believe that the results of studies on minimally invasive interventions and developments in imaging technologies will enable us in detecting pathological glands more accurately and focused surgery will be performed by physicians on a more substantial number of cases.

What Can We Learn from This Case?

- Primary HPT is initially diagnosed biochemically, and the treatment of choice is surgery.
- Solitary adenoma is the most common cause of primary HPT, and MIP yields good outcomes.
- Minimally invasive surgery can be feasible when the pathological glands are detected using various imaging methods. USG has a high diagnostic yield when used together with scintigraphy by an experienced radiologist.
- Problems encountered in identifying the pathological gland in some cases may be resolved using PTH washout fluid, IPM, and perioperative USG. The most useful technique must be selected as per the conditions of the given institution.
- In the last 20 years, many MIP methods have been described and performed. Although these methods have unique features, they offer lower morbidity rates and similar success rates compared with conventional methods (bilateral exploration).
- Another crucial element that influences the surgical success and treatment process is the surgeon. Provided that the case and surgical technique has been accurately selected, those experienced in endocrine surgery can safely perform open MIP.

74.4.1 Clues for Physicians for Performing Focused/MIP Surgery

Superior parathyroid glands may be developmentally located on the posterior aspect of the recurrent laryngeal nerve or behind the inferior gland. The superior parathyroid gland may be found on the inferior thyroid artery and the intersection of carotid and recurrent laryngeal nerve at a distance <1 cm.

The superior parathyroid gland may also be located under the thyroid capsule, and to reveal it, the thyroid capsule should be opened during surgery.

The thyroid capsule or parathyroid gland with abnormal localization should be considered within the tracheoesophageal groove.

References

1. Wilhelm SM, Wang TS, Ruan DT, Lee JA, Asa SL, Duh QY, et al. The American Association of Endocrine Surgeons Guidelines for definitive Management of Primary Hyperparathyroidism. JAMA Surg. 2016;15:959–68. PIMD:27532368.
2. Bilezikian JP, Cusano NE, Khan AA, Liu JM, Marcocci C, Bandeira F. Primary hyperparathyroidism. Nat Rev Dis Primers. 2017;2:16033. PMCID: PMC5385896.
3. Noureldine SI, Gooi Z, Tufano RP. Minimally invasive parathyroid surgery. Gland Surg. 2015;4:410–9. https://doi.org/10.3978/j.issn.2227-684X.2015.03.07. PMCID: PMC4561661.
4. Guerin C, Aoife L, Gabriel S, Castinetti F, Philippon M, Vaillant-Lombard J, et al. Preoperative imaging for focused parathyroidectomy: making a good strategy even better. Eur J Endocrinol. 2015;172:519–26. PIMD:25637075.
5. O'Doherty MJ, Kettle AG, Wells P, Collins RE, Coakley AJ. Parathyroid imaging with technetium 99m Sestamibi: preoperative localization and tissue uptake studies. J Nucl Med. 1992;33:313–8. PIMD:1531500.
6. Kim WW, Rhee Y, Ban EJ, Lee CR, Kang SW, Jeong JJ, et al. Is focused parathyroidectomy appropriate for patients with primary hyperparathyroidism. Ann Surg Treat Res. 2016;91:97–103. PMID:27617249.
7. Kuzu F, Arpacı D, Çakmak GK, Emre AU, Elri T, Ilıkhan SU, et al. Focused parathyroidectomy without intra operative parathormone monitoring. The value of PTH assay in preoperative ultrasound guided fine needle aspiration washout. Ann Med Surg. 2016;8:64–7. PIMD:26955476.
8. Clark OH, Duh QY. Primary hyperparathyroidism, a surgical perspective. Endocrinol Method Clin North Am. 1989;18:701.
9. Bakkar S, Matteucci V, Corsini C, Pagliaro S, Miccoli P. Less is more: time to expand the indications for minimally invasive video assisted parathyroidectomy. J Endocrinol Investig. 2017;40:979–83.
10. Gioviale MC, Damiano G, Altomare R, Maione C, Buscemi S, Buscemi G, et al. Intraoperative measurement of parathyroid hormone: a Copernican revolution in the surgical treatment of hyperparathyroidism. Int J Surg. 2016;28(Suppl 1):S99–102. PIMD:26708859.

11. Babunga ID, McHenry CR. Is intraoperative parathyroid hormone monitoring necessary for primary hyperparathyoidism with concordant preoperative imaging? Am J Surg. 2017;213:484–8. PIMD: 28017299.
12. Aspinall SR, Nicholson S, Bliss RD, Lennard TW. The impact of surgeon-based ultrasonography for parathyroid disease on a British endocrine surgical practice. Ann R Coll Surg Engl. 2012;94:17–22. PMID:22524912.
13. Singh-ospina NM, Rodriquez-Gutierren R, Maraka S, Espinosa de Ycaza AE, Jasim S, Castaneda-Guarderas A, et al. Outcomes of parathyroidectomy in patients with primary hyperparathyroidism: a systematic review and meta-analysis. World J Surg. 2016;40(10):2359–77. PMID:27094563.
14. Norman J, Lopez J, Politz D. Abandoning unilateral parathyroidectomy: why we reversed our position after 15,000 parathyroid operations. J Am Coll Surg. 2012;214(3):260–9. PMID:22265807.
15. Norlen O, Wang KC, Tay JK, Johnson WR, Gredski S, Yeung M, et al. No need to abandon focused parathyroidectomy: a multicenter study of long term outcome after surgery for primary Hyperpatathyroidism. Ann Surg. 2015;261:991–6. PIMD:25565223.
16. Tolley N, Garas G, Palazzo F, Prichard A, Chaidas K, Cox J, et al. Long-term prospective evaluation comparing robotic parathyroidectomy with minimally invasive open parathyroidectomy for primary hyperparathyroidism. Head Neck. 2016;38(Suppl 1):E300–6. PMID: 25545792.
17. Melfa GI, Rasponto C, Attard M, Cocorullo G, Attard A, Mazzola S, et al. Comparision of minimally invasive parathyroidectomy under local anaesthesia and minimally invasive video-assisted parathyroidectomy for primary hyperparathyroidism: a cost analysis. G Chir. 2016;37:61–7. PMID:27381690.
18. Agarwal G, Barraclough BH, Reeve TS, Delbridge LV. Minimally invasive Parathyroidectomy using the "focused" lateral approach. II surgical technique. ANZ J Surg. 2002;72:147–51.

75 Subtotal Glandectomy in Hyperparathyroidism

Mehmet Uludağ and Nurcihan Aygün

Abstract

Hypercalcemia was detected in a 52-year-old female while being investigated because of recurrent renal stones. Metabolic profile revealed hypercalcemia with hypophosphatemia and elevated parathyroid hormone level. No pathological focus was demonstrated neither on neck ultrasonography nor 99mTechnetium-MIBI scintigraphy with single-photon emission computed tomography. Bilateral neck exploration was performed with the diagnosis of primary hyperparathyroidism (pHPT). All four parathyroid glands were observed to be enlarged during the exploration. Subtotal parathyroidectomy (sPTX) was performed. PHPT is a common endocrine disorder characterized by the excess production of PTH, resulting in the dysregulation of calcium metabolism. The diagnosis of pHPT is established due to biochemical examination. Imaging studies are not used to confirm the diagnosis but should be used for localization of the pathologic glands and determine the surgical strategy. Negative preoperative localization studies are highly predictive of multiglandular disease (MGD) in sporadic pHPT. Parathyroidectomy is indicated for all symptomatic patients and should be considered for most of the asymptomatic patients. MGD may not be excluded before surgery. The possibility of MGD in pHPT should always be kept in mind. sPTX is the standard treatment approach for patients with sporadic pHPT, whose all parathyroid glands are enlarged.

M. Uludağ · N. Aygün (✉)
Şişli Hamidiye Etfal Training and Research Hospital, Department of General Surgery, Istanbul, Turkey

75.1 Case Presentation

Hypercalcemia was detected in a 52-year-old female while being investigated because of recurrent renal stones. The results obtained via laboratory examination were as follows: blood urea, 32 mg/dl; creatinine, 0.87 mg/dl; total protein, 7.2 mg/dl; albumin, 4.3 mg/dl; calcium, 11.1 mg/dl; phosphorus, 2.8 mg/dl; parathormone, 165 pg/ml (15–65); 25-OH vitamin D, 35 ng/ml; and 24-h urine calcium, 380 mg/d. The other biochemical tests revealed no abnormal finding. No pathological focus was demonstrated neither on neck ultrasonography (USG) nor 99mTechnetium-MIBI (methoxyisobutylisonitrile) scintigraphy with single-photon emission computed tomography (SPECT/CT). Bone densitometry measurement of the patient revealed T-scores of −2.9, −2.9, and −2.2 at the distal radius, femoral neck, and lumbar spine, respectively. Bilateral neck exploration (BNE) was performed with the diagnosis

T. Özülker et al. (eds.), *Thyroid and Parathyroid Diseases*, https://doi.org/10.1007/978-3-319-78476-2_75

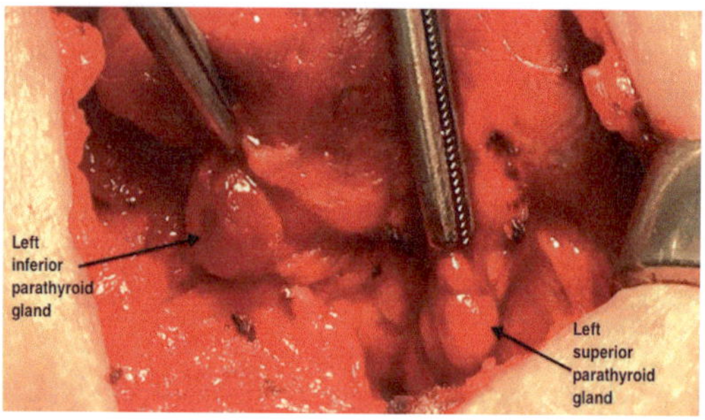

Fig. 75.1 The appearance of the enlarged left superior and inferior parathyroid glands during the surgery

of primary hyperparathyroidism (pHPT). All four parathyroid glands were observed to be enlarged during the exploration. The superior and inferior parathyroid glands on the right side were 1.1 × 0.8 × 0.4 cm and 1.5 × 1 × 0.3 cm, and those on the left side were 1.4 × 1 × 0.6 cm and 1.2 × 0.8 × 0.7 cm in size (Fig. 75.1) Subtotal parathyroidectomy (sPTX) was performed. A parathyroid remnant of 5 × 4 × 3 mm size was left behind in the right lower pole, and a clip was applied to it. Intraoperative parathormone (ioPTH) levels were 201 pg/ml before resection and 42 and 12 pg/ml at the 10th and 20th min after resection.

Calcium and parathormone levels were 9.2 mg/dl and 14 pg/ml, respectively, on the first postoperative day. Postoperative 6th-month calcium, PTH, and 25-OH vitamin D levels were 8,9 mg/dl, 37 pg/ml, and 45 ng/ml, respectively.

75.2 Discussion

75.2.1 Evaluation and Diagnosis

pHPT is a common endocrine disorder characterized by the excess production of PTH, resulting in the dysregulation of calcium (Ca) metabolism [1]. Women are affected more often than men by a ratio of nearly 3:1 and also incidence increases with age, rising dramatically after 50 years of age similar to our case of 52-year-old female [2].

The clinical presentation of pHPT varies from asymptomatic disease to classic symptomatic disease in which renal and/or skeletal complications are observed. Currently, at the time of diagnosis, most patients do not have classic symptoms or signs associated with pHPT and are often an incidental finding.

The patients with asymptomatic pHPT may not be truly asymptomatic as they may not carry diagnosed vertebral fractures, renal stones, and/or indistinct neuropsychiatric or neuromuscular symptoms, which may be related to the underlying pHPT. When properly evaluated, up to 80% of patients present with nonspecific symptoms of depression, fatigue, and lethargy, and they often are considered asymptomatic [3].

Once pHPT is suspected, or hypercalcemia is identified, biochemical confirmation is necessary. The differential diagnosis spectrum of hypercalcemia is quite broad. The most common cause of outpatient hypercalcemia remains pHPT, whereas that of hypercalcemia in hospitalized patients is malignancy [4].

Standard biochemical panel for the initial workup of suspected pHPT include the serum total and ionized Ca (hypoalbuminemic patients, borderline patient), PTH, phosphorus, creatinine, albumin, 25-OH vitamin D (nonclassical presentation or suspected vitamin D deficiency) and 24-h urinary calcium excretion (suggestive family history for familial hypocalciuric hypercalcemia) [4].

The diagnosis of the classic pHPT is verified by an elevated serum Ca level, with a concomitant inappropriately elevated intact PTH level excluding common causes of secondary HPT such as renal insufficiency, vitamin D deficiency, intestinal absorptive abnormalities, and renal leak syndrome [4].

Classic pHPT is defined with high serum Ca and PTH levels (Table 75.1).

Although the diagnosis is often straightforward, the biochemical evaluation may present a confusing picture. pHPT can also present with the normal serum PTH and/or Ca levels (Table 75.1). If normocalcemic pHPT is suspected, the diagnosis must be confirmed with normal albumin-adjusted total and ionized Ca concentrations [4]. On the other hand, in patients with hypercalcemia or Ca levels near the upper limit of the reference range, normal PTH levels do not rule out pHPT. An inappropriately normal

Table 75.1 The biochemical presentation of the pHPT

pHPT	Ca	PTH
Classic pHPT	High	High
Normocalcemic pHPT	Normal	High
Nonclassical pHPT (normohormonal or nonsupressed)	High	Normal

pHPT primary hyperparathyroidism, *PTH* parathyroid hormone, *Ca* calcium

(nonsuppressed) PTH level despite high level Ca is still indicative of an inappropriate negative feedback response to hypercalcemia and confirms the diagnosis of nonclassical pHPT. Nonclassical pHPT simply defines the pHPT that present with elevated serum Ca but inappropriately normal PTH (PTH 21–65 pg/ml) [4] (Table 75.1). A recently performed descriptive epidemiologic study showed that the number of patients with nonclassical pHPT nearly equaled the number of patients with classic pHPT [2]. However, the nonclassical pHPT rate is lower in clinical series (9%) [4]. Patients with pHPT, under the age of 40, should undergo genetic testing regarding familial diseases.

Causes include a single parathyroid adenoma in 80–85% of cases, double adenomas in 4–5%, multiglandular hyperplasia in 10–15%, and parathyroid cancer in less than 1% [1]. Most cases are sporadic and approximately 5% of cases are hereditary. MGD can be either sporadic or familial. In clinical practice, the majority of MGD are sporadic [5]. Hereditary syndromes with a pHPT component include multiple endocrine neoplasia (MEN) 2A, MEN 4, and hyperparathyroidism-jaw tumor syndrome. Prevalence of pHPT and its clinical properties differ among the various inherited syndromes [1]. pHPT may present without any syndromic association including familial isolated hyperparathyroidism, familial hypocalciuric hypercalcemia, severe neonatal hyperparathyroidism, and autosomal dominant moderate hyperparathyroidism [6].

The real incidence of MGD is difficult to be estimated, because it is influenced by several factors including the extent of parathyroid surgery (BNE or selective exploration), the experience of the operating surgeon to identify MGD, and also the experience of the pathologist to differentiate a (micro)adenoma from a normal gland [5].

Barczyński et al. summarize recent papers estimating a wide variable incidence of MGD ranging from 2.4 to 34%, arising a question about the clinical significance of these additional enlarged parathyroid glands.

It is now accepted that even in patients with concordant preoperative localization imaging demonstrating a single adenoma, further enlarged glands could be encountered if those patients undergo formal BNE [5]. Siperstein et al. reported unsuspected MGD identified in approximately 20% of patients who underwent BNE following the limited exploration [7].

If these additional enlarged glands would be hypersecreting, the failure rate of focused parathyroidectomy should be much higher than the reported numbers [5]. There are randomized prospective studies showing no difference in cure rate between focused parathyroidectomy and BNE [8].

Preoperative parathyroid imaging has become a standard preoperative procedure to locate abnormal parathyroid gland. Imaging studies should not be used in confirming or excluding the diagnosis of pHPT and selecting the patient for surgical indication. They should be only performed after deciding to proceed with parathyroidectomy to assist the surgeon while planning an appropriate parathyroid surgery. The mostly used imaging combinations are USG and 99mTc-sestamibi scintigraphy usually with SPECT/CT or scintigraphy and four-dimensional computed tomography [4D-CT]. Combined interpretation of scintigraphy and USG or scintigraphy and 4D-CT increases localization accuracy and improves sensitivity. MGD cannot be diagnosed preoperatively due to low accuracy, sensitivity, and specificity of any preoperative localization studies performed [5, 9, 10].

Negative preoperative localization studies are highly predictive of MGD in sporadic pHPT. Sebag et al. found that patients with negative preoperative study results had a high risk of MGD (31.6%), compared with patients with one positive study result (3.6%) and those with two concordant positive study results [11]. Negative or discordant imaging results are not a contraindication to parathyroid surgery.

Large series report similar cure rates for MGD and single adenomas. There is no data reported regarding more intense follow-up in sporadic MGD. In all cases, because of the risk of recurrent and/or new disease, a regular lifelong biannual serum testing for biochemical evidence of pHPT is recommended [5, 6].

75.3 Management

Today, surgery is the only curative therapy for pHPT, but it remains unclear whether all patients with pHPT require surgery [9]. Parathyroidectomy is indicated for all symptomatic patients and should be considered for most of the asymptomatic patients unless there are no significant comorbidities and contraindications to surgery. Surgery is more cost-effective than observation or pharmacological treatment. Parathyroidectomy diminishes the risk of nephrolithiasis and increases bone mineral density [3, 10].

Despite these findings and the establishment of expert guidelines that favor surgical treatment, only approximately one in four patients with pHPT is referred for surgery [8].

Cure rates are higher than 95% with a very low complication rate (<1–3%) when parathyroidectomy is performed by an experienced parathyroid surgeon. Surgery can be curative for the patient with a single adenoma that is seen in approximately 85% of pHPT patients. However, the recurrence risk is greater in the 15% of patients with hyperplasia who often require sPTHX. These patients are at higher risk of recurrent disease because the remnant parathyroid is defined to be abnormal and inclined to further growth [12]. Surgery performed by an experienced parathyroid surgeon from a high-volume center is the main factor in achieving the similar cure rates in patients with sporadic MGD when compared to those with single adenomas.

Although most patients with pHPT are ideal candidates for minimally invasive parathyroidectomy, some will require BNE due to MGD to achieve a biochemical cure. BNE in non-hereditary pHPT disease is indicated for patients with negative preoperative localization studies. Additionally, BNE should be planned for patients with the MEN-1 syndrome and inadequate decrease of intraoperative ioPTH level following removal of the image-indexed parathyroid lesion. Relative indications for BNE include history of lithium therapy, history of head and neck irradiation, discordant preoperative localization studies, isolated familial pHPT, and MEN-2 syndrome. Nevertheless, it should be taken into consideration that some grossly enlarged and histologically abnormal parathyroid glands can be nonfunctional, and BNE may lead to overtreatment in some patients with pHPT. IOPTH should be used to confirm that all enlarged hypersecreting glands have been identified and removed, but this technique is yet to be available in all units [5]. However, there is still a controversy over the utility of ioPTH in MGD. Hence, some do not use ioPTH with concerns that it cannot identify patients with double adenomas and provides false confidence leading to early concluding the operation leaving behind the abnormal parathyroid tissue.

MGD may not be excluded before surgery and is seen in approximately one in ten patients with sporadic pHPT [12]. Knowledge of parathyroid gland embryology and anatomy are critical for successful BNE and parathyroidectomy [13]. In BNE, all parathyroid glands are identified with the exploration of expected and, if necessary, ectopic cervical locations. When all four glands are enlarged, sPTX should be performed, leaving a viable remnant from the most normal-appearing gland and applying a clip to it [5, 9]. The lower gland is preferable because it is anterior to the recurrent laryngeal nerve and if re-exploration becomes necessary for persistent or recurrent disease, there will be less risk of injuring the nerve [13].

sPTX is the most recommended surgical approach for patients with MEN-1, MEN-4, and MEN-2A including all four glands enlarged, hyperparathyroidism-jaw tumor syndrome, familial isolated hyperparathyroidism, autosomal dominant moderate hyperparathyroidism, and lithium-associated pHPT [5, 6]. sPTX is also one of the standard treatment procedures in patients with surgical indication to secondary or tertiary HPT [14].

75.3.1 Future

It is impossible to diagnose MGD preoperatively. There is a limited data of histopathological findings to differentiate between adenoma and hyperplasia. Hyperplasia is usually associated with four glands. Currently and in the near future, the best clinical practice is likely a close cooperation between the pathologist and the surgeon. However, molecular biological methods may be a useful instrument in the future to distinguish and discriminate adenomas from hyperplasia.

What Can We Learn from This Case?

- The possibility of MGD in pHPT should always be kept in mind.
- Preoperative diagnosis of MGD is impossible. Negative preoperative localization studies are highly predictive of MGD in pHPT.
- The diagnosis of pHPT is established due to biochemical examination. Imaging studies are not used to confirm the diagnosis but should be used for localization of the pathologic glands and determine the surgical strategy.
- Negative preoperative localization imaging is not a contraindication to surgery. Surgical intervention of the patients with negative preoperative localization studies should not be delayed, and the patients should be conducted to an experienced parathyroid surgeon so that high cure rates can be achieved.
- BNE is still the gold standard surgical technique. sPTX is the standard treatment approach for patients with sporadic pHPT, whose all the parathyroid glands are enlarged.

References

1. Felger EA, Kandil E. Primary hyperparathyroidism. Otolaryngol Clin N Am. 2010;43:417–32. https://doi.org/10.1016/j.otc.2010.01.009.
2. Yeh MW, Ituarte PH, Zhou HC, Nishimoto S, Liu IL, Harari A, et al. Incidence and prevalence of primary hyperparathyroidism in a racially mixed population. J Clin Endocrinol Metab. 2013;98:1122–9. https://doi.org/10.1210/jc.2012-4022.
3. Bilezikian JP, Brandi ML, Eastell R, Silverberg SJ, Udelsman R, Marcocci C, et al. Guidelines for the management of asymptomatic primary hyperparathyroidism: summary statement from the Fourth International Workshop. J Clin Endocrinol Metab. 2014;99:3561–9. https://doi.org/10.1210/jc.2014-1413.
4. Wu JX, Yeh MW. Asymptomatic primary hyperparathyroidism. Diagnostic pitfalls and surgical intervention. Surg Oncol Clin N Am. 2016;25:77–90. https://doi.org/10.1016/j.soc.2015.08.004.
5. Barczyński M, Bränström R, Dionigi G, Mihai R. Sporadic multiple parathyroid gland disease—a consensus report of the European Society of Endocrine Surgeons (ESES). Langenbeck's Arch Surg. 2015;400:887–905. https://doi.org/10.1007/s00423-015-1348-1.
6. Iacobone M, Carnaille B, Palazzo FF, Vriens M. Hereditary hyperparathyroidism—a consensus report of the European Society of Endocrine Surgeons (ESES). Langenbeck's Arch Surg. 2015;400:867–86. https://doi.org/10.1007/s00423-015-1342-7.
7. Siperstein A, Berber E, Barbosa GF, Tsinberg M, Greene AB, Mitchell J, Milas M. Predicting the success of limited exploration for primary hyperparathyroidism using ultrasound, sestamibi, and intraoperative parathyroid hormone: analysis of 1158 cases. Ann Surg. 2008;248:420–8. https://doi.org/10.1097/SLA.0b013e3181859f71.
8. Elaraj D, Sturgeon C. Operative treatment of primary hyperparathyroidism: balancing cost-effectiveness with successful outcomes. Surg Clin North Am. 2014;9:607–23. https://doi.org/10.1016/j.suc.2014.02.011.
9. Callender GG, Udelsman R. Surgery for primary hyperparathyroidism. Cancer. 2014;120:3602–16. https://doi.org/10.1002/cncr.28891.
10. Wilhelm SM, Wang TS, Ruan DT, Lee JA, Asa SL, Duh QY, et al. The American Association of Endocrine Surgeons guidelines for definitive management of primary hyperparathyroidism. JAMA Surg. 2016;151:959–68. https://doi.org/10.1001/jamasurg.2016.2310.
11. Sebag F, Hubbard JG, Maweja S, Misso C, Tardivet L, Henry JF. Negative preoperative localization studies are highly predictive of multiglandular disease in sporadic primary hyperparathyroidism. Surgery. 2003;134:1038–41.

12. Khan AA, Hanley DA, Rizzoli R, Bollerslev J, Young JE, Rejnmark L, et al. Primary hyperparathyroidism: review and recommendations on evaluation, diagnosis, and management. A Canadian and international consensus. Osteoporos Int. 2017;28:1–19. https://doi.org/10.1007/s00198-016-3716-2.
13. Moalem J, Guerrero M, Kebebew E. Bilateral neck exploration in primary hyperparathyroidism--when is it selected and how is it performed? World J Surg. 2009;33:2282–91. https://doi.org/10.1007/s00268-009-9941-5.
14. Lorenz K, Bartsch DK, Sancho JJ, Guigard S, Triponez F. Surgical management of secondary hyperparathyroidism in chronic kidney disease--a consensus report of the European Society of Endocrine Surgeons. Langenbeck's Arch Surg. 2015;400:907–27. https://doi.org/10.1007/s00423-015-1344-5.

76 Success of Reoperative Neck Surgery in Persistent Hyperparathyroidism

Yeşim Erbil and Nihat Aksakal

Abstract

Sustained normocalcemia throughout postoperative 6 months is considered as a complete recovery achieved by surgery. Parathyroid hormone (PTH) and calcium levels not being reduced or becoming higher again during 6 months after the surgery are defined as persistent hyperparathyroidism, whereas hypercalcemia and high levels of PTH more than 6 months later are defined as recurrent hyperparathyroidism. The most common cause of persistent HPT is multiglandular disorder and ectopic adenomas. Persistent HPT occurs as a result of an insufficient surgery. The most critical factor that lowers the rate of HPT is surgical experience. In this article, we presented a case of 36-year-old woman with persistent hypercalcemia following an unsuccessful operation due to failure of localization of her parathyroid adenoma by conventional imaging modalities and became normocalcemic only after an operation guided by an 18F-choline PET/CT imaging spotting the adenoma in the mediastinum.

Y. Erbil · N. Aksakal (✉)
Division of Endocrine Surgery, İstanbul University, İstanbul, Turkey

76.1 Case Presentation

A 36-year-old woman presented with malaise, fatigue, and myalgia. The patient had had hypercalcemia in 2014, and the subsequent investigations resulted in the diagnosis of primary hyperparathyroidism (HPT). Neck ultrasonography (USG) had revealed a lesion in the lower left region of the thyroid that had been consistent with a parathyroid adenoma. However, no parathyroid adenoma had been found in surgical neck exploration. Frozen sections had been performed on structures that might be parathyroid; however, they had been identified as lymph ganglion. Left lobectomy and excision of the thymus had been performed for the possibility of an adenoma in the thyroid. The histopathologic examination had been negative for an adenoma. Patient's calcium and parathyroid hormone (PTH) levels had not decreased by the end of 24 h.

Neck USG was repeated in 2015, and the patient underwent Tc99m MIBI scintigraphy. The USG revealed a hypoechoic lesion posteromedially adjacent to the right lobe of the thyroid gland that could be a parathyroid pathology. There wasn't any pathology of the parathyroid in Tc99m MIBI. A second neck exploration was planned in the same year. Once again, no parathyroid pathology was detected during the exploration. Both surgeries involved the exploration of ectopic localizations in the neck, but there was not any adenoma present.

The patient was referred to our clinic with the diagnosis of persistent HPT. The followings were

T. Özülker et al. (eds.), *Thyroid and Parathyroid Diseases*, https://doi.org/10.1007/978-3-319-78476-2_76

the lab findings: calcium, 12.3 mg/mL (8.5–10.5); phosphorus, 2.2 mg/mL (2.7–4.5); and PTH, 430 pg/mL (15–65). Neck USG was reperformed by an experienced team of endocrine surgery and was negative for any pathologic lesions. SPECT-MIBI imaging did not suggest any pathologic uptake. CT scan of the neck and thorax showed a lesion in the aortopulmonary window which is considered to be primarily a lymph ganglion.

18F-fluorocholine PET study was planned for the patient whose pathologic parathyroid lesion was failed to be localized with any imaging studies. Choline PET spotted a nodular lesion in the mediastinum with the diameter of 1 cm that had a very high uptake of 18F-fluorocholine and thus suggested an ectopic parathyroid adenoma. Initially, the lesion was considered to be a lymph ganglion on CT due to its morphology in the aortopulmonary window in the mediastinum (Fig. 76.1).

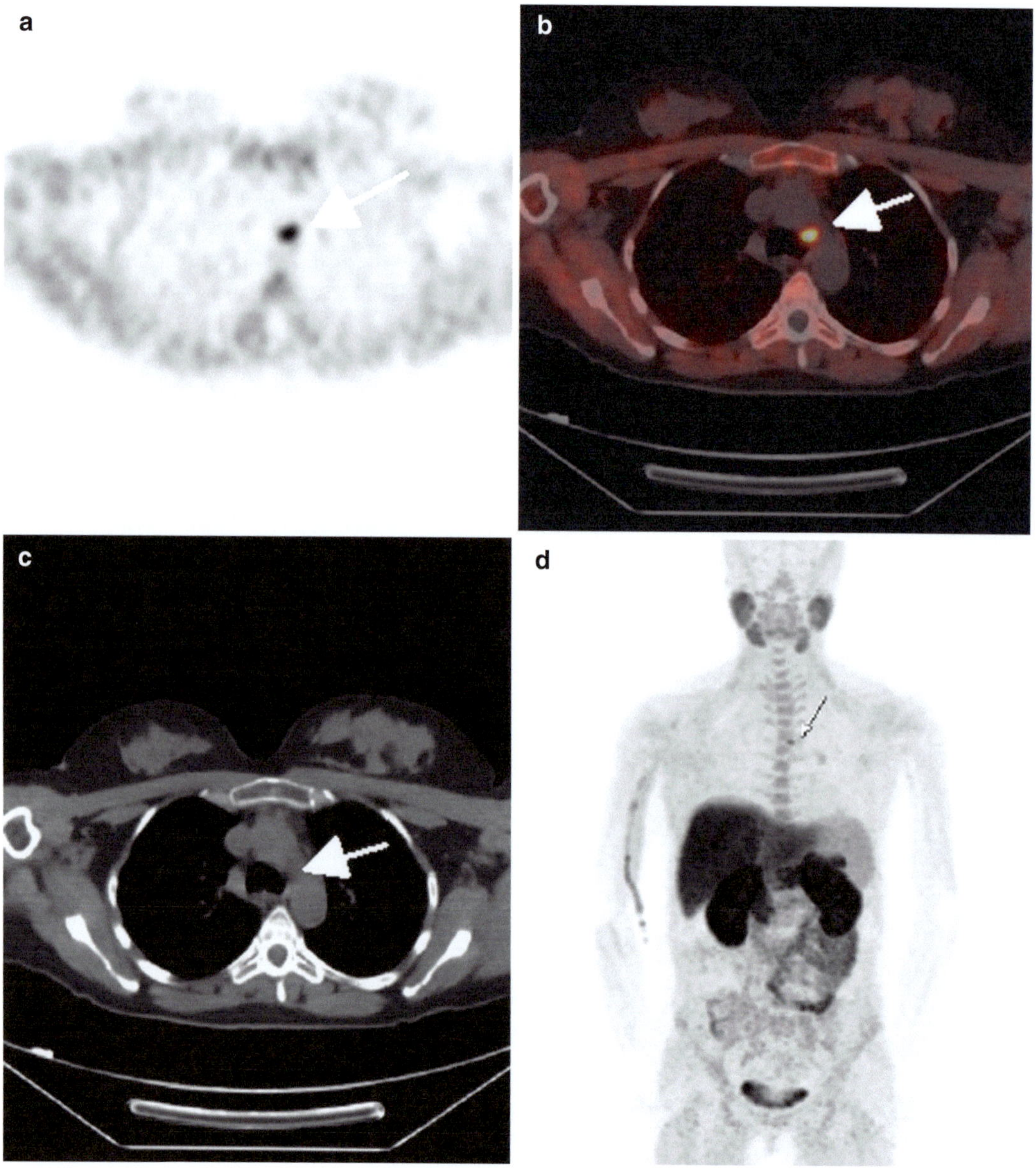

Fig. 76.1 ^{18}F-fluorocholine PET axial PET (**a**), fusion (**b**), CT (**c**) and MIP (**d**) images showing hypermetabolic focus corresponding to parathyroid adenoma at aortopulmonary window. (arrow)

Since the position of the lesion with pathologic uptake was not convenient for needle biopsy or PTH washout, exploration of the mediastinum via partial sternotomy was decided on. The thymus was excised in order to reach the aortopulmonary window where lymph ganglions were detected and excised. A protuberance with a diameter of 1 cm was noticed posteriorly to the aortic arcus. The adventitia over the protuberance was opened, and the pathologic parathyroid gland with a diameter of 1 cm was excised. The tissue was reported to be parathyroid gland in the frozen section examination. Quick PTH showed that patient's PTH levels decreased at a rate of 80% 30 min after the excision of the lesion.

The patient received parenteral calcium postoperatively and was discharged with oral calcium on the postoperative 4th day. The result of the pathological examination came out to be a parathyroid adenoma.

76.2 Discussion

76.2.1 Evaluation and Diagnosis

PHPT is a clinical entity that results from increased PTH secretion from parathyroid glands having one or more adenomas, hyperplasia, or rarely carcinomas [1]. Sporadic PHPT is caused by a single adenoma in 85–90%, hyperplasia in 10–15%, double-triple adenoma in 4–6%, and parathyroid cancer in 1% of the cases. The definitive treatment for the disease is surgery, and high rates of complete resolution are achieved by primary surgical intervention. Yet, persistent or recurrent disease in a subset of patients requires secondary and tertiary interventions even in experienced centers. Postoperative recurrence and persistent disease are reported in 1–10% and 2–22% of the patients, respectively [2–5].

Sustained normocalcemia throughout postoperative 6 months is considered as a complete recovery achieved by surgery. PTH and calcium levels not being reduced or becoming higher again during 6 months after the surgery are defined as persistent hyperparathyroidism, whereas hypercalcemia and high levels of PTH more than 6 months later are defined as recurrent hyperparathyroidism.

The most common cause of persistent HPT is multiglandular disorder and ectopic adenomas. Persistent HPT occurs as a result of an insufficient surgery. The most critical factor that lowers the rate of HPT is the surgical experience.

An undiagnosed multiglandular disorder which leads to the incomplete resection of the glands during the surgery is one of the most common causes of persistent disease. Siperstein et al. [6] performed limited exploration accompanied by preoperative scintigraphy, USG, and intraoperative PTH. Subsequently, they evaluated the ratio of the enlarged gland which can be left behind by standard bilateral exploration, prospectively. When USG and MIBI were congruent and focused surgery was performed, they noticed that enlarged glands were left behind at a rate of 20%. Adequate decreases in intraoperative PTH levels can just lower this rate to 16%. The investigators, therefore, stated that persistent or recurrent disease might develop from the results with early notice at a higher incidence. On the other hand, some studies have reported that the incidence of the multiglandular disorder is critically lower in the case series of focused surgery. These results may account for the fact that the patients are specifically selected for focused surgery [3, 4].

The prevalence of ectopic parathyroid glands been observed to be 28–42% in autopsy series, while 6.3–16% in surgical series of patients who underwent surgeries for primary hyperparathyroidism and 45% in cases who underwent re-exploration [2, 3].

The anterior mediastinum is the most frequent localization for ectopic inferior parathyroids which are usually embedded in the thymus gland, whereas superior parathyroids are commonly found in the posterosuperior mediastinum. Not so frequently, mediastinal parathyroid adenomas may be detected in the aortopulmonary window, and rarer localizations include the pericardium and right dome of the diaphragm [7, 8].

The treatment for persistent HPT is generally surgery. The diagnosis of HPT is reevaluated before the surgical intervention. The causes of hypercalcemia other than adenomas including, but not limited to, familial hypocalciuric hypercalcemia, use of medication that interfere with the metabolism of calcium such as thiazides and lithium, renal insufficiency, a renal calcium leak, gastrointestinal tract abnormalities, and vitamin D deficiency are investigated [3, 4].

Reoperative parathyroid surgery is harder due to scar formation and distorted anatomy, as well as having an increased risk of complications. Preoperative utilization of noninvasive and invasive techniques of localization would increase the surgical success.

USG is the lead noninvasive method. The range is wide for the sensitivity of USG in the literature (30–90%). USG is a fairly sensitive method for the localization of the parathyroid lesions that are intrathyroidal, adjacent to the carotid sheath, or located posteriorly to the thyroid gland. Despite this, the sensitivity is very low for revealing retroesophageal, retrotracheal, or mediastinal tumors. The most critical disadvantage of USG is its dependence on the performer and that it is affected by the presence of a thyroidal nodule or cervical lymphadenopathy. Moreover, the sensitivity is also low in multiglandular pathologies.

Other noninvasive imaging methods include technetium-99m sestamibi scans with a single-photon emission computerized tomography (SPECT), computerized tomography (CT) scans (4D is preferred), magnetic resonance imaging (MRI) scans, and sestamibi CT scans. Scintigraphic studies are more sensitive in localizing mediastinal parathyroid adenomas. All of the imaging studies are less reliable in the redo neck, and false-positive and false-negative results are commonly encountered [2, 3].

There have been limited number of studies reporting the identification of ectopic adenomas by 18F-choline PET when Tc99m-MIBI-SPECT fails to detect the lesion. Similarly, our patient's parathyroid adenoma was localized with 18F-choline PET, while all of the noninvasive imaging studies had failed. The parathyroid adenoma or hyperplasia exhibit increased cell proliferation, metabolism, and upregulation of choline kinase activity which leads to enhanced choline uptake. A choline analog is used for the evaluation of parathyroid adenomas based on the aforementioned theoretical mechanism 18F-choline [9].

Venous localization by a skilled angiographer may be applied in cases with failed noninvasive techniques [10]. Percutaneous parathyroid aspiration is a method that depends on USG while it clearly proves if the lesion comprises parathyroid tissue. The false positive and false negative rates of the method are significantly low [5, 11].

76.2.2 Management

Reoperative neck surgery, being a hard surgery due to scar formation and anatomic distortion, has higher rates of hypoparathyroidism and damage to the recurrent nerve compared to primary neck surgeries. For this reason, it is recommended that the operative adjuncts that may be of benefit for the reoperative surgery should be utilized and the surgery should take place in experienced centers. Operative adjuncts involve methods like nerve monitorization, intraoperative PTH assay, gamma-probed pathologic lesion, and bilateral internal jugular vein sampling for PTH during bilateral exploration. Diagnostic sensitivity of the intraoperative PTH assay is accepted to be low in multiglandular disorder.

The surgeon must master the embryology of the parathyroid glands and explore all possible ectopic positions in the cervical area since the most common causes of persistent and recurrent PHT are ectopic adenomas and multiglandular disease. Ectopic sites may include retropharyngeal, intrathymic, intrathyroid, retroesophageal, carotid sheath, retroclavicular, and mediastinal locations like the aortopulmonary window.

For pathologies of the parathyroid that are unable to be detected during exploration, a blind thyroid lobectomy on the same side with the missing gland, cervical thymectomy, and causing infarction of the occult parathyroid gland by means of ligating the ipsilateral inferior thyroidal artery are plausible approaches.

The ideal approach in reoperative parathyroid surgery should be to reveal whether HPT is a disease of a single gland or a multiglandular disorder, to localize the pathologic gland preoperatively, and to leave healthy parathyroid tissue present postoperatively.

Most mediastinal ectopic parathyroid adenomas can be removed by a cervical excision, whereas partial or complete median sternotomy and video-assisted thoracoscopic surgery are performed in certain cases.

Patients who reject the surgery or are not suitable for it receive bisphosphonates or cinacalcet as medical therapy.

76.3 Follow-Up and Outcome

Calcium and PTH levels of our patient, whose lesion was localized in the aortopulmonary window and excised through the adventitia posteriorly to the aortic arcus, achieved the levels of a normal range. Despite the use of all noninvasive imaging techniques, the lesion was managed to be localized with choline PET only. As was the case with this patient, choline PET is a legitimate option among imaging techniques to be tried in patients that are MIBI negative.

76.3.1 The Future

The most important fact that would increase the success of the reoperative parathyroid surgery is to localize the pathologic lesion. The sensitivity of localization becomes higher with the techniques of localization using advancing technology. There would be advancements in imaging techniques depending on the anatomical position and the function of the parathyroid lesion.

What Can We Learn from This Case?

- Sustained normocalcemia throughout postoperative 6 months is considered as a complete recovery achieved by surgery.
- PTH and calcium levels not being reduced or becoming higher again during 6 months after the surgery are defined as persistent hyperparathyroidism.
- The most common cause of persistent HPT is multiglandular disorder and ectopic adenomas. Persistent HPT is usually considered as a result of an insufficient surgery.
- An undiagnosed multiglandular disorder which leads to the incomplete excision of the glands during the surgery is one of the most common causes of persistent disease.
- Reoperative parathyroid surgery is harder due to scar formation and distorted anatomy, as well as having an increased risk of complications.
- Preoperative utilization of noninvasive and invasive techniques of localization would increase the surgical success.
- ^{18}F-choline PET/CT has proved to be useful in the localization of parathyroid adenomas, in case the other imaging modalities fail to detect.

Acknowledgment The authors would like to thank Assoc. Prof. Dr. Sait Sager for providing us with 18F-fluorocholine PET/CT image (Fig. 76.1) from the archive of Cerrahpasa School of Medicine, Department of Nuclear Medicine, İstanbul, Turkey.

References

1. Marx SJ, Stock JL, Attie MF, Downs RW Jr, Gardner DG, Brown EM, et al. Familial hypocalciuric hypercalcemia: recognition among patients referred after unsuccessful parathyroid exploration. Ann Intern Med. 1980;92:351–6. https://doi.org/10.7326/0003-4819-92-3-351.
2. Holt EH, Inzucchi SE. Physiology, and pathophysiology of the parathyroid glands and preoperative evaluation. In: Oertli D, Udelsman R, editors. Surgery of the thyroid and parathyroid glands. Heidelberg: Springer; 2008. p. 235–43.
3. Åkerström G, Juhlin C. Reoperation in primary hyperparathyroidism. In: Åkerström G, editor. Current controversy in parathyroid operation and reoperation. Austin: RG Landes Co.; 1994. p. 131–65.
4. Bilezikian JP, Khan AA, Potts JT Jr, Third International Workshop on the Management of Asymptomatic Primary Hyperparathyroidism. Guidelines for the management of asymptomatic primary hyperparathy-

roidism: summary statement of the Third International Workshop. J Clin Endocrinol Metab. 2009;94:335–9. https://doi.org/10.1210/jc.2008-1763.

5. Maser C, Donovan P, Santos F, Donabedian R, Rinder C, Scoutt L, et al. Sonographically guided fine needle aspiration with rapid parathyroid hormone assay. Ann Surg Oncol. 2006;13:1690–5. https://doi.org/10.1245/s10434-006-9180-z.
6. Siperstein A, Berber E, Barbosa GF, Tsinberg M, Greene AB, Mitchell J, et al. Predicting the success of limited exploration for primary hyperparathyroidism using ultrasound, sestamibi, and intraoperative parathyroid hormone: analysis of 1158 cases. Ann Surg. 2008;248:420–8.
7. Hu J, Ngiam KY, Parameswaran R. Mediastinal parathyroid adenomas and their surgical implications. Ann R Coll Surg Engl. 2015;97:259–61. https://doi.org/10.1308/003588415X14181254789088.
8. Noussios G, Anagnostis P, Natsis K. Ectopic parathyroid glands and their anatomical, clinical and surgical implications. Exp Clin Endocrinol Diabetes. 2012;120:604–10. https://doi.org/10.1055/s-0032-1327628.
9. Hodolic M, Huchet V, Balogova S, Michaud L, Kerrou K, Nataf V, et al. Incidental uptake of 18F-fluorocholine (FCH) in the head or in the neck of patients with prostate cancer. Radiol Oncol. 2014;48:228–34. https://doi.org/10.2478/raon-2013-0075.
10. Sugg SL, Fraker DL, Alexander R. Prospective evaluation of selective venous sampling for parathyroid hormone concentration in patients undergoing reoperations for primary hyperparathyroidizm. Surgery. 1993;114:1004–9.
11. Udelsman R, Aruny JE, Donovan PI, Sokoll LJ, Santos F, Donabedian R, et al. Rapid parathyroid hormone analysis during venous localization. Ann Surg. 2003;237:714–21. https://doi.org/10.1097/01.SLA.0000064363.21261.36.

Postoperative Hyperparathyroidism in Differentiated Thyroid Cancer

77

Burcu Esen Akkaş and Gülin Uçmak

Abstract

The coexistence of non-medullary thyroid carcinomas and primary hyperparathyroidism is very rare. The incidental diagnosis of thyroid carcinomas during or after the treatment of parathyroid disease, mostly in the pathology specimens, is common. However, parathyroid adenomas detected after total thyroidectomy may represent a clinical and diagnostic problem. In this chapter, a patient with parathyroid adenoma diagnosed after total thyroidectomy is reported with an emphasis on differential diagnosis of residual neck lesions and clinical awareness of concomitant thyroid and parathyroid pathologies.

77.1 Case Presentation

A 67-year-old female patient with multifocal thyroid papillary carcinoma was referred to Nuclear Medicine Department for radioactive iodine ablation after total thyroidectomy. On routine clinical exploration, a small residual thyroid tissue was observed on the right thyroid lobe bed on postoperative thyroid scintigraphy. Serum thyroglobulin was 0.2 ng/mL, whereas TSH was 90 mIU/mL, and anti-thyroglobulin antibody level was significantly elevated (350 IU/mL). Postoperatively serum calcium levels were slightly high (10.8 mg/dL) where the normal range was 8.2–10.5 mg/dL. Neck ultrasound (USG) findings were in accordance with scintigraphy apart from a hypoechogenic heterogeneous lesion located in the inferior medial aspect of the left lobe. Taking elevated levels of serum calcium into account, parathyroid adenoma was considered in the differential diagnosis, and elevated PTH level of 184 pg/mL was found (normal range: 10–65 pg/mL). On dual-phase Tc99m-methoxyisobutylisonitrile (MIBI) scintigraphy performed after the i.v. injection of 20 mCi Tc-99m MIBI, focal uptake in the inferior aspect of thyroid bed associated with the defined mass lesion on ultrasound was observed (Fig. 77.1). The most likely pre-diagnosis was parathyroid adenoma; even the defined lesion could associate with both residual thyroid nodule and parathyroid adenoma. Consequently, the patient underwent surgical re-exploration, and the mass in the thyroid bed was resected. Histopathology was consistent with parathyroid adenoma.

B. E. Akkaş (✉) · G. Uçmak
Department of Nuclear Medicine, University of Health Sciences (SBÜ) Dr. Abdurrahman Yurtaslan Ankara Oncology Training and Research Hospital, Ankara, Turkey

T. Özülker et al. (eds.), *Thyroid and Parathyroid Diseases*, https://doi.org/10.1007/978-3-319-78476-2_77

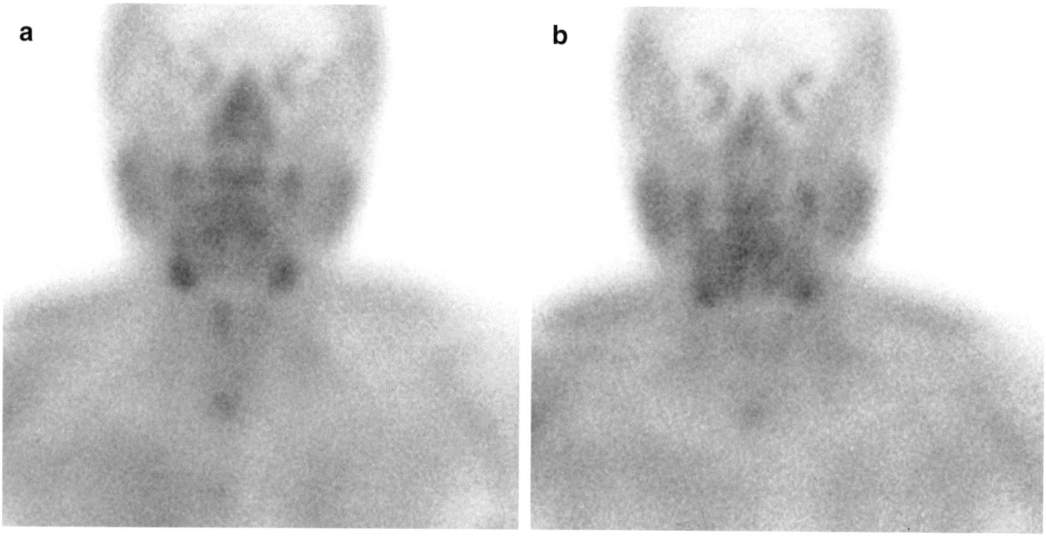

Fig. 77.1 Anterior planar neck images of dual phase Tc99m-methoxyisobutylisonitrile (MIBI) scintigraphy are shown. In (**a**) 20 min postinjection image, faint uptake in thyroid gland residue is seen. In addition, focal uptake in the inferior aspect of thyroid bed associated with the defined mass on neck ultrasound is noted. In (**b**) 2 h postinjection images demonstrate activity retention in the defined localization with physiological washout from the thyroid tissue

77.2 Discussion

Primary hyperparathyroidism (PHPT) is usually accompanied by underlying thyroid pathology. The rate of coexistence of primary hyperparathyroidism with thyroid diseases has been reported within a range of 22–70% in the literature [1, 2]. The reason for this association is controversial. Some researchers have shown this concomitance as coincidental, whereas other authors have explained elevated endogenous calcium levels or probably growth factors, such as epithelial growth factors and insulin-like growth factors, as goitrogenic factors [3, 4].

The concomitant appearance of medullary thyroid cancer and hyperparathyroidism in hereditary and sporadic multiple endocrine neoplasia syndromes is a well-known clinical situation. Nevertheless, the coexistence of non-medullary thyroid carcinomas and primary hyperparathyroidism are very rare and reported as 2.4–5.6% in the literature in isolated case reports [5, 6].

In general, parathyroid adenomas and thyroid tumors are diagnosed simultaneously. Incidental detection of thyroid tumors, especially papillary microcarcinoma is not an uncommon finding during parathyroid adenectomy. The reverse is also true. Today, most clinicians agree on the need to evaluate the thyroid gland before all parathyroid procedures, and thyroid surgery should be considered at the same operation with parathyroid surgery where necessary.

A careful neck examination before surgery may generally provide incidental diagnosis of parathyroid and thyroid diseases, and when detected, it does not represent a complicated clinical problem. However, parathyroid adenomas may develop years after total thyroidectomy and may represent a challenging situation. In the literature, isolated cases with parathyroid adenomas seen years after the treatment differentiated thyroid carcinoma (DTC) patients have been reported [6].

On follow-up of DTC patients, neck lesions detected after thyroidectomy is a clinical problem. The differential diagnosis of neck lesions must include residual thyroid nodules preferentially as well as parathyroid lesions on clinical management of patients with DTC. Although the recurrence of the primary tumor may account for the majority of cases, the possibility of an incidental appearance of parathyroid adenoma should not be neglected.

The presented case addresses several important points in the clinical follow-up of patients with DTC and in the differential diagnosis of neck lesions after thyroidectomy. Neck USG, magnetic resonance imaging, and molecular imaging techniques including positron emission tomography may have limitations in the differentiation of recurrent thyroid tumor from incidental parathyroid adenoma. Although a fine needle aspiration biopsy is needed for a definitive diagnosis, a proximate pre-diagnosis can be achieved if all radiological findings are supported with laboratory findings such as serum thyroglobulin, anti-thyroglobulin antibody, calcium, and parathormone levels.

Monitoring serum calcium levels is crucial after thyroid surgery, mainly for the early diagnosis of iatrogenic hypocalcemia. The incidence of transient and permanent hypocalcemia after thyroidectomy ranges between 19–38% and 1–3%, respectively [7]. Direct injury to parathyroid gland, devascularization, obstruction of venous drainage, or inadvertent excision of the parathyroid glands after thyroidectomy may account for the causes of hypoparathyroidism after thyroidectomy [8].

Serum calcium levels must be measured during clinical follow-up of patients with DTC principally for the possibility of hypocalcemia. However, despite the lack of a common embryologic cell origin, the existence of ensuing parathyroid gland hyperplasia and adenomas must also be kept in mind. In addition, primary hyperparathyroidism does not always manifest with significantly elevated serum calcium levels, and patients may not present with symptoms of hypercalcemia. It is recognized for many years that both clinical symptoms and complications of primary hyperparathyroidism may occur at all calcium levels, even when the serum calcium concentration is only mildly increased. Although clinicians may tend to choose a more conservative clinical approach that depends on "watch-and-wait" for patients with asymptomatic or mildly symptomatic hyperparathyroidism, the argument that patients with severely symptomatic hyperparathyroidism are sicker than their counterparts may not reflect the truth. Patients with only mild hypercalcemia are reported to have the same rates of every measure of disease severity and surgeons recommend treating these and contrast to recommend nonoperative management just because of the less impressive biochemical profile [9].

This report illustrates the need for clinical awareness for concomitant hyperparathyroidism with non-medullary thyroid tumors. The coexistence of PHPT and differentiated thyroid carcinoma is not well-known. Parathyroid adenomas may present years after thyroid carcinoma treatment, may be asymptomatic, and may mimic tumor recurrence.

77.3 Follow-Up and Outcome

Serum Ca levels decreased to normal levels following surgery. The patient is free of both thyroid cancer and parathyroid pathology. Serum Ca levels remained within normal ranges on follow-up.

What Can We Learn from This Case?

- Parathyroid adenomas may also be seen concomitantly with non-medullary thyroid carcinomas and may manifest years after the treatment of thyroid malignancy.
- Careful physical and radiological examination of the neck is crucial for patients with DTC both preoperatively and on follow-up. On differential diagnosis, coexisting parathyroid pathologies must also be kept in mind.
- Primary hyperparathyroidism does not always manifest with significantly elevated serum calcium levels, and patients may not present with symptoms of hypercalcemia.

References

1. Regal M, Páramo C, Luna Cano R, Pérez Méndez LF, Sierra JM, Rodríguez I, et al. Coexistence of primary hyperparathyroidism and thyroid disease. J Endocrinol Investig. 1999;22:191–7.
2. Sidhu S, Campbell P. Thyroid pathology associated with primary hyperparathyroidism. Aust N Z J Surg. 2000;70:285–7.
3. Burmeister LA, Sandberg M, Carty SE, Watson CG. Thyroid carcinoma found at parathyroidectomy: association with primary, secondary, and tertiary hyperparathyroidism. Cancer. 1997;79:1611–6.
4. Maiorano E, Ambrosi A, Giorgino R, Fersini M, Pollice L, Ciampolillo A. Insulin-like growth factor 1 (IGF-1) in multinodular goiters: a possible pathogenetic factor. Pathol Res Pract. 1994;190:1012–6.
5. Leitha T, Staudenherz A. Concomitant hyperparathyroidism and nonmedullarythyroid cancer, with a review of the literature. Clin Nucl Med. 2003;28:113–7.
6. Akkaş BE, Vural GU, Tan G. Parathyroid adenomas seen in the clinical follow-up of patients with differentiated thyroid carcinoma: a diagnostic dilemma. Clin Nucl Med. 2009;34:70–1. https://doi.org/10.1097/RLU.0b013e318192c525.
7. Almquist M, Hallgrimsson P, Nordenstrom E, Bergenfelz A. Prediction of permanent hypoparathyroidism after total thyroidectomy. World J Surg. 2014;38:2613–20. https://doi.org/10.1007/s00268-014-2622-z.
8. Cho JN, Park WS, Min SY. Predictors and risk factors of hypoparathyroidismafter total thyroidectomy. Int J Surg. 2016;34:47–52. https://doi.org/10.1016/j.ijsu.2016.08.019.
9. Boone D, Politz D, Lopez J, Mitchell J, Parrack K, Norman J. Concentration of serum calcium is not correlated with symptoms or severity of primary hyperparathyroidism: an examination of 20,081 consecutive adults. Surgery. 2017;161:98–106. https://doi.org/10.1016/j.surg.2016.09.012.

MIX
Papier aus verantwortungsvollen Quellen
Paper from responsible sources
FSC® C105338

If you have any concerns about our products,
you can contact us on
ProductSafety@springernature.com

In case Publisher is established outside the EU,
the EU authorized representative is:
Springer Nature Customer Service Center GmbH
Europaplatz 3, 69115 Heidelberg, Germany

Printed by Libri Plureos GmbH
in Hamburg, Germany